History and Physical Examination

A COMMON SENSE APPROACH

Mark Kauffman, DO, MS (Med Ed), PA
Assistant Dean of Graduate Studies
Associate Professor of Family Medicine
Lake Erie College of Osteopathic Medicine
Erie, Pennsylvania

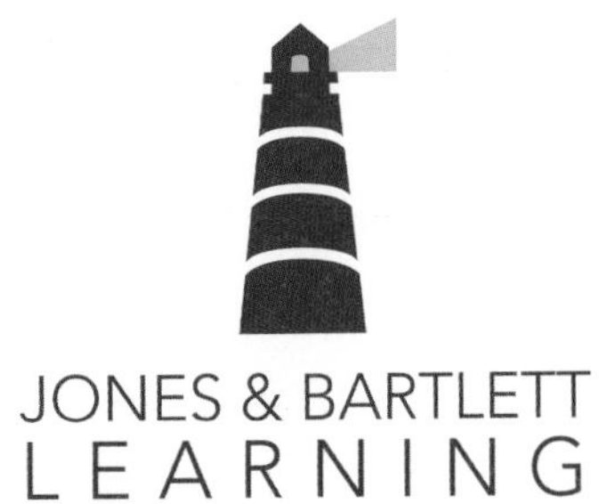

World Headquarters
Jones & Bartlett Learning
5 Wall Street
Burlington, MA 01803
978-443-5000
info@jblearning.com
www.jblearning.com

Jones & Bartlett Learning books and products are available through most bookstores and online booksellers. To contact Jones & Bartlett Learning directly, call 800-832-0034, fax 978-443-8000, or visit our website, www.jblearning.com.

Substantial discounts on bulk quantities of Jones & Bartlett Learning publications are available to corporations, professional associations, and other qualified organizations. For details and specific discount information, contact the special sales department at Jones & Bartlett Learning via the above contact information or send an email to specialsales@jblearning.com.

Copyright © 2014 by Jones & Bartlett Learning, LLC, an Ascend Learning Company

All rights reserved. No part of the material protected by this copyright may be reproduced or utilized in any form, electronic or mechanical, including photocopying, recording, or by any information storage and retrieval system, without written permission from the copyright owner.

History and Physical Examination: A Common Sense Approach is an independent publication and has not been authorized, sponsored, or otherwise approved by the owners of the trademarks or service marks referenced in this product.

Some images in this book feature models. These models do not necessarily endorse, represent, or participate in the activities represented in the images.

The screenshots in this product are for educational and instructive purposes only. All trademarks displayed are the trademarks of the parties noted therein. Such use of trademarks is not an endorsement by said parties of Jones & Bartlett Learning, its products, or its services, nor should such use be deemed an endorsement by Jones & Bartlett Learning of said third party's products or services.

The author, editor, and publisher have made every effort to provide accurate information. However, they are not responsible for errors, omissions, or for any outcomes related to the use of the contents of this book and take no responsibility for the use of the products and procedures described. Treatments and side effects described in this book may not be applicable to all people; likewise, some people may require a dose or experience a side effect that is not described herein. Drugs and medical devices are discussed that may have limited availability controlled by the Food and Drug Administration (FDA) for use only in a research study or clinical trial. Research, clinical practice, and government regulations often change the accepted standard in this field. When consideration is being given to use of any drug in the clinical setting, the health care provider or reader is responsible for determining FDA status of the drug, reading the package insert, and reviewing prescribing information for the most up-to-date recommendations on dose, precautions, and contraindications, and determining the appropriate usage for the product. This is especially important in the case of drugs that are new or seldom used.

Production Credits
Publisher: William Brottmiller
Senior Acquisitions Editor: Katey Birtcher
Associate Editor: Teresa Reilly
Associate Production Editor: Jill Morton
Marketing Manager: Grace Richards
V.P., Manufacturing and Inventory Control: Therese Connell
Composition: Publishers' Design and Production Services, Inc.
Cover Design: Scott Moden
Cover Images: Left to right, (A doctor and patient) © auremar/ShutterStock, Inc., (A doctor examines a patient) © Jupiterimages/Thinkstock, (Doctor examining eyes of patient) Courtesy of Mark Kauffman, (A doctor checks pressure) © Alexander Raths/ShutterStock, Inc., (Doctor examining glands of patient) © Blend Images/ShutterStock, Inc.
Printing and Binding: Courier Companies
Cover Printing: Courier Companies

To order this product, use ISBN: 978-1-4496-6026-0

Library of Congress Cataloging-in-Publication Data
Kauffman, Mark, DO.
History and physical examination : a common sense approach / by Mark Kauffman.
p. ; cm.
Includes bibliographical references and index.
ISBN 978-1-4496-5727-7 — ISBN 1-4496-5727-3
I. Title.
[DNLM: 1. Physical Examination. 2. Diagnosis, Differential. 3. Medical History Taking. WB 200]
616.07'5—dc23
2012044932

6048

Printed in the United States of America
17 16 15 14 13 10 9 8 7 6 5 4 3 2 1

Dedication

This book is dedicated to our daughter Jade.
Our love for you had no beginning and has no end, only a life in and of itself.
You are amazing.

Contents

About the Author

Mark Kauffman, DO, MS (Med Ed), PA, did his undergraduate studies at St. Francis University (Loretto, Pennsylvania) in the physician assistant program. He earned his Doctor of Osteopathic Medicine and Master of Science in medical education degrees at Lake Erie College of Osteopathic Medicine (LECOM). He is board certified in family medicine. Dr. Kauffman is assistant dean of graduate studies at LECOM. He developed and is director of the Accelerated Physician Assistant Pathway, an innovative three-year medical school curriculum for physician assistants who seek to obtain DO degrees, and the history and physical examination curriculum.

Introduction

The best way to learn how to obtain accurate, detailed patient histories, perform problem-specific physical examinations, devise essential differential diagnoses, construct evidenced-based treatment plans, and ultimately perform complete history and physical examinations leading to maximal care of your patient is to incorporate them into the study of medicine from the very beginning.

As you develop familiarity with the practice of medicine, logical thinking takes over, with intuition leading the way. With familiarity comes the risk of complacency and often the habit of taking shortcuts. When the day comes in which you mechanically listen to a patient's heart, begin to walk away, realize you might have heard something, and listen again, only to discover the nearly missed murmur, let it be a valuable lesson to you to humbly go back to your roots and the basics of your medical knowledge.

If there is one goal for this text, it is to encourage you to use common sense in your approach to patient care, hence the title. There are some classic memory aids, such as "On Old Olympus' Towering Top," for the cranial nerves, and you will undoubtedly invent some of your own, but when you resort to your logic, you are more apt to understand the material instead of memorizing it. Though at first you will need to memorize the physical exam flows, you will encounter them so often when you begin your clinical training that they will become standard procedure without effort, allowing only your patient's body to guide you through the exam.

Chapter 1, *Clinical Competencies*, discusses the competency-based educational movement and its potential to improve patient health by lessening unnecessary and unexplained variation in the process of clinical care. Students in healthcare professions must have the education and experience to assure the highest-quality patient care and public safety. The competencies are a calling of the healthcare professional and represent accountability to ourselves, our peers, and, of ultimate importance, our patients.

Chapter 2, *Interpersonal and Communication Skills*, is an exploration of the thought processes and actions behind obtaining a history. This includes what one does prior to walking into a patient room that will lead to a more accurate patient history. The medical provider may be able to ask all the right questions, but without competence within the humanistic domain, compassion, empathy, and professionalism, the bond of trust is difficult to forge.

Chapter 3 introduces the mnemonic CODIERS SMASH FM, an essential tool that allows the gathering of a detailed historical account of the patient's presenting complaint, and guides you through the patient's medical history, where buried clues, when unearthed, dramatically affect the outcome of the case. It further discusses techniques involved with clinical history taking. Why is history so important? It has been said that 90% of diagnoses are made through the history alone. If the patient is not asked the right questions, the correct diagnosis is much more likely to be missed.

Chapter 4 comprises history flows that represent patient case presentations. Each encounter is designed for you and a partner: schoolmate, friend, family member, or anyone you can compel to act as your patient. Armed with only your patient's primary reason for seeking your counsel, you must obtain the medical history from your patient, who provides you with scripted answers. Acute attention will allow you to identify those hidden clues that require further exploration to enable you to reach the correct conclusions. Early on you may not get the correct diagnosis, but you must still propose what is most likely, as this is the very essence of why we take histories. As your medical studies progress, your goal should be to expand your impressions to include several possible diagnoses: the differential diagnosis.

Chapter 5 introduces physical examination and approaches the body in a logical progression, essentially head to toe. The physical examination flows, presented in the head-to-toe fashion, encourage the student to allow the patient's body to dictate the order of examination and to repeat the exam in precisely the same fashion from patient to patient. This order, however, is provider dependent, meaning that once you master the exam techniques, you will perform these exams in the order that you find most logical. For example, after completing an abdominal exam, you may immediately feel for the femoral pulses, which lie right below the abdomen in the inguinal area. From there, you may complete the rest of the peripheral vascular exam, and then switch over to the musculoskeletal system, examining the extremities first. If, on the other hand, you reach the bottom of the abdomen and it makes you logically think of the longest nerve in the body—the vagus—then you may choose to perform the neurologic examination next. There is no right or wrong method, only completeness.

Chapters 6 through 15 then break down physical examination by system. Each chapter ends with a physical examination flow that guides the student through a comprehensive examination of the patient. Interweaving the techniques of examination with the head-to-toe, front-to-back approach allows the provider to develop a standardized approach to examination that becomes ingrained with practice, removing the need to memorize what should be done.

Chapter 16 brings history taking and physical examination together through the comprehensive flow, which represents the typical 15-minute patient encounter. Providers combine history taking with the performance of a problem-specific physical examination, allowing the development of a differential diagnosis and working with the patient to develop a plan of treatment.

Chapters 17 and 18 look at the approaches to history taking and examination of pregnant and pediatric patients, respectively.

Chapter 19 is a summation of documentation of patient encounters. The proper mindset required for appropriately documenting an encounter should be visualized as the patient's chart being read 5 years from the encounter by someone unfamiliar with the patient. If, by reading about the encounter, that person can understand the patient's story, visualize the patient in his/her mind, understand the thought process that led to the diagnosis, and evaluate the treatment plan to assure that the standard of care was followed, you have succeeded in proper documentation. This chapter guides you through the structure of the most common form of medical documentation, the SOAP note, as well as the documentation of standard admission and progress notes, and the full physical examination.

Becoming a great provider requires astute observation skills and heightened awareness of intuition. Learning from your peers and patients is a lifelong experience. Study hard but retain the ability to laugh at yourself. Humility is a wise teacher.

Early in my medical training, I was sitting in a crowded room where a lecture on emergency bleeds was to be presented. A physician came in and remarked that the topic was appropriate because a patient had just arrived in the emergency room with bleeding varices that were life threatening. Perplexed, I quietly leaned over to my supervisor and asked how someone could die from a bleed in the scrotum. How she refrained from laughing when she explained to me that the patient had *esophageal varices*, not a *scrotal varicocele*, is beyond me. With humbleness, we should all embark down the trail of the study of medicine.

Features of This Text

History and Physical Examination: A Common Sense Approach incorporates a number of engaging pedagogical features to aid in the student's understanding and retention of the material. Each chapter begins with **Objectives** and **Key Terms**, to guide learning and provide reference for the most important points covered in the chapter.

OBJECTIVES

At the conclusion of this chapter, the student will be able to

1. Discuss the evolution of the competency-based medical education movement in the United States
2. Define *competent* and relate it to the continuum of learning as described by Dreyfus and Dreyfus
3. Discuss the competency-based medical education movement in countries outside of the United States and in professions outside of medicine
4. Define each of the major competencies used in medical education in the United States and list behaviors expected of competent providers for each competency
5. Describe some of the issues that will face medical educators as the competency-based medical education movement continues to evolve

KEY TERMS

Competency-based education
Competencies
Medical knowledge
Patient care
Professionalism
Interpersonal and communication skills
Systems-based practice
Practice-based learning and improvement
Evidence-based medicine
Medical quality

Where this icon appears, visit **go.jblearning.com/HPECWS** to view the video.

EXTERNAL EXAMINATION

The Distant Exam

It is also important to evaluate the patient for symmetry. From 3 or 4 feet away, evaluate the position of the upper eyelids for ptosis (CNIII). With an open eye, lid margins typically touch the top and bottom edges of the iris. An upper lid droop indicates the presence of ptosis with possible CNIII deficiency. Sclera visible above and below the iris may be caused by exophthalmus, protrusion of the eye that may be found with hyperthyroidism or space-occupying lesions.

8-5 Also check for symmetry of brow creases and facial droop. To check for eye misalignment or strabismus, shine a light directly in the eyes. Assess the symmetry of the position of the light reflex within the pupil. Any asymmetry of the reflex within the pupil could indicate strabismus.

Cranial nerves III, IV, and VI are assessed by evaluating extraocular muscle motility, termed **extraocular movements** (EOMs). This is performed by holding a fixation target such as a pen or your finger 12 to 14 inches away and having the patient follow it with his/her eyes through all nine positions of gaze. Be sure to hold the upper eyelids if necessary to evaluate inferior ocular movements. Have the patient fixate on the target and check for nystagmus, which can indicate a cranial nerve VIII dysfunction.

The Close Exam

Evaluation of the anterior anatomic structures of the eye is performed from approximately 1 foot in front of the patient. The conjunctiva can be inspected for hyperemia, pallor, exudate, or hemorrhage. Hyperemia of the conjunctival vasculature may be caused by an allergy, virus, or bacterium. An exudative discharge is often associated with a bacterial infection. The sclera should be evaluated for signs of dilated vasculature, lesions, or icterus, yellowing of the sclera as a result of hyperbilirubinemia often associated with bile duct obstruction or liver disease. The iris should be inspected for lesions and excessive heterochromia.

The **cornea** should be evaluated for signs of opacity, edema, or foreign body. A pterygium is an abnormal growth of conjunctival tissue that may progress to involve the cornea. It is usually triangular-shaped and inflamed, typically occurs on the nasal aspect of the eye, and is found most commonly in tropical climates. Metal foreign bodies in the cornea may cause corneal edema, anterior chamber inflammation, and a rust ring. Rust rings must be removed completely and carefully to minimize the potential for scarring.

Sudden opacification of the cornea can be a sign of increased intraocular pressure. This dulling of the otherwise crystal-clear cornea may indicate an acute angle-closure attack. Acute angle-closure glaucoma is a true ophthalmic emergency and requires immediate treatment. To assess the depth of the anterior chamber, shine a light from the temporal side of the head parallel to the plane of the iris (see FIGURE 8-13). Determine how much of the nasal iris is in shadow. If greater than two-thirds of the nasal iris is in shadow, then a shallow anterior chamber should be suspected (see FIGURE 8-14). Further evaluation of the cornea can include evaluating the sensory component as supplied by cranial nerve V (trigeminal). This is done by dragging a wisp of cotton, from either a cotton ball or the tip of cotton-tipped applicator formed into a point, gently across the corneal surface.

8-6 Pupillary evaluation should include inspection of the pupil for both the direct and consensual response as well as symmetry of size and shape. The direct **pupillary reaction** is performed by

Extraocular movements: movement of the eyes through nine positions of gaze as an assessment of cranial nerves III, VI, and VI

Cornea: the most ventral surface of the eye, appearing as a transparent mound lying directly over the pupil, iris, and anterior chamber

Pupillary reaction: reaction of the pupils when a light is shown into the eyes as an assessment of cranial nerves II and III

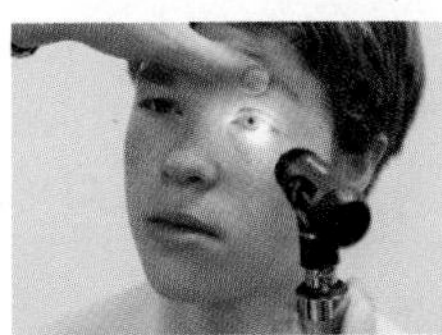

FIGURE 8-13 Assessment of the depth of the anterior chamber with the light source projected tangentially over the iris.

Throughout the text, key points are illustrated and important information is highlighted to ensure comprehension and to aid the study of critical material. **Key Terms** are bolded throughout the chapter, and shaded boxes in the margin provide the full definition for student reference and review. A colorful and engaging layout enables easy reading and supports the retention of important concepts. Additionally, almost 600 full-color photographs and illustrations provide valuable insight into proper procedure and accurate anatomy, as well as visual reinforcement of the material.

Video content is also a key element of this valuable resource. Footage of illustrative exams is included with every new print copy of *History and Physical Examination* on the **Companion Website** and embedded in the online, JBL eFolio edition, also available for purchase.

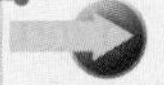

Where this icon appears, visit **go.jblearning.com/HPECWS** to view the video.

The *History and Physical Examination* **Companion Website** also includes useful study activities, practice quizzes, flashcards, and more. To redeem the Access Code Card available with your new copy of the resource, or to purchase access to the website separately, visit **go.jblearning.com/HPECWS**.

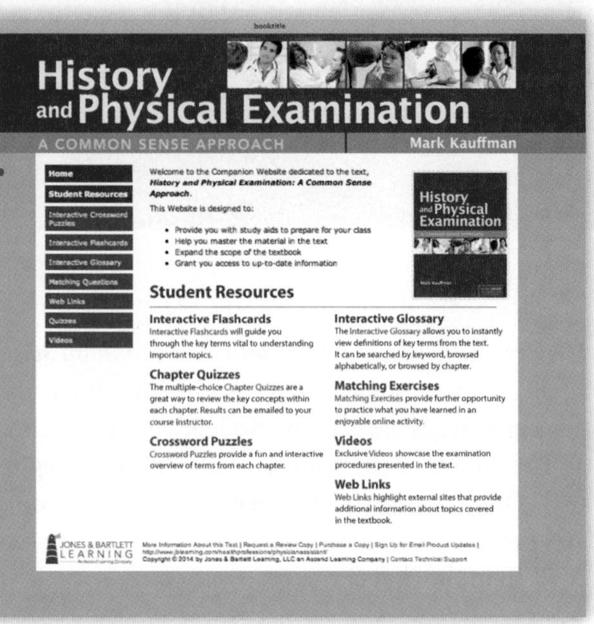

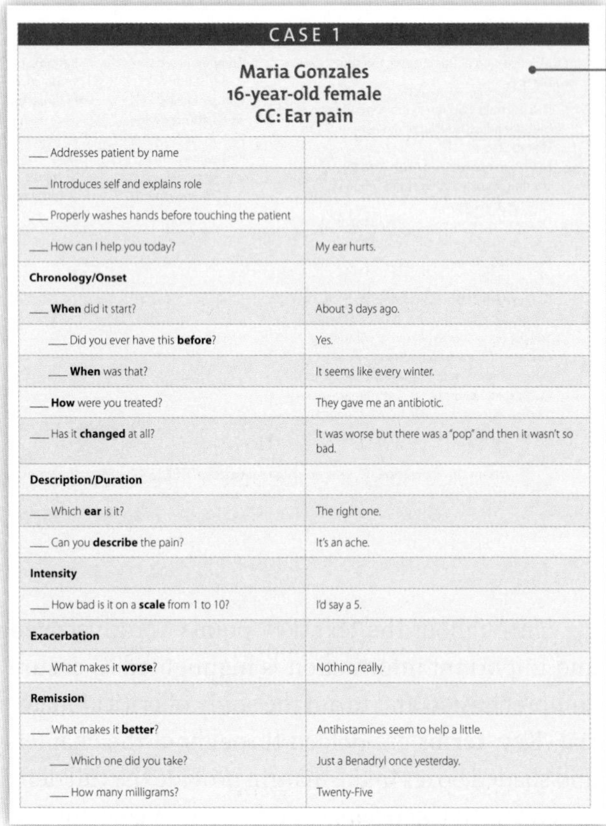

CASE 1

Maria Gonzales
16-year-old female
CC: Ear pain

___Addresses patient by name	
___Introduces self and explains role	
___Properly washes hands before touching the patient	
___How can I help you today?	My ear hurts.
Chronology/Onset	
___**When** did it start?	About 3 days ago.
___Did you ever have this **before**?	Yes.
___**When** was that?	It seems like every winter.
___**How** were you treated?	They gave me an antibiotic.
___Has it **changed** at all?	It was worse but there was a "pop" and then it wasn't so bad.
Description/Duration	
___Which **ear** is it?	The right one.
___Can you **describe** the pain?	It's an ache.
Intensity	
___How bad is it on a **scale** from 1 to 10?	I'd say a 5.
Exacerbation	
___What makes it **worse**?	Nothing really.
Remission	
___What makes it **better**?	Antihistamines seem to help a little.
___Which one did you take?	Just a Benadryl once yesterday.
___How many milligrams?	Twenty-Five

In Chapter 4, *The History Flows* and culminating in Chapter 16, *Comprehensive Flows*, **Clinical Cases** provide crucial, applied practice for the foundational content. To foster comfort and repetition, memory tools and **Patient Data Sheets** are included for student use in utilizing the cases, following the CODIERS SMASH FM mnemonic tool presented in Chapter 3 and utilized throughout the resource.

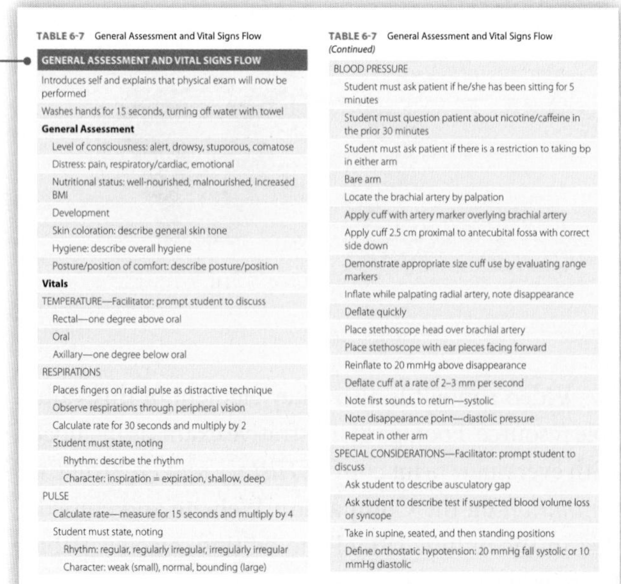

TABLE 6-7 General Assessment and Vital Signs Flow

GENERAL ASSESSMENT AND VITAL SIGNS FLOW
Introduces self and explains that physical exam will now be performed
Washes hands for 15 seconds, turning off water with towel
General Assessment
Level of consciousness: alert, drowsy, stuporous, comatose
Distress: pain, respiratory/cardiac, emotional
Nutritional status: well-nourished, malnourished, increased BMI
Development
Skin coloration: describe general skin tone
Hygiene: describe overall hygiene
Posture/position of comfort: describe posture/position
Vitals
TEMPERATURE—Facilitator: prompt student to discuss
Rectal—one degree above oral
Oral
Axillary—one degree below oral
RESPIRATIONS
Places fingers on radial pulse as distractive technique
Observe respirations through peripheral vision
Calculate rate for 30 seconds and multiply by 2
Student must state, noting
Rhythm: describe the rhythm
Character: inspiration = expiration, shallow, deep
PULSE
Calculate rate—measure for 15 seconds and multiply by 4
Student must state, noting
Rhythm: regular, regularly irregular, irregularly irregular
Character: weak (small), normal, bounding (large)

TABLE 6-7 General Assessment and Vital Signs Flow *(Continued)*

BLOOD PRESSURE
Student must ask patient if he/she has been sitting for 5 minutes
Student must question patient about nicotine/caffeine in the prior 30 minutes
Student must ask patient if there is a restriction to taking bp in either arm
Bare arm
Locate the brachial artery by palpation
Apply cuff with artery marker overlying brachial artery
Apply cuff 2.5 cm proximal to antecubital fossa with correct side down
Demonstrate appropriate size cuff use by evaluating range markers
Inflate while palpating radial artery, note disappearance
Deflate quickly
Place stethoscope head over brachial artery
Place stethoscope with ear pieces facing forward
Reinflate to 20 mmHg above disappearance
Deflate cuff at a rate of 2–3 mm per second
Note first sounds to return—systolic
Note disappearance point—diastolic pressure
Repeat in other arm
SPECIAL CONSIDERATIONS—Facilitator: prompt student to discuss
Ask student to describe auscultatory gap
Ask student to describe test if suspected blood volume loss or syncope
Take in supine, seated, and then standing positions
Define orthostatic hypotension: 20 mmHg fall systolic or 10 mmHg diastolic

Beginning after Chapter 5, *Introduction to Physical Examination*, and included for each body system and specialized type of exam conτvered, logical **Physical Exam Flows** are provided for reference and head-to-toe, front-to-back coverage. These valuable tables provide a critical checklist to ensure comprehensive, replicable, and reliable exams.

Qualified professors can also receive the full suite of **Instructor Support Resources**, including PowerPoints, TestBanks, and Instructor's Manual. To gain access to these valuable teaching materials, contact your Health Professions representative through **www.jblearning.com**.

Contributors

Rizwan Aslam, DO, MS, FACS
Clinical Assistant Professor of
Otolaryngology–HNS
Tulane University School of Medicine
New Orleans, LA

Hershey S. Bell, MD, MS, FAAFP
Professor, Vice President for Academic Affairs,
and Dean
Lake Erie College of Osteopathic Medicine
Erie, PA

John Czarnecki, MD, MPA, MPH
Assistant Professor of Family Medicine
Lake Erie College of Osteopathic Medicine
Erie, PA

William Donohue, PhD
Professor
Department of Communication
Michigan State University
East Lansing, MI

Frank Fatica, DO
Assistant Clinical Professor
Lake Erie College of Osteopathic Medicine
Erie, PA

Blake Hoppe, DO, MS (Med Ed)
Clinical Assistant Professor of Neurology
Lake Erie College of Osteopathic Medicine
Erie, PA

Mark Kauffman, DO, MS (Med Ed), PA
Assistant Dean of Graduate Studies
Associate Professor of Family Medicine
Lake Erie College of Osteopathic Medicine
Erie, PA

Krystle Lappinen, MD
Resident
Obstetrics and Gynecology Department
Western Pennsylvania Hospital
Pittsburgh, PA

Scott J. M. Lim, DO, FAOCD
Assistant Clinical Professor
Lake Erie College of Osteopathic Medicine
Erie, PA

Theodore Makoske, MD
Assistant Professor of Anatomy
Lake Erie College of Osteopathic Medicine
Erie, PA

Lynn McGrath, MSN, CRNP
Director SPEC Program
Lake Erie College of Osteopathic Medicine
Erie, PA

Janet Newcamp, RNC, MN, CNS, CCE
Assistant Professor of Nursing
Edinboro University
Edinboro, PA

Michele Roth-Kauffman, JD, PA-C
Professor and Chair
Physician Assistant Department
Gannon University
Erie, PA

Andrea Skomo, DO
Resident
Obstetrics and Gynecology Department
Western Pennsylvania Hospital
Pittsburgh, PA

Reviewers

Frank A. Acevedo, PA-C, MS, DFAAPA
Academic Coordinator, Assistant Professor, and Associate Program Director
New York Institute of Technology
Old Westbury, NY

Mary Carcella Allias, MPAS, PA-C
Assistant Professor
Physician Assistant Studies Program
University of Pittsburgh
Pittsburgh, PA

Renee Andreeff, MS, MPAS, RPA-C
Academic Coordinator and Clinical Assistant Professor
Physician Assistant Program
D'Youville College
Buffalo, NY

Natalie J. Belle, MD
Professor
Cleveland State University/Cuyahoga Community College
Parma, OH

SECTION I

Competencies

CHAPTER 1

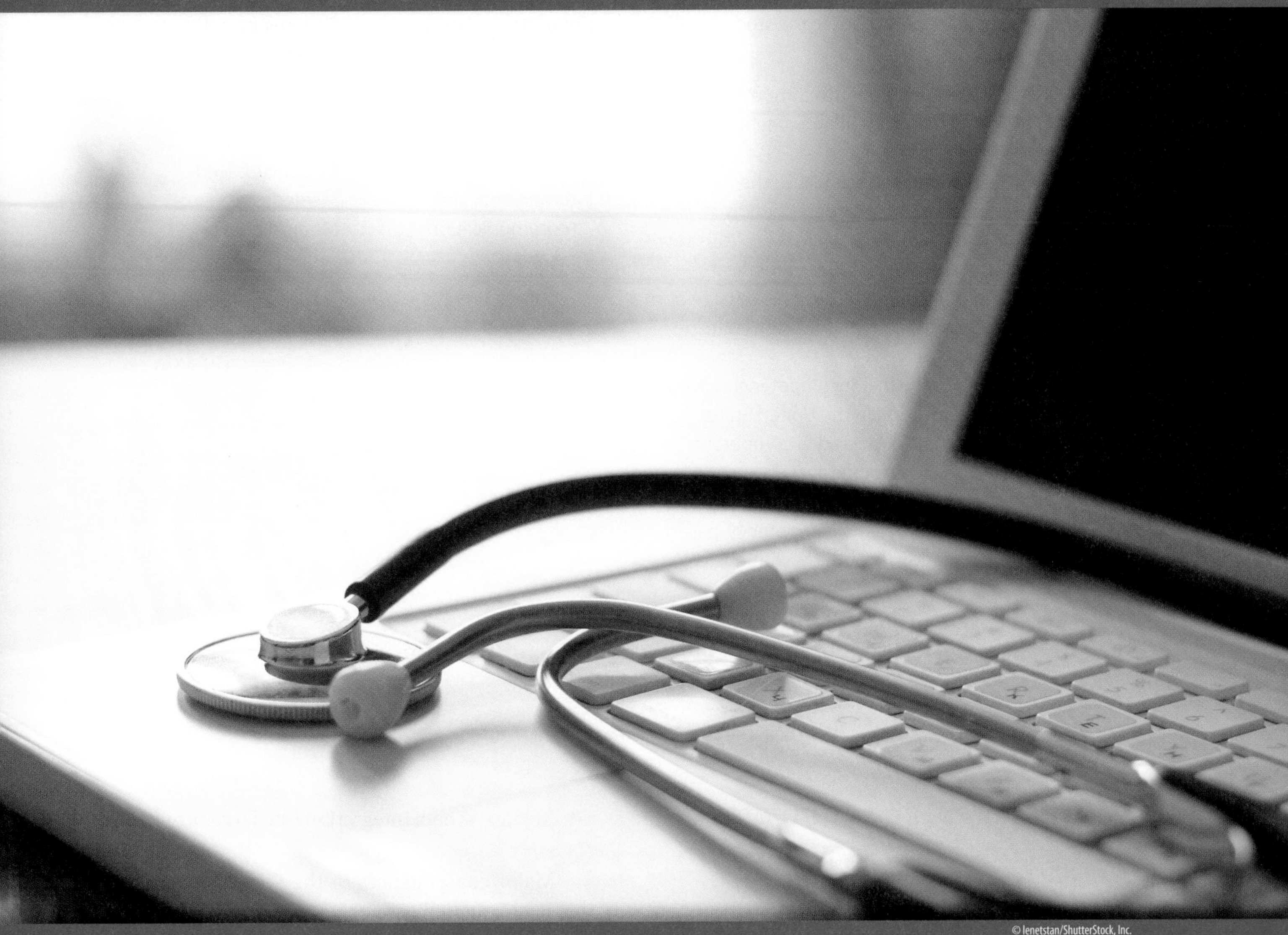

© lenetstan/ShutterStock, Inc.

Clinical Competencies

Hershey S. Bell, MD, MS, FAAFP
William Donohue, PhD

OBJECTIVES

At the conclusion of this chapter, the student will be able to

1. Discuss the evolution of the competency-based medical education movement in the United States
2. Define *competent* and relate it to the continuum of learning as described by Dreyfus and Dreyfus
3. Discuss the competency-based medical education movement in countries outside of the United States and in professions outside of medicine
4. Define each of the major competencies used in medical education in the United States and list behaviors expected of competent providers for each competency
5. Describe some of the issues that will face medical educators as the competency-based medical education movement continues to evolve

KEY TERMS

Competency-based education
Competencies
Medical knowledge
Patient care
Professionalism
Interpersonal and communication skills
Systems-based practice
Practice-based learning and improvement
Evidence-based medicine
Medical quality

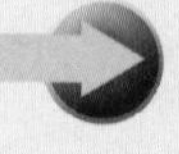
Where this icon appears, visit **go.jblearning.com/HPECWS** to view the video.

The History of the Competency-Based Education Movement in Medical Education

In 1910, Abraham Flexner produced his famous "Flexner Report," which called for major reforms in medical education.[1] While praising a number of schools in the United States and Canada, Flexner singled out Johns Hopkins as the model for all of medical education. Almost half the medical schools in the United States closed and those that remained open adopted a standardized approach to medical education that remains in effect to this day. Among the changes were:

Competency-based education: a method of education based on instruction and assessment centered around specified behavioral outcomes

- Standardized admissions requirements
- Four years of medical education
- Medical school integration into larger universities

Major consequences of the Flexner report were the close adherence to the scientific method in the educational process, the grounding of education in biochemistry and physiology, and the development of rigorous scientific research. While the overall impact on quality care increased substantially, as early as 1926 there were concerns that this new breed of scientifically trained providers may be lacking some essential ingredients of what we today refer to as competence.

In his address to Harvard Medical School students, later published in the *Journal of the American Medical Association* as "The Care of the Patient," Francis Weld Peabody lamented, "The most common criticism made at present by older practitioners is that young graduates have been taught a great deal about the mechanism of disease, but very little about the practice of medicine—or, to put it more bluntly, they are too 'scientific' and do not know how to take care of patients."[2] He concluded with one of the most famous and oft-quoted passages in the medical literature: "The good provider knows his patients through and through, and his knowledge is bought dearly. Time, sympathy and understanding must be lavishly dispensed, but the reward is to be found in that personal bond which forms the greatest satisfaction of the practice of medicine. One of the essential qualities of the clinician is interest in humanity, for the secret of the care of the patient is in caring for patients."

This general concern for the production of the complete provider surfaced again in the 1980s and 1990s. Merenstein and Schulte, in their task force report "Residency Curriculum for the Future," for the Society of Teachers of Family Medicine, called for the creation of a competency-based curriculum to address the myriad factors involved in the training of a family provider.[3] In 1997, Bell, Kozakowski, and Winter published "Competency-based Education in Family Practice," which called for education and evaluation around 26 core competencies for family providers, organized into five domains:[4]

- Clinical Acumen (how you "do" medicine)
- Interpersonal Skills (how you do medicine "with others")
- Organizational Skills (how you do medicine so that you "get it done")
- Business Practices (how you do medicine so that you can "keep doing it")
- Personal and Professional Growth and Development (how you do medicine so that you keep "doing it better")

The authors acknowledged, as Peabody did seven decades previously, that a great deal of medical knowledge is taught in family medicine residency education; however, there exists a cohort of providers who cannot or will not apply that knowledge in the most effective way to enable the highest-quality outcomes because of lack of attention to these concerns in the day-to-day process of learning.

In 1999, a watershed moment occurred in medicine in the United States with the publication of the Institute of Medicine's report "To Err Is Human: Building a Safer Health System."[5] The report estimated that between 44,000 and 98,000 people die each year as a result of medical errors, and called for a comprehensive effort by healthcare providers, government, consumers, and others. In 2001, the Institute of Medicine released "Crossing the Quality Chasm: A New Health System for the 21st Century."[6] This report called for six areas of improvement in the healthcare system:

- Safety
- Effectiveness
- Patient-centeredness
- Timeliness
- Efficiency
- Fairness

At approximately the same time, Leach and colleagues at the Accreditation Council for Graduate Medical Education (ACGME) decided to adopt changes to the required general requirements for residency education in the United States to address the concerns raised by the Institute of Medicine.[7] The Outcomes Project, a 10-year comprehensive effort designed to improve patient outcomes through education, was undertaken. Representatives from the 27 recognized specialty boards worked together to craft six core competencies that were to be studied by, and evaluated in, all resident and fellowship providers. The six **competencies** are:

- **Medical Knowledge**
- **Patient Care**
- **Professionalism**
- **Interpersonal and Communication Skills**
- **Systems-based Practice**
- **Practice-based Learning and Improvement**

A short while thereafter, the American Osteopathic Association (AOA) adopted these same

Competencies: a set of behaviors expected of all providers to be minimally prepared for the practice of medicine

Medical knowledge: as a competency, the application of medical sciences to the care of the individual patient

Patient care: as a competency, applying compassionate, necessary, and expert care to the patient, his/her family, and the community in which they live

Professionalism: as a competency, applying the values and ethics of the professional oath to each and every patient care situation

Interpersonal and communication skills: as a competency, applying the ingredients of effective communication (oral, written, and other) and teamwork to the care of the patient

Systems-based practice: as a competency, acknowledging the larger system of care in which the physician cares for the individual patient

Practice-based learning and improvement: as a competency, collecting and analyzing data from practice experience in order to continuously improve the quality of care

six competencies and added "the first competency," osteopathic philosophy and osteopathic manipulative medicine.[8]

What the ACGME and AOA efforts had in common was a desire to improve quality health care by lessening unnecessary and unexplained variation in the process of care used by clinicians. While the art of medicine is essential to the effective practice of medicine, there exists a need to ensure that every clinician demonstrates a core set of behaviors as a minimum standard. There should be little variation in the demonstration of the core behaviors described for each of the competencies regardless of a provider's specialty, scope of practice, or geographic location.

Today these competencies are part of the general education of all providers in the United States and beyond, and have become a driving force in medical school education and continuing medical education. While the full effects of the effort on patient care are not yet known, there is general agreement in the community of medical educators that value has been added to the educational process.

THE ACGME AND THE AOA COMPETENCIES

In 2001 the ACGME began its 10-year Outcomes Project to introduce learning and refine education around six core competencies in graduate medical education. The project included four phases:

- Forming the initial response (July 2001–June 2002)
- Sharpening the focus and definition of the competencies (July 2002–June 2006)
- Fully integrating the competencies with learning and clinical care (July 2006–June 2011)
- Developing models of excellence (July 2011 and beyond)

Leach and Swing from the ACGME partnered with Dreyfus and Dreyfus (learning experts) and Batalden (quality expert) to develop a model for competency-based education within graduate education that would drive the Outcomes Project. In their paper "General Competencies and Accreditation in Graduate Medical Education," they outlined the Dreyfus Model of Knowledge Development, in which medical learners progress through five distinct stages of development:[9]

- Novice (e.g., the freshman medical student learns the process of the history and physical examination using memorization)
- Advanced beginner (e.g., the junior medical student begins to see aspects of common situations, and maxims emerge)
- Competent (e.g., the resident provider learns to plan the approach to each patient's situation. Because the resident has planned the care, the consequences of the plan are knowable to the resident and offer the resident an opportunity to learn)
- Proficient (e.g., the specialist provider early in practice struggles with developing routines that can streamline the approach to the patient)
- Expert (e.g., the midcareer provider has learned to recognize patterns of discrete clues and to use intuition)

One implication of this model is that undergraduate medical education must prepare the learner to reach the advanced beginner stage so that the task of graduate medical education can be the assurance of competence by completion. Competence is therefore a *minimum standard* necessary for independent practice.

Another implication of this model is that competence is not necessarily something to be measured across each distinct competency. Rather, competence is a set of knowledge, skills, and attitudes that are habitually applied across many and varied situations. Because residents and fellows are in a position to experience the consequences of their decision and actions, a measure of competence can be the degree to which the graduate medical education student acts fully in accord with patient-centeredness—that is, the alignment of one's words, actions, thoughts, decisions, and plans in accord with the belief that *everything* is done on behalf of the patient, his/her family, and the community in which the patient lives. Said another way, graduate medical students can be deemed competent when they are consistently acting in accord with the idea that they *know* that patients' lives are on the line with every action and decision they make.

Epstein and Hundert captured this notion of competence in their article "Defining and Assessing Professional Competence."[10] They proposed that professional competence is "the habitual and judicious use of communication, knowledge, technical skills, clinical reasoning, emotions, values and reflection in daily practice for the benefit of the individual and community being served."

In 2003, the AOA published the Report of the Core Competency Task Force. Gallagher and colleagues acknowledged the impact of the Institute of Medicine and the work undertaken by the ACGME. The Task Force was asked to define, using measurable criteria, each of the seven competencies adopted by the AOA Board of Trustees. The Board of Trustees chose to adopt the six ACGME competencies and added Osteopathic Philosophy and Osteopathic Manipulative Medicine. The ACGME and AOA competencies are discussed in detail in this chapter.

COMPETENCIES FOR THE PHYSICIAN ASSISTANT PROFESSION

The physician assistant profession similarly embraced the challenge to define clinical competencies to meet the need for public accountability. In 2004, the National Commission on Certification of Physician Assistants (NCCPA) was joined by the Accreditation Review Commission for Education of the Physician Assistant (ARC-PA), the Association of Physician Assistant Programs (APAP), and the American Academy of Physician Assistants (AAPA) to create a consensus document: "Competencies for the Physician Assistant Profession."[11]

The defined competencies included the same six areas proposed by the ACGME and adopted by the AOA. In addition, the document cites "an unwavering commitment to continual learning, professional growth and the physician-PA team, for the benefit of patients and the larger community being served."

NURSE PRACTITIONER CORE COMPETENCIES

Core competencies for the nurse practitioner profession were defined by the National Organization of Nurse Practitioner Faculties and National Panel in 2006 to be consistent with the recommendations of the Institute of Medicine's report "The Future of Nursing."[5] Content within the competency headings aligns with that of other medical professional competencies. The following nine core competencies are identified:[12]

- Scientific Foundation Competencies
- Leadership Competencies
- Quality Competencies
- Practice Inquiry Competencies
- Technology and Information Literacy Competencies
- Policy Competencies
- Health Delivery System Competencies
- Ethics Competencies
- Independent Practice Competencies

Competency Statements from Other Countries

Efforts at defining provider competence for use in medical education have been described outside the United States.

In Canada, the CanMEDS (Canadian Medical Education Directions for Specialists) framework (see **FIGURE 1-1**) was created to address the question posed by the Royal College of Providers and Surgeons of Canada: "How can we best prepare providers to be effective in this environment and truly meet the needs of their patients?"[13] In the CanMEDS framework (depicted in the diagram below), there is acknowledgment of the provider as medical expert. The diagram then demonstrates the interconnectedness of the other "roles":

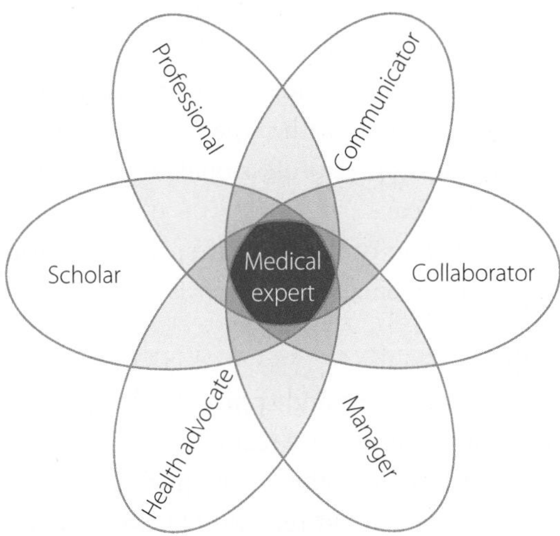

FIGURE 1-1 Medical experts.
Courtesy of: Canadian Medical Education Directions for Specialists

Communicator, Collaborator, Manager, Health Advocate, Scholar, and Professional.

Each of the roles has a list of Key Competencies. (Enabling competencies that are stated for each key competency is beyond the scope of this chapter. They can be found in the CanMEDS framework document.)

ROLES

Medical Expert

1. Function effectively as a consultant, integrating all of the CanMEDS Roles to provide optimal, ethical, and patient-centered medical care
2. Establish and maintain clinical knowledge, skills, and attitudes appropriate to their practice
3. Perform a complete and appropriate assessment of their practice
4. Use preventive and therapeutic interventions effectively
5. Demonstrate proficient and appropriate use of procedural skills, both diagnostic and therapeutic
6. Seek appropriate consultation from other health professionals, recognizing the limits of their expertise

Communicator

1. Develop rapport, trust, and ethical therapeutic relationships with patients and families
2. Accurately elicit and synthesize relevant information and perspectives of patients and families, colleagues, and other professionals
3. Accurately convey relevant information and explanations to patients and families, colleagues, and other professionals
4. Develop a common understanding on issues, problems, and plans with patients and families, colleagues, and other professionals to develop a shared plan of care
5. Convey effective oral and written information about a medical encounter

Collaborator

1. Participate effectively and appropriately in an interprofessional healthcare team
2. Effectively work with other health professionals to prevent, negotiate, and resolve interprofessional conflict

Manager

1. Participate in activities that contribute to the effectiveness of their healthcare organizations and systems
2. Manage their practice and career effectively
3. Allocate finite healthcare resources appropriately

Health Advocate

1. Respond to individual patient health needs and issues as part of patient care
2. Respond to the health needs of the communities that they serve
3. Identify the determinants of health of the populations that they serve
4. Promote the health of individual patients, communities, and populations

Scholar

1. Maintain and enhance professional activities through ongoing learning
2. Critically evaluate information and its sources, and apply this appropriately to practice decisions
3. Facilitate the learning of patients, families, students, residents, other health professionals, the public, and others, as appropriate
4. Contribute to the creation, dissemination, application, and translation of new medical knowledge and practices

Professional

1. Demonstrate a commitment to their patients, profession, and society through ethical practice
2. Demonstrate a commitment to their patients, profession, and society through participation in profession-led regulation
3. Demonstrate a commitment to provider health and sustainable practice

Good Medical Practice

In addition to these educational documents, two noteworthy papers exist to guide the development of physician competency. Good Medical Practice for General Practitioners published by the Royal College of General

Practice in the UK sets out the standards for the revalidation of general practitioners.[14] The report outlines seven broad categories for Good Medical Practice:

- Good medical care
- Maintaining good medical practice
- Relationship with patients
- Working with colleagues
- Teaching and training, appraising and assessing
- Probity
- Health and the performance of other doctors

In the United States, Good Medical Practice–USA (GMP-USA) "is a tool that has been developed to describe desirable characteristics of competent providers licensed to practice medicine in the United States."[15] GMP-USA follows the same six competencies defined by the ACGME, which are translated into six key principles. Good providers:

- Care for patients
- Maintain knowledge and skills
- Actively learn from their practices
- Exhibit excellent interpersonal and communication skills
- Exhibit commitment to the ethical and professional standards of the medical profession
- Practice effectively in systems of health care

Competencies

MEDICAL KNOWLEDGE

The medical knowledge competency requires *a demonstration of knowledge about established and evolving biomedical, clinical, and cognate (e.g., epidemiological and social-behavioral) sciences and the application of this knowledge to patient care.* Behaviors expected include:

- Demonstrating an investigatory and analytical-thinking approach to clinical situations
- Knowing and applying the basic and clinically supportive sciences that are appropriate to the provider's discipline

The competency of medical knowledge includes knowing basic medical science and social and behavioral sciences, and then correctly applying this knowledge.

ACQUIRES BASIC MEDICAL KNOWLEDGE

The foundation of medical knowledge is a deep, thorough understanding of the structure and function of the body, including the genetic, molecular, cellular, and biochemical mechanisms underlying the healthy development, structure, and function of its major organ systems. Equally important to this competency is knowledge of the various possible causes (genetic, metabolic, microbiologic, toxic, autoimmune, neoplastic, and traumatic) of adverse health outcomes.

Although medical knowledge is specialty-specific, there are a number of overarching principles of competence and the acquisition of skills that apply to all specialties. Many of these principles are embodied within the **evidence-based medicine** paradigm, which represents a shift in how providers learn and practice medicine.[16] These principles include:

Evidence-based medicine: the science of applying the best available literature to the care of the individual patient and his/her specific circumstance

- Using information derived from systematic, empirical research to determine the usefulness of diagnostic tests and the efficacy of therapy
- A thorough understanding of the rules of evidence required to evaluate and effectively apply the medical literature
- An understanding of and commitment to using decision analysis as a tool for solving difficult problems in clinical medicine

Acquires Social-Behavioral Knowledge

While medicine is considered a biological science, patients are social-behavioral beings who contract diseases. It is highly likely that a disease will affect the patient personally, and that the personality of the patient will affect the disease itself. Thus, the more social-behavioral knowledge clinicians have about patients, the greater their ability to apply scientific medical knowledge to improving the patient's health and welfare. Effective communications—questioning, observing, interacting, and interpreting—are the bedrock skills for acquiring social-behavioral knowledge about patients.

Perhaps the most effective strategy for incorporating social-behavioral knowledge into patient care involves adopting the biopsychosocial (BPS) model for medical diagnosis and treatment. This model, founded on the work of Dr. George Engel, is both a philosophy of clinical care and a practical clinical guide.[17] The BPS model represents a complex combination of the biological condition of the patient (i.e., the disease or pathological state); the psychological condition of the individual (i.e., native personality and reactions to the disease or primary psychopathology as a cause of somatic disease); and the social condition or cultural origins, which often define the patient's economic, religious, and attitudinal reactions to disease and prevention. These three dimensions are integrated in the patient as a whole greater than the sum of its parts: biological, psychological, and social.

The provider-patient interview is essential to acquiring necessary psychological and social knowledge. During the interview, the provider and patient exchange information in a fact-finding and analytic process to arrive at a diagnosis and treatment plan. Accordingly, the more the provider knows about the social and behavioral dimensions of the patient, the greater his/her ability to specify a treatment plan tailored to the patient's needs.

Providers must be skilled in social-behavioral knowledge to properly diagnose and treat any patient with a disease, whether medically or psychologically derived.

Applies Medical Knowledge

Medical and social-behavioral knowledge must be applied effectively to the clinical situation at hand. The process of evidence-based medicine is an important guide to the application of this knowledge. It is also a way of ensuring that clinical practice is based on the best evidence available. Key clinical questions must be formed that ultimately direct the patient care process. A five-step process forwarded by leading proponents of EBM includes:[16]

- Crafting a clinical question
- Searching the literature and selecting the best studies
- Critically appraising and interpreting the studies
- Applying the studies to the individual patient scenario
- Evaluating the performance with this patient

Key points pertaining to the medical knowledge competency are:

- Skilled providers have made a commitment to a lifelong process of advancing their medical knowledge through the systematic identification, evaluation, and application of the best available information.
- Providers must be skilled in social-behavioral knowledge to properly diagnose and treat any patient with a disease, whether medically or psychologically derived.
- The practice of medicine is not just about how much a clinician knows. To effectively manage medical cases and provide optimal care for patients, clinicians must also be able to apply systematic research and critical thinking processes to what they already have learned.

Providers who exemplify the medical knowledge competency demonstrate these behaviors:

- Have practical skills in acquiring, integrating, and implementing foundational knowledge in the biomedical sciences.
- Understand the pathophysiology of common conditions and diagnoses
- Understand the indications, contraindications, and complications of various tests and procedures
- Routinely demonstrate an investigatory and analytical-thinking approach to clinical situations
- Can consistently critique medical literature and locate the "best data" most applicable to the patient
- Understand the concepts of evidence-based medicine and are able routinely to apply these principles to patient care
- Understand that the medical knowledge base has layers of technical proficiency, practical (common) sense, and wisdom, and that it deepens with experience
- Demonstrate a nonjudgmental attitude toward gathering information about psychosocial factors and biological diseases

- Establish rapport, becoming a partner with the patient
- Understand the impact of the illness on the patient
- Develop mutual plans for diagnosis, treatment, and follow-up

PATIENT CARE

The patient care competency requires *the provision of patient care that is compassionate, appropriate, and effective for the treatment of health problems and the promotion of health.*

Behaviors expected include:

- Communicating effectively and demonstrating caring and respectful behaviors when interacting with patients and their families
- Gathering essential and accurate information about the patients
- Making informed decisions about diagnostic and therapeutic interventions based on patient information and preferences, up-to-date scientific evidence, and clinical judgment
- Counseling and educating patients and their families
- Using information technology to support patient care decisions and patient education
- Competently performing all medical and invasive procedures
- Providing healthcare services aimed at preventing health problems or maintaining health
- Working with healthcare professionals, including those from other disciplines, to provide patient-focused care

The patient care competency involves gathering information effectively, developing and implementing effective patient care plans, and providing effective patient education and counseling in a compassionate and empathic manner.

Effectively Gathers Information

The ability to gather relevant information and organize it into a patient care plan is at the heart of quality care. This information will be documented in patient records and shared with the healthcare team and the patient. Errors can often be traced to incomplete or disorganized information-gathering or failing to communicate findings in a clear and prioritized fashion—regardless of whether the information is oral or written.

According to Donabedian, patient care has two components: technical and interpersonal.[18] The technical component is always interwoven with the interpersonal and is effectively completed only if there is a trusting and informed relationship between provider and patient. Eliciting information is essential not only for diagnosis but also for clinical management, which considers patient preferences and participation in the process.

Like and Steinert, in their article "Medical Anthropology and the Family Provider," discuss the need to elicit four components of the patient's experience in order to effectively gather information about the patient's desire to seek care:[19]

- Explanatory models (the patient's meaning [understanding] of illness)
- Prototypical experiences (the patient's experience of the illness in him-/herself and others)
- Hidden agendas (special concerns the patient has that are difficult to voice)
- Requests (specific hopes and desires the patient has of his/her clinician and the health system)

Develops and Implements Effective Patient Care Plans

High-quality patient care requires gathering complete and relevant information and using this information in a reciprocal exchange that will assist in selecting diagnostic studies and treatment options. Billings and Stoeckle created a comprehensive model that organizes the clinical encounter into seven tasks:[20]

- Opening the interview
- Establishing a professional and supportive relationship
- Obtaining essential information for diagnosis and management
- Formulating a diagnosis
- Formulating an initial patient care plan
- Implementing the patient care plan
- Documenting information for the patient record

Gathering information leads to the development of the patient care plan, which includes three key dimensions: differential diagnosis, diagnostic evaluation, and therapeutic interventions. Each of these is described elsewhere in this text.

Provides Effective Patient Education and Counsel

Finally, once the care plan is in place, the provider must provide effective patient education and counsel to allow the plan to be enacted. Clinical care has been evolving toward a more patient-centered model in which patients are actively involved in their own care and providers design care plans suited to the patient's individual needs and preferences. From the patient's point of view, the provider who provides skilled clinical care:

- Treats him/her with dignity and respect
- Listens carefully to the questions
- Is easy to talk to
- Takes his/her concerns seriously
- Spends enough time with him/her

Studies such as the Kaiser Health Tracking Poll reveal that patients express frustrations.[21] They want information, they want to be heard, and they want to participate in systems of care that respond to their needs. This view was reaffirmed by the Institute of Medicine in the landmark report "Crossing the Quality Chasm," which included patient-centered care as one of the six primary aims for twenty-first-century health care, alongside improving patient safety, reducing healthcare disparities, and working from an evidence base.[6]

The patient-centered provider strives to understand the impact of the patient's family and work environments, his/her coping behaviors, and lifestyle and social support in ameliorating or aggravating the illness. The goal of patient-centered care is finding common ground in three key areas: the nature of the problem and priorities, the goals of treatment, and the roles of the provider and the patient.

A final component of patient-centered care involves conscious attention to the patient-provider relationship. At every visit patient-centered clinicians strive to build an effective long-term relationship with each patient as a foundation for their work together—recognizing that the relationship itself has healing potential.

The National Healthcare Quality Report, published by the Agency for Healthcare Research and Quality, uses four indicators to measure patient-centeredness:[22]

- Did the healthcare provider listen carefully?
- Did the healthcare provider explain things clearly?
- Did the healthcare provider show respect for what the patient had to say?
- Did the healthcare providers spend enough time with the patient?

Only slightly more than half of all patients reported that their healthcare provider always listened carefully, always explained things clearly, and always showed respect for what they had to say. Those who reported their health as fair or poor were more likely to report that they were not shown respect. Slightly less than half of patients felt that their providers spent enough time with them.

Various studies have shown that attending to these behaviors through a greater focus on patient-centeredness may lead to greater patient satisfaction and increase the likelihood that patients have access to essential medical and preventive health information, which in turn improves the chances of medical conditions' being properly diagnosed.

Key points pertaining to the patient care competency are:

- All of patient care is dependent on the initial collection of data that will inform each subsequent step in diagnosis and management. The method used should always be systematic, accurate, and relevant to the requirements of the clinical encounter.
- Once information is gathered, the provider must begin to define the potential active disease processes. The resulting "list" is the differential diagnosis. The diagnostic evaluation helps to sort the likelihood of the various possible conditions. Finally, the provider designs therapeutic interventions to address the better-defined condition or diagnosis.
- The once-prevalent idea of the detached clinician who keeps a safe emotional distance is being replaced with the patient-centered model.

Providers who exemplify the patient care competency demonstrate these behaviors:

- Utilize a standardized approach to data gathering, which leads to a problem list, identification of chief complaint, a history of present illness, the patient's medical history, medications, allergies, social and family history, review of relevant systems that will impact care, performance of an appropriate physical examination, and review of imaging and laboratory data if available
- Develop broad differential diagnoses that consider likely conditions as well as life-threatening conditions
- Rapidly narrow a broad differential diagnosis to a limited differential diagnosis
- Effectively diagnose and treat life-threatening conditions, emergent conditions, and chronic disease
- Synthesize all clinical and laboratory data into a treatment strategy that improves the patient's condition
- Create diagnostic and monitoring plans
- Understand the limitations of diagnostic studies as well as the risks and complications of any medication ordered or procedure performed
- Keep clear and accurate documentation
- Effectively and precisely communicate medical orders
- Provide effective strategies and education for disease and injury prevention and control
- Seek to understand patients' ideas about what is wrong with them
- Are sensitive to patients' feelings, especially fears about being ill
- Are responsive to patients' expectations about what should be done
- Counsel patients and their families regarding medical conditions and treatment plans

INTERPERSONAL AND COMMUNICATION SKILLS

The interpersonal and communication skills competency requires *a demonstration of interpersonal communication skills that result in effective information exchange and teaming with patients, the patients' families, and professional associates.* Expected behaviors include:

- Creating and sustaining a therapeutic and ethically sound relationship with patients
- Using effective listening skills and eliciting and providing information using effective nonverbal, explanatory, questioning, and writing skills
- Working effectively with others as a member or leader of a healthcare team or other professional group

The interpersonal communication skills competency includes the dimensions of providing precise, effective instruction to staff and patients, effectively seeking feedback, and demonstrating attentiveness when communicating.

Provides Precise, Effective Instruction to Staff and Patients

Providers who are effective in giving precise instructions take great care in explaining their diagnoses, informing patients and staff members about the medical situation, and justifying their decisions. They assess what information people need, when they need it, and the level of detail required for a carefully crafted message that individuals are likely to find instructive. The goal is not just to give information but also to connect with the patient and then instruct and explain clearly and precisely.

A review article in the *Annals of Internal Medicine* written by Weiner indicated that optimal communication skills involve relationship building, asking open-ended questions, using verbal encouragement, avoiding interruptions, providing patient education, expressing personal warmth, and eliciting patient concerns.[23] More importantly, when providers use these skills, patient outcomes improve. Patients report greater satisfaction, lower stress, stricter medication adherence, better blood-pressure control, and success in smoking cessation.

Travaline and his colleagues outlined an effective strategy for giving instructions to either patients or staff.[24] Their nine strategies are:

- Assess what the patient already knows
- Assess what the patient wants to know
- Be empathic

- Slow down
- Keep it simple
- Tell the truth
- Be hopeful
- Watch the patient's body and face
- Be prepared for a reaction

Cultural issues may cause problems in cross-cultural encounters. Some patients and staff members may have trouble with authority, physical contact, communication styles, gender, sexuality, and/or family. Misra-Hebert recommends that providers try three things to manage these differences:[25]

- Build the relationship to establish trust by speaking slowly and avoiding jargon. Give information in a structured way, step-by-step so as to enhance learning.
- Assess the patient's understanding of health problems to determine how he/she is experiencing or making sense of the condition.
- Manage the patient's problems by acknowledging and respecting the role of the family, inquiring about the use of alternative treatments, and providing patient education materials in the language the patient can understand.

Effectively Seeks Feedback

Providers who are open to feedback are generally more effective than those who resist listening to others' views. Feedback creates collaboration, and seeking feedback signals a willingness to work collaboratively as part of the team to share information, opinions, and strategies. The Institute of Medicine emphasized the need for effective teamwork in reducing many medical errors.[6] Fewer errors occur when members know their responsibilities, trust one another, and share information. Soliciting and accepting feedback from other team members, patients, and their families creates a communication safety net that protects the patients.

Seeking feedback gives patients a chance to participate in their own care and lessens patient anxiety and the likelihood of medical malpractice claims. Nodding, reflective facial expressions, and continued eye contact constitute the most essential nonverbal signals that the provider is open to feedback and genuinely wants the patient to be a partner in his/her treatment.

Students of medicine should be able to incorporate feedback from the beginning of their training. Papadakis and colleagues found that medical students who did not listen to and incorporate feedback had a threefold-higher risk of having medical licensure issues as compared with their peers.[26]

Demonstrates Attentiveness When Communicating

Listening and attentiveness are essential to collecting detailed medical information and to interacting with healthcare professionals in busy, noisy, and often stressful clinical settings. Not only is listening a patient safety issue, but being attentive to patients and staff members is perhaps the single most important communication feature in building productive, trusting relationships. Remaining attentive both verbally and nonverbally sends a message that the provider cares about the patient's needs and goals.

In a document titled "The Kalamazoo Consensus Statement," a group of 21 experts in the field of medicine identified seven essential components of communication.[27] The seven elements are:

- Establishes rapport
- Opens discussion
- Gathers information
- Understands the patient's perspective of illness
- Shares information
- Reaches agreement on problems and plans
- Provides closure

There are three main components to effective listening:

- The first element is paying attention by demonstrating appropriate nonverbal cues that you value the other person's contribution. These include eye contact, body posture, allowing the person to complete their thoughts without interruption, providing occasional verbal acknowledgment that you are listening, and using open-ended questions.
- The second element of effective listening is summarizing or paraphrasing the other's comments or key phrases. This communicates both empathy and understanding.
- The third skill is asking questions or providing comments that are clearly focused on the other's

topic. Giving the "topic control" to the other demonstrates empathy and shows support for his/her perspective. It honors the other's point of view, which is pivotal in building a lasting relationship. Perhaps more importantly, it stimulates even more self-disclosure.

Key points pertaining to the interpersonal and communication skills competency are:

- Delivering precise, step-by-step instructions enhances learning and increases patient safety.
- Actively soliciting feedback builds a collaborative team culture, creates effective relationships with patients and staff, and reduces medical errors.
- Providers who avoid chronic interruptions and focus on the speaker are significantly more likely to be judged as competent communicators.

Providers who exemplify the interpersonal and communication skills competency demonstrate these behaviors:

- Provide information in a detailed, friendly manner
- Adjust the message to the listener's needs, level of emotion, and medical literacy
- Work to establish credibility through the demonstration of knowledge and trustworthiness, and seek to understand patient and staff perspectives on issues
- Demonstrate a concern for patient safety
- Contribute to the creation of a team atmosphere
- Are perceived as being friendly and accessible
- See issues from the other's perspective
- Empathize with the other's condition and circumstance
- Maintain eye contact and an open body posture
- Paraphrase key elements of the other's contributions

PROFESSIONALISM

The professionalism competency requires *a demonstration of a commitment to carrying out professional responsibilities, adherence to ethical principles, and sensitivity to a diverse patient population.* Expected behaviors include:

- Demonstrating respect, compassion, and integrity; a responsiveness to the needs of patients and society that supersedes self-interest; accountability to patients, society, and the profession; and a commitment to excellence and ongoing professional development
- Demonstrating commitment to ethical principles pertaining to provision or withholding of clinical care, confidentiality of patient information, informed consent, and business practices
- Demonstrating sensitivity and responsiveness to patient's culture, age, gender, and disabilities

The professionalism competency includes the domains of demonstrating ethical behavior, showing sensitivity and compassion, and taking responsibility.

Demonstrates Ethical Behavior

Providers who act professionally consistently put the needs of patients and their families, societies, and the medical profession itself ahead of their own needs. They weigh every action they take, both while engaged in active practice and while participating in all other aspects of their lives. Attention to ethical behavior is a key component of the demonstration of professionalism. Lack of attention to professionalism and ethical behavior is not only the number one cause that state medical boards cite for taking action against providers; it is also a key factor in medical error and patient safety concerns. Providers who fail to act ethically create barriers to communication, teamwork, and quality patient care.

"Project Professionalism," a major report from the American Board of Internal Medicine, cites altruism, accountability, excellence, duty, service, honor and integrity, and respect for others as the aspirations of professionalism.[28] The authors state that professionalism is compromised by the abuse of power, arrogance, greed, misrepresentation, impairment, lack of conscientiousness, and conflicts of interest.

The Tavistock Principles move the conversation of ethical conduct beyond the individual provider-patient relationship and into the realm of global ethics.[29] The principles include:

- Attention to the basic human right to health care
- The importance of the health of populations

- Medicine's obligations to end suffering, minimize disability, and prevent disease and promote health
- A need for cooperation
- To do no harm
- To be open, honest, and trustworthy as healthcare providers

Chervenak and McCullough draw attention to the relationship between ethics and leadership in medicine by introducing the concept of the provider-leader as the "moral fiduciary of the patient."[30] The virtues that follow from this stance include self-effacement, self-sacrifice, compassion, and integrity. Vices that undermine the moral culture of professionalism include unwarranted bias, primacy of self-interest, hard-heartedness, and corruption.

Shows Sensitivity and Compassion

The professionalism competency encourages providers to increase their sensitivity to the specific needs of patients and staff no matter who they are.[31] Diversity covers issues such as religion, sexual orientation, gender, race, disability, social class, education, income, and age. When working with patients, it is important to think of them not only as biological systems, but as people with diverse backgrounds that strongly shape their beliefs regarding health, illness, and medicine. Approximately 1 million immigrants per year come to the United States, mostly from Latin America and Asia. Roughly one in every three people in this country belongs to an ethnic minority group.

People of European ancestry remain the largest ethnic group in the United States. In 2002, the Hispanic, or Latino, population became the largest minority group, composing 13% of the population. The African American population composes about 12% of the total population. About 2% of the population identifies themselves as belonging to more than one ethnic group.

Cultural beliefs associated with ethnicity shape patients' responses to symptoms, health, and health care. Cultural factors influence a person's tendency to seek treatment.

Age and gender also influence the quality of health care a person receives. Older Americans and females, the latter even after accounting for visits for maternal care, report more symptoms and seek more care than their younger male counterparts. Older Americans and females also experience unique barriers to health care, such as financial factors and the perception of the role of emotional issues.

Responsibility

To serve implies that the needs of the person being served have primacy over the needs of the person providing that service. In medicine this means that the provider must possess the ability to correctly identify the needs of the patient and then choose actions that are generated on behalf of the patient. The litmus test for professionalism is the determination of the root of the behavior. If the behavior is rooted in conversations generated on behalf of the patient, that behavior is deemed professional. If the behavior is rooted in conversations generated on behalf of the provider, then that behavior is deemed unprofessional.

Placing the patient's needs first means that when you are acting within your professional role, you make decisions and choose actions solely on behalf of your patient's well-being. It also means that you represent your profession well by your personal decisions and actions.

Among the considerations for providers operating from the primacy of patient needs are their personal appearance, the appearance of their practice site, the behavior of their staff, the manner in which they schedule patients, the systems they use for collecting and tracking medical information and providing follow-up to patients, the telephone and other communications systems that are used, the telephone or email message for assuring access to care after hours, and the manner in which they bill for services. The literature supports the idea that attention to professional appearance increases the effectiveness of the care delivered.

Key points pertaining to the professionalism competency are:

- You will be known as an ethical provider based on your actions, rather than on your words. The actions that are most important are those that demonstrate your willingness to serve your patient, your patient's families, and society in general.
- Professionalism means tailoring interventions to patients' diverse backgrounds. These backgrounds

influence their perception of illness, interactions with their provider, trust and satisfaction, adherence, and ultimately outcomes.

- The "litmus test" for professionalism requires asking the question, "On whose behalf am I considering this action?" If the answer suggests that anyone other than the patient, their family, or society is being served, the professionalism of the choice must be questioned.

Providers who exemplify the professionalism competency demonstrate these behaviors:

- Put the best interests of their patients ahead of self-interest
- Honor their commitments, duties, and responsibilities to their patients
- Commit to excellence by exceeding ordinary expectations and partaking in lifelong learning
- Demonstrate their humanism via respect for others
- Are honest and trustworthy
- Demonstrate their integrity by the consistency of their behavior
- Respect the rights of patients by being fully involved in decision making
- Recognize the limits of their professional competence
- Do not abuse their position or status as providers
- Avoid using condescending language and behaviors that are biased in terms of race, ethnicity, culture, age, gender and sexual orientation, or social class
- Treat patients as individuals
- Seek greater understanding of their patients' and coworkers' diverse backgrounds, beliefs, and behavior
- Dress and groom in accord with patient expectations
- Arrive on time or early for scheduled activities
- Create a safe, professional appearance and healing environment of care
- Ensure that all necessary tasks surrounding patient care are accomplished in a timely, organized, and professional manner
- Follow through on promises and commitments to patients and their families
- Arrange for coverage, or alternate avenues of care, when they will not be personally available to their patients
- Bill patients fairly and appropriately for services rendered, referring those who need help to those properly assessed
- Give back to the profession by honoring the oath to teach students and residents who are learning the profession

SYSTEMS-BASED PRACTICE

The systems-based practice competency requires *a demonstration of an awareness of and responsiveness to the larger context and system of health care and the ability to effectively call on system resources to provide care that is of optimal value.* Expected behaviors include:

- Understanding how patient care and other professional practices affect other healthcare professionals, the healthcare organization, and the larger society, and how these elements of the system affect the provider's practice
- Knowing how types of medical practice and delivery systems differ from one another, including methods of controlling healthcare costs and allocating resources
- Practicing cost-effective health care and resource allocation that does not compromise quality of care
- Advocating for quality patient care and assisting patients in dealing with system complexities
- Knowing how to partner with healthcare managers and healthcare providers to assess, coordinate, and improve health care, and knowing how these activities can affect system performance

The systems-based practice competency encompasses the realms of understanding system complexities, working with other healthcare professionals, and practicing cost-effectiveness.

Understands System Complexities

Systems-based practice is an awareness of and responsiveness to the larger context and system of health care. It is the ability to effectively call on the system's resources in order to provide care of optimal value.

The Institute of Medicine focused national attention on the performance of health systems through two major publications: "To Err Is Human: Building a Safer Health System" and "Crossing the Quality Chasm: A New Health System for the 21st Century."[5,6] The Institute concluded that fundamental changes are needed in the organization and delivery of health care. The purpose of these changes should be to "reduce the burden of illness, injury, and disability to improve the health and functioning of the people of the United States." Six specific improvement aims were proposed:

- Safety
- Effectiveness
- Timeliness
- Efficiency
- Patient-centered care
- Care that is equitable

The Institute proposed that healthcare organizations must redesign their care processes, develop effective teams, manage clinical knowledge and skills, and make effective use of information technologies.

Systems-based practice is immediately grounded by our primary responsibility for the individual patient. However, it simultaneously recognizes the critical need for direct attention to navigating the complex healthcare system in order for providers to provide successful and effective patient care. Systems-based practice requires a thinking approach that recognizes that organizational structure drives interdependencies and behavior, that cause and effect are separated by time and space, and that one individual's actions within a system can have unintended consequences. Specific aspects of the system that are critical to understand include:

- The environmental context in which we practice. It is forever changing and its key drivers are federal and state government legislation, environmental regulations, reimbursement and insurance agencies, advancing technologies, and alternate treatment options, as well as the aging demographics of the U.S. population
- The specific macro-organization ("the system"). Organizational governance, strategic planning and decision making, and overall mission, vision, goals, and strategies all have an impact on health care. The strengths and style of the organization's leadership can create proactive or reactive decisions that can impact the quality of care in the community.
- The micro-system ("the practice"). This involves the referral network for a particular practice, policies and procedures, available technologies, and which members of the team are involved in direct care.
- The patient and the community. The healthcare decisions made by a provider should account for the patient's ability to understand and carry through instructions, his/her ability to withstand the treatment, what type of additional support is available within his/her community, and the cost-benefit considerations for the patient.

Working with Other Healthcare Professionals

The nature of health care is changing as patients experience chronic conditions that require coordinated care by a variety of healthcare professionals.

Wagner defines a patient care team as "a group of diverse clinicians who communicate with each other regularly about the care of a defined group of patients and participate in that care."[32] The organization and interaction of patient care teams can be conceptualized along the continuum from multidisciplinary (practitioners contribute individually to the care of a patient) to interdisciplinary (practitioners work together closely and communicate regularly about the course of care, usually to solve a series of problems, which draws upon the individual knowledge of the team members) to transdisciplinary (where team member roles are blurred to the point that duties overlap).

Teams need to function in a way that encourages collaborative action and purpose among individuals on the team. There are five key elements that effective clinical teams incorporate:

- Establishing clear goals
- Utilizing and/or designing clinical systems to facilitate workflow
- Designing and assigning specific tasks and roles
- Training individuals to perform roles
- Developing clear processes for communication

Other important factors include a focus on teamwork principles including establishing the team's mission, values, and goals; understanding the nature of the group process; developing communication, role-negotiation, conflict-management, problem-solving, and decision-making skills; and recognizing other factors involved with patient care.

Practices Cost-effectiveness

Healthcare costs have climbed steadily and yet the nation's health care has not improved. Cost-effectiveness analysis has not demonstrated benefit for many conditions. The greatest contributors to escalating healthcare costs are drugs, medical devices, and other medical advances. Rising provider expenses account for approximately one-fifth of the overall increase. Government mandates and regulations account for approximately 15% of the overall increase in healthcare costs. Increased consumer demand adds approximately 2% annually to healthcare costs, accounting for 15% of the increased cost. The aging population, as well as the consumerism movement, have also contributed to the cost escalation. Litigation risk management contributes approximately 7% of the increase in healthcare costs.

Key points pertaining to the systems-based practice competency are:

- A provider practicing within the larger healthcare system knows his/her role and acts accordingly in the treatment of his/her patients and with other members of the healthcare team.
- Working in patient care situations requires teamwork and partnering with other healthcare professionals to provide patient care that is both effective and efficient. As such, it will be imperative that you are aware of key teamwork components and how your role or expertise integrates with other team members.
- Providers will be called upon to measure the performance of clinical and administrative processes, improve systems of care to reduce costs, and streamline operations.

Providers who exemplify the systems-based practice competency demonstrate these behaviors:

- Recognize and appropriately utilize available healthcare delivery systems that include multidisciplinary and managed care models to provide optimal patient care
- Demonstrate respect for and appreciation of other healthcare professionals within the system and appropriately call upon their skill and training
- Empathize with patients and how they must navigate the system, and willingly assist patients in dealing with system complexities
- Anticipate barriers to patient care that can include insurance approvals, costs, and test turnaround times
- Apply excellent time-management skills, including in scheduling patient appointments
- Maintain a positive, professional attitude while working within the system and do not become frustrated by issues one provider cannot change
- Seek opportunities to contribute to the improvement of the overall system
- Use a patient-centered approach to patient care
- Provide clear and precise communications with other team members, both verbal and nonverbal
- Use appropriate conflict management skills
- Are willing to assess self and team performance
- Realize the importance of calling on system resources to provide optimal-value care
- Formulate treatment plans that include both short- and long-term goals involving the patient, support systems, and interdisciplinary collaboration
- Are meticulous in the accuracy and timeliness of documentation and coding
- Identify and coordinate services and resources necessary to implement the plan
- Carry out ongoing evaluation of the effectiveness and appropriateness of the services throughout the spectrum of care
- Advocate for appropriate, cost-effective services to ensure quality care and goal attainment

PRACTICE-BASED LEARNING AND IMPROVEMENT

The practice-based learning and improvement competency requires *an ability to investigate and evaluate patient care practices, appraise and assimilate scientific evidence, and improve patient care practices.* Expected behaviors include:

- Analyzing practice experience and performing practice-based improvement activities using a systematic methodology

- Locating, appraising, and assimilating evidence from scientific studies related to the patient's health problems
- Obtaining and using information about the provider's own population of patients and a larger population from which his/her patients are drawn
- Applying knowledge of study designs and statistical methods to the appraisal of clinical studies and other information on diagnostic and therapeutic effectiveness
- Using information technology to manage information, access online information, and support the provider's own education
- Facilitating the learning of students and other healthcare professionals

The practice-based learning and improvement competency encompasses the realms of performing an effective analysis of the patient care process, facilitating professional learning, and using information technology effectively.

Conducts an Effective Analysis of the Patient Care Process

Keeping up to date on new treatments, new medications, new reimbursement guidelines, etc., is one of the greatest challenges in modern medicine. Analyzing the patient care process requires the use of information technology, a focus on continuous practice improvement, and an ability to critically appraise the literature and assimilate this information into patient care. This is all aided by fostering an environment of teaching and learning.

The speed of progress in medicine is astounding and can be overwhelming for many providers. The constant stream of new information has been accelerated by the movement to practice evidence-based medicine. Research has demonstrated the difficulty of teaching and practicing evidence-based medicine in a busy practice. The process can be made more effective by:

- Receiving training in critical appraisal of the literature
- Consulting scientific evidence to get answers to questions, as a part of the daily routine
- Making "real time and real world" searches for information
- Having the ability to search literature available at the point of care

In addition to the use of evidence-based medicine, there must be a culture of continuous quality improvement, also known as total quality management. Improvements to patient care require the effective use of evidence-based medicine and a commitment to continuous quality improvement.

Facilitates Professional Learning

Facilitating the professional learning of others (students, residents, and other staff), as well as a commitment to lifelong learning, is critical to success in facilitating one's own professional learning. Facilitating professional learning of others requires skills in a number of areas, including knowledge of the subject matter, working knowledge of effective teaching practices, the ability to stay current with recent clinical studies, and a commitment to lifelong learning. Wipf, Pinsky, and Burke concluded, "As clinical experience increases, clinical knowledge becomes more tightly compiled and interconnected."[33] Good teachers are able to break down all of these connections to facilitate learning in others.

Studies have identified the following to be important factors in teaching:

- Medical knowledge/keeping up to date
- Assessing learner knowledge and learning needs
- Providing constructive feedback
- Knowledge of practical teaching skills such as micro skills and case-based teaching.

Uses Information Technology Effectively

A provider's ability to use information technology can have a profound effect on the cost and quality of health care. It can help make diagnosis and treatment more effective, make the work of the cross-functional care team more productive, and potentially save time and other resources for all involved. Information technology also helps a clinician tap into a vast array of resources and provides a means for continual learning.

When the Department of Health and Human Services introduced its plan to build a national electronic health information infrastructure in the United States, the intent of the plan was to "achieve always current, always available electronic health records for Americans."

Advantages from using modern information technology in medical practice include:

- Availability of current medical information whenever and wherever the patient and health professionals need it
- Improved quality of care through minimization of errors
- Decision-support
- Cost savings
- Access to the best quality care for the medically underserved

The five electronic health record features found most beneficial to users' practices are:

- Quick access to patient records
- Managing medication lists
- Managing clinical documents and notes
- Searching for data
- E-prescribing

It is also vitally important for providers to have access to current information because patients now have unlimited access to health information via the Internet. Providers can help guide patients to the most accurate and most helpful information while steering them away from misleading and inaccurate information.

Key points pertaining to the practice-based learning and improvement competency are:

- To best serve your patient's needs, you must keep up with all scientific evidence and make wise changes to the patient care process. Your challenge is to find ways to do this efficiently and routinely, using all the resources available.
- One cannot underestimate the potential impact of a skilled practitioner on other healthcare professionals' learning. Providers who practice alone find it more difficult to maintain their professional competence.
- Now and in the future, information technology will be an integral part of the healthcare environment. Effective use of information technology is no longer optional for providers. It is expected.

Providers who exemplify the practice-based learning and improvement competency demonstrate these behaviors:

- Routinely locate clinical studies relevant to their patients and use information from the studies to inform patient care decisions
- Critically evaluate research design and results of clinical studies
- Continually analyze the practice experience
- Possess a desire to teach and to improve teaching skills
- Use knowledge of new information and discussions with others to help keep them up-to-date
- Demonstrate a commitment to lifelong self-directed learning
- Understand and fully utilize information technology resources
- Communicate with colleagues and patients via electronic means
- Carry and routinely use a handheld device
- Efficiently get answers to clinical questions at point of care
- Use information technology resources to manage patient and practice information

COMPETENCY ISSUES SPECIFIC TO OSTEOPATHIC MEDICINE

In distinction to the six competencies developed by the Accreditation Council for Graduate Medical Education (ACGME), the American Osteopathic Association (AOA) has added the "first competency" of osteopathic philosophy and principles and manipulative treatment and has asked its trainers *not* to evaluate this competency separately; rather, they should evaluate its appearance through the other six competencies.[34] The underlying message is that osteopathic medicine is not simply allopathic medicine plus osteopathic philosophy and principles and manipulative treatment. Osteopathic medicine requires incorporation of osteopathic philosophy and principles and

TABLE 1-1 Competencies and Required Elements

Competency	Required Elements	Examples of Associated OPP Competencies*
Medical Knowledge and Its Application to Osteopathic Medical Practice	1. The understanding and application of clinical medicine 2. Knowledge and application of the foundations of clinical and behavioral medicine	• Participating in CME offered by osteopathic organizations • Demonstrating understanding of somato-visceral relationships and the role of the musculoskeletal system in disease • Participating in OMT/OPP training • Demonstrating the treatment of people rather than symptoms
Osteopathic Patient Care	1. Gathering accurate and essential information 2. Competently performing diagnostic, osteopathic, and other treatment and procedures 3. Provision of healthcare services consistent with osteopathic philosophy, including preventive medicine and health promotion	• Performing OMT • Using listening skills, caring, compassionate behavior, and touch with patients
Interpersonal and Communication Skills and Osteopathic Medicine	1. Developing appropriate provider-patient relationships 2. Effective listening, written, and oral communication skills	• Demonstrating knowledge of behavior in accordance with the Osteopathic Oath and the AOA code of ethics
Professionalism in Osteopathic Medicine	1. Respect for patients and families and advocates for the primacy of patient's welfare and the economy 2. Adherence to ethical principles 3. Awareness and proper attention to issues of culture, religion, age, gender, sexual orientation, and mental and physical disabilities 4. Awareness of one's own mental and physical health	• Completing OMT computer educational modules • Self-adherence to preventive care • Establishing a routine form of physical activity
Osteopathic Medical Practice-based Learning and Improvement	1. Using the most up-to-date information 2. Self-evaluation of clinical practice patterns and practice-based improvement activities using a systematic methodology 3. Understanding research methods, medical informatics, and the application of technology	• Participating in AOA Clinical Assessment Program • Critically appraising OMT/OPP literature
System-based Osteopathic Medical Practice	1. Understanding national and local healthcare delivery systems and medical societies and how they affect patient care and professional practice and relate to advocacy 2. Advocate for quality health care	• Assuming increased responsibility for the incorporation of osteopathic concepts in patient management

*Many of the associated OPP competencies appear in more than one competency and more than one element. For more information, please visit the website of the American Osteopathic Association.

Adapted from: American Osteopathic Association.

manipulative treatment, where appropriate, into all that the osteopathic provider does.

The first competency of osteopathic philosophy and principles and manipulative treatment states:

> *. . . an expectation to demonstrate and apply knowledge of accepted standards in OPP/OMT* ***appropriate to the specialty.*** [Emphasis in the original.] *The educational goal is to train a skilled and competent osteopathic practitioner who remains dedicated to lifelong learning and to practice habits in osteopathic philosophy and manipulative medicine.*

The remaining six competencies (2 to 7) are:

2. Medical knowledge and its application to osteopathic medical practice
3. Osteopathic patient care
4. Interpersonal and communication skills and osteopathic medicine
5. Professionalism in osteopathic medicine
6. Osteopathic medical practice–based learning and improvement
7. System-based osteopathic medical practice

Each competency (2 to 7) is broken down into several required elements, and within each element are listed the essential ingredients for success for all providers as well as the essential ingredients for success specific to osteopathic medicine. Examples of the latter are presented in **TABLE 1-1**.

Future Directions

When the competency movement began in the late 1990s and early 2000s, its ultimate aim was to improve the quality of health care in the United States by lessening unnecessary and unexplained variation in the process of care. The Institute of Medicine shed light on where individual practitioners, hospitals, healthcare systems, and medical and allied health professions education must focus in order to eliminate this needless variation that accounts for our inability to achieve the highest levels of quality. In both medical practice and medical education, the unwanted variation that existed was in the area of the demonstration of clinical competencies discussed in this chapter. With time, it is fully expected that the evidence will emerge that demonstrates that when providers, healthcare systems, and all allied healthcare professionals adhere to behaviors consistent with what the competencies call for, the quality of care will indeed improve. In fact, while the competency movement is only a decade old, already evidence is emerging to demonstrate the impact of competency-based behaviors on quality healthcare outcomes.

With respect to medical education, Aron and Headrick utilized Reason's model of medical error to demonstrate where unnecessary and unexplained variation are creating quality issues.[35] The model suggests that in order to produce a provider who cannot effectively offer high-quality medical care, the educational system must fail at many levels. Reason's model depicts layers of Swiss cheese—the analogy is that each slice of Swiss cheese acts as a barrier against educational system failure. However, if the student is able to pass through the holes in all of the pieces of Swiss cheese, the system will fail and will produce a provider who cannot improve care and safety.

Fortunately, efforts are underway in each of the five key areas described in the model, which have the potential to continue to move the U.S. healthcare system toward the highest-achievable-quality outcomes. These efforts are:

- Entrance requirements. The MR5 is the fifth comprehensive review of the Medical College Admission Test (MCAT).[36] The preliminary recommendations include:
  - Reporting on four distinct sections: molecular, cellular, and organismal properties of living systems; physical, chemical, and biochemical properties of living systems; behavioral and social science principles; and critical analysis and reasoning skills.
  - Testing on research methods and statistics that are most important for success in medical education
  - Testing on the foundations of the behavioral and sociocultural determinants of health
  - Testing on the ability to analyze and reason through passages in ethics and philosophy, cross-cultural studies, population health, and a wide range of social sciences and humanities disciplines to ensure that students possess the

necessary critical thinking skills to be successful in medicine

- Curriculum. Although the competency-based education movement began in residency education, competencies for medical schools and for continuing education are now available to ensure that attention to mastering behaviors critical to producing high-quality outcomes are available across the continuum of medical education. More recently, several health professions including medical, pharmacy, dental, public health, and nursing have described competencies for interprofessional education and practice.[37] Recognizing the key importance of interprofessional education practice was a major focus of the Institute of Medicine.
- Organizational Culture and Professionalism. Research by Hafferty, Hafler, and Haidet has drawn attention to the importance of the hidden curriculum—the context in which health professions education occurs—in affecting the behaviors of medical school graduates.[38,39,40] More attention is being given to the educational environment and the behaviors of professors and preceptors in accord with the understanding of how these behaviors can shape the actions and thoughts of developing professionals. As well, attention to professionalism in schools has been heightened primarily due to landmark research produced by Papadakis and her colleagues, which demonstrated that unprofessional behaviors left unchecked in medical school can have consequences for **medical quality** as well as career-threatening implications down the road.[26]

Medical quality: the science of lessening unexpected and unnecessary clinical variation that could negatively impact the outcomes of care

- Student assessment. While stating competencies expected of medical school graduates is a start, Bell and colleagues argue that in order to be certain that we are graduating providers who can actually demonstrate the necessary behaviors incumbent in the competencies, a shift from summative toward formative evaluation is necessary.[4] Traditionally medical schools and residencies rely on periodic overall assessments that rate performance on a continuum from excellent to poor. Competency-based education, as originally described by Carroll, Bloom, and others, relies on formative evaluation that provides real-time information to students with an intention to correct behaviors that are not working and to reinforce behaviors that are working. Bell has described the "FED Model of Formative Evaluation," which includes:[41]
  - F (Feedback): providing information to learners intended to highlight areas of needed improvement that may be known or unknown to the learner.
  - E (Encouragement): providing feedback in a way that "heartens" the learner toward competency and mastery as opposed to providing feedback that humiliates, discourages, and "disheartens" learners. (The root of the word "encouragement" is the French word for heart, "coeur.")
  - D (Direction): the competencies, and the associated patient-centered behaviors as described in this chapter, provide a roadmap for success. All feedback should be linked to the outcomes expected of learners.
- Program accreditation. Accreditors have acknowledged that their prior emphasis on measuring what a school, program, hospital, or health system was doing was not a good method for assuring quality. In the last decade, there has been a powerful shift toward outcomes assessment. By measuring the outcomes of the educational and practice processes, the public can have more faith that accreditors are looking more carefully at the issues that truly affect quality care and patient safety. It is no surprise that many accreditors, including the Joint Commission, have also stated specific competencies that they expect for practitioners, hospitals, and health systems.

Summary

The *outcome that matters* in health professions education and practice is the assurance of high-quality patient care that represents the best practices available today and protects the public's safety. The development of competencies for providers in the late 1990s and early 2000s was a watershed event in the history of medical education. The competency-based educational movement has the potential of improving the health of all Americans in a profound and lasting way by lessening unnecessary and unexplained variation in the process of clinical care.

The authors, Dr. Bell and Dr. Donohue, would like to acknowledge those who contributed to the development of the Medical Professional Performance Systems Assessment and Development Tool for Resident Providers, which supplied information germane to the sections of this chapter on the six ACGME competencies. In addition, they would like to thank those who participated in authoring dimension reports for use with osteopathic medical students at the Lake Erie College of Osteopathic Medicine. These individuals are:

Kenneth Alonso, MD

Mark Andrews, PhD

Michael Barnes, MD

Megan Becker, PhD

Mark Best, MD, MBA, MPH

Anthony Ferretti, DO

Naushad Ghilzai, PhD

Laura Griffin, DO

Rasheed Hassan, DO

Rebecca Henry, PhD

Blake Hoppe, DO

Hannah Howell, PharmD

Mohamed Hussein, PhD

Abir Kahaleh, PhD

Gary Laco, PhD

Tracey Larson, MA

Ross Longley, PhD

Theodore Makoske, MD

Norman Miller, MD, JD

Ali Moradi, MD, MPH

Kristen Nardozzi, DO

Rachel Ogden, PharmD

Allison Ownby, PhD

Stephanie Peshek, PharmD

Teresa Pettersen, MD

Tom Quinn, DO

Earl Reisdorff, MD

Stephen Sharkady, PhD

Laura Stevenson, PharmD

Bojana Stevich, PharmD

Richard O. Straub, PhD

Ronald Trale, DO

Joshua Tuck, DO

References

1. Flexner A. *Medical Education in the United States and Canada: A Report to the Carnegie Foundation for the Advancement of Teaching.* Bulletin No. 4. New York, NY: Carnegie Foundation for the Advancement of Teaching; 1910:346. OCLC 9795002, http://www.carnegiefoundation.org/publications/medical-education-united-states-and-canada-bulletin-number-four-flexner-report-0. Accessed April 5, 2012.
2. Peabody F. The care of the patient. *JAMA.* 1927;88:877–882.
3. Merenstein JH, Schulte JJ. A residency curriculum for the future. The STFM Task Force on Residency Curriculum for the Future. *Fam Med.* 1990;22(6):467–473.
4. Bell HS, Kozakowski SM, Winter RO. Competency-based education in family practice. *Fam Med.* 1997;29(10):701–704.
5. Kohn L, Corrigan J, Donaldson M. *To Err Is Human: Building a Safer Health System.* Washington, DC: Institute of Medicine; 1999.
6. Corrigan J, Donaldson M, Kohn L, Maguire S, Pike K. *Crossing the Quality Chasm: A New Health System for the 21st Century.* Washington, DC: Institute of Medicine; 2001.

7. Swing S. The ACGME outcome project: retrospective and prospective. *Med Teach.* 2007;29:648–654.
8. Gallagher M (Chairman). *Report of the Core Competency Task Force.* Chicago, IL: American Osteopathic Association; 2003.
9. Batalden P, Leach D, Swing S, Dreyfus H, Dreyfus S. General competencies and accreditation in graduate medical education. *Health Aff.* 2002;21(5):103–111.
10. Epstein RM, Hundert EM. Defining and assessing professional competence. *JAMA.* 2002;287:226–235.
11. Competencies for the Physician Assistant Profession. http://www.nccpa.net/pdfs/Definition%20of%20PA%20Competencies%203.5%20for%20Publication.pdf. Published 2004. Accessed July 8, 2012.
12. National Association of Nurse Practitioner Faculties. Nurse Practitioner Core Competencies. http://www.nonpf.com/associations/10789/files/NPCoreCompetenciesFinal2012.pdf. Published 2012. Accessed July 11, 2012.
13. CanMEDS Framework. http://www.collaborativecurriculum.ca/en/modules/CanMEDS/CanMEDS-intro-background-01.jsp. Published 2005. Accessed April 5, 2012.
14. Good Medical Practice. http://www.gmc-uk.org/static/documents/content/GMP_0910.pdf. Published November, 2006. Accessed April 5, 2012.
15. GMP-USA. http://gmpusa.org/Docs/GoodMedicalPractice-USA-V1-1.pdf. Published March 9, 2009. Accessed April 5, 2012.
16. Sackett DL, Rosenberg WC, Gray JAM. Evidence-based medicine: what it is and what it isn't. *BMJ.* 1996;312:71–72.
17. Engel GL. The need for a new medical model: a challenge for biomedicine. *Science.* 1977;196:129–136.
18. Donabedian A. The quality of care: how can it be assessed. *JAMA.* 1988;260(12):1743–1744.
19. Like RC, Steiner RP. Medical anthropology and the family provider. *Fam Med.* 1986;18(2):87–92.
20. Billings JA, Stoeckle JD. *The Clinical Encounter: A Guide to the Medical Interview and Case Presentation.* 2nd ed. St. Louis, MO: Mosby; 1998.
21. Kaiser Health Tracking Poll. http://www.kff.org/kaiserpolls/8251.cfm. Published October, 2011. Accessed April 5, 2012.
22. National Healthcare Quality and Disparities Reports. http://www.ahrq.gov/qual/qrdr10.htm. Published March, 2011. Accessed April 6, 2012.
23. Weiner SJ, Barnet B, Cheng TL, Daaleman TP. Processes for effective communication in primary care. *Ann Intern Med.* 2005;142:709–714.
24. Travaline JM, Ruchinskas R, D'Alonzo GE. Patient-provider communication: why and how. *JAOA.* 2005;105:13–18.
25. Misra-Hebert AD. Provider cultural competence: cross-cultural communication improves care. *Cleve Clin J Med.* 2003;70:289–303.
26. Papadakis MA, Teherani A, Banach MA, et al. Disciplinary action by medical boards and prior behavior in medical schools. *NEJM.* 2005;353:2673–2682.
27. Duffy FD, Gordon GH, Whelan G, et al. Assessing competence in communication and interpersonal skills: the Kalamazoo II report. *Acad Med.* 2004;79(6):495–507.
28. Stobo JD (Project Chair). *Project Professionalism.* Philadelphia, PA: American Board of Internal Medicine; 1995.
29. Berwick D, Davidoff F, Hiatt H, Smith R. Refining and implementing the Tavistock principles for everybody in healthcare. *BMJ.* 2001;323:616.
30. Chervenak FA, McCullough LB. The moral foundation of medical leadership: the professional virtues of the provider as fiduciary of the patient. *Am J Obstet Gynecol.* 2001;184:875–880.
31. Brennan T (Chair). Medical professionalism in the new millennium: Project of the ABIM Foundation, ACP-ASIM Foundation, and European Federation of Internal Medicine. *Ann Intern Med.* 2002;136(3):243–246.
32. Wagner EH. The role of patient care teams in chronic disease management. *BMJ.* 2000;320:569–572.
33. Wipf JE, Pinsky LE, Burke W. Turning interns into senior residents: preparing residents for their teaching and leadership roles. *Acad Med.* 1995;70(7):591–596.
34. American Osteopathic Association. Program Director's Annual Evaluation Report. http://www.osteopathic.org/inside-aoa/accreditation/postprovideral-training-approval/Documents/core-competency-compliance-program-part-3-program-director-report.pdf. Unpublished data. Accessed April 5, 2012.
35. Aron DC, Headrick LA. Educating providers prepared to improve care and safety is no accident: it requires a systematic approach. *Qual Saf Health Care.* 2002;11:168–173.
36. MR5: 5th Comprehensive Review of the Medical College Admission Test (MCAT). https://www.aamc.org/initiatives/mr5/. In press. Accessed April 5, 2012.
37. Interprofessional Education Collaborative Expert Panel. *Core Competencies for Interprofessional Collaborative Practice: Report of an Expert Panel.* Washington, DC: Interprofessional Education Collaborative; 2011.
38. Hafferty FW. Beyond curriculum reform: confronting medicine's hidden curriculum. *Acad Med.* 1998;73(4):403–407.
39. Hafler JP, Ownby AR, Thompson BM, et al. Decoding the learning environment of medical education: a hidden curriculum perspective for faculty development. *Acad Med.* 2011;86:440–444.

40. Haidet P, Stein HF. The role of the student-teacher relationship in the formation of providers: the hidden curriculum as process. *J Gen Int Med*. 2006;21(suppl):S16–S20

41. Bell HS. Encouragement: giving "heart" to our learners in a competency-based education model. *Fam Med*. 2007;39(1):13–15.

CHAPTER 2

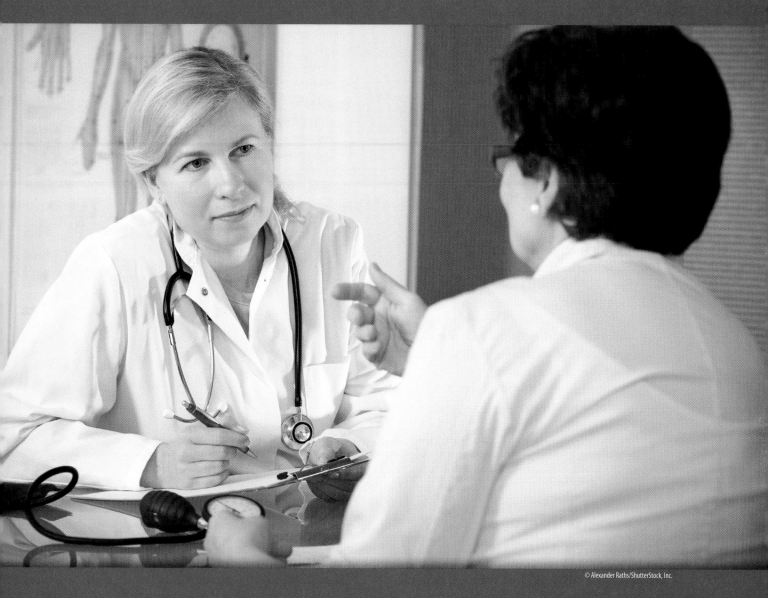

© Alexander Raths/ShutterStock, Inc.

Interpersonal and Communication Skills

Michele Roth-Kauffman, JD, PA-C
Mark Kauffman, DO, MS (Med Ed), PA

OBJECTIVES

At the conclusion of this chapter, the student will be able to

1. Understand the importance of proper mindset prior to seeing patients
2. Recognize personal prejudices that may inhibit quality patient care
3. Distinguish between open-ended and closed-ended questioning and know when to use each during the patient interview
4. Identify components of each skill set of the Humanistic Domain
5. Incorporate Humanistic Domain skills into patient encounters
6. State interviewing techniques that demonstrate respect for the patient
7. Demonstrate professionalism in actions
8. Define Health Literacy
9. Tailor education and instruction of the patient to age, level of socioeconomic status, level of education, ethnicity
10. Recognize the goals and tools of cultural competency training

KEY TERMS

Patient interview
Mindset
Prejudice
Humanistic Domain
Verbal skills
Open-ended questions
Closed-ended questions
Listening skills
Respect
Empathy
Professionalism
Confidence
Confidentiality
HIPAA
Medical ethics
Health Literacy
Culture
Cultural competency in health care
Cultural humility
Ask Me 3
4 Cs

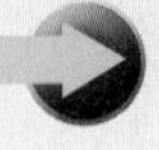 Where this icon appears, visit **go.jblearning.com/HPECWS** to view the video.

The Patient Interview: More Than Asking Questions

Gathering the medical history from a **patient interview** is not simply asking questions and receiving an answer. Interpretation of the patient's true complaint requires intuition and the skill to observe as much of what is *not* said as of what is. Interviewing therefore truly is an art. The asking of questions may in fact be the easiest part of the interview. A detailed, thorough history can be obtained through the use of memory tools, and the area requiring the most deduction will be the symptoms associated with the primary concern of the patient. Heightened skills of observation, where the patient's nonverbal response is assessed as much as the uttered word, allow the provider a depth of understanding far beyond that of data collection.

Patient interview: the process of gathering historical data surrounding the patient's medical concern while employing humanistic principles

Gaining the trust of patients and encouraging them to become invested in their own care require humanistic skills that infuse the brief encounter shared between you and your patient with empathy, respect, and professionalism. This can be no easy feat to achieve with the pressures of time-limited patient encounters. As we practice medicine and become intimate with its daily needs, we must guard against the drift of complacency and avoid the shortcuts we are tempted to undertake. When you have looked in the one-thousandth ear for a routine physical and have found nothing, you will be tempted to remove the otoscopic exam from future physicals. Be assured that the one-thousand-and-first patient will have a cholesteatoma, a destructive ear canal tumor that can result in permanent hearing loss, even intracranial abscess, if not detected.

Your guiding principle should be this: If at the end of your day, you cannot honestly say that you treated each and every patient in the same manner and with the same recommendations as you would wish to see your father, mother, siblings, or children be treated, you have not treated them correctly—assuming, of course, that you like your family.

MINDSET

Long before you enter your patient's room, your encounter has been prejudiced. You were on call last night with sleep being interrupted on an hourly basis. When you rounded at the hospital, one of your patients needed to be transferred to the intensive care unit. You arrived at your office a half hour late, nearly caught up when you had a "no-show," slid behind again with three "double-books," then skipped lunch arguing with an insurance company about the need for an MRI for your patient with a knee injury, as they insisted on a trial of physical therapy while your exam revealed that the anterior cruciate ligament was in tatters. Your day is ending. You have but one more patient and then a stack of paperwork to clean off your desk. You grab the chart. It's a new patient with dizziness. You know the possible complexities only too well. How easy it would be to sink into the depths of despair.

What is the purpose of seeing a patient? Is it not to take care of the patient's needs and address his/her concerns? This may be as simple as a patient needing a physical examination for a driver's license, having a cold, or wanting you to examine a mole that just doesn't look right. Or it may be as complex as fatigue or shortness of breath.

In any case, your goals during the interview are not only to gather information but also to gain the trust of the patient. Gaining trust allows you to gather information that the patient may not otherwise share. This is not achievable by allowing your current mood to paint a morose mask upon your face, slump your shoulders, thin your patience, or cut short your greeting. Your patient has failed to find relief from his pain for many years. He had heard you were different, that you gave everyone a chance, that you were honest, competent, and caring. Will he now think that he heard wrong?

So no matter how bad your day has been, the patient you are about to see deserves your time, patience, sincerity, and empathy. Your **mindset** is indeed that: yours. You must have control of it and be able to reset it at each and every encounter. The key to successfully doing this is mindfulness of one's self, something often easier said than done. A first step is recognizing your prejudices.

Mindset: a state of mind or attitude that influences patient-provider encounters

PREJUDICES

We all bring our personal experiences along with us into the care of our patients. The tendency to do so is unavoidable as these experiences shape our knowledge and character, as a potter molds a vase. Some of these experiences help our patients, as when they allow us to recognize disease or dysfunction through the memory of seeing other patients in similar situations. But some of these experiences have the potential of inhibiting patient care. Take, for example, the family member with addiction. When you spend your life watching the destructive power addiction has, not only on the addict but on those surrounding them, you could easily develop intolerance toward a patient with such a condition. It is our duty to recognize prejudices that we have and aggressively act to prevent them from influencing the patient encounter.

Ask yourself the following questions:

- What kind of people do I avoid?
- What behaviors grind on my nerves?
- What experiences with people have left a bad taste in my mouth?

These are some of the questions that will help you identify patients at risk of being treated in a biased fashion . . . by you. Consciously identifying your **prejudices** is the first step in avoiding mistreatment of these patients.

Prejudices: a preconceived attitude, opinion, or feeling

Humanistic Domain: The component of the patient–provider interaction that seeks to engage the patient holistically through appropriate use of verbal, listening, educational, and instructional skills and the demonstration of respect, empathy, and professionalism

THE HUMANISTIC DOMAIN

Humanism in patient care focuses on the relationship between the provider and the patient, and in particular the ability of the provider to communicate properly with the patient. The **Humanistic Domain** is the component of the patient–provider interaction that seeks to engage the patient holistically through appropriate use of verbal, listening, educational, and instructional skills and the demonstration of respect, empathy, and professionalism. Communication only begins with the spoken word, but it transcends this basic level of verbalization, requiring mastery of the ability to listen, educate, and instruct your patient at a level where comprehension is achieved to a degree that demonstrates understanding of the significance of diagnosis and intended outcomes of each treatment or nontreatment option. Communication must be woven with the threads of respect, empathy, and professionalism to gain the full trust and investment of the patient in his/her own care.

Verbal Skills

Verbal skills are essential to the ability to obtain a thorough medical history. At the most rudimentary level, one must speak clearly and with a level of volume appropriate to the patient's needs. Recognition of diminished hearing should prompt the speaker to lower the frequency of voice rather than increase the volume, recognizing that high-frequency hearing loss is the most common type.

The patient's level of education must be considered in order to avoid speaking above or below his/her level of comprehension. If one speaks above a patient's level of comprehension, the patient may readily express understanding to avoid appearing unknowledgeable. Use of medical jargon should be avoided. Conversely, speaking below a patient's level of comprehension may result in feelings of undesired paternalism, even belittlement. Should your patient have training in a medical field, use of medical terminology may be appropriate, as it tells the patient that you acknowledge his/her level of education and expect a higher level of collaboration in providing his/her care.

Verbal skills: the ability to communicate with the patient both mechanically and tactically so that the patient is encouraged to concisely disclose his/her medical history

Open-ended questions: questions posed during the clinical encounter that prompt the patient to answer in his/her own words, knowledge, and feelings

Closed-ended questions: questions posed during the clinical encounter that narrow patient responses to "yes," "no," or a specific selection of choices

OPEN-ENDED VS. CLOSED-ENDED QUESTIONING

Verbal skills also include presenting questions in **open-ended** format. Asking the patient, "What brings you in today?" or "How may I help you?" invites the patient to tell their story in their own words. If you were to say instead, "I see you're here for stomach pain," you would immediately limit the response of the patient to that one complaint. The use of open-ended questioning is akin to your patient answering an essay question instead of one in multiple-choice format. For example, "Could you describe the pain?" requires the patient to consider the pain and use his/her own words describe it. When the product of open-ended questions becomes less fruitful, the transition to **closed-ended questions** is appropriate and preserves the momentum of the interview. After several attempts of asking the patient to describe the pain have resulted in "I don't know. It just hurts," it is time to reformulate the question into closed-ended format:

- Interviewer: "Could you describe the pain?" (open-ended)
- Patient: "It just hurts."
- Interviewer: "Could you be more specific and describe what it feels like?" (open-ended)
- Patient: "It just feels really bad."
- Interviewer: "Would you say the pain is sharp, dull, throbbing, burning . . . ?"

This approach of asking open-ended questions and only moving to closed-ended questions allows the patient to choose the descriptive term that fits his/her perception of it most accurately.

THOUGHT COMPLETION

Your flow of thought must be logical and you should strive to complete one line of questioning before moving to another. One answer from a patient often leads to the next question. Never abandon a question for which you have received an incomplete answer. If someone admits to having had the same abdominal pain twice in the past, ask about those past occurrences. When were they? How long did they last? How were they treated? What were the outcomes? The same is true for medications. It is not enough to discern that the patient is taking a medication for his gout. What is the name of the medication? How often does he take it? How many milligrams at a time? How long has he been on it? Does he have any side effects from it?

Another task of the provider is to keep the patient's narrative in line with the current concern. This may be a challenge when a patient begins to deviate from the current topic. It takes artful redirection to gently guide a patient back to the topic at hand without appearing uninterested or rushed.

VERBAL SKILLS CHECKLIST

- Speak clearly with an appropriate level of volume.
- Lower your voice for patients with hearing loss instead of increasing volume.
- Speak at the appropriate level of education for the patient.
- Avoid medical jargon.
- Begin lines of inquiry with open-ended questions, moving to closed-ended questions only as needed.
- Gently redirect patients who drift too far away from the topic of concern.

Listening Skills

Skills in active listening refer to more than noting an answer to a posed question. In truth, to excel we must listen with our eyes as much as we do with our ears. Nonverbal clues can reveal subtle components of the patient's story and shed light on underlying meaning.

Listening and documenting patient responses set the foundation of the history to be built upon. The first several questions you ask a patient regarding any complaint serve as a starting point for simple data collection. These are used to define the patient's concern and reveal time frames surrounding it, such as the onset of symptoms, how symptoms have changed since onset, and prior history of similar symptoms. Early on, responses to one question should clue the mind to possible diagnoses. The astute listener catalogs the clue and explores associated signs and symptoms.

For instance, a patient presenting with abdominal pain admits that it occurs after eating. The differential may at least include peptic ulcer disease, cholelithiasis, mesenteric ischemia, lactose intolerance, or celiac sprue. Knowing the disease characteristics of each allows the provider to consider each one in an attempt to define which is most likely. In this case, it is not enough to know that the symptom is associated with eating; one should logically ask which type of food is most likely to cause the pain. Upon hearing that milk products are the major culprits, lactose intolerance comes to the forefront, the others not necessarily being discarded, but lessened in likelihood. Further questioning may completely eliminate some possibilities from the differential. This describes the fluidity of building a list of possible diagnoses called the differential diagnosis: a modeling and remodeling of causes of the patient's condition.

Silence often has the unyielding power to force the provider to continue speaking if only to fill the void. As providers first begin interviewing patients, a pause of 15 seconds feels like an eternity. Our minds falter as we worry that our patients will mistake our inability to proceed with a line of questioning for incompetence. We worry that the patient will see through us and think that we haven't got a clue as to what is going on. In truth, we may indeed not know the exact diagnosis, but a list of possibilities is building.

Providers should become comfortable with short periods of silence. As a patient begins to relate the story that prompted his/her visit to you, avoid the impulse to interject too quickly. As long as the patient is relating pertinent information, allow the story to unfold naturally. Should the patient pause, it may not be necessary to pose a new question. Instead, prompt minimization, such as "I see," "That's interesting," or even "Hmm," allows the patient to continue without interruption. Only when the patient's dialogue strays too far from pertinence should you draw him/her back to center by returning to focused questions.

If you find that you need time to consider possibilities, do not hesitate to share your intent with the patient. Saying "Let me think about that" or "I'm considering the possibilities" allows the patient to appreciate your contemplation. If this is presented correctly, the patient will perceive careful consideration of your concern, not a lack of competence.

Listening skills: the ability of the provider to observe, promote, and interpret verbal and nonverbal communication throughout the patient interview

FOLLOW-UP QUESTIONS

Listening skills include being able to perceive clues from the patient dialogue and properly respond to them. When a historical clue is encountered, it must be explored by asking appropriate follow-up questions. Often in our early patient encounters we tend to ask questions and simply record the answers we hear rather than listen to the answer themselves.

- Provider: "Did anything make it worse?"
- Patient: "Standing too long on it."
- Provider: "Did anything make it better?"
- Patient: "Not really."

The provider should have asked what the patient does that requires them to stand for long periods of time. Is it their occupation, modes of travel, or activities of daily living? By following up in this way, the provider will be able to assess if any changes can be made that would lessen the impact of those behaviors.

At some point in all of our careers, we find ourselves asking a patient the same question that we asked but a few short minutes ago. It is not difficult to read frustration and cynicism on a patient's face. The patient may feel that you are mechanically going through a checklist of questions without really paying attention. Indeed, the patient may wonder if you have actually heard a word that he/she has said.

- Provider: "How did this happen?"
- Patient: "I was bit by a dog while delivering the mail."
- Provider: "When was that?"
- Patient: "Two days ago."

Followed later by:

- Provider: "What do you do for a living?"
- Patient: "I'm a dentist. I just deliver the mail as a hobby."

When you find yourself in this situation, acknowledge your mistake immediately: "I'm sorry; I've already asked that question, haven't I?" Attempt to recognize the reason for your lapse. Were you in too much of a hurry? Was your mind racing through symptoms associated with a possible diagnosis that dashed through your mind? Were you simply writing down a response to a prior question and weren't prepared to listen to the answer to the next? Whatever the reason, share it with your patient. Express your regret. Refocus and pay close attention: "I'm really sorry. I know I already asked that question. I'm afraid I was moving too fast. Let me slow down and give you my full attention."

Patients may express concerns regarding a diagnosis or treatment plan vaguely instead of directly. This may especially be true with a treatment plan that was dictated to the patient instead of built with his/her collaboration. The astute provider should be on alert for both verbal and nonverbal clues that suggest a patient may not agree with what he/she is being told. Avoidance of eye contact by the patient despite verbal assurances of compliance should trigger concern from the provider. There are many reasons a patient may avoid discussing concerns.

Disagreement with the presented diagnosis or treatment is one. You explain to your patient that she has a viral upper respiratory tract infection for which you prescribe rest, keeping well-hydrated, symptomatic relief with an antihistamine, and the passage of time. She, on the other hand, knows that she has sinusitis and will not get better without an antibiotic.

Embarrassment may prevent a patient from voicing his/her concerns. When a young mother is handed a prescription for her child, she haphazardly stuffs it into her purse with a look of despair in her eyes. Directly discussing your observation with her, you learn that she has neither insurance nor money to pay for the prescription no matter what the cost.

A patient's doubt of his/her ability to comply with the treatment plan can also play a role. You have just advised your patient with high cholesterol that he needs to eat a low-fat, high-fiber diet and exercise one hour a day for the next three months and then you will recheck his blood work. As a long-haul truck driver who eats his meals on the road and drives for up to 12 hours a day, he knows it won't happen, but he says, "Sure." Had you asked him how he would like to work on lowering his cholesterol, he would have asked for a pill. Do not disregard these vague clues as figments of your imagination.

When you recognize patient or family concerns, discuss them openly. This legitimizes the concern and allows for further discussion of the treatment plan with consideration of alternatives where appropriate, risks and complications, and reinforcement of expectations of both the patient and the provider.

LISTENING SKILLS CHECKLIST

- Closely observe the patient for use of nonverbal clues.
- Actively model and remodel the differential diagnosis with each answer received.
- Encourage spontaneity of patient storytelling through prompt minimization.
- Recognize and respond to historical clues.
- Collaborate with the patient and gauge his/her responses to treatment plans.
- Avoid repeating questions that were already answered.
- Legitimize patient concerns.

Respect

Building trust begins with mutual **respect** between the patient and the provider. Though each must earn the respect of the other, it may be that the preponderance of the earning of respect is shouldered by the provider. To earn our patient's respect we must demonstrate a solid foundation in medical knowledge, utilize standard of care in our treatment plans, be unbiased in our approach, and show compassion and empathy.

Conversely, respect for our patients must be granted from the outset, given freely and unconditionally. The patient's duty is to retain it. A new patient presents to your office and it is soon evident that he has sought the council of multiple providers before you. He is convinced that exposure to a chemical agent in the military has resulted in his poor health. He is frustrated by the "incompetence" of his prior providers and states that no one will help him get the disability claim he deserves. Despite the urge to paint the patient in negative light, we have the responsibility to begin anew with the patient, offer respect and unbiased consideration. It is not being naive to begin each new patient encounter with this approach. Explaining to the patient that you recognize his/her frustration and that you intend to wipe the slate clean and start at the beginning lays a solid foundation upon which to begin building. This demonstration of regard and consideration defines respect for the patient.

Respect: the demonstration of giving high regard, consideration, politeness, and kindness without bias

Respect as a component of humanism must be genuine. A patient who feels that it is being offered disingenuously will quickly develop distrust for the provider. It is easy to become cynical in the practice of medicine, yet the best physician is one who leaves prejudice at the door while walking through its frame.

Respect begins with politeness. When you encounter a new patient, introduce yourself using your name and title. If you are in training and another provider will be interacting with the patient, clarify that you are a student and explain your role in his/her visit. When greeting the patient, use his/her title and last name, then ask the patient how he/she would like to be addressed. Thanking the patient at the end of the encounter shows that you value his/her time as much as you value your own.

Sensitivity can be shown by demonstrating kindliness. Demonstrate warmth by shaking the patient's hand. When preparing to perform an examination, ask permission from the patient to do so. When finishing an abdominal examination, don't just walk away and tell the patient to sit up, allowing him/her to flounder. Help the patient with any position change regardless of his/her age. Demonstrate concern for the patient's dignity by properly gowning and draping the patient during the examination. If a patient is asked to lower his/her gown to expose the chest for an examination, once the exam is completed the gown should be replaced immediately before moving on to another area of examination. Likewise, cover the lower extremities with a sheet when performing an abdominal examination. This allows the gown to be raised to expose the abdomen while keeping the sheet in place over the pelvic region and lower extremities.

Patient autonomy refers to the patient's right to choose. It is easy for providers to have a tendency toward being autocratic when devising treatment plans: "This is what you have and this is what I want you to do about it. Have a nice day." Respect for the autonomy of the patient has been lost.

For example, when you identify a patient as a tobacco smoker, before you simply advise the patient to quit, you must first ask if he/she has considered

Empathy: verbal and nonverbal expression of understanding, sympathy, and compassion

stopping. They may not have any intention to do so. That does not mean that the topic stops there. It is our duty to then inform the patient of the risks associated with tobacco use. However, once we have done so, the patient's autonomy in choosing whether to continue smoking remains. You may go so far as to ask the patient if you may bring up the topic at each visit as you consider it of vital importance to their health. If the patient would rather that you didn't, you may still intermittently broach the topic but will avoid aggravating or demoralizing the patient by your persistent barrage.

If a patient does expresses interest in quitting, you must explore what attempts the patient has made in the past and how well they worked. Explaining treatment options allows the patient to make informed decisions. Further asking the patient what he/she thinks will work best will lead to the highest levels of success.

Respect for cultural differences and backgrounds must also be displayed. A Middle Eastern couple comes to your clinic. The husband has been explaining that his wife has a cough. You are a male physician and recognize that you need the permission of the husband to examine his wife. He will not allow it. Do you get angry and say you can't treat her without listening to her chest, or do you find an alternative, such as asking your female office partner to perform the examination?

RESPECT CHECKLIST

- Begin each new patient encounter with unbiased consideration.
- Be polite.
- Introduce yourself by name, title, and role.
- Greet the patient by title and last name.
- Ask how the patient would like to be addressed.
- Shake the patient's hand unless prohibited by culture.
- Demonstrate kindness.
- Help the patient with position changes.
- Gown and drape the patient to preserve dignity.
- Ask permission before examining or exposing the patient.
- Respect the patient's right to choose.
- Respect differences in culture and background.

Empathy

Synonyms for **empathy** include understanding, sympathy, and compassion. Empathy can be expressed both verbally and nonverbally. Eye contact is important in developing a bond with the patient. The expression "the eyes are the windows to the soul" reflects on our ability to communicate with our eyes alone. Patients typically like eye contact about 50% of the time, but this should be based on the individual encounter. Elderly patients may desire more, younger patients less. Making initial eye contact on entering the room forges an early bond the patient. Staring at your paper or computer screen as you take notes may make you appear distant, mechanical, and lacking compassion.

To demonstrate compassion and empathy, the provider must not only hear the patient but must listen to what is being said. Mr. Jones had his gallbladder removed last year. Since that time, fatty foods have caused him to have episodes of urgent diarrhea. Twice he has been eating out and couldn't make it to a restroom before soiling himself. Though eating out was a great pleasure for him, he has stopped doing so. Hearing what the patient is saying leads you to diagnose postcholecystecomy syndrome with diarrhea related to the removal of the gallbladder. Listening to the patient, however, means that you empathize with the embarrassment and restrictions in activity and lifestyle that this is causing the patient.

The provider must show genuine interest in the patient's condition. Telling the patient "It's just a cold virus. You'll get better" shows very little investment on the part of the provider. Patients have invested a great deal to come to see you. They have scheduled an appointment, taken a day off work, waited in a crowded waiting room with sick people all around them, remained calm when you were running an hour late, and have waited in the exam room for another half hour. You may be correct that the patient just has a virus that it will run its course in a few days, but there are different ways to relate this to the patient.

Obviously the condition is a concern for the patient. What symptoms can you treat? Does the patient need a decongestant or cough suppressant? Would osteopathic manipulation benefit the patient? Does he/she need a day or two off from work so that the virus isn't spread to others?

Acknowledging the patient's life situation also demonstrates empathy. Eugene has injured his rotator cuff. This condition is aggravated by his occupation as a roofer. You advise Eugene that he needs to take a week off from his work to allow his shoulder to begin healing. He replies, "A week off?! Doc, roofing doesn't happen in the wintertime. If I don't work now, I don't get paid. We don't have sick time."

Your initial recommendation failed to take the patient's life situation into account. Had you instead involved the patient in the decision-making process from the onset, you would not have had to backtrack to try to remedy the situation. Knowing that a rotator cuff injury requires rest and rehabilitation should lead the provider to inquire how the injury will affect the patient's activities of daily living, including work, exercise, recreation, and the ability to care for himself. Investigating these areas allows you to acknowledge and demonstrate understanding of how the current condition affects your patient's life.

Ms. Wagaman is 93 years old and just fractured her right wrist. Did you know she lives alone? Did you ask her how she was going to drive back home and take care of herself once she got there? Ask the patient if there is anyone you can call to discuss her condition and needs. She has three children in town—could she live with anyone while she recovers?

EMPATHY CHECKLIST

- Demonstrate compassion and sympathy.
- Make appropriate eye contact, speaking with the eyes.
- Move beyond hearing the patient—listen to him/her.
- Show interest in the patient's condition, making clear that it is important to you.
- Demonstrate investment of time and concern.
- Acknowledge the patient's current life situation.
- Recognize how the condition impacts the patient's work, exercise, recreation, and ability to care for him-/herself.

Professionalism

Professionalism is a competency that must not only be maintained while providing skillful medical care but also shadows the provider into his/her private life. Epstein and Hundert define professional competence as the habitual and judicious use of communication, knowledge, technical skills, clinical reasoning, emotions, values, and reflection in daily practice for the benefit of the individual and community being served.[1]

In the clinical setting, patients and their families judge the level of professionalism of their providers largely on the outcomes of the clinical care they receive, how information is shared with them, and how they are treated. The behavior of the provider is also assessed: Is the provider friendly, does he/she appear energetic, does he/she demonstrate respect for coworkers, is he/she overheard in the hallway discussing other patients, does he/she possess an ego? Further, they also base their impressions on their provider's physical appearance.

PROFESSIONAL DRESS

Physical appearance is the first thing the patient sees when you enter the room. Patient impressions of competence in care directly relate to physical appearance. The better-dressed the provider, the higher the quality of care is perceived to be. When required to round on inpatients on weekends for only a few hours, it is tempting for the provider to don jeans and sneakers, slip into the hospital and then back out. Yet those who do are deemed to be less competent than their peers who wear khakis and dress shirts. Adding a tie and dress pants further increases the patient's perception of competence. To be regarded as the most competent, add a clean, wrinkle-free white coat to the attire. Women's clothing should be conservative. Short skirts and revealing blouses should be avoided. Jewelry should be modest, limiting the number of rings, earrings, and necklaces. Facial piercings should also be avoided.

Patients prefer that men who do not have beards to be cleanly shaven. Beards should be well kempt. Hair should be neatly combed or brushed. Shorter hair length on men is preferred over longer styles. Heavy colognes, perfumes, and makeup should be avoided.

Professionalism: the habitual and judicious use of communication, knowledge, technical skills, clinical reasoning, emotions, values, and reflection in daily practice for the benefit of the individual and community being served

Communication with patients often occurs in tight quarters; therefore hygiene is important. This condition is one that may not be perceived by the provider him-/herself. The presence of body odor may be interpreted as lack of self-care. Patients may question the level of care they will receive if the provider seems unable to care for him-/herself. This is not dissimilar to a provider who smokes counseling his patient on smoking cessation. The discussion of malodor may pose an uncomfortable and embarrassing situation between colleagues, but when approached with honest concern and intent to share awareness that may be lacking, benefit can be derived.

CONCERN FOR THE PATIENT

The demonstration of humane concern for the patient begins with kindness. Identifying the patient's medical condition is only the beginning. Eliciting a complaint of pain and ranking it on a scale of severity is simply mechanical if concern is not shown for the findings. Once a component of pain is recognized, validate it directly so that the patient understands it is a priority for you as well for him/her: "Mrs. Green, I can see that you are in a lot of pain. I'll help you as quickly as I can."

The psychological components of the patient must also be considered. A longtime patient of yours, Mr. Kendall, who is 87 years old, just lost his wife of 63 years. Though he is seeing you for monitoring of his high blood pressure, your concern for his loss should share equal importance. How is he coping with the loss of his wife? Is he able to care for himself? What did his wife do for him that he must now do for himself? Does he have the support of family and friends? Has he isolated himself? Beyond grief, is he depressed or even suicidal? Not all of these questions may need to be asked, but the conversation must begin and be tailored to his needs.

Confidence: assurance and belief in oneself and abilities

Confidentiality: the tenent of professionalism assuring that information given by the patient will be kept in strictest confidence and privacy

HIPAA: The Health Insurance Portability and Accountability Act of 1996 (HIPAA) was designed to protect the private health information of patients

CONFIDENCE

Patients must be able to discern an air of **confidence** in their provider. Confidence should be displayed but egotism avoided. Displaying confidence is uncomplicated in cases where the diagnosis and standard of care are immediately known. Rarely do providers find themselves without at least some suspicion or a list of possible diagnoses from which to work. Even when a diagnosis is not at hand, the patient still has symptoms that provide a basis for investigation. When the provider is truly at a loss, the feeling of disequilibrium may stifle his/her ability to proceed. Honesty and humility are the keys to a successful outcome. Portraying omniscience when knowledge is lacking is detrimental to the forging of trust.

When seeing a patient with a presentation for which an immediate diagnosis cannot be made, do not be hesitant to share this information with the patient. Confidence does not need to be lost. Instead it can be portrayed to the patient by the demonstration of commitment to finding the answers. Fulfilling your obligation to the patient may require research, testing, or referral. Reassuring the patient of your intent demonstrates your perseverance. Being willing to say to a patient, "I do not know but let's find out" and pulling a reference text from a bookcase can add a level of mutual respect to the relationship.

CONFIDENTIALITY

The tenets of professionalism dictate that **confidentiality** is inherent to the patient-provider relationship. Not only is the maintenance of confidentiality another key to building trust, it is a legal requirement. The Health Insurance Portability and Accountability Act of 1996 (**HIPAA**) was designed to protect the private health information of patients and carries heavy civil and criminal penalties if information is disclosed without the consent of the patient.

Much more common than intentional disclosure of a patient's private information is inadvertent disclosure. Patient information should never be discussed in common areas where other patients, staff, or healthcare workers may overhear these discussions. Though providers may take precautions to avoid using patient names, discussion of the case alone may be enough to result in inadvertent dissemination of confidential information. A patient in a semiprivate room is seen by his surgeon during morning rounds and is told he is scheduled for 10 AM. After the surgeon leaves, the wife of the man in the bed next to him asks why he was in the hospital. He simply replies that he is having a minor procedure done, preferring not to share his personal information. Still, she is able to learn with some likelihood what the gentleman is having done when, while riding in the elevator, she overhears the same surgeon tell his medical student to read up on penile implants for his/her 10 AM case.

Establishing confidentiality early on in the encounter supports the development of trust and gives patients the opportunity to share more information with their provider than they may otherwise do. Though the majority of encounters will not require this discussion, there may be times to assure the patient directly that any information he/she shares with you will be kept confidential. These times often surround sensitive topics such as sexuality, infectious disease, abuse, dependency, and mental health issues. You should ask patients if there is anyone that they would like you to talk to about their condition. This reassures them that unless they give you permission, you will not share the information with anyone.

There are times when providers are legally required to report information. Some examples of these include when patients state that they intend to harm themselves or others, when there is suspected abuse of a minor or elder in the care of another, or when the diagnosis of HIV is made. Laws covering mandated disclosure vary from state to state, and providers must familiarize themselves with the requirements in the area of their practice. Should providers find themselves in a situation where they are legally required to share information with others, trust can be maintained by being forthcoming as soon as the possibility is identified during the encounter.

Mrs. Gearhart brings her 16-year-old daughter Jennifer in to see you because of persistent headaches. She is concerned because Jennifer, who had previously been a straight-A student, is missing significant amounts of time at school and her grades have dropped to the point where she may need to repeat the year. After initial questioning and a physical exam, you are concerned about the vagueness with which Jennifer answers your questions. You explain to Mrs. Gearhart that Jennifer is becoming a young lady and that this is a chance to develop a relationship and trust with a physician. You ask if you could summarize the history with just her daughter alone, if it is all right with Jennifer, assuring both of them that no physical examination will be performed and an assistant can come into the room if either of them prefers. Mrs. Gearhart consents and leaves the room. The conversation should start with an explanation of why you wished to speak with her alone. Assurances of strict confidentiality, however, cannot be made, as some situations may require you to share the information.

"Jennifer, I'm concerned that these headaches you're having are being caused by something going on in your life. I wanted to speak with you in private because I know as you get older there are some things that you may not feel comfortable sharing with your mother. You are my patient and there are some things that we can talk about that I won't be required to share with your mother unless you ask me to, like alcohol, drugs, or if you've become sexually active. But there are other things that I would be required to share, like if you were being sexually or physically abused, or if you had intentions to hurt yourself or others. In any case, I will do whatever I can to help you. That being said, is there anything you can share with me that can help me figure out where headaches are coming from?"

At this point, the patient has the ability to determine what information she is willing to share. Whether or not she does so, you have not made the mistake of ensuring confidentiality only to later find that you are required to report what you have learned, losing you the trust of your patient.

MEDICAL ETHICS

We have chosen a profession that often places our families second. When the patient walks in at 4:45 on a Friday afternoon, we must strive to provide the same level of care, concern, and commitment that was shown to the first patient on Monday morning.

Medicine as a profession demands stewardship and vigilance in ethical behavior long after the day is completed. Our social networking must protect the profession and its moral code. Confidentiality does not dissolve on the weekends. It is very difficult to gain the trust of our patients and the community when we preach one word but speak another.

Whether it is documentation, billing, or the self-reporting of errors, we are called to the highest levels

Medical ethics: moral principles and rules of conduct in the practice of medicine

Health Literacy: the degree to which individuals have the capacity to obtain, process, and understand basic health information and services needed to make appropriate health decisions

of morality. All professions are meritorious but when an accountant makes a mistake, amendments can be made. When we make a mistake, we affect the lives and well-being of our patients, their families, and ourselves. Vigilance in upholding **medical ethics** through our moral code can be found in maintaining awareness of our calling and our duty.

PROFESSIONALISM CHECKLIST

- Wear professional attire.
- Maintain good hygiene and grooming.
- Prioritize patient concerns by verbally acknowledging them.
- Demonstrate compassion and kindness.
- Be confident but avoid egotism.
- Assure and preserve confidentiality.
- Adhere to the highest ethical standards.
- Avoid participating in behaviors that you would not want patients to emulate.

Educational and Instructional Skills

The skills required to provide exceptional care to your patient go beyond the ability to make the correct diagnosis. If the patient fails to understand the diagnosis, treatment options, and risks and benefits of each, he/she will have little invested in reaching for successful outcomes. Your ability to involve the patient and gain a commitment from him/her relies heavily on your ability to educate and instruct the patient at appropriate levels.

HEALTH LITERACY

Healthy People 2010 defines **Health Literacy** as "the degree to which individuals have the capacity to obtain, process, and understand basic health information and services needed to make appropriate health decisions."[2] And yet, as reported by the Institute of Medicine in *Health Literacy: A Prescription to End Confusion*, nearly one-half the population in the United States has difficulty understanding and using health information.[3]

Health information is frequently shared with patients in the form of printed materials that require a tenth-grade or higher level of reading comprehension. Contradictory to this practice is the finding that most adults in the United States read at the eighth- or ninth-grade level.[4] Printed instructions or results given or mailed to patients should therefore be written at the sixth-grade level.[5]

Therefore, the art of educating and instructing patients must be based on their ability to:

- Understand the diagnosis they are being presented
- Grant informed consent after considering the identified benefits, risks, and alternatives of each treatment option
- Participate in building a treatment plan based on recognizing treatment options, including that of declining treatment
- Understand and follow verbal and written provider directions, including those on self-care, health maintenance, taking medications, patient-based medical literature, and follow-up instructions
- Articulate objectives, questions, and concerns
- Seek out additional information to aid in decision making
- Make decisions

There are many factors that influence the level at which education and instruction of the patient should occur. Early and advanced age, lower socioeconomic status, learning and cognitive disabilities, experience with chronic medical conditions, and immigrant and minority ethnicity are but a few factors that contribute to vulnerability of patient populations.

AGE OF THE PATIENT

Sharing diagnoses with preadolescent patients should be appropriate to their level of comprehension. For example, after examining a 5-year-old with a low-grade fever, clear runny nose, and sore throat, you might share, "You have a cold" instead of, "You have a viral upper respiratory tract infection." Even downplayed to the level of "You have a virus" is likely beyond their comprehension. The responsibility of adhering to a prescribed treatment plan is delegated completely to the caregiver from infancy through the toddler stage and drifts consistently toward the patient the closer the patient advances toward adolescence. However, moving the entire responsibility too swiftly toward the caregiver should be avoided. The recently potty-trained, 4-year-old female with recurrent urinary tract infections may be quite capable of understanding the need to wipe from front to back after urinating in order to help prevent infections.

Similarly, when the adolescent patient is seen but ignored while the discussion of the diagnosis and treatment plan is shared with the parent, the provider misses the opportunity to recognize the developing independence of the patient and the chance to build trust while deepening the patient-provider relationship.

Adults with learning deficits or cognitive deficiencies may always require caregiver assistance throughout their lives to ensure success. However, attempts at independence may reveal unsuspected ability to adhere to treatment plans, allowing for greater autonomy for the patient.

Many adult patients will demonstrate comprehension and cognitive abilities that allow one-on-one discussion of the diagnosis and treatment plan solely with the patient. However, it is prudent to ask patients if anyone else should be involved in the discussion. Inclusion of family members, significant others, or even friends at the consent of the patient should be explored. Though many will likely decline the offer, providers may be surprised when the offer to include others is accepted and acted upon.

Cognitive function begins to decline with advanced age and includes the ability to accurately read, interpret, and follow written instructions, patient-based medical literature, and directions on how to take prescriptions. It is important to assess patient understanding at each patient visit. As the encounter is concluding, ask the patient to relate what his/her understanding of the diagnosis is and have the patient recount the steps in the treatment plan. This approach ensures that both the patient and the provider have shared understandings of what is required for the best outcomes.

LOWER SOCIOECONOMIC STATUS

Socioeconomic status typically comprises the level of education attained, occupation, and income, and commonly correlates with the health status of our patients. These three components have direct effects on health care, healthcare choices our patients make, and environmental exposures.[6]

Healthy food choices are aligned with increased costs; therefore choices are restricted for our patients with lower levels of income. It is easy enough to recommend a balanced diet consisting of lean meats, fruits, and vegetables, but our patients may lack the means to acquire them. Still, educating the patient on the avoidance of known offenders such as fast-food burgers and fries is vital.

Lower educational levels are associated with increased rates of smoking. It seems contradictory, then, that those with the lowest levels of education, who have lower levels of income, choose to spend their limited resources on the expense of purchasing cigarettes with the known associated health risks. Patients with lower levels of education also have higher risk factors for the development of cardiovascular disease, including high blood pressure and elevated cholesterol levels.[7] Lower socioeconomic status has also been shown to be associated with low birthweight, arthritis, diabetes, and cancer.[6]

LEVEL OF EDUCATION

Learning disabilities and the attained level of education must be considered when educating and instructing the patient. Recognition of learning disabilities may require the provider to seek further support services available to the patient or to devise alternative instruction methods, such as use of illustrations. The level of education achieved by your patient should be assessed and documented at the first comprehensive visit. At times, providers may overlook details that may seem obvious to themselves but that can be quite confusing for the patient. For example, patients have commented that suppositories are difficult to swallow and birth control pills have a tendency to slip out of the vagina.

When prescribing medications, it is important for the provider to explain exactly how the medication should be taken, including the name of the medication, the amount, frequency, and route. Written instructions on medication labels should be supplemented with handwritten instructions when appropriate.

Culture: a dynamic and creative phenomenon, some aspects of which are shared by large groups of people and other aspects of which are the creation of small groups and individuals resulting from particular life circumstances and histories

Cultural competence: the ability of systems to provide care to patients with diverse values, beliefs, and behaviors, including tailoring the delivery of care to meet patients' social, cultural, and linguistic needs

When writing for a prescription medication, both brand and generic names should be given. This is evident when the arthritic patient with gastric ulcers is advised to stop taking Motrin, but when seen in the emergency room three days later confirms that she stopped the Motrin and switched to ibuprofen because she needed something for her pain. Motrin and ibuprofen are the same medication.

We cannot expect our patients to remember dosages of each medication they take, though we can encourage them to keep a written list with them at all times. When instructing the patient in dosage, units of administration such as 1 tablet, 1 teaspoon, and 1 puff are appropriate. Frequency should be specific. "One tablet twice a day" does not provide enough specificity. The patient may take the first tablet when awakening at 8 AM and the second at noon with lunch because he/she heard that you should always take medications with food. If the medication is meant to last for 12 hours, the patient will have inadequate drug levels from midnight until 8 AM.

Route of administration should also be provided, as well as any specific instructions related to using the medication. For example: "Mrs. Cook, because your blood pressure has been high for each of your last visits, we are going to start that new medication that we talked about, hydrochlorothiazide. Some people just call it HCTZ. These will be in tablet form with each tablet having 25 mg of the medication. This medication typically makes you urinate more frequently, so you should take one tablet each morning. That way you won't be up all night going to the bathroom. You should link taking it to something you do about the same time every day, like when you first get out of bed, brush your teeth, eat breakfast, or watch the morning news."

ETHNICITY AND CULTURAL COMPETENCE

Primary care clinicians represent the front line in the delivery of effective health care and can play an important role in addressing racial and cultural disparities. The fact that 49.6 million Americans (18.7%) speak a language other than English at home, and 23 million Americans (8.4%) have limited English proficiency, highlights the importance of the need for **cultural competence.**[7,8]

Increasing recognition of well-documented disparities in health status, healthcare access, and healthcare service delivery by race, ethnicity, socioeconomic status, gender, age, sexual orientation, and other sociodemographic characteristics in the United States has resulted in a call for change.[9] One approach to address such disparities suggested by the Unequal Treatment report is to integrate cross-cultural education into the training of current and future health professionals to improve the quality of health care and healthcare communication.[9]

Lack of cultural awareness is believed to be a barrier to improving health care for minority patients, particularly when evidence suggests that patient race has a subtle but important influence on clinical decision making by physicians.[10]

Cultural competency training can provide insights into caring for a diverse patient population by increasing clinician awareness of the need to improve care for patients from diverse backgrounds.[10]

Culture can be defined as a "dynamic and creative phenomenon, some aspects of which are shared by large groups of people and other aspects which are the creation of small groups and individuals resulting from particular life circumstances and histories."[11] It can be viewed as a process that links the past to the present and is shaped in part by social, historical, and political context. Culture shapes lifestyles and beliefs that ultimately impact on one's risk for and subsequent response to health and illness.[11,12]

Unhealthy habits may not be exclusively an individual or personal matter. They are often related to learned social behaviors. People from various cultural orientations view sickness and health differently.[12] As such, culture can affect decisions about choosing healthcare providers, describing symptoms, and considering treatment options.[11]

Culture also influences the choice to obtain medical treatment and to follow treatment recommendations. Although often viewed narrowly, culture is broader than race or ethnicity. It extends to other areas, including language, gender, class, age, sexual orientation, and religion.[9,11] For example, African American patients report more lower-quality care experiences with physicians than do white patients, and often perceive bias in healthcare delivery.[10] Infant mortality rates are twice as high among African American infants as whites, and Hispanics are less likely to receive smoking cessation messages.[13]

It is believed that socioeconomic status accounts for much of the observed racial disparities in health outcomes. Minorities more often lack health insurance and a primary care physician.[13] Uninsured individuals are less likely to have a regular provider, are more likely to report delaying seeking care, and are more likely to report that they have not received needed care—all resulting in increased avoidable hospitalizations, emergency hospital care, and adverse health outcomes.[13]

Cultural competency in health care is defined as "the ability of systems to provide care to patients with diverse values, beliefs, and behaviors, including tailoring the delivery of care to meet patients' social, cultural and linguistic needs."[14,15]

The underlying motivation for recognizing culture is that culture is intertwined with an individual's health beliefs, values, preferences, and practices.[12] Culturally sensitive care is essential to creating the optimal patient-centered experience; effective patient-provider communication; delivery of high-quality, evidence-based health care; achievement of positive treatment outcomes; and high patient satisfaction rates.[14,15]

Cultural humility "incorporates a lifelong commitment to self-evaluation and self-critique, to redressing the power imbalances in the patient-physician dynamic, and to developing mutually beneficial and nonpaternalistic clinical and advocacy partnerships with communities on behalf of individuals and defined populations."[16] Culture should be considered a factor (if relevant to the patient) in health care.[15]

The goals of cultural competency training include:

- Understanding attitudes such as mistrust, subconscious bias, and stereotyping that practitioners and/or patients may bring to the clinical encounter
- Attaining knowledge of the existence and magnitude of health disparities, including their multifactorial etiologies and the multiple solutions required to eliminate them
- Acquiring the skills to effectively communicate and negotiate across cultures, including trust-building and the use of key tools to improve cross-cultural communication and relationship building[13]

Several tools have been developed in an effort to facilitate clear communication between patients and physicians. The ***Ask Me 3*** pamphlet takes a simple patient-centered approach to improving health outcomes, by encouraging patients to understand the answers to three simple but essential questions in every healthcare interaction:

1. What is my main problem?
2. What do I need to do?
3. Why is it important for me to do this?[16]

These questions serve as an activation tool encouraging patient participation in the healthcare visit and decision making while establishing good interpersonal relations and facilitating information exchange.[16] It can aid in the reduction of health disparities. Research has found that patients find the questions to be a useful framework for engaging in conversation with their physicians.[16] Another tool that can be used by practitioners to improve communications is the **4 Cs**.[17] This tool can be used to help patients articulate their preferences and understand the needs of a diverse patient population:

- Call: What do you call your problem?
- Cause: What do you think has caused or contributed to your problem?
- Concern: What concerns you most that we need to be sure to address?
- Cope: What are you currently doing to cope with your problem?

Cultural humility: the lifelong commitment to self-evaluation and self-critique, to redressing the power imbalances in the patient-physician dynamic, and to developing mutually beneficial and nonpaternalistic clinical and advocacy partnerships with communities on behalf of individuals and defined populations

Ask Me 3: tool to facilitate clear communication between patients and physicians that takes a simple patient-centered approach to improving health outcomes by encouraging patients to understand the answers to three questions: (1) What is my main problem? (2) What do I need to do? and (3) Why is it important for me to do this?

4 Cs: tool used to improve communications by helping patients articulate their preferences through the use of four questions: (1) Call: What do you call your problem? (2) Cause: What do you think has caused or contributed to your problem? (3) Concern: What concerns you most that we need to be sure to address? and (4) Cope: What are you currently doing to cope with your problem?

Listening is a simple practice that can enhance the health and well-being of patients in a number of ways:

1. It is a mechanism for ascertaining details of a patient's concerns, attitudes, circumstances, and belief system that are essential to appropriate treatment.
2. Patients who experience listening may develop a higher level of trust with their caregivers.
3. Patient compliance and outcomes may improve.
4. New solutions may be discovered.[18]

Enhanced active listening skills such as nodding when talking to another person, asking clarifying questions, paraphrasing another person's statements, using of proper posture and eye contact, paying attention, and refraining from judging the patient can enhance patient communications.[18]

Learning about each patient's experience and culture, and empowering him/her to ask questions, will improve the patient's healthcare experience.[18] Human interactions should be rooted in recognition of the innate equality, dignity, and worth of every person.[18] Providers should honor the integrity and authority of each individual and support their patient's right to decide what treatment option will best serve his/her needs.[18]

There is value in learning to pay attention, to listen to what is not being said (or to what is being said but minimized), and to learn the art of "waiting" and "asking the right questions" rather than having the right answers.[18] The practitioner should make inquiries that elicit information, clarify ideas, and encourage involvement in healthcare decision making.[18]

Betty Cheng, LCSW, chief operating officer at the Charles B. Wang Community Health Center in New York, stated, "I know I have no way of being able to understand everyone's cultures, so the key is to listen to each patient and let them teach you about their culture."[18]

Healthcare providers should develop practical skills such as listening and relationship building that can be applied to all cultures, while learning the values, attitudes, behaviors, and spiritual beliefs of those multiethnic patients whom they serve.[19]

Things to consider include hiring trained, full-time interpreters, educating language-competent staff members in interpretation techniques, and accurately tracking patients requiring language assistance.[14]

It is recommended that services be customized to meet the unique needs of specific populations to whom you will be providing health care. This will result in reduced barriers to care. Health disparities can be addressed through staff education, physical environment redesigns (including the use of universal symbol signage), and interest in patients' religious practices, opinions about healthcare institutions, and death and dying rituals across the different cultural groups that you will serve.[14] If you can, learn a few words from your patient's native language. Speaking the same language as the patient automatically makes the patient feel more at home.[8]

Ask employees from the appropriate backgrounds to teach one another important cultural concepts, such as whether you shake hands or nod your head as a greeting, what questions you can ask in front of other family members, how much eye contact to make, and how close to stand. Contact the language or other appropriate department of a local college or university to find someone who is familiar with the culture, behavior, and beliefs of the ethnic groups for whom you provide medical care. Develop cultural fact sheets and diversity workshops for your practice.[8]

Browning and Waite advise that "patients are the experts on themselves. We will never know more about people or their culture than they do. They have to tell us who they are, and we need to listen to what they want."[18]

Providing patient-centered care is one approach to improving communication and reducing health disparities.[17] Evolving one's education and practice to achieve true cultural competency requires a lifelong process of learning and reflection.[12] Online training resources include the following:

http://culturalmeded.stanford.edu/
http://www.nhlbi.nih.gov/training/
http://culturalmeded.stanford.edu/teaching/unnaturalcausesresource.html
https://implicit.harvard.edu/implicit/

PROVIDING THE DIAGNOSIS AND BUILDING THE TREATMENT PLAN

When patient outcomes are poor, it is convenient for providers to call patient compliance into question. The last prescription you wrote for a cholesterol-lowering medication was a 30-day supply that should have lasted the patient only until his follow-up appointment. He returns to your office three months later having missed the earlier appointment, without improvement in his cholesterol level or having called in for a refill. In this case, doubting compliance would be justified. How tempting to confront the patient by saying, "No wonder your cholesterol hasn't improved. You ran out of medication two months ago!" Before you do so, perhaps you should ask yourself what factors may have contributed to lack of compliance. Did the patient experience an adverse side effect? If so, did you instruct the patient on which side effects to expect and what to do if they did occur? Was the patient unable to afford the medication? Did a family crisis prevent him from returning earlier? Did you properly educate the patient on the importance of the medication?

The building of a treatment plan is a cooperative effort between the patient and the provider. Though patients seek the guidance, knowledge, and experience of the provider, it is important to avoid dictating a course of action without input from the patient. Patients who are asked to contribute to their own health care are invested to a deeper degree and demonstrate increased compliance. This process begins with sharing the diagnosis with the patient.

The majority of diagnoses are accurately obtained through detailed and concise history taking. Physical examination functions to confirm the diagnosis and may lead to other diagnoses that were unsuspected, such as finding a heart murmur in a patient who denies ever having one. At other times, the diagnosis is elusive and requires further investigation. In such cases the provider constructs a list of the possible diagnoses, called the differential diagnosis. Recognizing early in your medical career that we as providers do not always know the diagnosis allows you to approach the patient with honesty and sincerity when discussing your suspicions.

It is always important to provide your patient with a proposed diagnosis, even if you are not sure of what the exact diagnosis is. For example, a patient presents with a chronic cough. After taking a thorough history and performing a physical examination, you suspect gastrointestinal reflux disease (GERD) as the primary cause. However, the social history reveals that the patient has smoked for 20 years, having successfully stopped two years prior. In your differential you suspect GERD as the most likely diagnosis, but you also consider chronic obstructive pulmonary disease (COPD) and even lung cancer as other possibilities.

Sharing this information with your patient requires educational skill. Skill in educating your patient requires that you share your suspicions with her and yet avoid causing stress or anxiety.

Though the following would seem intuitively inappropriate, there would be few providers who could deny observing similar conversations:

- "Mrs. Smith, I think your cough is coming from acid reflux although your history of smoking bothers me. You could have chronic lung changes from all of that smoking you did, even lung cancer. Might not be but I'll check it out."

Though a diagnosis was proposed, no skill in its presentation was apparent. It lacked both empathy and concern for the anxiety it may have induced in the patient. The tone is accusatory, immediately putting the patient on the defensive instead of drawing her in as a collaborator in her own health care. The same information can be shared with the patient in a completely different, nonconfrontational, empathetic way:

- "Mrs. Smith, coughing such as you describe very frequently comes from acid reflux. There are some other possibilities that I am thinking about. I'm very impressed that you stopped smoking two years ago. You did the best thing you could have done for yourself. There could have been some injury to your lungs from the smoking, so we'll need to check that out. I would recommend a test that measures how well you breathe and an x-ray of your chest. How do you feel about that?"

Here you shared the diagnosis that you felt was most likely, but openly expressed that there were other possibilities that must be explored. Instead of criticizing the patient for her smoking and blaming her for the condition she was in, you provided encouragement and positive reinforcement for her successful smoking cessation and bolstered her self-esteem. Part of your evaluation included testing to rule out the other diagnoses. You did not simply dictate that these tests needed to be done; you explained why they should be. Saying, "We'll need to check that out" includes the patient as part of "we," the investigating team. "Need" implies the necessity of the action. Finally, though you built the differential diagnosis through your knowledge of medicine and recommended the appropriate evaluation, you also asked the patient for her input and gave her the opportunity to ask questions, seek clarification, or even object to the proposal.

It is important to clearly explain the diagnosis. The practitioner must determine the level of detail to present. Examining the pathophysiology from the previous example of GERD, we see the movement of gastric fluids in a retrograde fashion from the stomach into the esophagus. This is usually prevented from occurring by a lower esophageal sphincter that constricts, and is aided by the anatomical design of the gastroesophogeal (GE) junction with abnormalities such as that associated with a hiatal hernia allowing reflux to occur.

Providing this level of information to the patient would rarely be warranted unless the patient is knowledgeable in the practice of medicine. Instead the discussion might go as follows: "We have acid in our stomachs that helps to break down foods and kill bacteria. That acid is supposed to stay in the stomach but sometimes goes back up into the esophagus. If that happens repeatedly, it can cause injury, which might be felt as 'heartburn.' Our goal in treatment is to prevent the injury from happening." This would provide the diagnosis in a short, simple format using terminology the patient can understand.

Building a plan of treatment involves our clinical expertise but must involve the patient in the treatment decision making. A patient needs a medication for high cholesterol but has not tried dieting and exercise, which may be recommended as the first line of treatment. Ask the patient which route he would like to take. You may discover that the patient would rather start the medication now, since he knows he will be noncompliant in restricting his diet and exercising because his occupation requires long days at work and eating on the road. Conversely, a second patient "hates to take medication" and would much rather make an honest effort at balancing his diet and beginning an exercise program. In either case you have involved the patient in his treatment plan, which means he is more likely to feel invested in his path to success, as he now "owns" it.

Treatment plans must be easy to understand and logical. This may require writing the information down for the patient. Following your description of the diagnosis of reflux, you explain the options for the plan of treatment. First is a discussion on behavioral aspects that allow stomach acid to slide back up into the esophagus, such as use of tobacco and alcohol, and eating before lying down. Avoidance of these things alone reduces reflux.

Next you may discuss the different types of medication that are used for the condition. "Mrs. Smith, there are several classes of medications that we can use to treat reflux. We often use a stepwise approach, trying milder medications first and then advancing if symptoms fail to improve. Some of these medications are over-the-counter, and some require a prescription. Do you have any thoughts or concerns about this?" Giving the patient the opportunity to express concerns and options again encourages adherence to the treatment plan and ultimately an investment in the outcome, as the patient was instrumental in its formation.

Mrs. Smith advises you that her finances are fairly tight at the moment and that she would prefer the least costly alternative as her insurance does not cover prescription medications. You may now discuss the options found among the various over-the-counter medications, which, when combined with the changes in behavior, have proven efficient in the treatment of reflux.

Consideration for including others in the development of a treatment plan should be tailored to the individual patient. A 24-year-old male with a wart would not likely prompt the provider to inquire if the patient would like anyone else involved in the decision making. The opposite is true when a very independent 86-year-old man is suffering from vertigo. His restrictions on driving and his high risk of falling necessitate the development of a treatment plan that includes an assessment of the types of support the patient has through family and friends. Though he may be hesitant at the consideration of loss of some of his independence, reassurance that support is necessary while he works at recovering his balance and will likely speed his recovery and return to independence will ease the transition.

Summarize the visit by asking the patient to restate the plan of treatment. This assures that the plan was presented logically and that the patient fully understands it.

EDUCATIONAL AND INSTRUCTIONAL SKILLS CHECKLIST

- Use the principles of Health Literacy when educating and instructing patients.
- Recognize disparities in medical outcomes presented by low socioeconomic status.
- Identify ethnic populations within your practice setting and explore related cultural beliefs and preferences concerning health care.
- Clearly explain diagnoses, avoiding medical terminology.
- Invest the patient in the outcome by including the patient in the development of his/her plan of treatment.
- Inquire if others should be included in developing a plan of treatment.
- Assure that the treatment plan is logical and easily understood.
- Have the patient restate the treatment plan to assure understanding.

Interviewing a patient is an art that goes far beyond simply asking historical questions surrounding a medical complaint. The encounter begins with the provider's mindset and mindfulness in avoiding prejudice. Adherence to the Humanistic Domain requires expertise in verbal, listening, and educational/instructional skills, while displaying empathy, respect, and professionalism. Patient encounters must account for diversity of cultures and Health Literacy.

References

1. Epstein RM, Hundert EM. Defining and assessing professional competence. *JAMA*. 2002;287(2):226–235.
2. National Network of Libraries of Medicine. Health Literacy. http://nnlm.gov/outreach/consumer/hlthlit.html. Published 2012. Accessed September 17, 2012.
3. Institute of Medicine. Health Literacy: A Prescription to End Confusion. http://www.iom.edu/Reports/2004/Health-Literacy-A-Prescription-to-End-Confusion.aspx. Published 2004. Accessed July 13, 2005.
4. Kirsch I, Jungeblut A, Jenkins L, Kolstad A. Adult literacy in America: A First Look at the Findings of the National Adult Literacy Survey. Washington, DC: National Center for Education Statistics, U.S. Department of Education, 1993. http://nces.ed.gov/pubs93/93275.pdf. Accessed December 31, 2012.
5. Institute of Medicine. Health Literacy: A Prescription to End Confusion. http://www.iom.edu/Reports/2004/Health-Literacy-A-Prescription-to-End-Confusion.aspx. Published 2004. Accessed July 13, 2005.
6. Adler NE, Newman K. Socioeconomic disparities in health: pathways and policies. *Health Aff.* 2002;21(2):60–76. http://sph.umich.edu/sep/downloads/Adler_Newman_Socioeconomic_Disparities_in_Health.pdf. Accessed January 2, 2012.
7. Winkleby MA, Jatulis DE, Frank E, Fortmann SP. Socioeconomic status and health: how education, income, and occupation contribute to risk factors for cardiovascular disease. *Am J Public Health.* 1992;82(6):816–820. http://www.ncbi.nlm.nih.gov/pubmed/1585961. Accessed September, 17, 2012.
8. Levoy B. How multicultural is your practice? *Podiatry Manag.* March 2011:59.
9. Carter-Pokras O, Bereknyei S, Lie D, Braddock III C. Surmounting the unique challenges in health disparities education: a multi-institution qualitative study. *J Gen Intern Med.* 2010;25(suppl 2):S108–S114.
10. Sequist T, Fitzmaurice G, Marshall R, et al. Cultural competency training and performance reports to improve diabetes care for black patients. *Ann Intern Med.* 2010;152:40–46.
11. Waite R, Calamaro C. Culture and depression: a case example of a young African American man. *Perspect Psychiatr Care.* 2009;45(3):232–238.
12. Simon M, Chang ES, Dong XQ. Partnership, reflection and patient focus: advancing cultural competency training relevance. *Med Educ.* 2010;44:540–542.
13. Ross P, Cene C, Bussey-Jones J, et al. A strategy for improving health disparities education in medicine. *J Gen Intern Med.* 2010;25(suppl 2):S160.
14. Gertner E, Sabino J, Mahady E, et al. Developing a culturally competent health network: a planning framework and guide. *J Healthc Manag.* 2010;55(3):109–204.
15. Chun M. Pitfalls to avoid when introducing a cultural competency training initiative. *Med Educ.* 2010;44:612–620.

16. Michalopoulou G, Falzarano P, Arfken C, Rosenberg D. Implementing Ask Me 3 to improve African American patient satisfaction and perceptions of physical cultural competency. *J Cult Divers*. 2010;17(2):62–67.
17. Wilkerson LA, Fung CC, May W, Elliott D. Assessing patient-centered care: one approach to health disparities education. *J Gen Intern Med*. 2010; 25(suppl 2):S86–S90.
18. Browning S, Waite R. The gift of listening: JUST listening strategies. *Nurs Forum*. 2010;45(3):150–158.
19. Thompson G. Cultural competency: Haiti and at home [editorial]. *Br J Community Nurs*. 2006;15(3):109.

SECTION II

History Taking

CHAPTER 3

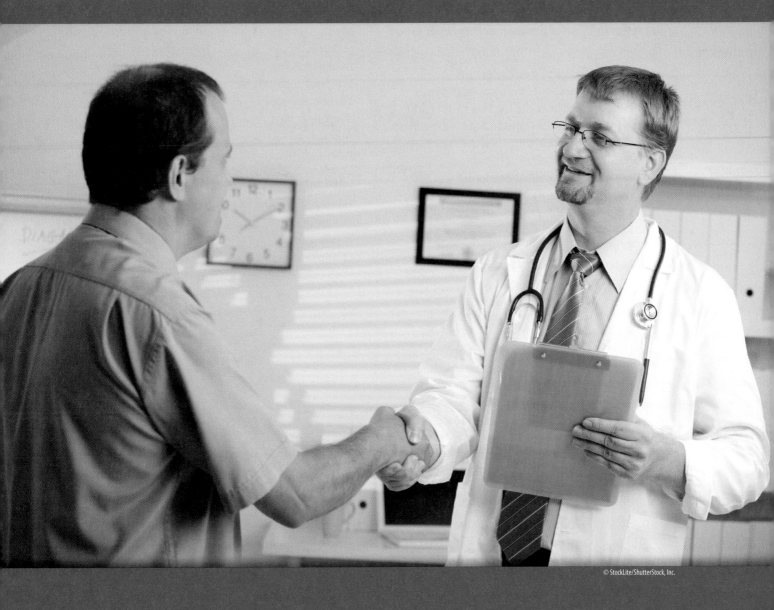

© StockLite/ShutterStock, Inc.

History Taking

OBJECTIVES

At the conclusion of this chapter, the student will be able to

1. Use problem and medication lists to identify interconnections between the current complaint and medical history and identify unrelated comorbidities and health maintenance issues
2. Relate the pre-encounter screen to urgency of the patient encounter and early development of the differential diagnosis
3. Differentiate Reason for Visit from Chief Complaint
4. Begin the patient interview by properly entering the room and providing introductions
5. Demonstrate competency in hand hygiene techniques in prevention of disease transmission
6. Use appropriate opening questions to prompt the patient to begin relating the medical history
7. Recognize appropriate points for transitioning from open-ended to closed-ended questioning
8. Know the components of the history taking mnemonic CODIERS SMASH FM
9. Differentiate between Review of Systems and Symptoms Associated
10. Know the components of the social history mnemonic, FED TACOS

KEY TERMS

Medical history
Problem list
Medication list
Pre-encounter screen
Demographics
Reason for Visit
Admission Ticket
Hand hygiene
Opening question
Chief complaint
History of present illness (HPI)
Redirection
CODIERS SMASH FM
Chronology
Intensity
Exacerbating factor
Remitting factor
Review of Systems (ROS)
Symptoms associated
Anatomy-based questioning
FED TACOS
Menstrual history
Gravida
Para

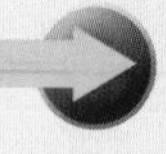
Where this icon appears, visit **go.jblearning.com/HPECWS** to view the video.

The **medical history** is a collection of data that is used to rule in or rule out particular diagnoses. It comprises the rudiments surrounding the current condition of the patient as well as medically related elements in the patient's past. The goal of achieving competence in obtaining a medical history during a patient encounter can be accomplished by developing a systematic, thorough, yet logical approach to questioning that can be consistently repeated with little variation.

Medical history: a systematic, thorough collection of data surrounding the patient's current condition and medically related elements in the patient's past used to build a differential diagnosis

Chart Review: On the Outside, Looking In

The history taking and physical examination of a patient begin outside the patient's room. Except in the case of emergency, the provider typically has access to at least some patient information prior to the actual clinical encounter. In the emergency room, it may be as simple as a one-line complaint and the vital signs.

In the inpatient setting the patient's chart contains a full history and physical examination, laboratory data, imaging results, consultation reports, nursing notes, vital sign graphics, medication administration history, and daily notes describing the patient's progress (the progress note), just to name a few.

In the outpatient setting, however, you may have years of medical history in your hands. The patient chart is a historical medical record and should contain patient demographics (age, sex, race), a problem list, medication list, prior office visit notes (the SOAP note), laboratory data, imaging results, patient correspondence, referral reports, and billing and insurance information.

Before entering the examination room, the provider should review the chart. This review begins with the patient's name. If the patient is new to you, nothing can scream disinterest and unpreparedness to a patient like the provider's entering the room and fumbling with the chart looking for a name. "Nice to meet you . . . um . . . Mr. . . . um . . . Jones." Spending a few moments with the chart prior to entering the room allows you to tell the patient that you see him/her as an individual with concerns and not as just the next appointment on the list.

Even patients new to a medical practice may have had the forethought to have their records sent to the new practice location prior to the visit. It can be very frustrating for a patient to take the time, effort, and often financial expense to have records precede his/her visit only to quickly realize that the provider never looked at them.

If you have seen the patient in the past and a relationship has already been established, a mere glimpse of the name can allow the patient's medical history to spill forth unabated and paint the canvas with the often complex artistry of his/her medical past.

THE PROBLEM LIST

A **problem list** is an inventory, often on a single page, that quickly allows you to identify medical conditions that the patient currently has or has had in the past (see TABLE 3-1). Each diagnosis should have a date of onset and date of resolution. Briefly reviewing this list allows for quick identification of recurrences of prior conditions, continuity of chronic conditions, and possible relations of new concerns with conditions of the past.

Problem list: an inventory of current or past medical conditions located in the patient chart that includes dates of onset and dates of resolution, which allow the provider to quickly identify recurrences of prior conditions, provide continuity of care in chronic conditions, and relate new concerns to conditions of the past

When the 16-year-old girl presents with dysuria—burning on urination suggestive of a urinary tract infection (UTI)—a review of the problem list may show anatomically related vesicoureteral reflux, the retrograde passage of urine from the bladder into the ureters, with an average of three similar UTIs a year since birth. Conversely, the lack of a prior UTI may suggest new onset of sexual activity resulting in the first UTI the patient has ever had.

Review of the problem list also allows the provider to quickly scan the patient's last several visits. Tim Johnson, a 35-year-old male, presents at this visit for ankle pain. His last visit, two months prior, was for a physical examination that was required for his application to obtain a license to drive a truck. During that exam you noticed a suspicious lesion on his back. Suspecting melanoma, you referred the patient to a dermatologist but cannot recall that you ever received anything from the consultant regarding the referral; nor does the chart contain any documents. This is not typical for the dermatologist to whom you refer. After addressing the patient's current concern, you inquire about the lesion only to learn that he was too busy to go to the appointment and has yet to reschedule the appointment.

TABLE 3-1 Sample Problem List

PROBLEM LIST		
Date	**Description**	**Problem Resolved**
12/3/1999	Hypertension	
10/17/2002	Sinusitis	10/30/2002
11/27/2010	Cholelithiasis—required cholecystectomy	1/15/2011
3/2/2012	Hyperlipidemia—3-month diet/exercise trial	

Medication list: an inventory of medications located in the patient chart that outlines which medications the patient has taken in the past or currently takes and includes the name, dose, and frequency of the medication, the amounts of medication to be dispensed by the pharmacy, and the dates originally ordered and when refills were authorized

Pre-encounter screen: a preliminary patient evaluation typically completed by a medical assistant or nursing staff prior to being seen by the provider that provides information about the patient's current needs and status and commonly contains patient demographics, Reason for Visit, and vital signs

Demographics: the patient's age, sex, and race used in development of the differential diagnosis and introduced early in the documentation of the encounter

THE MEDICATION LIST

The **medication list** is another valuable tool to review prior to entering the room (see **TABLE 3-2**). This list, again often only a page or two long, provides a linear outline of medications the patient currently takes or has taken in the past. It comprises the name, dose, and frequency of the medication that was prescribed. Also valuable to the provider are the amounts of medication that were to be dispensed by the pharmacy, the dates when the medication was originally ordered, and when refills were authorized.

When a patient presents with dizziness, a review of the current medications shows that she is on atenolol. This beta blocker, often used for high blood pressure, hypertension (HTN), has dizziness as a known significant adverse reaction occurring in up to 10% of the people prescribed it.

Another patient with HTN is seen in follow-up but shows severe elevation of the blood pressure despite being prescribed three medications to help control it. A review of the refill dates shows that although the patient was only prescribed enough medication for one month as you attempted to control his blood pressure, he has not been in to see you for three months and has not called for refills. Your suspicion that he is not taking his medications as directed would be warranted.

The Pre-encounter Screen

Each new visit begins with the completion of a **pre-encounter screen**, which is typically completed by a medical assistant or nursing staff prior to the patient's being seen by the provider. The screen provides information about the patient's current needs and status, and it commonly contains the following:

- Patient name
- Date and time of visit
- Demographics: age, sex, race
- Reason for current visit
- Vital signs

The process of constructing a differential diagnosis, a list of possible diagnoses listed in order of most to least likely, is fluid. As the provider moves through each component encountered during the patient demographics, prior records, history, and physical examination, the list of possible diagnoses grows and shrinks, twists and rearranges, fades and grows bolder until the silt settles, the waters clear, and the diagnosis bobs to the top.

DEMOGRAPHICS

Patient **demographics** include age, sex, and race. The age of the patient puts the reason for the visit into context. Chest pain in a 75-year-old man has a much greater likelihood of being a heart attack caused by hardening of arteries (atherosclerosis) than it does in a 7-year-old girl. A vesicular rash in the 7-year-old girl

TABLE 3-2 Sample Medication List

MEDICATION LIST						
Name	**Dose**	**Frequency**	**Date**	**Date**	**Date**	**D/C Date**
HCTZ	25mg	Daily	12/3/1999 #30, R 1	1/10/2000 #90, R 1	5/25/2000 #90, R 3	11/27/2000
Amoxicillin	500mg	BID	10/17/2002 #14, R 0			
HCTZ	50mg	Daily	11/27/2000 # 90, R 1	4/1/2001 #90, R 3	9/30/2001 #90, R 3	

is much more likely to be chickenpox (varicella zoster, a primary infection caused by a herpes virus) than is a vesicular rash in the 75-year-old man, who likely has shingles, a reactivation of the same virus, which has lain dormant in his nervous system for seven decades.

Knowing the prominent age of disease predilection helps narrow the diagnostic possibilities just as sex and race does. A 12-year-old African American boy who presents with severe abdominal pain is much more likely to be having sickle cell crisis than is a 12-year-old Caucasian female. Likewise, medications used in treatment may have better or worse efficiency in treating patients of one ethnic background versus another, such as avoiding monotherapy with angiotensin converting enzyme inhibitors (ACEI) in the treatment of African Americans with hypertension.

REASON FOR VISIT

When calling in for an appointment or when being screened prior to seeing the provider at the visit, patients will typically be asked for the reason they are seeking care: the **Reason for Visit**. This information is placed on the pre-encounter screen and has not come to you directly from the patient but rather through a support staff team member. It is often documented in only a word or two:

"Cough"
"Diabetes follow-up"
"Slammed hand in car door"

After the provider sees the patient and documents the encounter in a SOAP note, the reason for the patient visit is titled the Chief Complaint. Usually the two are synonymous, but that may not always be the case and the Reason for Visit may not be the true reason the patient is seeking care. Patients may be embarrassed, wish to share the reason for their visit only with the provider, or have some secondary gain in mind, like a few days off from work.

"**Admission Ticket**" is a term that is used when patients intentionally provide a Reason for Visit that is not consistent with what they actually have. Embarrassment, confidentiality, or secondary gain may lead the patient. Only a few patients would readily provide a Reason for Visit such as:

- "Hemorrhoids flaring up"
- "Unable to maintain an erection"
- "Wants STD testing, husband cheated on her"

Instead, the patient may offer a less revealing, partially factual, or completely unrelated Reason for Visit, with the true reason coming to light only during the provider interview:

- "Itch"
- "Discuss medications"
- "Abdominal pain"

Reason for Visit: explanation provided by the patient to a screening member of the healthcare team that may or may not be the true reason the patient is seeking care

Admission Ticket: term used when patients provide a Reason for Visit that is not the true reason for seeking care

Patients may offer a diagnosis as the Reason for Visit and may be correct, as when the patient with migraine headaches begins to suffer yet another. The offered diagnosis, however, may not be the correct one:

- "I have pneumonia" is actually a viral upper respiratory tract infection (URI)
- "I have an urinary tract infection" is actually polypuria secondary to undiagnosed diabetes mellitus
- "Abdominal pain" is actually a somatic presentation of depression

Each of these represents an unintentional misrepresentation of a diagnosis that the patient presents in good faith.

The Reason for Visit can have a powerful effect on the provider, one which may be bad or good. You have a love for office-based procedures. When you look at the pre-encounter screen for the next patient, you see "funny looking mole" and nearly salivate anticipating the possibility of a full thickness excision.

The next pre-encounter screen you see causes the exact opposite effect: "Oh no, not another dizziness. I hate these workups!" The longer one is in clinical practice and the more patients one sees, the more likely compassion and empathy can slowly be replaced with cynicism. Do not let yourself become biased before you see the patient. No matter how discouraging the last encounter was, each patient must be approached with respect and dedication.

Do not allow a person's race, gender, sexual orientation, substance abuse, "frequent flyer" status, mental illness, or any other characteristic cloud your judgment. A known patient with schizophrenia presents to the emergency room (ER) with back pain. She is known to visit an ER every Saturday morning, rotating through the four hospitals in the area so that she visits each one only once a month. On this particular Sunday, she states she was seen at the two biggest hospitals in town, one on Friday and one on Saturday. She had been seen and discharged with mild analgesics for her complaint of left-sided back pain. The provider recognizes that something about the story was different. She never went to more than one hospital on a weekend. A thorough exam revealed weakness in flexion of her left leg and the CT scan showed she had a staghorn kidney stone that was so big it had eroded through her left kidney and caused an abscess to form in the psoas muscle.

Approach each patient with unclouded vision.

MINDFULNESS OF YOUR SURROUNDINGS

Prior to entering the room, there may be multiple opportunities to observe the patient before the actual encounter. Sitting at your desk, you're looking out the window as you speak on the phone. You observe a patient as he is getting out of his car. He grabs his pant leg with both hands, lifting his left foot out the door, then pulls himself up and out of the car. As he walks toward the door you notice the right foot lift effortlessly off the ground about six inches with each step while the left foot barely leaves the ground. Your impressions and differential diagnoses begin to form immediately.

Other opportunities exist to observe patients before the actual encounter as the patient speaks with the receptionist, sits in the waiting room, slips into the bathroom, stands on the scale, or makes his/her way to the exam room.

Standing right outside the exam room as you prepare to enter, you may hear coughing, crying, arguments, anger, or laughter, all of which can impact your diagnosis. The same is true should you need to leave the room, return, or finish an encounter. A 5-year-old is brought to the ER with a laceration to the back of his head. His father says he wasn't in the room when it happened but heard him bouncing on the bed when he fell and struck his head on the bedpost. After cleaning the wound, stapling it shut, and covering it with a bandage, you leave to get the discharge instructions. Realizing you forgot to tell the man to change his son's bandage once a day, you turn back and overhear the young boy say to his father, "Where's the five dollars you promised me?" How does this change the diagnosis?

Hand hygiene: steps taken to remove pathogens from the hands prior to the patient encounter intended to lessen disease transmission

Entering the Room and Introductions

You have noted the patient's name, age, and sex; have briefly reviewed the problem list, medication list, last visit, and pre-encounter screen; and have already begun to form an idea of what his needs may be. You knock and enter the room.

Typically the first thing the patient will notice is your facial expression. Do you appear fatigued, enthusiastic, distracted, friendly, or hurried? A genuine smile is not only welcoming; it invites trust and has been equated with higher levels of perceived clinical competence. Eye contact should be made with the patient immediately upon entering the room. The provider should not be looking through the chart or at his/her watch.

And now we come to the first conundrum. It is common in the United States for two people to greet each other by shaking hands. This gesture is the beginning of trust. It reflects equality and a balance in the patient-provider relationship.

HAND HYGIENE

Unfortunately, one of the greatest and most preventable modes of disease transmission is through direct contact. Thus proper **hand hygiene** is at the forefront of disease prevention. In the practice of medicine, this transmission is termed healthcare-associated infection (HCAI) and occurs in approximately 5% of hospitalized patients in the United States.[1] In other words, 1 in every 20 patients in the hospital has increased morbidity or mortality due to an infection that was preventable. The best way to prevent this occurrence is proper hand hygiene.

Two accepted methods of hand hygiene are with soap and water or with an alcohol-based handrub based on the conditions shown in **TABLE 3-3**. It is not

TABLE 3-3 Recommended Hand Hygiene Methods

Soap and Water	Alcohol-based Handrub
Hands visibly dirty	Before and after touching the patient
Hands visibly soiled with blood or body fluids	Before handling an invasive device for procedures
After using a bathroom	After contact with any body fluids
In prevention of spore-forming pathogens such as *C. difficile*	Before moving from a body site of contamination to any other areas on the same patient
	After contact with immediate surroundings of the patient
	After removing gloves
Before handling medication or preparing food	

Adapted from: World Health Organization. WHO Guidelines on Hand Hygiene in Health Care: A Summary. Published 2009. http://whqlibdoc.who.int/hq/2009/WHO_IER_PSP_2009.07_eng.pdf. Accessed January 7, 2012.

recommended to use both simultaneously. If handrub is not available, wash with soap and water.[1]

If you have not immediately washed your hands after seeing the last patient, you will need to rewash your hands prior to seeing the next. Just opening the door to the next patient's room poses a risk for contamination, as we don't know who touched the door handle last or if contamination could have occurred.

Now the conundrum: You are expected to wash your hands before touching the patient, but you are also expected to greet the patient with a handshake when walking into the room. If a patient is rather new to your practice, it may feel a bit awkward not to offer your hand immediately, but once a patient knows your habits, he/she will understand your purpose for a delay in handshake.

To avoid disease transmission, once you knock, smile, and enter the room, pause after taking a few steps into the room, maintaining steady eye contact, greet the patient by name, introduce yourself by name and title if you have not previously met, then simply excuse yourself to wash your hands, explaining your intent in doing so.

- "Hello, Ms. Green. I'm student doctor/physician assistant/nurse practitioner Kelly Thomas. Just let me wash my hands before I shake yours."

You then proceed to the wash station and cleanse your hands appropriately.

This 30- to 60-second procedure gives you a chance to bond with the patient. Avoid the inclination to jump directly into the medical concern of the patient by asking what brings him/her in today. Instead, begin a nonmedical conversation inquiring about their trip in, the weather, or a local topic. This short time invested in the patient as a person instead of a medical concern demonstrates your concern for the patient at multiple levels instead of just a purely medical one.

Handshaking is a common and even expected greeting in much of the United States; however, keep in mind that some cultures and religions do not allow handshaking in certain circumstances. For example, in Orthodox Judaism, physical contact between members of opposite sexes is prohibited, so a proffered hand may be rejected. This may take you by surprise if unprepared for the encounter because by tradition, refusing to shake a hand is insulting. Should you find yourself in this situation, default to recognizing that the patient may have beliefs or customs different from your own that must be respected. A direct, nonjudgmental inquiry made to enhance your understanding will gain your patient's respect.

Hand Hygiene Technique

The first obstacle to overcome in decreasing HCAI is compliance among healthcare workers. Physicians are notorious for being the greatest offenders in maintaining proper hand hygiene, but no healthcare workforce can claim 100% compliance. Only conscientious individuals can do so.

Many excuses are offered for noncompliance:

- I don't have enough time.
- My hands are sensitive.

- There's no soap or gel around.
- The patient doesn't have an infection.

And the list goes on and on.

Education has the greatest potential to increase compliance. Reminder boards outside patient rooms, inside bathrooms, and on patient charts help healthcare workers to become vigilant. In addition, notices in patient rooms, exam rooms, and hallways now encourage patients to ask their providers if they have washed their hands before they are examined. Some patients may take the initiative but others may feel intimidated or reluctant to do so. Healthcare workers may also feel hesitant to point out noncompliance in their coworkers, especially superiors, despite the potential consequences to the patients.

The ability to wash the hands appropriately sounds commonsensical; however, proper technique is important.

In an effort to increase compliance, many healthcare facilities now have alcohol-based handrubs located directly outside each patient room. Some of these are motion-activated to further reduce the chance of contamination. When using these handrubs, dispense at least a half-dollar-size amount in the center of one palm, then rub evenly over both hands, paying close attention to include the spaces between the fingers and the back of the hands and fingers. Continue to rub the hands until they are completely dry, a procedure that should last approximately 30 seconds.

Using soap and water is a bit more complex. When approaching a sink to perform a hand wash, first assure that a clean, single-use towel is accessible to dry with after completing the wash without causing contamination. For example, some older paper towel dispensers require the operator to turn a crank to advance the towel. Some dispensers designed to advance the next towel by a few inches after one is ripped off can malfunction, resulting in the need for the operator to turn a wheel to re-access the paper. Either of these causes contamination.

Once towel availability is confirmed, turn on the water and adjust to a comfortable level, avoiding overly hot water. Wet the hands completely, front and back, and then dispense a quarter-size amount of liquid soap into the hands. Bar soap should never be used. Lather the soap and rub over the entire hand, front and back and between the fingers. Now divide the hand into sections: palm, palmer fingers, dorsal fingers, dorsum of hand, thumb, and between the fingers. Using the right palm, rub the left palm in a circular motion for a count of five, the same count you will use for each section. Now move distally to the palmer surface of the fingers, repeating the motion, and flex the left fingers over the palm and rub. Now move proximally to the dorsum of the hand and repeat. Envision the thumb as having four surfaces—medial, lateral, dorsal, and ventral—and rub each. Finally, interlace the fingers, first with one fifth digit most laterally, then switching so that the other fifth digit is most lateral. Now repeat, using the left hand to wash the right. This 5-second-per-section method provides for a 60-second hand wash.

Now rinse your hands under the water, being careful not to touch any part of the sink. The water should be left running as you take a towel and dry your hands. When your hands are dry, throw away the towel you were using and take a clean towel. Use it to turn off the water, and dispose of that towel. Do not use it to dry your hands again after turning off the water, a mistake frequently observed.

FINALIZING THE INTRODUCTION

Immediately after washing your hands, shake the patient's hand and offer another greeting:

- Jim, it's nice to see you again."

Or, if the patient is new to you:

- "Ms. Green, it's really nice to meet you. How would you like me to address you?"

Though patients typically prefer to be called by their first names, you should not assume that is the case. Always use proper titles if meeting someone for the first time, such as Mr., Mrs., or Ms., as it denotes respect. You may then ask the patient what he/she would prefer to be called. If you are unsure of the pronunciation of a last name, simply ask the patient how to pronounce his/her name correctly.

- "I'm sorry, could you help me with the pronunciation of your name?"

Now you are ready to begin the medical interview.

SUMMARY OF ENTERING THE ROOM AND INTRODUCTIONS

- Knock.
- Smile.
- Enter the room and pause after taking a few steps.
- Maintain steady eye contact.
- Greet the patient, using the last name for new patients or the preferred name for established patients.
- Introduce yourself to new patients by name and title.
- Excuse yourself to wash your hands.
- Bond with small talk during the hand wash.
- Shake the patient's hand and offer another greeting.
- Sit down.
- Begin the medical interview.

Opening Question

One of the keys to obtaining an accurate history is to allow your patient to tell you his/her story first. When beginning the medical interview, do so with an **opening question** that is open-ended prompting the patient to start telling his/her story. The patient often does so by starting with the concern that is most significant to them. "Open-ended" means that the question cannot be answered with a yes-or-no response. It requires further explanation.

- "What can I do for you today?"
- "What brings you in today?"
- "How may I help you?"

Avoid an opening question that may be considered rude or offensive despite not having that intention:

- "What's your problem?"
- "So, you're back already?"

Providers are cautioned to avoid looking at the Reason for Visit and limiting the patient response by their opening question:

- "I see you have a sore throat."
- "So, you have a headache?"
- "Let's take a look at that blood pressure."

If the patient had other concerns that he/she had intended to address, the patient may now be distracted or feel uncomfortable to do so, such as with concerns that he/she finds embarrassing.

Jim, a 75-year-old, was embarrassed to tell the 20-year-old female nurse that he was having difficulty maintaining an erection, instead saying that he was having a problem with his cholesterol pill instead. The nurse documents "Problem with cholesterol pill" as the reason for the patient visit. As the physician enters:

- "Jim, it's nice to see you again. I see you have a concern with your cholesterol pill. What's going on?"

Jim, who is now embarrassed for misleading the nurse, spends the next 10 minutes discussing the mild fatigue he has after taking his pill. The physician performs an exam and discusses alternatives to Jim's current medication. As the physician is about to leave the room, Jim says:

- "One more thing Doc . . . you know . . . I've been having a difficult time maintaining an erection."

The provider now either recognizes that this was the main reason Jim was coming in for the appointment or feels pressured by the time spent and downplays the inquiry, telling Jim that they will discuss it in detail on his next visit, a disservice to the patient. This may have been avoided if the opening statement had been:

- "Jim, nice to see you again. What brings you in today?"
  - "Hi Doc, nice to see you too. It's a bit embarrassing but I'm here because I'm having a difficult time keeping up an erection."
- "I see the nurse also noted you were having a problem with your cholesterol pill too?"
  - "Well, I thought that might be contributing to the problem, but honestly, this has been going on longer than I have been on that pill."

Beginning the patient visit with an open-ended opening question and avoidance of restating the Reason for Visit provides an increased opportunity for accuracy and honesty as the patient provides his/her history.

Opening question: the first open-ended question posed to the patient during the encounter designed with the intent to prompt the patient to begin a narrative as to why he/she is seeking care

Chief complaint: response provided by the patient directly to the primary provider during the patient encounter in response to the opening question and may or may not be the same as the Reason for Visit provided to the screening healthcare team member

History of present illness: series of questions posed to the patient that investigate the concern or reason for which the patient is currently being seen

Chief Complaint

The response to your opening question becomes the patient's **chief complaint** when you document the visit. This is the reason the patient came in to see you and is typically the same reason that was giving during their pre-encounter screen. It is often and best documented in the patient's own words. The statement should be concise and describe the symptom, diagnosis, or other reasons for the encounter:

- "My toe hurts."
- "I have a urinary tract infection."
- "I'm following up about my diabetes."

When Miss Titus states, "I have a urinary tract infection," this is the perceived diagnosis in her eyes derived by past experience, advice given to her, or her own investigation into symptoms. It is put into parentheses to show that these are the quoted words of the patient. She may not actually have a urinary tract infection, but in her opinion, it is why she's come to see you. When a patient offers you a diagnosis, pay serious attention to it as quite often he/she is correct.

Duration

The chief complaint may also include duration of time. Including duration of the complaint may change the differential diagnosis significantly.

- "I have chest pain" × 3 hours
- "I have chest pain" × 3 years

The sense of urgency felt with a 75-year-old male presenting to the ER with three hours of chest pain varies greatly from that with the same patient had he indicated three years of chest pain. Both in fact may be having an acute coronary syndrome, but the likelihood in the first scenario is much greater than in the latter.

History of Present Illness (HPI)

The **history of present illness** (HPI) is a series of questions posed to the patient that investigate the concern or reason for which the patient is currently being seen. The HPI is a subjective story given to you by the patient in response to the questions you pose and is documented in the "Subjective" part of your SOAP note. "Subjective" means that the information provided is based on that person's opinions, and it may not be accurate.

For instance, Mrs. Ross is being evaluated for a total hip replacement. When asked about her pain, she says she doesn't have any. Her daughter who accompanies her informs the doctor that Mrs. Ross has pain daily and takes acetaminophen three times a day. Mrs. Ross has short-term memory loss. She responded to the question about pain with sincerity, but the answer was subjective (that is, based on her opinion) and was not accurate. It is helpful to remember that the information is "subjective" because it represents the patient's (that is, the "subject's") point of view, rather than objective, proven fact.

OPEN-ENDED QUESTIONING

The technique of using open-ended questioning should be followed throughout the HPI as it allows patients to use their own words instead of words we put into their mouths. If a response to the original open-ended question fails to give you enough details, it should be followed by another open-ended question or statement.

- "What brings you in today?" (Opening question)
  - "I have chest pain."
- "Could you tell me more about that?" (Open-ended question)
  - "My chest really hurts." (Does not add sufficient information)
- "Can you describe the chest pain?" (Open-ended question)
  - "I don't know. It's just painful." (Vague response)
- "Would you describe it as sharp, dull, achy, pressure, squeezing, burning . . . ?" (Closed-ended)

This demonstrates the correct progression from open-ended to closed-ended questions, those that allow the patient to pick from a list of provided answers or reply in yes-or-no fashion. When you do move to questioning that presents options from which the patient will choose, such as describing pain, avoid running too quickly through a list, instead offering each choice slowly so that the patient has a moment to associate the pain he/she is experiencing to the option that was presented.

REDIRECTION

Many patients prompted by an opening question will quickly provide a fairly extensive narrative that completes many of the components of the HPI without the need for the provider's frequent prompts.

Other patients answer in reserved fashion, providing short or even monosyllabic responses that answer only the exact question being asked. This requires the provider to ask many more questions, move to closed-ended questions, and ask follow-up questions to initial responses in order to get the appropriate level of detail needed.

A third type of scenario can be found with patients who diverge too far from the primary concern or begin to provide too much information that is irrelevant.

- "Evelyn, have you ever had chest pain like this before?"
  - "Oh, yes, the first time I had chest pain was back in 1962, when I was visiting my sister Gwendolyn in Florida. Lovely place she has, really. Her house was built back in the 1920s. She only paid ten thousand dollars when she bought the place and you can't touch the area now for less than a hundred thousand. A lot of retirees too there, you see. It's warmer in the winter and our old bones . . . "

Though the story may be interesting and we want to allow some time to bond with the patient, gentle **redirection** is required. Occasionally the flow of conversation from the patient is at such a rate that the provider actually has to interrupt. When you do so, do so with compassion and warmth.

- "I'm sorry to interrupt, Evelyn, and if we have time, I'd love to come back to that, but I'm really concerned about that chest pain. Can you tell me when you had the chest pain last?"

It may take several redirections in a case like this to keep the information on track. An earlier transition to the use of closed-ended questions would also help to limit divergence from the questions asked.

LOGICAL SEQUENCE

Several mnemonics are used to guide providers through the components of the HPI. When students of medicine first begin to participate in medical history taking, they may feel compelled to ask each question as a checklist just to be sure to get each point: ask one question, the patient answers, ask the next question. The procedure is mechanical and often the answer is heard but not truly comprehended.

- "Does anything make the pain worse?"
  - "Smelling fumes."
- "Does anything make the pain better?"

Here the provider missed the possible connection of environmental exposure to fumes causing the patient's headaches. Instead of moving on to ask what made the pain better, the prior answer should have been contemplated and judged for its effect on the likely diagnosis. Most patients do not have frequent exposure to fumes. When she offers this response it leads to a completely different question than the one that was next on the list.

The provider role is to keep the patient on track while exploring the chief complaint and gaining sufficient information to obtain an accurate diagnosis. The provider's stream of questioning moves through different thought processes behind your questions as shown in **TABLE 3-4**. In this conversation, the impression of the provider changes from thinking the person may have alcohol dependency to recognizing the potential cardiovascular benefits of moderate alcohol consumption. As the interview continues, if you were to discover that the patient had been in rehab six times over the last two years for alcohol abuse, you would immediately return to your original opinion that drinking on a daily basis is not appropriate for this patient.

Never abandon a question for which you have received an incomplete answer. If someone admits to

Redirection: the technique of politely bringing the patient interview back to the topic of concern once discussion has strayed from pertinence

TABLE 3-4 Stream of Questioning

	Dialogue	Thought Process
Provider	Do you drink alcohol?	Social history screening.
Patient	Yes.	Positive screen.
Provider	How often do you drink?	Follow-up question to positive.
Patient	Every day.	That's pretty frequent.
Provider	How much do you drink in a day?	Quantifier.
Patient	Oh, only one glass of wine a day.	Well, that reduces cardiovascular risk.

CODIERS SMASH FM: history taking mnemonic used during the patient encounter to guide the provider while obtaining a logical, thorough, and concise medical history

having had the same abdominal pain twice in the past, ask about those past occurrences. When were they? How long did they last? How were they treated?

Providers must be careful not to stray too far from the main course of questioning or follow one path into too much detail. For example, if a 35-year-old male patient presents with a possible ligamental injury to the knee incurred while playing basketball, a detailed family history is unnecessary as it does not contribute to the case.

Components of the History of Present Illness: CODIERS SMASH FM

Developing a stepwise yet logical approach to history taking is the key to obtaining a complete, concise history. As students of medicine begin taking patient histories, utilizing a mnemonic is helpful to assure that comprehensive yet relevant histories are acquired. This early exposure has the potential to become the default even of experienced providers, increasing competence and accuracy throughout their careers and allowing them to provide better patient care.

We begin patient histories and allow the story to emerge in logical sequences based on the patient's answers, with us redirecting if the patient strays too far away from the topic at hand or bringing back the patient to partially answered questions that have gaps.

The fact that there is no set sequence does not mean that the questions are not in a logical order. For example, when a patient presents with dizziness, one of the first questions that may be asked is, "Can you describe what you mean by dizziness?" However, there are many other options for the next question, such as, "When did you first have this dizziness?" or "Have you ever had this before?"

Despite a lack of set sequence, having a mnemonic to fall back on is a valuable tool that puts the provider back on track should he/she get confused while taking the history. This mnemonic is **CODIERS SMASH FM** (see **TABLE 3-5**).

Early on the student should write this mnemonic down on a note sheet and make notations next to each entry as each component is explored. As the provider finds he/she is running out of questions and if the provider has written down the mnemonic, a brief glance at the paper will show which areas have not yet been discussed.

C
O
D
I
E
R
S

S
M
A
S
H

F
M

For example, the first "M" in SMASH is Medical History. Your patient is a 20-year-old male who presents with chest pain while playing basketball. It is associated with shortness of breath. There is no radiation of the pain. With the history you have taken so far, you have included spontaneous pneumothorax and musculoskeletal etiologies in your differential diagnosis. As the patient is only 20 years old and appears athletic, you may inadvertently put less thought into prior medical history and a contributor to his current condition, maybe even assuming none exists. When you glance at your paper and see the blank next to the "M" for medical history, you are prompted to ask,

- "Do you have any medical conditions?"
  - "I have Marfan's syndrome"

Instantly, you add dissecting thoracic aortic aneurysm as a possible diagnosis and move it up to the top of your differential diagnosis as the most likely, increasing the sense of urgency in the patient evaluation.

CODIERS

Chronology/Onset

The mnemonic is a guide, not an absolute order in which questions should be asked. CODIERS groups

TABLE 3-5 CODIERS SMASH FM Mnemonic

Mnemonic	Overview	Specific Questions
C—Chronology	Time frame showing the sequence of events	**Have you ever had this BEFORE?** With a positive: When was that? When was the first time you had it? How often does it occur? How long does it last? Did you seek intervention? Was there a prior diagnosis? What was the prior treatment? What was the prior outcome? **How has it CHANGED?** **What was the order of symptoms?**
O—Onset	Occurrence	**When did the current symptoms start?**
D—Description	Describe it Location Radiation	**Can you DESCRIBE it to me?** What does it FEEL like? Where is it located? Does it go anywhere?
I—Intensity	Scale How bad is it?	**On a scale from 1 to 10, how bad is the pain?** How has the symptom affected your activities of daily living? What can't you do anymore?
E—Exacerbating factors		**What makes it worse?**
R—Remitting factors		**What makes it better?**
S—Symptoms associated	Concurrent findings	For a cold, question about the presence of fever, chills, runny nose, sinus pressure, headache, nasal congestion, a sore throat, cough, etc.
S—Social history	FED TACOS	Food (diet), exercise, drugs, tobacco, alcohol, caffeine, occupation, and sexual history
M—Medical history		Prior medical conditions (acute or chronic), immunizations, health maintenance?
A—Allergies		Food, environmental, drug—what happens?
S—Surgical history		What? When?
H—Hospitalization		What? Where? When?
F—Family History		Mother, father, siblings, family tendencies
M—Medications		Name, dose, frequency?

Chronology: the time frames of the patient's symptoms, consisting of three major areas: onset of the current concern, how the concern has changed since onset until currently being interviewed, and prior history of similar concerns or conditions

together all of the aspects of the current complaint, whereas SMASH FM pertains to the general medical and social history of the patient. Generally the patient's story comes together with more cohesiveness by exhausting CODIERS prior to advancing to SMASH FM. This rule, however, should not interrupt the flow of the case. If a patient presents stating, "I think I'm having an allergic reaction to my medication!" likely your very first and most appropriate question would be, "Which medication?" Here, jumping to the last "M" in the mnemonic makes complete sense and one simply has to return to CODIERS should logical flow dry up.

Timing of an event has many components, which are represented by both "C—Chronology" and "O—Onset." Chronology is the first item in the mnemonic; however, Onset would typically come first within clinical questioning. Alyson, a 16-year-old female, presents complaining of headaches:

- "Alyson, when did this headache start?" (O—Onset)
  - "About a week ago."

Chronology represents the time frame of the patient's symptoms and consists of three major areas outside of the onset:

1. Prior history of the same complaint
   - "Have you ever had a headache like this before?"
     - "No"
2. How the complaint has changed since onset
   - "Has anything changed about the headache?"
     - "It felt like it started behind my right eye, but now the whole right side of my head hurts."
3. Order of symptom presentation when multiple symptoms are present
   - "When this starts, which symptom do you get first?"
     - "First I see this fuzzy, bright spot and then I get a throbbing headache that makes me want to throw up."

Chronology should make you think of two separate time sequences. The first is from the onset of when the current complaint started—"about a week ago" until now, the time you are seeing the patient. Within this period of time we want to know if there has been any change to the symptoms since its onset. "It felt like it started behind my right eye, but now the whole right side of my head hurts" suggests progression of the symptom and worsening of severity.

The second time sequence is only found if the patient has had similar episodes in the past. If this has occurred, exploring the prior history of the complaint can give us valuable clues. If you find a positive for a patient having a prior history of the same complaint, you should thoroughly investigate it:

- When the patient first had it
- How often it occurs
- How long it lasts
- Did the patient seek intervention?
- Was there a prior diagnosis?
- What was the prior treatment?
- What was the prior outcome?
- Is there any change in the pattern of occurrence?

Using this line of questioning for Alyson's headaches:

- "Have you ever had headaches like this before?" (C-Chronology)
  - "Yes"
- "When was that?"
  - "I started getting them two years ago."
- "Did you see anyone for them?"
  - "I saw the pediatrician I had before we moved here."
- "Were you told what was causing them?"
  - "She said I was having migraines."
- "How were you treated?"
  - "She wanted to give me some pills, but I gag when I take pills so instead she said we could try to find out if anything I was eating might be causing them. She gave me a diary to keep track of what I ate."
- "Did you find out what was causing them?"
  - "It did seem that I'd get them more frequently when I ate chocolate."
- "What did you do then?"
  - "I cut out the chocolate and they did seem to go away for a while."
- "So now you are getting them even though you're not eating chocolate?"
  - "Um, well, I might have slipped a bit on that."

By exploring the chronology and finding that the patient had similar headaches in the past, not only did you find the likely diagnosis, but you also found out how to treat the patient. Instead of placing her on an expensive medication with possible side effects, trigger avoidance seems most appropriate.

Mr. Cook is another case that emphasizes the need for thorough exploration of past similar complaints. Mr. Cook, a 93-year-old, stops in at the office of his primary care provider at 4:15 on a Friday afternoon asking to be seen. As his provider begins the interview, he learns that Mr. Cook is experiencing dizziness, a complaint associated with a complex range of possibilities and intensities of evaluation, and a differential diagnosis alarm is set off inside the provider's head. It looks like a long week has just gotten longer. Would this patient need to be admitted to the hospital? Would he need a cardiac monitor? Was it even safe for him to drive home? Despite the daunting possibilities and the likely delay to ending the workweek, the provider begins the medical history without abandoning CODIERS SMASH FM:

- "Mr. Cook, what brings you in today?" (Onset)
  - "I'm really dizzy. Almost falling down."
- "Have you ever had this before?" (Chronology)
  - "Yes, last year." (Positive response)
- "Did you see someone for it?" (Follow-up to positive prior history of same)
  - "Yes." (Positive response)
- "What did they do for you?" (Follow-up to positive prior intervention)
  - "They washed out my ears and fixed it just like that."

The differential diagnosis just got a lot smaller. While continuing the questioning, the provider looks into the patient's ears and is met by a plug of cerumen. Two minutes and a water evacuation later, Mr. Cook walks up and down the hall stating that the dizziness is completely resolved. A thorough history commonly leads to a quick, definitive diagnosis and treatment.

Description/Duration

"D" should prompt the provider to ask the patient to "Describe" the symptom. A 78-year-old male patient presents with a chief complaint of chest pain. Description of the pain could easily alter or enhance a presumed diagnosis.

- "Can you describe the chest pain?"
  - "It's like someone is sticking a knife in my chest."

  OR
  - "It feels like an elephant is sitting on my chest."

Which of these descriptive answers is more likely to represent an acute coronary syndrome? Musculoskeletal chest pain is more often associated with sharp, stabbing chest pain, whereas chest pain from cardiac ischemia is visceral and more often described as pressure or heaviness.

The complaint of dizziness, in the case above, provides another example of description helping to narrow the diagnosis. Upon being asked to describe his dizziness, Mr. Cook stated that he just felt "off balance." Other clues could have altered the differential had he described vertigo, the perception of the room spinning around (possible inner ear dysfunction), lightheadedness (possible anemia), or near syncope, the perception of the room getting dark or nearly passing out (possible cardiac arrhythmia).

Description would also include the location of the patient complaint.

- "Alyson, where's your headache located?"
  - "It's the right side of my head."
- "The entire right side?"
  - "Yes, I think so."
- "Could you show me?"
  - She runs her hand from the right forehead back to the occiput.
- "With one finger, could you show me where the pain is the worst?"
  - She touches the right parietal area.
- "Does the pain go anywhere else?"
  - (Holding the right cervical area) "It does go down into my neck a bit."

Intensity

Intensity is the patient's perception of the severity of the symptom. A typical pain scale will range from 0 to 10, with 0 being no pain and 10 being the worst pain imaginable.

Intensity: the assignment of severity of symptoms or conditions often documented through a defined scale or by the effect on the patient's activities of daily living

Exacerbating factor: anything that makes a symptom or condition worse

Remitting factor: anything that makes a symptom or condition better

Many patients will rate their pain without delay given that brief description. Further clarification may be needed in a case where you have a patient rank his/her pain at a level of 10 although the patient has been smiling throughout the interview. You might first clarify that a 10 is the worst imaginable pain, the kind that the patient would seek hospitalization to help treat.

In cases of chronic or severe pain, the use of printed numerical and facial grimace scales helps patients more accurately assign the level of pain intensity they are experiencing. If a pain scale is not available, you might describe a typical scale to a patient as:

- "A 0 means that you have no pain at all."
- "A 1 would mean that you have pain but that sometimes you actually have to think about it to notice it."
- "A 5 would be a moderate amount of pain for which you would take something to help the pain fairly regularly or several times a day."
- "An 8 is pain in the severe range for which you would need to take something on a very regular basis."
- "A 10 is the worst possible pain imaginable. It is so bad that you would seek admission to the hospital to get help in reducing the pain."

Not all histories will have every component of CODIERS SMASH FM. Intensity is one of those common areas that may be missing. For example, if someone is complaining of a runny nose, you would not ask him/her to rate the runny nose on a scale from 0 to 10 with 10 being the worst runny nose imaginable. You could assess the runny nose in general terms by asking, "How runny is it?" to which the patient might respond, "My nose is cracked and bleeding from wiping it so much."

Intensity can also be assessed by the effect the symptom has on the patient's activities of daily living (ADLs). Mr. Cook presents for dizziness. You may be able to assign an imprecise intensity such as being so dizzy that he has fallen or so dizzy that the patient couldn't go to work that day. A scale, however, would likely not be used.

Exacerbating and Remitting Factors

These questions are straightforward. **Exacerbating factors** refer to anything that makes the symptom worse, and **remitting factors** refer to anything makes the symptom better. There are common errors that are encountered when asking these questions.

One such error is to ask the patient both questions in one sentence.

- "Does anything make your chest pain better or worse?"

Some patients may be able answer both questions without delay.

- "Spicy sauces and wine seem to make it worse. Antacids seem to make it better."

Other patients, especially the elderly, will have a tendency to answer only the second half of the question, that which they hear last.

- "Does anything make your chest pain worse or better?"
  - "Antacids seem to tame it down a bit."

More precise information can be obtained by asking each question separately and giving the patient enough time to contemplate and answer each question individually.

- "Does anything else make it better?"
  - "Antacids seem to tame it down a bit."
- "Does anything make it worse?"
  - "Spicy sauces and wine seem to make it worse."
- "Anything else?"
  - "It's worse if I eat right before going to bed."

This example is an improvement over the combined question; however, another common mistake was made by moving away from the line of questioning too quickly. When getting a positive answer to the inquiry, you must follow that line of thought to completion:

- "Does anything make your chest pain better?"
  - "Antacids seem to tame it down a bit." (Positive remitting factor)

- "What is the name of the antacid?" (Name of medication)
  - "Whatever I get a hold of, mostly Tums."
- "Just over-the-counter medications or prescription medications as well?"
  - "Just over-the-counter."
- "Are they always the chewable kind or do you take liquids and pills as well?"
  - "Just the chewable ones."
- "How often do you take antacids?" (Frequency)
  - "Every day."
- "How many times a day?"
  - "Oh, four or five." (Frequency)
- "How many do you take at a time?"
  - "Oh, three or four." (Dose)

With this approach, more precise information was obtained. It can be deduced that even though the patient is not completely sure of the names of each medication that has been tried, only the chewable kind has been tried. This is likely a calcium-based antacid. With this information the provider can avoid prescribing the same class of medications and move on to the next class of medications recommended.

Symptoms Associated: The Problem-Specific Review of Systems

Diagnosis-Based Questioning.

Review of Systems (ROS) is a technique used while performing complete history and physical examinations wherein the provider uses an inventory-like approach, going through each body or organ system and inquiring if the patient has or had symptoms related to that system. **Symptoms Associated** is another form of the ROS but one that is problem-specific, where the symptoms asked help confirm or rule out possible diagnoses that the provider has compiled based on the questions posed in the HPI.

While working through CODIER toward symptoms associated, the provider is building a list of possible diagnoses, the differential diagnosis. Each answer received has the ability to add more or less weight to a diagnosis or to add previously unconsidered possibilities to the differential. Some providers ask symptoms associated regarding a specific diagnosis as soon as they consider it a possibility. Others, especially early in their medical training, build the differential and then ask symptoms associated only after reaching it in the mnemonic. With increased experience, most will ask immediately upon considering a diagnosis.

Mary is a 75-year-old female presenting with shortness of breath (SOB). As you work your way through CODIERS, you find out that she has had these symptoms before. The last occurrence was one year ago when she was admitted to the hospital and treated for pneumonia. Immediately upon hearing this, you consider another episode of pneumonia as a possible diagnosis and add it to your differential. You must ask yourself, "What are the other symptoms of pneumonia?" This would prompt to you inquire about fever, chills, cough, sputum production, and chest pain.

However, there are many conditions that cause SOB. The next diagnosis that you entertain is acute coronary syndrome. Ask yourself, "What are the other symptoms of a heart attack?" You would then ask the patient if she is experiencing any sweating, nausea, pain going into the arms or neck, or numbness or tingling.

As quickly as a new diagnosis enters your thoughts, the questions to prove yourself right or wrong should be asked. Mary admits that she has smoked two packs a day for the last 40 years, an 80 pack-year smoking history. You add acute exacerbation of COPD (AECOPD) to your growing list of possible diagnoses. Ask yourself, "What are the other symptoms of AECOPD?" Then ask the patient if she can tell you if she has more problems getting the air in or getting it out. You also ask if she has been wheezing. Other symptoms associated with AECOPD, such as fever, have already been asked when considering other diagnoses and do not need to be repeated.

When going through the patient's medications, you learn that she takes both an ACE inhibitor and furosemide, a loop diuretic. These medications are commonly

Review of Systems: a technique used while performing complete history and physical examinations wherein the provider uses an inventory-like approach, going through each body or organ system and inquiring if the patient has or had symptoms related to that system

Symptoms Associated: an abbreviated Review of Systems (ROS) that is problem-specific, where the provider inquires only about symptoms related to a developing differential diagnosis to help confirm or rule out possible diagnoses

Anatomy-based questioning: a method for determining the appropriate symptoms associated to ask the patient based on anatomic location of the complaint

used to treat heart failure. Though the patient denies a history of heart failure, you must add it to your differential. To rule it out, you must ask about difficulty breathing while lying flat (orthopnea), sudden shortness of breath while sleeping (paroxysmal nocturnal dyspnea), dyspnea on exertion, and peripheral edema.

Anatomy-Based Questioning.

A second method for determining the appropriate symptoms associated to ask can be based on anatomy and becomes practical to use in situations where you are unsure of the diagnosis. By identifying the area of complaint, you should work through organ involvement within the area.

Gwen is a 40-year-old female who presents with right upper quadrant abdominal pain. Taking the history, you have considered cholelithiasis as a possible diagnosis, and have therefore asked about exacerbation after eating fatty foods, radiation of the pain into the right shoulder blade, and clay-colored stools, but are not convinced that this is the diagnosis.

Imagine approaching the anatomy as an arrow passing straight through the right upper quadrant directly from anterior to posterior, and consider which organs the arrow would touch as it passed through the body. The first point of contact would be the skin. Ask yourself what conditions could cause pain of the skin in the right upper quadrant location. Herpes zoster, shingles, is a possibility, even though Gwen is not in the typical age group. What are the symptoms associated with shingles?

- "Did you have any tingling in the area before this started?"
- "Does the pain wrap around to the back? "
- "Do you have a rash or blisters?"

The next point of contact would be the subcutaneous tissues and the rib cage. Could this be a rib dysfunction or costochondritis?

- "Do you have any pain with deep breaths?"
- "Does movement or deep inspiration cause pain?"
- "Have you had any trauma?"
- "Do you have any shortness of breath?"

We then touch the parietal pleura. Is there an acute peritonitis such as could occur with a rupturing gallbladder?

- "Do you have any fever?"
- "Nausea?"
- "Vomiting?"
- "Does it hurt to press in on your abdomen?"

Continuing with the thoughts of perforated viscous, could this be a duodenal or gastric ulceration?

- "Have you had any heartburn?"
- "Have you noticed any dark or sticky stools?"

The transverse colon stretches across both upper quadrants. Could this be colitis?

- "Have you had any changes to your stool?"
- "Diarrhea?"
- "Blood in your stools?"
- "Mucous?"

We have already considered the gallbladder, but let us consider the rest of the biliary system. Could this be distal obstruction, such as from a gallstone or pancreatic head cancer? We have already asked the questions about the gallbladder, but is there pancreatic involvement? You would add:

- "Have you had any weight loss?"
- "Night sweats?"
- "Lightheadedness?"
- "Left upper quadrant pain?"
- "Pain going into the back?"

Next we encounter the liver. Is it possible the patient has acute hepatitis? Many symptoms overlap what we have already asked, such as clay-colored stools, nausea, and vomiting. What else can we ask?

- "Have you noticed any yellowness in your eyes or skin?"

- "Have you been in contact with anyone with hepatitis?"
- "Have you traveled recently?"
- "Have you had any exposure to blood or body fluids?"
- "Have you eaten any raw shellfish?"

Passing through the liver, we encounter the right kidney. Is this pyelonephritis? This is less likely as the pain is usually perceived to be in the back; however it is still a possibility even though it has low probability. We have already asked about fevers and back pain.

- "Do you have any chills?"
- "Flank pain?"
- "Blood in your urine?"
- "Cloudy urine?"
- "Burning with urination?"
- "Foul-smelling urine?"

Finally we pass through the inferior lobe of the right lung. Could this be pneumonia?

- "Do you have a cough?"
- "Sputum production?"

Because the pain is anterior, pneumonic etiologies are also lower in likelihood, but can quickly be considered. Further atypical etiologies exist, such as a right upper quadrant appendix, but again are less likely.

It is important to reinforce that Symptoms Associated are part of the history and as such are documented under the Subjective part of the note. **TABLE 3-6** contains

TABLE 3-6 Symptoms Associated: The Problem-Specific Review of Systems (ROS)

System	Symptoms
Constitutional	Fever, chills, weight loss or gain, night sweats, fatigue
Eyes	Blurred vision or loss of vision, double vision, eye pain, injection, discharge, deviation
Ears, nose, mouth, and throat	Ear pain, discharge, hearing loss, epistaxis, nasal congestion, lesions, tooth pain, dysphagia, tinnitus, sore throat
Cardiovascular	Palpitations, chest pain, peripheral edema, claudication, irregular heartbeats, murmur, orthopnea
Respiratory	Shortness of breath, dyspnea on exertion, coughing, wheezing, chest pain, paroxysmal nocturnal dyspnea, hemoptysis
Gastrointestinal	Dyspepsia, nausea, vomiting, diarrhea, constipation, eructation, bloating, hematemesis, hematochezia, abdominal pain, change in caliber of the stools, bright red blood per rectum, melena, food intolerances
Genitourinary	Hesitancy, flank pain, dysuria, hematuria, urgency, frequency, decrease in force of stream, vaginal or penile discharge, dyspareunia, hematospermia
Musculoskeletal	Arthralgia, myalgia, bone deformity, weakness, range of motion limitation
Integumentary/breast	Changes in pigmentation or texture, rashes, lesions, pruritus, hair loss or change in hair texture, nail changes, dimpling of the breast, change in direction of the nipples, discharge
Neurologic	Facial asymmetry, memory loss, paresthesias, weakness, slurred speech, imbalance, changes in gait, dysphagia
Psychiatric	Depression, anxiety, suicidal or homicidal ideation, hallucinations, phobias
Endocrine	Polyuria, polyphagia, polydipsia, heat or cold intolerances
Hematologic/lymphatic	Easy bruising or bleeding, anemia, transfusion history, syncope, lymphadenopathy
Allergic/immunologic	Allergies, recurrent infections, eczema, nasal polyps

examples of symptoms associated for each body area but may be expanded.

SMASH FM

SMASH FM represents a survey of the medical and social history of the patient. Again, logical flow and following clues from the patient's answer to lead you to the next question is most appropriate. For example, SMASH FM puts medications at the end. You will likely find yourself asking about medications much earlier in the patient interview as a historical clue prompts you to ask about them. The patient interview is fluid, meaning that you will find yourself jotting down answers that skip back and forth between CODIERS and SMASH FM as the story unfolds. Utilizing the mnemonic while taking the history allows you, once the flow of logic ebbs, to glance at your note sheet and see the remaining the gaps. Filling in the gaps will allow you to complete a most detailed history.

FED TACOS: a history-taking mnemonic used during the patient encounter to guide the provider while obtaining a social history

Social History

The second mnemonic to write on your paper is "**FED TACOS**," which can be added horizontally across from the "S" in SMASH.

C
O
D
I
E
R
S

S—F E D T A C O S
M
A
S
H

F
M

This "S" stands for Social History. Not every component in the social history mnemonic is appropriate to ask. As a memory prompter, the provider should consider each component, ask if it relates to the current condition, and ask it only if appropriate. For example, if a 27-year-old male roofer presents with shoulder pain from grabbing a bucket full of nails as it slid off the roof, you would likely not need to inquire about his diet, represented by "F—Food."

However, his "E—Exercise" habits might indeed be very important, as would his "O—Occupation." How is this injury going to affect his ability to play on the softball team, and when will he be able to return to work?

The FED TACOS mnemonic is shown in **TABLE 3-7**.

When approaching the social history, begin with the least sensitive questions first and advance into the more sensitive areas. For example, you are taking a history from Alyson, the 16-year-old with ear pain. Although she is presenting only for ear pain, it is important to perform the social history screen and consider preventive health measures during the visit. Utilizing FED TACOS, we inquire first about "F—Food," asking about her diet. This is important in that dietary behavior in an adolescent may influence eating patterns throughout her life; likewise for "E—Exercise."

Next in the mnemonic would be "D—Drugs." The defenses of this 16-year-old may fly up if the next question you ask is, "Do you use any drugs?" She may not see the association with ear pain and may feel that you are prying or accusing her of something.

Begin with the least offensive question of "C—Caffeine" use, followed by "T—tobacco" and "A—Alcohol," ending with the inquiry about drugs. The approach should be matter-of-fact and may even begin with an explanation of why you are asking.

- "Alyson, I'm going to take a social history from you. I ask the same questions of everyone. How much caffeine is in your diet, such as coffee, pop, or chocolate?"
  - "I drink a pop or two a day but it's decaffeinated."
- "Do you use any tobacco?"
  - "I smoke a little?"
- "How much is a little?"
  - "One or two cigarettes a day."
- "Only one or two?"

TABLE 3-7 Social History Mnemonic: FED TACOS

		Examples of Pertinence
F	Food	Nutritional Balance—weight loss Restrictions—sodium in hypertension carbohydrates in diabetes cholesterol in coronary artery disease fats in cholelithiasis
E	Exercise	Obesity Cardiac rehabilitation Musculoskeletal injury Health maintenance
D	Drugs	Street drugs—recreational use Prescription drug abuse—chronic pain syndromes
T	Tobacco	Smoking—shortness of breath Smokeless tobacco (chewing tobacco)—mouth lesions
A	Alcohol	Abdominal pain—pancreatitis Cough and shortness of breath—aspiration pneumonia Depression—abuse Dyspepsia—reflux esophagitis
C	Caffeine	Coffee, tea, pop, chocolate—tachycardia, insomnia
O	Occupation	Etiologies Shortness of breath—asbestosis Rash—contact dermatitis Limitations—when can the patient return to work?
S	Sexual History	Obstetrical history Menarche Menopause Menstruation FDLMP—First day last menstrual period Sexually transmitted diseases Pregnancy planning and prevention

  - "Yes. I never buy them. My friends all smoke so when they drive me to school they give me a cigarette and then they give me one on the way home too."
- "How long have you been doing that?"
  - "Just this year."
- "Do you drink any alcohol?"
  - "No."
- "Do you use any street drugs or prescription drugs?"
  - "Nope."

By starting with the most benign questions such as that about caffeine, you are more likely to get honest answers, and as you progress the patient feels that these are just screening questions, not accusations. This screen allows you to be proactive and address preventive issues during the visit. You may be able to relate positive findings to the current concern as well, such as smoking leading to inflammation of nasal mucosa, obstructing the inner ear canal, and contributing or being the cause of her ear pain. You can then make recommendations for smoking cessation as part of your plan.

"O—Occupation" should be screened for two primary reasons. First, is the chief complaint directly related to the patient's occupation? You may assume Alyson, being 16 years old, is a student and is not working, or you may doubt that her occupation has anything to do with her ear pain; however, asking her about occupation you find out that she is a lifeguard. A little further questioning about her lifeguarding reveals that after she finishes her shift at the pool, she soaks in the hot tub for an hour. Worse yet, you learn that she submerses her head in the water. You should now consider pseudomonas otitis externa as part of your differential diagnosis. Perhaps Occupation was an appropriate question to ask after all.

The second reason to review occupational history comes into play when constructing your plan of treatment. You diagnose your patient with pinkeye. Occupational history reveals that she works at a day-care facility. You would not send her back to work with pinkeye until the infection has cleared and she is no longer contagious. Knowing what the patient's occupation is will allow you to assess whether restrictions on working should be placed.

Menstrual history: history of menses including onset, frequency, duration, flow, and cessation

Gravida: the number of times the patient has been pregnant

Para: the number and result of pregnancies defined through the mnemonic sentence "Florida Power And Light" (FPAL), where "F" stands for full term at delivery, "P" stands for preterm delivery, "A" stands for abortions, which includes miscarriages and elective abortions, and "L" stands for living children such that a woman who carried two pregnancies to full term, had no preterm deliveries, had 1 miscarriage, and has 3 living children would be P2013

Sexual history will likely be the most skipped area of questioning. If Mrs. Dunley, an 83-year-old, presents with a cough, you would not ask her if she is sexually active. However, if the same patient presents with vaginal discharge, it is an appropriate question.

Very frequently, the only sexual history question pertinent to the case will be inquiring about the patient's first day of last menstrual period (FDLMP), as this should be a consideration in both diagnostics and treatment options. Again, with a complaint of cough, we wouldn't ask Mrs. Dunley when her last period was. If, however, she presented with vaginal bleeding, we would.

Some providers may choose to put Obstetrical History here under "S—Sexual History." More commonly it is asked as a subsection of Medical History. There is no right or wrong about where it is placed as long as the provider includes it when appropriate in the evaluation.

Medical History

The first "M" in SMASH FM is Medical History. This may include obstetrical history, as just discussed, but should also include acute and chronic medical conditions, injuries, and immunizations as appropriate.

Some ways to pose these questions:

- "Do you have any current medical conditions?"
- "Have you been treated for any medical issues in the past?"
- "Are you being treated for any medical problems?"
- "Have you had any injuries?"

Obstetrical History.

Obstetrical History can be approached on two fronts, menstrual history and pregnancies.

Menstrual history.

- Menarche—age of onset of menses
  - "How old were you when you got your first period?"
- Menopause—age at cessation of menses
  - "How old were you when you had your last period?"
- Cycle frequency—number of days between menses
  - "How many days are there from one period to the next?
- Duration—number of days of menses
  - "How many days does your period last?"
- Flow—amount of blood lost during menses
  - "How many tampons or pads do you use per day of your period?"

Pregnancies. The history of pregnancies includes **gravida**, the number of times the patient has been pregnant despite the outcome of the pregnancy, and para, the number of times the patient has delivered. **Para** is further defined through the mnemonic sentence "Florida Power And Light" (FPAL), where "F" stands for full term at delivery, "P" stands for preterm delivery, "A" stands for abortions, which includes miscarriages and elective abortions, and "L" stands for living children. This information is documented such as G2P1001. This would indicate that the patient has been pregnant twice, had delivered one full-term infant, had not had any preterm deliveries, miscarriages, or abortions, and has one living child. Therefore, the patient is currently pregnant.

Gravida represents each pregnancy, not the number of fetuses, so that a pregnancy with multiples, twins, triplets, etc., only adds one to gravida. G1P0303 would indicate that the patient has had only one pregnancy in which their babies were born preterm, but all survived and are living.

G4P2021 would indicate that the patient has been pregnant four times, delivered two babies at full term, had two miscarriages or abortions, and only has one living child, meaning that one of the babies born at full term is no longer living. This would prompt further historical inquiry as to how old the child was when she died and the cause of death. This information may have also been obtained in the Family History.

- "Have you ever been pregnant?"
  - "Yes."
- "How many times?"
  - "Two."
- "Did you carry the babies to full term?"
  - "Only one of them. The other was born at 36 weeks."
- "Other than those two pregnancies, have you ever had a miscarriage or abortion?"
  - "I did have a miscarriage when I was 20."
- "How old are your children now?
  - "Ten and seven."

Documentation for this patient's pregnancy history would be G2P1112. This conversation could lead to many more questions, such as if there were any complications with the deliveries, if she was told why she went into labor early for one of the pregnancies, and further investigation of the miscarriage. Again you can see overlap, in that the sex and health history of her children could be explored here or under family history.

Immunizations.

A general inquiry into status of immunizations may be posed as, "Are your immunizations up to date?"

However, immunization history is much more specific based on the given situation. For example, a patient who presents to the ER with a laceration should be asked about the date of his/her most recent tetanus booster. Records of immunizations should be requested for any patients new to the practice. Other immunizations require frequent updating, such as yearly influenza vaccination.

Allergies

Allergy history should investigate three categories of allergies: foods, drugs, and environmental allergies. For each reported allergy, the reaction experienced by the patient should be investigated.

- "Do you have any food allergies?"
  - "Yes, I'm allergic to bananas."
- "What happens?
  - "I can't breathe."

This represents a true anaphylactic reaction and you must ensure that the patient has an up-to-date prescription for an EpiPen.

- "Are you allergic to any medications?"
  - "Penicillin."
- "What happens?"
  - "I'm not sure. My mother just always told me never to take it."

Without records or further description of the witnessed accounts, a true allergy cannot be confirmed. The provider should still document the possible allergy and avoid the use of penicillin as a first-line treatment, but allergy testing could be considered.

- "Are you allergic to any medications?"
  - "Aspirin."
- "What happens?"
  - "It upsets my stomach."

This is not a true allergic reaction, but rather an adverse reaction. Perhaps the patient has only tried non-enteric-coated aspirin at higher doses. If the patient has diabetes, a trial of low-dose, enteric-coated aspirin would be appropriate as daily aspirin as indicated.

Surgical History

Use a chronological approach to obtain surgical history. Inquire as to the type of surgery performed and the date of the procedure. Emergent surgery or injury can result in blood transfusions, which can also be asked about. If appropriate, more specific detail such as the symptoms prompting the need for surgery, complications, and the outcome can be assessed.

Kathy, a 32-year-old, presents with abdominal pain and fever:

- "Have you had any prior surgeries?"
  - "Yes."
- "What did you have done?"
  - "I had my appendix taken out."
- "When was that?"
  - "About 10 years ago."

We now know the problem is not her appendix, and with a 10-year gap, it would not likely be a complication related to the surgery. Changing the scenario with the same patient:

- "Have you had any prior surgeries?"
  - "Yes."
- "What did you have done?"
  - "I just had a baby."
- "When was that?"
  - "About five days ago."
- "Was it a vaginal delivery or caesarean section?"
  - "Vaginal."

We would consider complications of the delivery, including retained placenta.

Hospitalization History

Under Hospitalization History, create a list of the approximate dates, reasons for admission, treatments undergone, and outcomes.

Family History

General screening for family history typically focuses on first-degree relatives: parents, siblings, and children. Given advancing life spans, avoid asking the age at which parents have died. Jim, an 81-year-old, has moved to Arizona and is seeing his new primary care physician for the first time.

- "How old was your mother when she passed away?"
  - "Mom died!? When did that happen?"

Mom is 98 and moved to Arizona with him. Instead assess each first-degree relative's age and health status.

- "Is your mother living?"
  - "Yes."
- "How old is she?"
  - "98."
- "Does she have any medical conditions?"
  - "She has osteoporosis and a little Alzheimer's."

As a general screen, after repeating the process for all other first-degree relatives, inquire if any conditions are common in the family, including history of heart attack or stroke at age 50 or younger, and history of colon cancer or polyps.

When disease presentation suggests genetic properties, detailed family history should be expanded beyond first-degree relatives.

Medications

The last "M" in SMASH FM stands for medications. List the name, dose, and frequency of each medication the patient takes, both regularly and as needed. Include prescription medications, over-the-counter medications, herbals, and vitamins.

William, a 78-year-old, presents with knee pain.

- "Are you on any medications?"
  - "No. I don't like to take medications."
- "Did you take anything to try to make it better?"
  - "I took some ibuprofen. It didn't do a dang thing."
- "How much did you take?"
  - "Two of them little brown pills."
- "How often did you take them?"
  - "Just that once. Like I said, they didn't do much for it."
- "When did you take them?"
  - "A couple of days ago."

This frequency of dosing does not represent a therapeutic failure, but rather a failure to treat at appropriate doses and does not exclude nonsteroidal anti-inflammatory drugs as a treatment option.

Utilization of these two mnemonics will help assure thoroughness and consistency in the gathering of the medical histories.

References

1. World Health Organization. WHO Guidelines on Hand Hygiene in Health Care: A Summary. http://whqlibdoc.who.int/hq/2009/WHO_IER_PSP_2009.07_eng.pdf. Published 2009. Accessed January 7, 2012.

CHAPTER 4

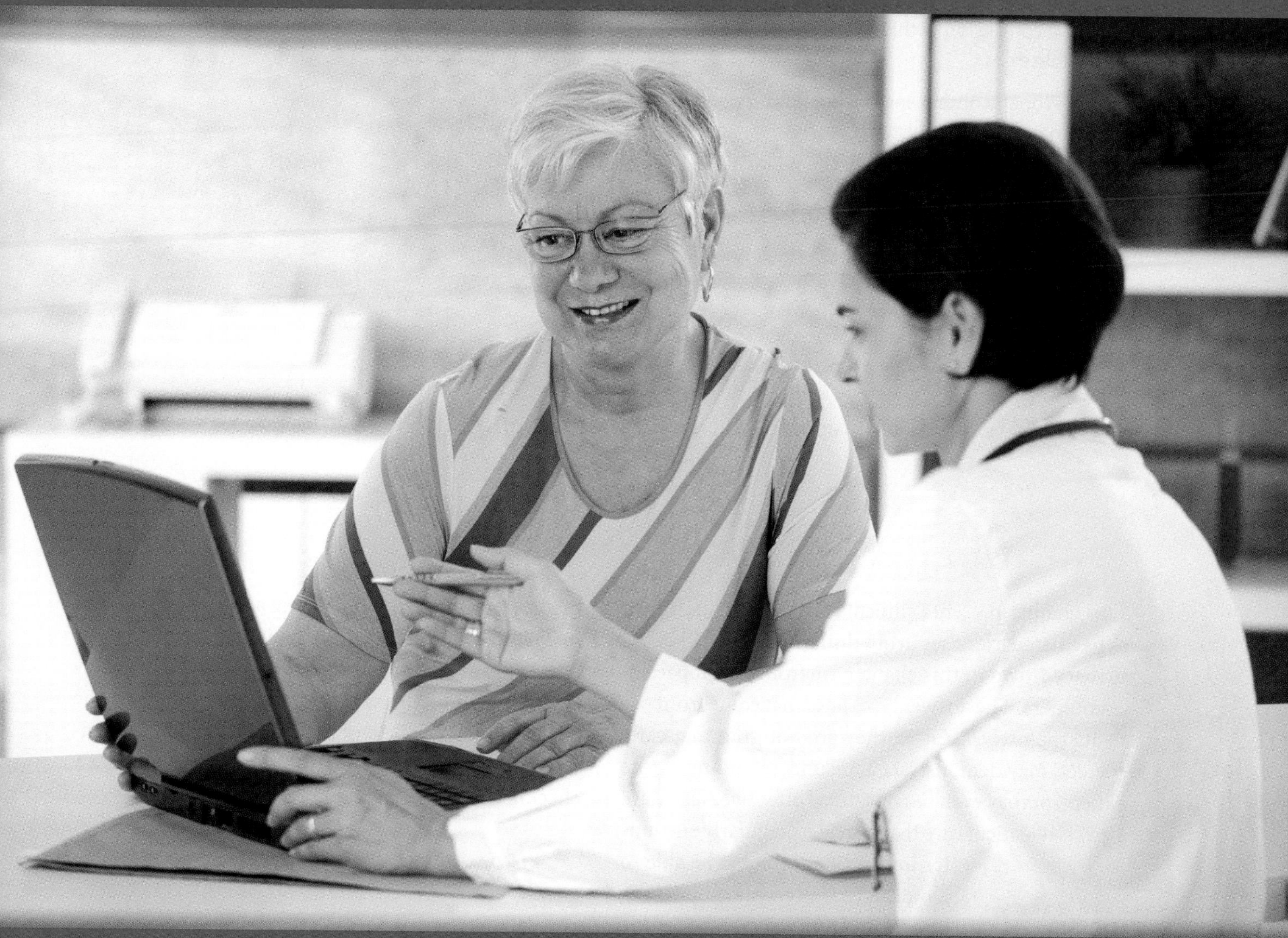

© StockLite/ShutterStock, Inc.

The History Flows

OBJECTIVES

At the conclusion of this chapter, the student will be able to

1. Properly obtain and document complete patient clinical histories
2. Recognize and tailor interviewing techniques for difficult patients
3. Incorporate humanistic qualities in the patient interview
4. Begin to relate signs and symptoms to differential diagnoses
5. Produce a structurally correct SOAP note encounter based on a patient encounter

KEY TERMS

History flow
Differential diagnosis
SOAP note

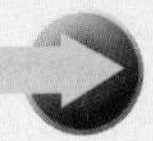
Where this icon appears, visit **go.jblearning.com/HPECWS** to view the video.

This chapter presents clinical cases that are designed as partnered exercises in obtaining histories. All of the **history flows** in this chapter are from actual patient encounters. The answers are those that came from patients themselves. Often they are not grammatically correct, may demonstrate a misunderstanding by the patient, or may even be considered offensive. These are aspects of patient care that providers regularly encounter in practice and must be able to handle efficiently while preserving respect and professionalism for the patient.

History flow: clinical case scenarios designed as partnered exercises where "providers" presented with patient demographics, vital signs, and a chief complaint attempt to obtain a complete medical history from the "patient"

Differential diagnosis: a list of possible etiologies (diagnoses) for patient complaints or concerns that demonstrates fluidity as the most likely diagnosis changes throughout the patient encounter based on questions asked and examination performed

The best way to achieve competence in taking patient histories is to practice them over and over again. If used in conjunction with a formal history and physical examination class, peer partners should be assigned and rotated so that each experience is enhanced by the difference in personalities. If you are practicing these flows outside the classroom, enlist your family members, friends, or study partners to act as the patient for each case. The patient dialogue requires no medical training, though having a flair for acting can make the cases that much more interesting.

At the beginning of your medical career, it is likely that you will focus on trying not to miss any of the questions that you believe need to be asked. The downfall of this is that, early on, the approach is more of a checklist:

- Provider thought: O is Onset.
- Provider: "When did this start?"
- Patient: "About a week ago"
- Provider thought: Yes, I got that point.

Be cognizant of this tendency and pause with each question to really listen to the answer and not just think about the next question. With continued experience, you will become less reliant on the mnemonic and will begin to *think* instead of remember.

After achieving competence in identifying the components of the medical history, your major goal is to develop a **differential diagnosis**, the list of possible etiologies for the patient's complaints arranged in an order with the most likely diagnosis presented first. As you become adept at taking histories, you will begin to formulate the diagnoses even before seeing the patient.

Standing outside the examination room you hear the patient sneeze. Your differential diagnosis begins to form immediately: upper respiratory tract infection, environmental allergies. You open the chart and see that your patient is a 32-year-old female who was last seen for a lesion on her back six months earlier. Perhaps she is just here for a follow-up and the sneeze was incidental. Her problem list shows that she is a smoker. Hopefully she is ready to take you up on the offer to help her with smoking cessation. Looking at her medication list you see that her only medication is birth control pills. She could be presenting for her yearly exam and medication refill. Finally you read the chief complaint as documented by the medical assistant: "Cough × 1 week." The differential morphs once more, adding bronchitis to your list, and yet you haven't seen the patient. What if she has chest pain and shortness of breath? Could she be having a pulmonary embolism? Her risk is increased because she is a smoker and on birth control pills.

This example demonstrates the constantly fluctuating possibilities of diagnoses and with experience occurs spontaneously and nearly subconsciously over a span of only a few seconds. When you start the interview your questions will either rule in or rule out each possible diagnosis. No shortness of breath or chest pain? She's likely not having a pulmonary embolism. She admits to a runny nose; itchy, watery eyes; and a tickle in the throat. Allergic rhinitis moves up the list.

Flow Orientation

For these cases each partner is assigned to a role as either the provider or the patient. Mindset is important for each role. The participants should avoid going out of the role. For example, the provider should never say, "If you were a real patient, I would . . . "

After the case is chosen, the provider should review the patient data sheet to note the office setting, patient's name, demographics, chief complaint, and vital signs. While this is occurring, the patient should read the answers to the historical questions in order to become familiar with the answers. The patient, of course, would not be expected to remember all of the answers but will at least have a general idea of the storyline and where to look for the answer, allowing for a smoother, more natural presentation. With practice, the repetitive nature of the location of answers will become second nature.

There are many more questions that could have been asked for each case but an attempt has been made to limit them to those of highest yield. If a question is asked that does not have an answer, the patient should default to negative answers or provide a simple answer that will have little effect on the outcome of the case, avoiding "I don't know." This is most common for the symptoms associated. For example, if the patient is asked if they have any wheezing, but the answer is not in the flow, they should answer, "No."

When the patient indicates that he/she is ready, the provider begins the case with an introduction that includes the patient's name, title, role, and an open-ended introductory question:

"Hello, Mrs. Humphry, I'm Student Doctor Stuart Dent. I'm with Dr. Thomas. If it's all right with you, I'll be taking your history and performing a short exam and then we'll have Dr. Thomas come in. How can I help you today?"

This clearly provides the patient with your name and level of education. The patient is aware of your role and this reassures the patient that, as a student, you will not be making management decisions on your own but will be discussing the patient with an advanced provider. The open-ended question that follows allows the patient to begin his/her story with the chief complaint. The provider is now ready to elicit the HPI and all of its CODIER SMASH FM components.

As you first begin taking histories, you will be learning simply how to take a history and not the intricacies of medicine. Thus, your "symptoms associated" category is likely to be short. Your task will be to develop a logical sequence to your interviews. Concentrate on the time frame: What symptom developed first, had it ever occurred before, and how has it changed? Never let a question be answered incompletely.

- Provider: "Describe the pain."
- Patient: "It just hurts."

This does not answer the question. You are no further ahead in finding the cause of the pain than you were before you asked the question.

As your history-taking skills and the depth of your medical knowledge increase, you will be able to intricately weave the components of the HPI together. When a 23-year-old woman presents with right knee pain, undoubtedly you will not take a sexual history. Why would you? Later, however, you will recognize that knee pain in a sexually active female may be monoarthropathy caused by gonorrhea.

When practicing with a peer partner, do one case as the provider and then switch roles and do another case as the patient. There is no "right" order to the questions, only one question leading to the next.

Timing

When first starting these flows you should not strictly limit your time. As you advance, your skills, begin to limit each history-taking encounter to 7 minutes. This mimics a true patient encounter, which typically is a 15-minute appointment. You have 15 minutes to take the patient's history, perform the problem-specific exam, and complete an assessment and plan while educating your patient and involving the patient in his/her own treatment—a seemingly daunting task.

Flow Summary

1. Pick a history flow to perform.
2. The provider reviews the patient data sheet.
3. The patient reviews the answers and indicates when ready to begin.
4. The provider:
   a. knocks
   b. enters the room
   c. addresses patient by name
   d. introduces self by name and title
   e. explains the role he/she will be playing
   f. washes his/her hands before shaking hands with the patient
   g. asks the first open-ended question
5. As the provider asks a question
   a. the patient provides the answer
   b. the patient checks the question off on the history flow
6. When the provider has no further questions, the provider
   a. thanks the patient
   b. asks if the patient has any questions
7. Review the case with the patient to determine areas that were missed.
8. The provider should now document the case with a SOAP note.

Documentation: The SOAP Note

The first case is followed by sample SOAP notes. Following completion of each flow, the case should be

Subjective (S):

Date:
Time:
Chief complaint:
HPI (CODIERS): Demographics followed by CODIERS in paragraph form
SMASH FM (bulleted format)

- Social Hx (FED TACOS)
  - Food (diet)
  - Exercise
  - Drugs
  - Tobacco
  - Alcohol
  - Caffeine
  - Occupation
  - Sexual history
- Medical Hx
- Allergies
- Surgical Hx
- Hospitalizations
- Family Hx
- Medications

Objective (O): Not completed for history flow

Assessment (A): Differential diagnosis in order of likelihood

1) Primary diagnoses
2) Rule out (r/o) diagnoses
3) Doubtful diagnoses

Plan (P): (MOTHRR)

1) Medications
2) OMM
3) Testing
4) Holistic/Humanistic
5) Referral
6) Return plan

Legible signature

FIGURE 4-1 SOAP note format.

documented in the standard **SOAP note** format. For the history flows, no objective section of physical findings will be included. Remember that each SOAP note starts with the date and time of encounter. The Subjective section of SOAP, "S," summarizes the medical history. Start this section with the Chief Complaint (CC) followed by CODIERS, which represents the history of present illness (HPI), in paragraph format. The time frame should be developed using a logical flow. Pertinent positives and negatives of the symptoms associated should be grouped, remembering that negatives are equally important to demonstrate diagnoses that were considered but ruled out. SMASH FM can then be presented in bulleted format for ease of reading. If one question should lead to another, the follow-up question will be inset (see **BOX 4-1**).

When you are first beginning to take patient histories, you may choose to ask every question in the mnemonic, such as shown in Case 1, to gain experience. However, with increasing medical knowledge, only appropriate questions should be asked.

SOAP note: standardized documentation format for patient encounters consisting of four sections: subjective, objective, assessment, and plan

Just as in clinical practice, not every case has a pure diagnosis but rather a differential. Following each flow, the main historical clues are discussed. The flows progressively become more clinically advanced as you progress through the chapter (see **FIGURES 4-1** to **4-4**).

BOX 4-1 Follow-up Questioning

Provider's Question	Patient's Answer
"Do you smoke?"	"Yes."
"How much a day?"	"About a pack and a half."

Subjective (S):

Objective (O):

Assessment (A):

Plan (P):

FIGURE 4-2 SOAP note template.

SAMPLE CASE

Mark Onyer
37-year-old male
CC: Tingling in the right hand

Vital signs

Blood pressure: 122/68

Respirations: 16 per minute

Pulse: 72 bpm

Temperature: 98.6 degrees F

Weight: 175 lbs

Height: 6′1″

Student writes:

C

O

D

I

E

R

S

S – F E D T A C O S

M

A

S

H

F

M

FIGURE 4-3 Sample patient data sheet.

CASE 1

Clinical Setting: Family Practice Office
Maria Gonzales—16-year-old female
CC: Ear pain

Vital Signs

Blood pressure: 112/58

Respirations: 12 per minute

Pulse: 70 bpm

Temperature: 99.9 degrees F

Weight: 115 lbs

Height: 5′6″

CASE 1	
Maria Gonzales **16-year-old female** **CC: Ear pain**	
___ Addresses patient by name	
___ Introduces self and explains role	
___ Properly washes hands before touching the patient	
___ How can I help you today?	My ear hurts.
Chronology/Onset	
___ **When** did it start?	About 3 days ago.
___ Did you ever have this **before**?	Yes.
___ **When** was that?	It seems like every winter.
___ **How** were you treated?	They gave me an antibiotic.
___ Has it **changed** at all?	It was worse but there was a "pop" and then it wasn't so bad.
Description/Duration	
___ Which **ear** is it?	The right one.
___ Can you **describe** the pain?	It's an ache.
Intensity	
___ How bad is it on a **scale** from 1 to 10?	I'd say a 5.
Exacerbation	
___ What makes it **worse**?	Nothing really.
Remission	
___ What makes it **better**?	Antihistamines seem to help a little.
___ Which one did you take?	Just a Benadryl once yesterday.
___ How many milligrams?	Twenty-five.

Symptoms associated	
___ **Drainage**?	Yes, there is.
___ What **color is it**?	It's yellow or green and smells funny.
___ **Stuffy/runny nose**?	Yes.
___ What **color** is it?	It's just clear.
___ **Fever or chills**?	No.
___ **Sore throat**?	No.
___ **Hearing loss** or **dizziness**?	No.
___ **Toothache**?	No.
SMASH FM	
Social History (FED TACOS)	
___ Could you describe your **diet**?	My dad cooks most of the meals.
___ Do you **exercise**?	I play soccer and swim.
___ Do you drink **caffeine**?	Not too much. I don't like pop.
___ Have you ever used **tobacco**?	I kind of smoke a little bit.
___ **How much a day**?	One or two cigarettes.
___ **How long**?	Just since school started this year.
___ Do you drink **alcohol**?	No.
___ Do you use any **drugs**?	No.
___ Do you **work**?	I'm a lifeguard.
___ When was the **FDLNMP**?	About a week ago.
___ Do you have any **medical** conditions?	No.
___ Do you have any **allergies**?	No.
___ Any prior **surgeries**?	I had tubes in my ears when I was younger.
___ Any prior **hospitalizations**?	No.

___ Anyone in the **family** with the same?	No.
___ Are you on any other **medications**?	No.

Case 1 Review

In this case, we have a 16-year-old female with ear pain, and although middle ear infections–otitis media—are more commonly found in younger children, any age group can develop them, especially if they have a prior history of the same condition. It is also an age where adolescents frequently go swimming or use hot tubs, which leads one to consider an external ear infection, otitis externa. In this case the patient swims and is a lifeguard.

These diagnoses are from the chief complaint only. She does have a prior history of ear pain that occurs mostly in the winter, which lessens the likelihood of an external ear infection and increases the likelihood of a middle ear infection because this is more common in the winter season. The key to diagnosis is the description by the patient of the sudden release of pain, likely the tympanic membrane rupturing, which correlates with the discharge from the ear that seems to be bacterial from the color and odor characteristics.

Questions to determine the other symptoms associated are in regard to what organs are likely to be affected also; these would include the nose and throat as well as fever and chills as signs of infection. SMASH FM adds little to our diagnosis except that the patient may be more prone to infection as she is a smoker. What should draw your attention is why she smokes only one to two cigarettes a day. With further questioning you may have discovered that she rides to school with friends who smoke and who give her one on the way home. This would be a good time for intervention before it becomes a habit.

12/29/12 15:35
S:
CC: Ear pain × 3 days
16 y/o Hispanic female presents with right ear pain × 3 days. She describes the pain as an ache, which had been of greater intensity but is now at a level of 5/10 following a sudden release of pressure. Nothing has made the pain worse, and antihistamines have helped somewhat. She has had similar pain in the past, occuring mostly in the winter months. She admits to a yellow or green malodorous drainage from the right ear and nasal congestion with clear exudate. She denies fever, chills, or sore throat.

- **Social Hx (FED TACOS)**

Food (diet) – Dad cooks	Alcohol – denies
Exercise – plays soccer and swims	Caffeine – denies
Drugs – denies	Occupation – Student and lifeguard
Tobacco – 1 to 2 cigs/day from friends	Sexual history – FDLMP 1 week ago

- **Medical Hx** – denies
- **Allergies** – none
- **Surgical Hx** – history of e-tubes
- **Hospitalizations** – none
- **Family Hx** – non-contributory
- **Medications** – none

O (Objective):	The physical exam (PE) would follow here.
A (Assessment):	Right acute otitis media
P (Plan):	Right otitis media: amoxicillin 250 mg qid × 10 days Increase fluids. Return to school in 2 days. Return to clinic in 2 weeks for recheck. Call earlier with no improvement, increase in pain, fever, or discharge. Stuart Dent, OMSI

FIGURE 4-4 Sample SOAP note.

Lastly, all women should be asked when the first day of last normal menstrual period (FDLNMP) occurred, as you are likely going to be giving this patient an antibiotic and would not want to harm a fetus.

Note: Although both FDLMP (first day of last menstrual period) and "LMP" (last menstrual period) are often used as acronyms, there is a recent advancement toward a more precise delineation of the exact date. This is why we use the longer but more categorical "FDLNMP" acronym has been used here.

From the history alone our differential diagnosis would have right acute otitis media as the primary diagnosis. Less likely diagnoses may include right otitis externa and upper respiratory tract infection (URI). Once examination is added to the encounters, the diagnosis would be limited by physical findings. For the history flows you should expand the differential diagnosis to include several possibilities, listing them in order of likelihood.

Possible differential diagnosis for the note above:

1. Right acute otitis media
2. Right otitis externa
3. Upper respiratory tract infection

CASE 2

Clinical Setting: Urgent Care Center
Ritchey Kinn—12-year-old male
CC: Rash

Vital Signs

Blood pressure: 102/52

Respirations: 16 per minute

Pulse: 78 bpm

Temperature: 98.2 degrees F

Weight: 90 lbs

Height: 4′8″

CASE 2	
Ritchey Kinn **12-year-old male** **CC: Rash** **Presents with his mother**	
___ Addresses patient by name	
___ Introduces self and explains role	
___ Properly washes hands prior to touching patient	
___ How can I help you today?	I have a rash.
Chronology/Onset	
___ **When** did you first notice it?	A couple of days ago.
___ Ever **had it before**?	I think, maybe last summer.
___ How did you treat it?	It just went away.
___ Has it **changed** in appearance?	I think it's spreading.
Description/Duration	
___ **Where** is it (**location**)?	All over.
___ Where did you **get it first**?	It started on my legs.
___ Then where did it go?	My arms and stomach.
Exacerbation	
___ Does anything make it **worse**?	The heat makes it itch more.
Remission	
___ Does anything make it **better**?	A cool bath helped a little.
Symptoms associated	
___ **Itch**?	Like crazy.
___ **Sore throat**?	No.
___ **Fever**?	No.

___ **Shortness of breath**	No.
SMASH FM	
Social History (FED TACOS)	
___ Anything new in your **diet**?	No.
___ Did you have any **exposures** to anything?	I don't know.
___ Were you out in the **woods or weeds** at all?	Probably.
___ Any **new** laundry **detergents/deodorants**?	**Mom:** No.
___ Have you been **bitten by anything**?	I don't think so.
___ Do you have any **medical** conditions?	**Mom:** He has ADD.
___ Do you have any **allergies**?	No.
___ Any prior **surgeries**?	No.
___ Any prior **hospitalizations**?	No.
___ Any **family or contacts** with a rash?	No.
___ Are you on any **medications**?	**Mom:** He just started taking Ritalin.
___ **When**?	**Mom:** Just this week.
___ Was he ever **on it before**?	**Mom:** No.
___ What is the dose?	**Mom:** One pill a day.
___ Do you know how many milligrams?	**Mom:** No.

Case 2 Review

Many times you will be attempting to interview a patient, but others in the room will be answering the questions. When evaluating an adolescent, attempt to direct questions to and keep as much eye contact with the patient as possible, although parents often like to answer for them. If the patient is unable to provide the answer, you can then look to the parent for the answer. This approach helps to develop trust and the patient-provider relationship as the adolescent approaches adulthood.

This seems like a fairly straightforward case. The patient developed a rash over the last several days. Location is important. Asking the patient where it started and the pattern of spread can help to differentiate the cause of the rash. For example, the rash associated with Rocky Mountain spotted fever (RMSF) usually starts on the wrists and ankles, and then spreads to the extremities and onto the trunk. The palms and soles are affected in RMSF but spared in other diseases.

The characteristic of pruritus suggests a possible contact dermatitis, prompting questioning of new detergents, outdoor activities, or other exposures. The fact that he had it last summer increases the suspicion of Rhus dermatitis (poison ivy or poison oak), but we would have been even more suspicious if his social history revealed that he had been camping in the last week. Sore throat is investigated in conjunction with viral syndrome.

This case demonstrates the importance of completeness. In a 12-year old, you may discount his past medical history, but finding that he has ADD and was just started on a new medication allows you to add "drug reaction" to the differential diagnosis. It was likely that shortness of breath would not have been asked as a symptom associated until the possibility of a drug or allergic reaction was entertained.

This is also a good case to demonstrate the need to follow up questions with positive answers. It is not enough to find out that the patient just started a new medication. You should also ask when it was started, if he had ever been on the same or similar medications in the past, what dose he is taking, and how often he is taking it.

Possible differential diagnosis:

1. Drug reaction
2. Rule out contact dermatitis
3. Doubt viral exanthema

CASE 3

Clinical Setting: Primary Care Office
Iris McCarty—23-year-old female
CC: Red eye

Vital Signs

Blood pressure: 108/54

Respirations: 16 per minute

Pulse: 68 bpm

Temperature: 99.2 degrees F

Weight: 128 lbs

Height: 5′5″

CASE 3	
Iris McCarty **23-year-old female** **CC: Red eye**	
___ Addresses patient by name	
___ Introduces self and explains role	
___ Properly washes hands prior to touching patient	
___ What brings you in today?	My eye is red.
Chronology/Onset	
___ **When** did it start?	Yesterday.
___ What were you **doing**?	I just noticed it in the bathroom mirror.
___ Have you ever had this **before**?	No.
___ Has it **changed** at all?	It's redder today.
Description/Duration	
___ Which **eye** is it?	My left one.
Exacerbation	
___ Does anything make it **worse**?	No.
Remission	
___ Does anything make it **better**?	A warm washcloth helps a little.
Symptoms associated	
___ **Pain**?	No.
___ **Photophobia**?	No.
___ **Visual changes**?	It's a little blurry until I get the goop out.
___ **Drainage/matting**?	Yes, there is.
___ What **color is it**?	It's crusty and a bit yellow.
___ **Itch**?	Yes, it does.

___ **Runny nose**?	No.
___ **Sore throat**?	No.
___ **Trauma/get anything in the eye**?	No.
___ Do you wear **contact lenses**?	No.
SMASH FM	
Social History (FED TACOS)	
___ Have you ever used **tobacco**?	Yes, I smoke.
___ **How much a day**?	Half a pack a day.
___ **How long**?	About 5 years.
___ Do you drink **alcohol**?	No
___ Do you use any **drugs**?	No
___ What is your **occupation**?	I work at a day-care center.
___ When was the **FDLNMP**?	About two weeks ago.
___ Do you have any **medical** conditions?	Just some seasonal allergies.
___ Do you have any other **allergies**?	No.
___ Any prior **surgeries**?	No.
___ Any prior **hospitalizations**?	No.
___ **Contact with other** with the same?	Some of the kids at work have it too.
___ Are you on any **medications**?	No.

Case 3 Review

When someone presents with a red eye, the diagnoses of viral and bacterial conjunctivitis immediately come to mind. The method of discovery by the patient, simply looking into the mirror and seeing that her eye was red, lessens the likelihood of trauma.

One of the commonly missed questions in this flow is, "Which eye?" The reason is that clinically, when a patient presents with a complaint of a red eye, it is quite easy for us to identify which eye by looking at the patient. The red eye jumps out at us. At first this seems a minor point to include with this case, but then wrong-site surgery comes to mind as a leading reason of medical errors. "Tragic" does not fully describe the young basketball player who was diagnosed with bone cancer and awoke from the surgery to find that the surgeon had removed the wrong leg. It is better practice to clarify which side the complaint is on now, ingraining the habit in your subconsciousness.

Matting and drainage correlate with conjunctivitis. The lack of photophobia and pain help to rule out acute glaucoma or iritis. This case demonstrates another incomplete answer. When you get a positive answer for drainage you must follow up with additional questioning. A good rule to follow is that when anything is noted to come out of the body you should describe what it looks and smells like.

In this case ask about the color of the drainage. Viral conjunctivitis may be clear and stringy, whereas bacterial conjunctivitis is often purulent. Quantifying the amount can also help in diagnosis. A smaller quantity such as this that dries and crusts in the morning is again common with conjunctivitis. If the patient described copious amounts of purulent drainage, bacterial conjunctivitis with gonorrhea as a possible diagnosis would lead the provider to ask a more detailed sexual history.

Important in patients who present with eye complaints is documenting the level of vision before your treatment is begun. Once we study the physical exam component, you will be able to assess visual acuity, but documenting the patient's report of diminished acuity or visual changes prior to treatment also clarifies that the loss was not a result of delayed or improper therapy.

In the holistic approach to patients, we ask every patient about tobacco use. The same could be argued for alcohol and drug use; however, many providers would feel this is inappropriate and would be uncomfortable doing so as it is not pertinent to the case at hand.

One thought is that these questions should be asked of every adolescent and young adult but reserved as case-appropriate for older adult populations. With this line of thought, the provider would likely not ask about alcohol and drug use. Others may argue that with a positive history of tobacco use the risk of use for these other substances warrants questioning. Finding that the patient smokes, you can address the issue during the current visit even though it was not a presenting concern.

Trauma is also a concern and should be directly asked early on. Consideration of trauma also relates to the social history and a review of occupation. If the patient is a metal worker, despite no known history of trauma, a foreign body in the eye should be considered. Other exposures should be considered as well. After discovering that this patient works in a day-care setting where conjunctivitis is notorious, it is important to ask if she has had any contact with others who have the same complaint or symptoms. This thought process also holds true for other infectious exposures. This is also where we ask about other members of the family who may be experiencing the same symptoms, recent visits to hospitals or nursing homes, coworkers with symptoms, and the like.

Possible differential diagnosis:

1. Bacterial conjunctivitis
2. Viral conjunctivitis
3. Allergic conjunctivitis

CASE 4

Clinical Setting: Primary Care Office
Michele Shore—26-year-old female
CC: Back pain

Vital Signs

Blood pressure: 128/74

Respirations: 16 per minute

Pulse: 88 bpm

Temperature: 98.4 degrees F

Weight: 152 lbs

Height: 5′4″

CASE 4

Michele Shore
26-year-old female
CC: Back pain

___ Addresses patient by name	
___ Introduces self and explains role	
___ Properly washes hands prior to touching patient	
___ What brings you in today?	I hurt my back.
Chronology/Onset	
___ **When** did you hurt it?	Last night at midnight.
___ What were you **doing** at the time?	Lifting a stack of anatomy textbooks.
___ Did you ever have this **before**?	No.
___ How has it **changed**?	It hasn't really.
Description/Duration	
___ **Describe** the pain.	It's a burning kind of pain.
___ **Where** is it?	Right here (points to right lumbar area).
___ Does it **radiate**?	A little into my right buttock.
___ Is it continuous or does it come and go?	It's continuous.
Intensity	
___ On a **scale** from 1 to 10, how would it rate?	A 5.
Exacerbation	
___ Does anything make it **worse**?	Yes, when I bend over or twist.
Remission	
___ What makes it **better**?	Ibuprofen made it a little better.
___ How much did you take?	A couple of tablets.
___ How often?	Twice, about 6 hours apart.

Symptoms associated	
___ **Numbness, tingling**?	No.
___ **Weakness**?	No.
___ Changes to **bowel or bladder** function?	No.
SMASH FM	
Social History (FED TACOS)	
___ Could you describe your **diet**?	It's OK. I eat a lot of pasta. It's easy to make.
___ Do you **exercise**?	Not regularly. I'm studying all the time.
___ What do you study?	I'm in med school.
___ Do you drink **caffeine**?	4 or 5 Cokes a day. It helps me stay awake.
___ Diet or regular?	Regular.
___ Have you ever used **tobacco**?	No.
___ Do you drink **alcohol**?	Not even a drink a month.
___ Do you use any **drugs**?	No.
___ Do you **work**?	I don't have time to work with my studies.
___ When was the **FDLNMP**?	About a week ago.
___ Do you have any **medical** conditions?	No.
___ Do you have any **allergies**?	Bee stings.
___ What reaction do you have?	I can't breathe.
___ Do you carry an EpiPen?	Yes.
___ Any prior **surgeries**?	I had my tonsils taken out when I was a kid.
___ Any prior **hospitalizations**?	Just for my tonsils.
___ Medical conditions in the **family**?	Nothing in particular.
___ Are you on any other **medications**?	I'm on the pill.

Case 4 Review

The answer to the introductory question, "What brings you in today," is answered by "I hurt my back," and not "My back hurts." From the outset, trauma is implied and immediately leads the provider in this direction.

This case demonstrates the importance of defining the time frame. When a patient tells you that a symptom started at a precise time, there must be reason that he/she knows it with such precision, again suggesting that something occurred exactly then. Knowing what a patient is doing when pain occurs also alters the differential diagnosis. This patient bends over and rotates simultaneously, a position that weakens the supporting ligaments of the spinal column and risks intervertebral disc bulge or herniation.

Past history of similar pain is extremely important. In this case, no prior history of trauma makes a less severe diagnosis like muscle strain or somatic dysfunction much more likely. If, however, the patient had a history of a motor vehicle accident with lumbar vertebral fracture, our differential would change, perhaps dramatically. How the pain changed since it first started finishes the chronology. Abdominal pain that starts at the umbilicus and moves into the right lower quadrant is characteristic of appendicitis; hence developing the pattern of pain can be the key to an accurate diagnosis. It is also important to identify other areas of pain and if the pain radiates anywhere. Pain from gallstones classically radiates into the right shoulder blade, pancreatitis to the area between the scapulae. In this case, the patient's back pain radiates into the buttock, which is a sign of L4 radiculopathy or irritation of the nerve.

When determining intensity, a scale must be provided for the patient, such as from 0 to 10, with 10 being the worst possible pain. This case also provides examples of asking the next logical question when it first presents itself and not strictly following the mnemonic. When asked if she exercises, she explains that she's studying all the time. The next logical question is "What are you studying?" which partially answers the question of occupation.

Why was it important to ask what type of Coke she drinks? Look at the patient data sheet again for the clue. Holistically we have to look at the whole patient. She is 26 years old, has new onset back pain, doesn't eat well or exercise, weighs 152 lbs, and is 5'4". This represents an opportunity for preventative medicine with an emphasis on a healthy lifestyle despite the demands of her studies.

Finally, you also identify that she has anaphylactic reactions to bee stings. She is likely living in the area to go to school. Though she is seeing you for her back pain, you've identified the risk she is under should a bee sting occur, meaning that you must confirm that she has an unexpired EpiPen at the ready—taking care of the whole patient and not just the complaint.

Possible differential diagnosis:

1. Lumbar somatic dysfunction
2. Intervertebral disc bulge
3. Doubt intervertebral disc herniation
4. Bee sting allergy

CASE 5

Clinical Setting: Primary Care Office
Scratch E. Trote—32-year-old male
CC: Sore throat

Vital Signs

Blood pressure: 114/64

Respirations: 16 per minute

Pulse: 68 bpm

Temperature: 98.5 degrees F

Weight: 190 lbs

Height: 6′1″

CASE 5	
Scratch E. Trote **32-year-old male** **CC: Sore throat**	
____ Addresses patient by name	
____ Introduces self and explains role	
____ Properly washes hands prior to touching patient	
____ How can I help you today?	I've got a sore throat.
Chronology/Onset	
____ **When** did it start?	About 2 or 3 days ago.
____ Did you ever have this **before**?	No.
____ Has it **changed**?	It's just getting worse and worse.
Description/Duration	
____ **Describe** how if feels.	It's really scratchy and sore.
____ Is it **continuous** or does it **come and go**?	It's continuous.
Intensity	
____ On a scale from 1 to 10, how bad is it?	An 8 or 9.
Exacerbation	
____ Anything make it **worse**?	Swallowing makes it really bad, especially in the morning.
Remission	
____ Anything make it **better**?	Throat spray helps a little.
Symptoms associated	
____ **Runny nose**?	No.
____ **Sinus pressure**?	No.
____ **Fever or chills**?	I have felt warm.

____ **Cough**?	Not really.
____ What do you mean by "Not really"?	Well, I cough a little in the morning but it goes right away.
____ Do you feel **really tired/fatigued**?	Yeah. The throat keeps me up at night.
____ **Wheezing**?	No.
____ **Ear pain**?	No.
____ **Heartburn**?	No.
SMASH FM	
Social History (FED TACOS)	
____ Could you describe your **diet**?	I lift, so I eat a lot of protein.
____ How often do you **exercise**?	I lift for an hour or so every day.
____ Do you drink **caffeine**?	Maybe an energy drink once a week.
____ Have you ever used **tobacco**?	No.
____ Do you **drink alcohol**?	Yes.
____ **How much** a day?	Not every day, maybe 2–3 a week.
____ **How many** at a sitting?	Just one or two.
____ Do you use any **drugs**?	No.
____ What is your **occupation**?	I'm a physical therapist.
____ Do you have any **medical** conditions?	I have reflux.
____ Do you have any **allergies**?	No.
____ Any prior **surgeries**?	No.
____ Any prior **hospitalizations**?	No.
____ Medical conditions in the **family**?	Just some high blood pressure.
____ **Contact with others** with the same?	I think my girlfriend had it last week.
____ Are you on any other **medications**?	I take ranitidine.
____ How many milligrams?	150.

___ How many times a day?	Twice.
___ Does it control your symptoms?	I don't have heartburn anymore.

Case 5 Review

The patient has a sore throat that has progressed in severity over the last two to three days. Our first real clues come into play when the patient identifies swallowing as making it worse but especially in the morning. This should draw the thought process along the lines of what occurs in the morning that could make a sore throat worse. Use anatomy to explore other possible associated symptoms that revolve around the upper respiratory tract, including the sinuses, ears, nose, and lungs. You might think of posterior nasal drainage and air breathing through the mouth due to nasal congestion with rhinosinusitis. Asking these questions in symptoms associated results in negative answers.

He has felt a little warm though he hadn't taken his temperature. After you press a little bit about "not really" having a cough, he does admit to one in the morning which he discounts as it goes away quickly. If you thought of a smoker's cough, you may have asked about tobacco use now.

A significant complaint of fatigue may clue you in to adding mononucleosis to your differential. He attributes his fatigue to the sore throat keeping him up at night, but could it be more than that? Thinking of EBV may prompt you to ask about contacts with similar symptoms, which seems at first to be the only appropriate contact or family history to explore. This would change, though, once the medical history of reflux is encountered, as reflux and Barrett's esophagus are at increased risk with family history.

Reflux can indeed cause sore throat as well as morning coughing and wheezing. Though he denied heartburn upon being asked about his medications we must ask if the other symptoms indicate poor control. Your exam will help you narrow down the diagnoses.

Possible differential diagnosis:

1. Pharyngitis
2. Rule out streptococcus
3. Rule out mononucleosis
4. Consider severe reflux esophagitis

CASE 6

Clinical Setting: Emergency Room
Abby Dominic—13-year-old female
CC: Abdominal pain

Vital Signs

Blood pressure: 114/64

Respirations: 24 per minute

Pulse: 118 bpm

Temperature: 102.5 degrees F

Weight: 98 lbs

Height: 5′2″

CASE 6	
Abby Dominic **13-year-old female** **CC: Abdominal pain** **Presents with her mother**	
____ Addresses patient by name	
____ Introduces self and explains role	
____ Properly washes hands prior to touching patient	
____ What's going on today?	My belly hurts.
Chronology/ Onset	
____ **When** did it **start**?	Yesterday afternoon.
____ What were you **doing** at the time?	Just watching TV.
____ Have you ever had this **before**?	No.
____ Have there been any **changes** in the pain?	Yes, it was up in the middle and now it's down lower.
____ Can you show me **where**?	Points to mid-abdomen then RLQ.
Description/Duration	
____ Can you **describe** the pain?	It's real sharp and burning.
____ Does it **radiate (go)** anywhere else?	No.
____ Is it **constant** or does it **come and go**?	Constant.
Intensity	
____ How bad is it, on a scale from **1 to 10**?	An 11.
Exacerbation	
____ Does anything make it **worse**?	Touching my belly or moving.
Remission	
____ Does anything make it **better**?	Mom gave me some Tylenol, but it didn't help.
____ How much did you take?	Two tablets.

Symptoms associated	
___ **Fever or chills**?	The nurse said it was 102.
___ **Nausea or vomiting**?	I feel like I could throw up.
___ **Diarrhea or constipation**	A little diarrhea this morning.
___ Any **blood or mucous**?	No.
___ **Burning with urination**?	No.
___ **Vaginal discharge or bleeding**?	No.
SMASH FM	
Social History (FED TACOS)	
___ Any changes to your **diet**?	I haven't felt like eating since yesterday.
___ How often do you **exercise/play sports**?	I don't really.
___ Have you ever used **tobacco?**	No.
___ Do you **drink alcohol**?	No.
___ Do you use any **drugs**?	No.
Sexual Hx	
___ Are you **sexually active**?	I don't think so. (Mom: You don't think so!?)
___ Do you know what sexually active means?	Not really.
___ When was the **FDLNMP**?	I don't know.
___ Have you had your first **period** yet?	Yes.
___ When was that?	When I was 12.
___ Did you have a period last month?	I think so.
___ Do you have any **medical** conditions?	No.
___ Do you have any **allergies**?	No.
___ Any prior **surgeries**?	No.
___ Any prior **hospitalizations**?	No.

___ Medical conditions in the **family**?	Mom: Her twin sister had the same thing last year.
___ What did they find?	Mom: She needed her appendix taken out.
___ **Contact with others** with the same?	No.
___ Are you on any other **medications**?	No.

Case 6 Review

In this flow we again have an adolescent patient who is quite adept at answering her own questions, though with the level of pain reported you might have needed to direct more questions to her mother if the patient hadn't been able to answer. You'll be surprised how many times a parent will try to tell you what the child's pain feels like.

The patient was watching television when the pain started, which lessens the concern for trauma. Chronology is very important in this flow, specifically in how the pain has changed. The classic presentation for appendicitis is onset of pain around the umbilicus with progression to the RLQ.

Although we offer a pain scale and explain its meaning, you will still find patients who respond with a number that is outside the scale. In this case if you could see the patient's guarding position and facial expression you would doubt very little that she really means 11 out of 10. Other patients who say it's a 15 with a smile on their face should be redirected. A good tool for clarification in these cases where you doubt sincerity is to define 10 out of 10 as pain that is so bad it would require hospitalization.

Sharp, burning, constant pain that is worse with movement or touching suggests possible peritoneal signs. You could further this line of questioning by asking about jarring motions making it worse, such as the car ride to the hospital.

The symptoms associated include some of the other classic signs of appendicitis: anorexia, fever, nausea, vomiting, and diarrhea. Thinking of other organ systems in the right lower quadrant such as the colon, we are also led to ask about diarrhea and constipation. With an affirmative answer for diarrhea, we question further to ask about blood or mucous: Could she have inflammatory bowel disease or infectious colitis?

We should also consider the female reproductive organs of the RLQ. Here we run into a small roadblock. With Mom in the room we were hesitant to ask about sexual activity but did so anyway. When the patient replies, "I don't think so," you're probably not surprised by her mother's response, but the provider must ask what circumstances would make her reply in such a way. It may just be her level of understanding, thinking perhaps that kissing boys is being sexually active; she may not want to answer in front of her mother; or she might just be unable to answer more questions, with the pain she is in. It may be hard to readdress her indecision as to whether she is sexually active, but by questioning her about her basic understanding, you put the mother's mind at ease at least a bit. In the acute pain setting, it may not be the appropriate time to ask her mother if she has had any discussions with her daughter, but knowing the answer may help you to measure the patient's level of understanding in other less urgent cases, and discussing what her mother or her school has taught her might open the door to developing trust and providing vital preventive education. Mom may either say, "No, we haven't discussed this. She is too young and we homeschool her." Or she may say, "Please, I didn't know how to bring this up, tell her everything!"

Another stumbling block is reached when asking her FDLNMP. Maybe she just truly doesn't keep track of it. Start at the beginning by asking about prior menses. If she hasn't had one, perhaps she has an imperforate hymen and is having her first menses now, which could result in the pain she is having. If she has been menstruating, try to narrow down the time frame to rule out pregnancy. No matter what she tells you, a pregnancy test is appropriate in any case.

Possible differential diagnosis:

1. Appendicitis
2. Rule out ectopic pregnancy
3. Doubt inflammatory bowel disease

CASE 7

Clinical Setting: Family Medicine Clinic
Melvin Noma—24-year-old male
CC: Mole

Vital Signs

Blood pressure: 110/62

Respirations: 14 per minute

Pulse: 68 bpm

Temperature: 99.4 degrees F

Weight: 168 lbs

Height: 6′

CASE 7	
Melvin Noma **24-year-old male** **CC: Mole**	
___ Addresses patient by name	
___ Introduces self and explains role	
___ Properly washes hands prior to touching patient	
___ What brings you in today?	I have this mole my girlfriend doesn't like the color of.
Chronology/Onset	
___ **When** did you first notice it?	Ever since I can remember.
___ Has it **changed** in appearance?	She said it's bigger and has changed colors.
___ What **color** is it?	Brown and black.
Description/Duration	
___ **Where** is it?	On my back.
Exacerbation	
___ Does anything **irritate it**?	No.
Symptoms associated	
___ Does it **itch**?	Maybe, a little.
___ **Bleed**?	No.
SMASH FM	
Social History (FED TACOS)	
___ How often do you **exercise/play sports**?	I run 5 miles a day.
___ Have you ever used **tobacco**?	No.
___ What is your **occupation**?	I work for the power company.
___ **Outdoors**?	Most of the time.
___ Have you had any **sunburns**?	Yes, until I tan up.

___ Have you **blistered**?	Yes.
___ Do you use **sunscreen**?	I forget most of the time.
___ Do you have any **medical** conditions?	No.
___ Do you have any **allergies**?	No.
___ Any prior **surgeries**?	I had another mole taken off.
___ **When**?	A couple of years ago.
___ What did it show?	They said it was dysplastic.
___ Any prior **hospitalizations**?	No.
___ Any **family history of skin cancer/moles**?	My dad had something taken off.
___ Did he require further treatment?	No.
___ Are you on any **medications**?	No.

Case 7 Review

Some patients will have very limited complaints. Avoid the tendency to skip the questions and just look at the mole immediately. Chronology reveals a mole that the patient believes he has had for his lifetime but about which his girlfriend is concerned. The patient is relating secondhand history, as the mole is on his back and not easily amenable to self-examination. You may have asked within chronology if he has had other moles in the past. If this was skipped due to the lifelong history, you would then have had another opportunity to discover other moles through the surgical history. Once the positive is found, follow up with what was done and found at the time. If the other mole had been a melanoma, his risk for another would increase.

The patient's exercise and occupational history suggest sun exposure. Follow through with the questions about factors that would put him at increased risk for skin cancer. Ask about sunburns and blistering, which again increase risk and will allow for preventive education when developing the treatment plan with the patient. Much of the other social history would not contribute to his current complaint. Begin to think about each question and consider whether it is appropriate to ask. Would asking about diet, caffeine, drug use, and sexual history add value to this case? If you can answer yes, then ask the questions.

Melanoma also has familial tendencies so that a family history of melanoma would heighten suspicion.

Possible differential diagnosis:

1. Nevus
2. Rule out melanoma
3. Rule out atypical nevus

CASE 8

Clinical Setting: Emergency Room
Rita Gonner—34-year-old female
CC: Knee pain

Vital Signs

Blood pressure: 130/82

Respirations: 20 per minute

Pulse: 92 bpm

Temperature: 101.5 degrees F

Weight: 128 lbs

Height: 5′4″

CASE 8	
Rita Gonner **34-year-old female** **CC: Knee pain**	
____ Addresses patient by name	
____ Introduces self and explains role	
____ Properly washes hands prior to touching patient	
____ What brings you in today?	I have pain in my knee.
Chronology/Onset	
____ **When** did it **start**?	About 3 days ago.
____ What were you **doing** when it started?	I just noticed it when I woke up.
____ Was there any history of **trauma**?	No.
____ Have you **had this before**?	No.
____ Has there been any **change in the pain**?	It's been getting worse.
Description/Duration	
____ **Describe** the pain.	It's a deep ache.
____ **Which knee** is it?	The right one.
____ **Where in the knee** is it?	(Points to right knee inferior patella.)
____ Does it **radiate (go)** anywhere?	Not really.
____ Is it **constant** or **does it come and go**?	It's constant.
Intensity	
____ How severe is it on a scale from **1 to 10**?	About a 7 or 8.
Exacerbation	
____ What makes it **worse**?	If I put any weight on my leg at all.
Remission	
____ Did you try anything to make it **better**?	A heating pad helped a little.

Symptoms associated	
___ **Redness**?	Yes.
___ **Swelling**?	Yes.
___ **Fever or chills**?	I think so.
___ **Pain with movement of the leg**?	Yes.
___ **Pain in the calf**?	No.
___ **Sore throat**?	No.
___ **Vaginal discharge**?	Yes, actually I do.
___ **Abdominal pain**?	No.
___ **Burning with urination**?	Just when it starts.
SMASH FM	
Social History (FED TACOS)	
___ Do you **exercise**?	I walk a lot.
___ Have you ever used **tobacco**?	Yes, I smoke.
___ **How much** a day?	One pack a day.
___ **How long** have you smoked?	I started when I was 16.
___ Do you **drink alcohol**?	Yes.
___ **How many** drinks a day?	Two or three.
___ Do you use any **drugs**?	No.
___ What is your **occupation**?	I'm a cashier.
___ Do you **stand** a lot?	All day.
___ Are you **sexually active**?	Yes.
___ **How many partners** in the last month?	2 or 3
___ Did any of them have any discharge?	Not that they said.
___ Have you ever had an STI?	Yes.

___ What infection was it?	Chlamydia.
___ When was that?	Last year.
___ **FDLNMP**?	Last week.
___ Do you have any **medical** conditions?	No.
___ Do you have any **allergies**?	No.
___ Any prior **surgeries**?	No.
___ Any prior **hospitalizations**?	No.
___ Medical conditions in the **family**?	Some sugar diabetes.
___ Are you on any **medications**?	No.

Case 8 Review

The patient presents with isolated right knee pain and no prior history of a similar complaint or injury. Patients who present with a known injury, such as the football player who has a knee injury, greatly limit the diagnostic possibilities to the anatomical damage that has occurred. In this case the patient awakened with the knee pain, so we can include injury even if the patient cannot remember any particular incident, but we cannot limit ourselves to it.

The pain is described as an ache of significant intensity aggravated by weight bearing. The area of pain must be questioned precisely. As we are only in the history-taking stage, we limit ourselves to questions, wherein an actual clinical setting we would have the benefit of laying our hands on the patient to discern if and where we elicit pain. Think anatomically around the site. Asking about calf pain briefly entertains the idea of a deep vein thrombosis but is found to be negative.

As we approach the symptoms associated, we can begin with basic musculoskeletal findings. She admits to redness and swelling. Some may argue incorrectly that you would not need to ask these questions, as when you examined the patient you would note these findings. This, however, fails to account for redness and swelling that were present but have since resolved, a very common finding with edema that progresses throughout the day but resolves as the patient is supine through the night.

Along the musculoskeletal lines, pain with movement should also be inquired about. You may have found yourself struggling to find other symptoms associated at this point. Careful examination of the patient data sheet provides a clue in the fever, to which the patient admits. What is fever a sign of? Most commonly the answer is infection, but what infection could cause knee pain in a young woman?

The bothersome part of the history is precisely the fact that she has had no injury. Anatomically, what else could be causing the pain? Her young age and short duration of complaint make osteoarthritis unlikely. Could she have rheumatoid arthritis? Along this line of thought is infectious arthritis. Gonorrhea could account for this presentation, and so monoarticular large joint pain in women of reproductive age must include this as a possible diagnosis. Evidence of concurrent infection elsewhere should be sought, hence the questions about sore throat, vaginal discharge, and abdominal pain, as would be found with pelvic inflammatory disease (PID).

With this line of thought our social history can focus on risk factors for STI. Begin with a general screen by asking the patient if she is sexually active. Since the answer is positive, you need to expand. Providers should refrain from being judgmental, as we do not and usually cannot understand the intricacies of what makes our patients who they are. Being nonjudgmental is the only way to truly ask sensitive questions that are not prejudiced.

Her number of partners, history of STI, and tobacco and alcohol use increase the risk of STI.

Possible differential diagnosis:

1. Septic arthritis
2. Rule out gonorrhea arthritis
3. Doubt rheumatoid arthritis

CASE 9

Clinical Setting: Family Medicine Clinic
Diana Betty—24-year-old female
CC: Urinary tract infection

Vital Signs

Blood pressure: 134/84

Respirations: 14 per minute

Pulse: 60 bpm

Temperature: 98.5 degrees F

Weight: 178 lbs

Height: 5′4″

CASE 9

Diana Betty
24-year-old female
CC: Urinary tract infection (UTI)

___ Addresses patient by name	
___ Introduces self and explains role	
___ Properly washes hands prior to touching patient	
___ What brings you in today?	I have a urinary tract infection.
Chronology	
___ Have you had urinary tract infections before?	Yes.
___ When was the last one?	A couple of years ago.
___ What did they do for you then?	They gave me an antibiotic and a yeast infection.
Onset	
___ **When** did you first notice it?	A couple of weeks ago.
Description/Duration	
___ Can you **describe** what you mean by UTI?	I just pee all the time.
___ **How often** is "all the time"?	It seems like every half hour.
___ Times you get up through the night to urinate?	4 or 5.
___ About how much at a time?	A lot.
Exacerbation	
___ Does anything make it **worse**?	Nothing I noticed.
Remission	
___ Did you try anything to make it **better**?	Cranberry juice, but it didn't work.
Symptoms associated	
___ **Burning** with urination?	No.

___ **Difficulty starting** to urinate?	No.
___ Urinary **urgency**?	No.
___ **Cloudy or foul-smelling** urine?	No.
___ **Blood** with urination?	No.
___ **Abdominal pain**?	No.
___ **Fever**?	No.
___ **Thirsty or hungry** a lot?	Yes, I am thirsty all the time.
___ **Lightheadedness or dizziness**?	No.
___ **Weight loss or gain**?	I've actually lost about 20 pounds.
___ Over what **period of time**?	Three months.
___ Have you been trying to lose weight?	I think I've actually been eating more.
___ **Fatigue**?	Yes, I'm tired all the time.
SMASH FM	
Social History (FED TACOS)	
___ What type of **foods** do you prefer?	I like pasta and breads.
___ Do you **exercise**?	I'm too tired to exercise.
___ Have you ever used **tobacco**?	No.
___ Do you drink **alcohol**?	No.
___ What is your **occupation**?	I'm an administrative assistant.
___ **FDLNMP**?	I should be getting it any day now.
___ Are you **sexually active**?	Not for the past 6 months or so.
___ Do you have any **medical** conditions?	No.
___ Do you have any **allergies**?	No.
___ Any prior **surgeries**?	No.
___ Any prior **hospitalizations**?	No.

___ Medical conditions in the **family**?	Both of my parents have diabetes.
___ Are you on any **medications**?	No.

Case 9 Review

Providers quickly become wary of patients who present with a diagnosis in hand, especially with availability of the internet. In some cases, however, it may be helpful, as with a young man presenting in the emergency room with abdominal pain and known inflammatory bowel disease. He had been through this type of pain many times before and knew exactly what was happening again.

If a patient presents with a proposed diagnosis, you should include it in your differential, as the patient is indeed often correct, but it should not limit other possibilities. The remainder of your questions should prove or disprove the patient's assumption.

When this patient stated she had a "urinary tract infection," the immediate next thought should be, "How do you know it's a urinary tract infection?" You can ask this question without being condescending by asking the patient to describe what symptoms she has that make her think she has a UTI. Perhaps she has had UTIs in the past and knows what one feels like.

Her isolated complaint of urinary frequency is the clue that something else may be going on. Urinary tract infections rarely present with just urinary frequency; they also have associated dysuria, cloudy or foul-smelling urine, and suprapubic discomfort. In addition, urgency, hesitancy, hematuria, fever, and even back pain may be present.

When a patient makes a statement such as that she urinates "every half hour," be sure to quantify it. Is she voiding out of behavior or need? If she is only voiding small amounts, perhaps it is more consistent with a UTI. Getting up at night suggests true polyuria.

At this point you have to ask yourself what else causes someone to urinate all the time. We have to wonder then how much she is drinking. If a diagnosis hadn't come to mind to this point, when you asked family history you quickly realized the association with diabetes, illustrating the importance of asking these screening questions despite not always knowing the immediate association. Now that you suspect diabetes, the other symptoms associated questions may be much more obvious: polydipsia, polyphagia, fatigue, and weight loss.

The social history comes into play with patient education, as her diet is heavy in carbohydrates. When the date of last menses is a little vague, go further to see if pregnancy should be considered.

Finally, take the hint from the patient about the outcome of her last treatment with antibiotics. She obviously wasn't happy with the resultant yeast infection. She wasn't being funny when she said they gave her an antibiotic and a yeast infection. She was saying that if you give her an antibiotic you should plan to treat the yeast infection she is expecting to get as a result. Are patients with diabetes more prone to yeast infections? Add another clue.

Possible differential diagnosis:

1. Polyuria
2. Rule out diabetes mellitus
3. Rule out diabetes insipidus

CASE 10

Clinical Setting: Family Medicine Clinic
Stubb Dupt—46-year-old male
CC: Cold

Vital Signs

Blood pressure: 144/88

Respirations: 14 per minute

Pulse: 62 bpm

Temperature: 99.5 degrees F

Weight: 230 lbs

Height: 6′4″

CASE 10

Stubb Dupt
46-year-old male
CC: Cold

___ Addresses patient by name	
___ Introduces self and explains role	
___ Properly washes hands prior to touching patient	
___ How can I help you today?	I've got a cold.
Chronology/Onset	
___ **When** did it start?	About 3 days ago.
___ Did you ever have this **before**?	Yes.
___ **When** was the **last time**?	About a year ago.
___ How was it treated?	I bought some cough medicine.
___ **How often** does it happen?	About once a year.
Description/Duration	
___ **Describe** what you mean by a "cold."	I have a stuffy nose, a sore throat, and a cough.
___ Did they all start at the same time?	No. I had a runny nose first, then the sore throat and cough started today.
___ What **color** is the drainage from your nose?	It was clear, but now it's green.
___ **Bringing anything up** with the cough?	Yes, a little.
___ What **color** is it?	Same green as my nose.
Intensity	
___ Have you **missed work/school**?	Yes, I took off today.
Exacerbation	
___ Does anything make it **worse**?	Coughing makes my throat worse.

Remission	
___ Does anything make it **better**?	A shower clears my nose a little, but Theraflu didn't help this time.
___ How much did you take?	You mix a pouch into hot water.
___ How often did you take it?	At least 3 or 4 times.
Symptoms associated	
___ **Fever or chills**?	No.
___ **Sinus congestion/pressure**?	Yes, especially below my eyes.
___ **Itchy or watery eyes**?	No.
___ **Ear pain**?	No.
___ **Shortness of breath (SOB)**?	No.
___ **Eating and drinking all right**?	It just hurts to swallow a bit.
___ **Vomiting or diarrhea**?	No.
___ **Fatigue**?	Just tired of working.
SMASH FM	
Social History (FED TACOS)	
___ Have you ever used **tobacco**?	Yes.
___ What type?	I chew snuff.
___ **How much a day**?	A can.
___ Do you drink **alcohol**?	Sure.
___ How many a day?	Just 2 or 3 beers on the weekend.
___ What is your **occupation**?	Road maintenance.
___ Do you have any **medical** conditions?	My blood pressure's a bit high.
___ Do you have any **allergies**?	Ah, a little seasonal stuff.
___ Any prior **surgeries**?	No.
___ Any prior **hospitalizations**?	No.

____ Medical conditions in the **family**?	Blood pressure and cholesterol.
____ **Contact** with others with similar symptoms?	Yes, my sister had her brats up last week. They all had the crud.
____ Are you on any **medications**?	HCTZ.
____ How many **milligrams**?	Fifty.
____ How many **times a day**?	Just in the morning.

Case 10 Review

When this patient presents with a "cold," the first goal is to define what symptoms constitute a cold to this patient. In clinical practice it is simple enough to say, "What symptoms are you having?" For you as the student, this shortcut will not work for your practical exams, where you must ask each question individually.

Did you notice the slight variation in the patient's answers about nasal drainage? When you asked him to describe the cold, he stated, "stuffy nose," but when you asked which symptoms started first, it was "runny nose." You may have chosen to clarify which was more prominent. Time frame is important. We note that the first symptom was rhinorrhea that has indeed changed from a clear discharge to one that is green, which combined with stuffy nose may suggest bacterial infection. The rhinorrhea is admittedly associated with sinus pressure and we perhaps should have went further to quantify the amount of exudate.

The time frame suggests that the sore throat is likely from postnasal drainage, as the runny nose started first and then the sore throat, but pharyngitis remains in the differential diagnosis. Using anatomy as your guide, ask about involvement of other HEENT organs. No other organ systems seem to be involved to any great extent.

Notice that we try to get a description of the expectorant. Be aware that some patients, especially women, will be less than willing to give a description, because often they just don't look at it, while others may take great pleasure in describing the color, consistency, etc., in great detail.

The patient had contact with others with similar symptoms, reinforcing the likely infectious nature of the diagnosis.

Another example in this case is the phrasing for tobacco use. If you asked this patient if he smoked, the answer would have been, "No," and you would have missed his smokeless tobacco use. Now think about that sore throat again. Do you want to add any possible diagnoses?

Possible differential diagnosis:

1. URI
2. Viral rhinosinusitis
3. Rule out bacterial rhinosinusitis

CASE 11

Clinical Setting: Emergency Room
Jennifer Atole—18-year-old female
CC: Burning on urination

Vital Signs

Blood pressure: 114/68

Respirations: 14 per minute

Pulse: 64 bpm

Temperature: 99.6 degrees F

Weight: 130 lbs

Height: 5'4"

CASE 11

Jennifer Atole
18-year-old pregnant female
CC: Burning on urination

___ Addresses patient by name	
___ Introduces self and explains role	
___ Properly washes hands prior to touching patient	
___ How can I help you today?	It hurts when I pee.
Chronology/Onset	
___ **When** did it **start**?	About 2 weeks ago.
___ Have you had this **before**?	Yes, twice.
___ **When** was that?	When I was 15.
___ Did you **see anyone** for it?	Yes.
___ Did they tell you **what it was**?	Bladder infections.
___ How did they **treat** you?	An antibiotic.
Description/Duration	
___ Can you **describe** the pain?	I have a lot of burning down there.
Exacerbation	
___ What makes it **worse**?	It's worse when I pee.
___ Do you have burning when you don't pee?	Yes.
Remission	
___ Did you try anything to make it **better**?	No.
Symptoms associated	
___ **Difficulty starting** to urinate?	Yeah, 'cause it burns when it starts.
___ Urinary **frequency**?	No.

___ Urinary **urgency**?	No.
___ **Cloudy or foul-smelling** urine?	No.
___ **Blood** with urination?	No.
___ **Abdominal pain**?	No.
___ **Fever or chills**?	No.
___ **Nausea or vomiting**?	No.
___ **Vaginal discharge or bleeding**?	Just a little clear drainage.
___ **Lesions** in the genital area?	I didn't look.
___ Any **tingling in the area**?	Yes, a couple of weeks ago.
Sexual/OB/GYN history	
___ When was the **FDLNMP**?	About 5 months ago.
___ Have you seen your OB doctor for this?	I moved here a couple of months ago and haven't seen one yet.
___ How many **times** have you been **pregnant**?	This is the first time.
___ Are you **sexually active**?	I'm pregnant, aren't I?
___ Are you sexually active during your pregnancy?	Yes.
___ **How many partners** in the last month?	Just one.
___ Does your **partner** have any **discharge or lesions**?	He's a little raw. He says he's not used to having sex so often.
___ Do you use **protection**?	No, I'm pregnant and I trust him.
___ How long have you been with him?	About a month.
___ Have you ever had an **STI**?	I had some warts.
___ When was that?	When I was 15.
SMASH FM	
Social History (FED TACOS)	
___ What kind of **foods** do you eat?	Whatever's easy to make; canned stuff.

___ Do you **exercise**?	With this belly?
___ How much **caffeine** in your diet?	A couple pops a day, I guess.
___ Have you ever used **tobacco**?	I bum a cigarette now and then.
___ Do you drink **alcohol**?	No.
___ Do you use any **drugs**?	No money for that.
___ What's your **occupation**?	I'm not working right now.
___ Do you have any **medical** conditions?	No.
___ Do you have any **allergies**?	No.
___ Any prior **surgeries**?	No.
___ Any prior **hospitalizations**?	No.
___ Medical conditions in the **family**?	They're drinkers.
___ Are you on any **medications**?	No.
___ Are you taking prenatal vitamins?	No.

Case 11 Review

The conversation in this case has been deemed offensive by some readers, but it is nearly word for word as it occurred and many, if not all, providers will encounter conversations like this one. This young lady had come from another town and recently moved into the area. Her chief complaint was that it "hurt to pee." UTI would come to the forefront as a possible diagnosis. Chronology reveals a prior history of UTI treated with antibiotics, which would make it quite easy to jump to it as a sole diagnosis.

She does have dysuria; however, when being asked about exacerbating factors she states that it is worse with urination. This should prompt the astute provider to ask if there is burning other than when she urinates, which is not consistent with typical UTIs. Exploring the differential you find she also lacked frequency, urgency, fever, chills, or abdominal or back pain. What else, then, can cause burning in the genital area that is worse with urination?

This case demonstrates the importance of speaking on the correct level with the patient. She refers to urination as "peeing," so you may refer to it in that way. The burning without urination makes one concerned about a sexually transmitted infection (STI), specifically herpes simplex with open ulcerations being irritated by urine when the patient voids. The patient has not looked for lesions, but one can still ask about tingling in the area as an additional symptom that typically occurs before the onset of lesions.

The social history should focus on behavior that will impact the pregnancy. An extensive sexual and OB/GYN history is important and shows that she has not had prenatal care. A detailed sexual history shows the patient has a new partner, has many risk factors for STI, and continues to have unprotected sex, an opportunity for education. Unfortunately, she might have to have a caesarean section if she has an outbreak when she is in labor. You should explore partner history. His being "raw" was most likely an active herpes outbreak. Although such frank language is perhaps not typical, it should not be a surprise.

This patient was referred to an OB/GYN with an appointment that afternoon; unfortunately, she failed to keep the appointment.

Possible differential diagnosis:

1. Herpes simplex virus type II
2. Rule out syphilis
3. Rule out chancroid
4. Doubt urinary tract infection

CASE 12

Clinical Setting: Family Medicine Clinic
Reed Flunks—24-year-old male
CC: Chest pain

Vital Signs

Blood pressure: 110/62

Respirations: 14 per minute

Pulse: 64 bpm

Temperature: 98.4 degrees F

Weight: 198 lbs

Height: 5′10″

CASE 12

Reed Flunks
24-year-old male
CC: Chest pain

___ Addresses patient by name	
___ Introduces self and explains role	
___ Properly washes hands prior to touching patient	
___ How can I help you today?	I have chest pain.
Chronology/Onset	
___ **When** did it **start**?	A couple of months ago.
___ What are you **doing** when it occurs?	It's usually after I eat.
___ Have you had this **before**?	No.
___ Have there been any **changes in the pain**?	It's been getting more frequent.
___ How frequently do you get it?	Almost every day.
Description/Duration	
___ **Describe** the pain.	It's a burning.
___ **Where** is it?	(Points to epigastria.)
___ Does it **radiate (go)** anywhere?	Sometimes a little up into my neck.
___ Where in the neck?	(Touches right side.)
___ Is it **constant** or does it **come and go**?	It comes and goes.
___ How long does it **last**?	A couple of hours.
Intensity	
___ How severe is it on a scale from **1 to 10**?	About a 4 or 5.
Exacerbation	
___ What makes it **worse**?	Eating before going to bed and certain foods.
___ What **kinds of foods**?	Spicy stuff.

Remission	
____ Did you try anything to make it **better**?	Mylanta helps for about an hour.
____ How often do you take it?	Once a day or so?
____ How much?	I just take a swig out of it.
Symptoms associated	
____ **Belching**?	It actually feels a little better when I do.
____ **Bad breath**?	Not that I've been told.
____ **Cough or wheezing**?	No.
____ **Nausea or vomiting**?	I'm a little nauseated sometimes.
____ **Changes to your stools**?	No.
____ **Blood or dark-colored stools**?	No.
____ **Sweating**?	No.
____ **Pain with exertion**?	No.
____ **Shortness of breath**?	No.
____ **Pain anywhere else**?	No.
SMASH FM	
Social History (FED TACOS)	
____ What kind of **foods** do you eat?	I like Mexican and Italian foods.
____ Do you eat before going to bed?	I lift after work so dinner is usually at 8.
____ Other **exercise**?	A half-hour bike on the weekends.
____ How much **caffeine** in your diet?	A couple coffees a day.
____ Have you ever used **tobacco**?	No.
____ Do you drink **alcohol**?	Yes.
____ **How many a day**?	A couple beers after dinner.
____ Do you use any **drugs**?	No thank you.

____ What's your **occupation**?	I drive for UPS.
____ Do you have any **medical** conditions?	Asthma, but only when I was a kid.
____ Do you have any **allergies**?	No.
____ Any prior **surgeries**?	No.
____ Any prior **hospitalizations**?	No.
____ Medical conditions in the **family**?	Some Alzheimer's.
____ Are you on any **medications**?	Just the Mylanta.

Case 12 Review

Notice how the complaint of chest pain brings to mind a markedly different differential diagnosis in a 24-year-old than in a 64-year-old. Before asking your first question, you should have already moved myocardial infarction way down on your differential. Is it still possible? Of course it is, but it is much less likely.

This flow demonstrates the power of an accurate chronological history. If you didn't follow up the onset by asking what he is doing when the pain occurs, you would have missed that it occurs after eating. At the top on our list of possibilities now are cholelithiasis, gastroesophageal reflux, and gastric or duodenal ulcer disease. His description of the pain as "burning" conforms, but do not be fooled by this characteristic, as cardiac pain can be described as burning in nature as well. Don't let the comment of the pain occurring more frequently go unchallenged: Ask how frequent it is.

Regarding location, the pain's pattern of radiation is particularly helpful as cholelithiasis classically radiates in the right shoulder blade, a dissecting aneurysm into the back, and reflux often centrally into the neck and throat.

When asking about exacerbating factors, follow through for more details. When you find out that food makes the symptoms worse, ask what kind of food. If dairy products were involved, we would have to add lactose intolerance to our differential and ask about the appropriate symptoms associated with it. What happens when we go to bed shortly after eating? The supine position encourages reflux. You could also ask if his symptoms are worse after eating large meals.

Though this picture seems straightforward, a good practice to get into is to ask what other diagnoses, if missed, would harm or even kill the patient. He is young but you must prove that he is not having a heart attack by asking the symptoms associated such as SOB and diaphoresis.

A middle-aged colleague was walking up a flight of stairs. When he reached the top, he complained about having heartburn. It was a short encounter but, in retrospect, walking up stairs is not a common aggravating factor for dyspepsia. One week later the gentleman had cardiac bypass.

Finally, determining alcohol intake gives you the opportunity to educate your patient. Your treatment plan will include educating your patient that alcohol loosens the gastroesophageal sphincter, resulting in more reflux, that he should avoid foods that make his symptoms worse, not to eat late a night, and to eat smaller meals.

Possible differential diagnosis:

1. Gastroesophageal reflux disease
2. Esophagitis
3. Gastritis
4. Rule out gastroduodenal ulceration

CASE 13

Clinical Setting: Emergency Room
Montane Numo—32-year-old male
CC: SOB

Vital Signs

Blood pressure: 110/58

Respirations: 36 per minute

Pulse: 118 bpm

Temperature: 98.4 degrees F

Weight: 198 lbs

Height: 6′5″

CASE 13

Montane Numo
32-year-old male
CC: SOB

___ Addresses patient by name	
___ Introduces self and explains role	
___ Properly washes hands prior to touching patient	
___ How can I help you today?	I can't catch my breath.
Chronology/Onset	
___ **When** did it start?	Last night.
___ **What were you doing** when it started?	I was playing basketball.
___ Did it start **suddenly or gradually**?	I was a little short of breath when I was playing, but then it got suddenly worse.
___ Did you ever have this **before**?	No.
___ Has it **changed** since last night?	It's much harder to breathe.
Description/Duration	
___ Is it **constant** or does it **come and go**?	It's constant.
Intensity	
___ How has it **affected your activities**?	I can't do anything but sit still.
___ Has it affected your **sleep**?	I woke up a lot, short of breath.
Exacerbation	
___ What makes it **worse**?	It's worse when I exert myself or if I lie on my right side.
Remission	
___ What makes it **better**?	Nothing.

Symptoms associated	
___ **Chest pain**?	Just when it suddenly got bad. I kind of heard a pop. Had to stop playing ball.
___ **Where** is the pain?	Right here (holds left upper thorax).
___ **How long** did it last?	Only a few seconds.
___ **Lightheaded**?	No.
___ Have you had a **cold** recently?	No.
___ **Wheezing**?	No.
___ **Cough**?	Yes.
___ **Sputum**?	A little.
___ What **color** is it?	Clear.
___ Did you bring up any blood?	Maybe a little streak of it.
___ **Leg pain, swelling, or redness**?	No.
___ **Trauma**?	No.
SMASH FM	
Social History (FED TACOS)	
___ Do you normally get **SOB with exercise**?	No, I play ball all the time.
___ Have you ever used **tobacco**?	I smoke when I'm out with the guys.
___ **How many** a day?	Probably 6 cigarettes a month.
___ Do you drink **alcohol**?	Yes.
___ **How many a day**?	Just weekends, maybe a six-pack.
___ Do you use any **drugs**?	No, I'd be off the team.
___ What's your **occupation**?	I'm studying forensics.
___ Do you have any **medical** conditions?	No.
___ Do you have any **allergies**?	No.
___ Any prior **surgeries**?	No.

___ Any prior **hospitalizations**?	No.
___ Medical conditions in the **family**?	My dad's brother died young, but I don't know what it was.
___ Are you on any **medications**?	No.

Case 13 Review

By this case, the questions should be coming to you more naturally. When this patient presents with shortness of breath (SOB), you naturally want to know when it started and how it has changed since starting. Again, what the patient was doing is important. Playing basketball is typically a strenuous activity requiring a high cardiopulmonary output, suggesting that we should focus on these organ systems first in our differential.

Considering the respiratory system, it is unlikely that the patient is suffering from pneumonia or any infectious process, as the onset was so sudden and the patient data sheet shows he is afebrile. He could have a pulmonary embolism but he lacks leg pain, swelling, or redness associated with a deep vein thrombosis, which is the most common cause of pulmonary embolism. Interestingly, the patient felt a pop in his chest, associated with a sudden worsening of SOB and some pain. What could have occurred?

Shortness of breath is difficult to assign a scaled intensity level to ("On a scale from 0 to 10, how short of breath are you?"). Intensity, however, can be reflected in how the symptom affects activities of daily living (ADLs)—that is, what the patient is and is not able to do.

Why would his breathing be worse when he is lying on his right side? Adding his body habitus to the history you obtained and the mysterious "pop," the possibility of spontaneous pneumothorax should be considered. The reason for the worsened SOB while lying on his right side is that he is dependent on the right lung for his respirations, so lying on the right side essentially restricts the ability to expand the right hemithorax.

Notice the follow-up questions to the inquiry of chest pain. The patient tells you when it occurred, so you have to ask him where it occurred and its duration. You basically perform another mini CODIERS on the pain itself.

Possible differential diagnosis:

1. Spontaneous pneumothorax
2. Rule out pulmonary embolism
3. Doubt dissecting aortic aneurysm

CASE 14

Clinical Setting: Ambulatory Clinic
Dee Vane—48-year-old female
CC: Leg swelling

Vital Signs

Blood pressure: 148/90

Respirations: 16 per minute

Pulse: 88 bpm

Temperature: 98.9 degrees F

Weight: 148 lbs

Height: 5′4″

CASE 14	
Dee Vane **48-year-old female** **CC: Leg swelling**	
___ Addresses patient by name	
___ Introduces self and explains role	
___ Properly washes hands prior to touching patient	
___ How can I help you today?	I have swelling in my leg.
Chronology/Onset	
___ When did it **start**?	3 days ago.
___ What were you **doing at the time**?	I noticed it putting my shoes on.
___ Did you ever **have this before**?	No.
___ How has it **changed**?	The swelling's gotten bigger.
Description/Duration	
___ **Where** is the swelling?	It's my right leg.
Intensity	
___ How swollen is it?	I'm wearing my slipper because I can't get my shoe on.
Exacerbation	
___ What makes it **worse**?	It gets worse as the day goes on.
Remission	
___ Does anything make it **better**?	No.
Symptoms associated	
___ **Pain**?	Yes.
___ **Describe** the pain.	It's a dull ache.
___ Does it **come and go or is it constant**?	It's there all the time.

____ **Intensity** on a scale of 1 to 10?	Not too bad, a 3.
____ **Redness**?	Yes, a little.
____ Increased **warmth**?	Yes.
____ **Shortness of breath**?	No.
____ **Chest pain**?	No.
____ **Trauma**?	Just a scratch I got last week in the garden.
____ **Recent travel**?	I visited my sister last week.
____ How far away is that?	We take our time, an 8-hour drive.
SMASH FM	
Social History (FED TACOS)	
____ Do you **exercise**?	Not so much.
____ Have you ever used **tobacco**?	I used to smoke.
____ When did you **quit**?	2 weeks ago.
____ **How much** did you smoke a day?	A pack.
____ **How long** did you smoke?	Maybe 40 years.
____ Do you drink **alcohol**?	No.
____ What's your **occupation**?	I'm a librarian.
____ Do you have any **medical** conditions?	No, I've been fortunate.
____ Do you have any **allergies**?	No.
____ Any prior **surgeries**?	I had a hysterectomy
____ When was that?	When I was 40.
____ What was the indication?	I was bleeding too much.
____ Any prior **hospitalizations**?	Just for my surgery.
____ Medical conditions in the **family**?	Dad had a heart attack.
____ Are you on any **medications**?	None. I just take estrogen.

___ How many milligrams?	I'm not sure.
___ How many pills a day?	Just the one.

Case 14 Review

Ms. Vane presents with swelling in her leg. Even before asking questions the differential diagnosis should include cellulitis, heart failure, venous insufficiency, deep vein thrombosis (DVT), and gout, just to name a few.

The swelling has been getting progressively worse and was noticed simply because she could not get her shoe on. The swelling gets worse as the day goes on, supporting dependent edema from venous insufficiency or an obstructive process. Perhaps she has a pelvic malignancy causing lymphatic drainage compromise, which would be consistent with unilateral swelling.

Considering heart failure (HF) leads us to ask about SOB, which she denies, and the swelling is unilateral whereas in HF it is usually bilateral. Had she admitted to SOB, we would have pursued questions of orthopnea, dyspnea on exertion, and paroxysmal nocturnal dyspnea.

Your concern for cellulitis is heightened when you learn she scratched her leg in the garden a week prior, which you learned by asking about trauma.

Knowing the patient is on estrogen, posthysterectomy, raises your concern for a DVT. DVTs place patients at risk for pulmonary embolism; therefore we ask about both local signs such as redness and increased warmth as well as SOB and chest pain. Now consider other factors that increase risk of DVT. Recent travel adds to your suspicion. You must ask the means of travel and its duration. A one-hour car trip is less worrisome than an eight-hour trip.

The patient's smoking history could easily have been missed if we hadn't posed the question as "Have you ever used tobacco?" This also demonstrates the importance of not walking away from a line of questioning. Her response, "I used to smoke," should lead you to ask when she quit, how long she smoked prior to quitting, and how much she smoked a day. If you walked away, you would have missed her smoking history, which is significant and may be contributing to her condition, as with DVT and tumor. Humanistically she should be congratulated on her success in having quit for two weeks already, and your plan should include ways to help her remain smoke-free.

Your physical examination will aid in your diagnosis. Restricted only to history here, our differential contains several possibilities, especially DVT and cellulitis. Your job now is to investigate each possibility to arrive at the correct diagnosis.

Possible differential diagnosis:

1. Cellulitis
2. Rule out DVT
3. Rule out lymphatic obstruction

CASE 15

Clinical Setting: Family Medicine Office
Albert Nemia—55-year-old male
CC: Nausea and vomiting

Vital Signs

Blood pressure: 140/88

Respirations: 16 per minute

Pulse: 68 bpm

Temperature: 98.3 degrees F

Weight: 180 lbs

Height: 5′10″

CASE 15

Albert Nemia
55-year-old male
CC: Nausea and vomiting

___ Addresses patient by name	
___ Introduces self and explains role	
___ Properly washes hands prior to touching patient	
___ How can I help you today?	I've been vomiting, Doc.
Chronology/Onset	
___ When did it **start**?	Last night.
___ What were you **doing** when it started?	Having some beers and wings.
___ How **many times** have you vomited?	4 or 5 times.
___ When was the **last time** you vomited?	About 6 hours ago.
___ When were you first **nauseated**?	For the last 3 or 4 days.
___ Did you ever **have this before**?	Yes.
___ **When** was that?	About 6 months ago.
___ Did you see anyone for it?	Yes, I went to the hospital.
___ What did they find?	Nothing. I was in pain and they wouldn't give me my pain pills so I just took off.
Description/Duration	
___ What does the vomit **look like**?	It's dark and looks like dirt.
___ Was there any **blood in it**?	I didn't see any.
Intensity	
___ Are you **lightheaded**?	You know, I am if I stand up too fast.
Exacerbation	
___ Anything make it **worse**?	Alcohol.

Remission	
____ Does anything make it **better**?	If I take a ton of antacids.
____ You have **heartburn**?	Oh yeah, for a long time.
Symptoms associated	
____ **Dark stools**?	Yes, for the last week.
____ **Blood in your stools**?	No.
____ **Pain anywhere**?	In my stomach (points to LUQ).
____ **Describe** the pain.	It's like a gnawing.
____ On **scale** from 1 to 10?	A 4.
____ **Weight loss or night sweats**?	No.
SMASH FM	
Social History (FED TACOS)	
____ Do any kinds of **foods** bother you?	Almost everything. I'm nauseated but hungry.
____ Have you ever used **tobacco**?	I smoke.
____ **How much** a day?	Pack, pack and a half.
____ **How long** have you smoked?	Since I was 15.
____ Do you drink **alcohol**?	Six-pack a day and a few shots.
____ Do you use any **drugs**?	No.
____ What's your **occupation**?	I raise dogs.
____ Do you have any **medical** conditions?	Arthritis, got it bad in the knees.
____ Do you have any **allergies**?	No.
____ Any prior **surgeries**?	Had my gallbladder out.
____ When was that?	Couple of years ago.
____ Any prior **hospitalizations**?	Just to have my gallbladder out.
____ Medical conditions in the **family**?	Blood pressure. Cholesterol.

___ Are you on any **medications**?	Just my pain pills.
___ What's the name of the pill?	Motrin.
___ How many milligrams?	200.
___ How many pills a day?	Three in the morning, 4 before bed or the arthritis keeps me up, and sometimes 3 in the afternoon if it's a bad day.
___ Are these prescribed?	No, I buy them myself.

Case 15 Review

The case demonstrates the rolling thought processes that occur as history gathering progresses. The patient presents with nausea for the last 4 or 5 days and vomiting of short duration having only started the night before. Early in chronology you learn that he was eating wings and drinking beer. The provider may question how bad the nausea was if the patient is still able to eat such a diet. Gastroenteritis should be considered for the differential. You may also consider food poisoning, though the timing would suggest it wasn't his last meal that would be responsible but a meal sometime earlier.

It is important to quantify the vomiting, as a patient who has vomited only once or twice likely will not have dehydration or an electrolyte imbalance, which could mean the difference between admitting a patient and discharging him/her to home. It is also necessary to know when the patient has last vomited. Here the patient has not vomited for about six hours, meaning he may have had a gastritis that is getting better already.

When probing for the character of the emesis, the patient describes the black coffee-ground appearance that the provider recognizes as being classic for UGI bleeding, but the patient should still be asked if he/she has seen any blood, which most often is visualized by the patient as being red. If he had been vomiting bright red blood, we would have been concerned about an urgent or emergent process such as bleeding esophageal varices or a Mallory-Weiss tear of the esophagus from his vomiting.

The patient has had this once before, six months prior. Upon asking about the outcome we learn that he went to the hospital but left before intervention because "they wouldn't give me my pain pills." The provider should be careful about jumping to conclusions of drug-seeking behavior and has two options: pursue the line of questioning immediately or continue with the history gathering, leaving the topic temporarily but planning to return. With this later method the patient may be less defensive, as he would likely expect that with his last comment he is about to be judged for his actions.

When you do ask about his pain medication, you find out that he takes Motrin, which he buys himself and takes at very large doses for arthritis of his knees. It appears a large gap in communication occurred at his last visit to the hospital. The hospital personnel likely recognized the role that the nonsteroidal was playing with his UGI symptoms, but this information was not shared with the patient in a timely enough fashion for him to understand that his pain pills were contributing to his problem. The provider is left to guess at what events truly occurred, including his condition on past presentation in regard to his admitted alcohol use. When the patient's amount of alcohol use is revealed, the provider adds alcohol abuse to the differential for two reasons: first, its association with the presenting complaint, and second, the stand-alone diagnosis of alcohol abuse. In this possibly emergent situation, stabilization of the patient should take precedence, but the provider should also consider further intervention of the alcohol use by employing the CAGE questionnaire and referring the patient for intervention as appropriate.

The symptoms associated point us toward a UGI bleed. Intensity for bleeds may be defined by symptoms that are associated with blood loss, such as dizziness, syncope, falls, palpitations, and SOB, and the physical exam will help to determine if he is actively bleeding or hemodynamically unstable. Here, his vital signs show a stable blood pressure and lack of tachycardia, which along with the cessation of vomiting suggest stability.

The patient's arthritis plays a pivotal role as it is a driving factor in his nonsteroidal abuse. Patient education will be paramount in a successful outcome.

Possible differential diagnosis:

1. Upper GI bleed
2. Rule out NSAID-induced ulceration
3. Doubt esophageal varices

CASE 16

Clinical Setting: Emergency Room
John Dish—46-year-old male
CC: Abdominal pain

Vital Signs

Blood pressure: 120/68

Respirations: 24 per minute

Pulse: 98 bpm

Temperature: 100.3 degrees F

Weight: 138 lbs

Height: 5′5″

CASE 16	
John Dish **46-year-old male** **CC: Abdominal pain**	
___ Addresses patient by name	
___ Introduces self and explains role	
___ Properly washes hands prior to touching patient	
___ What brings you in today?	My stomach really hurts.
Chronology/Onset	
___ When did it **start**?	Been going on the last couple of days.
___ Anything happen recently that might have caused it?	Nothing that I can think of.
___ Did it come on **suddenly or gradually**?	Gradually.
___ Did you ever **have this before**?	A couple of times.
___ **When** was that?	About twice in the last year, but it went away on its own after a couple of days.
___ Has the **pain changed** since it started?	It's just getting worse.
Description/Duration	
___ What does it **feel like**?	Hard to say, a deep ache.
___ Is it **constant** or does it **come and go**?	It's always there, but gets worse and then a little better.
Location	
___ **Where** is it?	In my stomach.
___ Can you show me, with one finger?	(Points to RUQ.)
___ Does it **radiate** anywhere?	It seems to go a little into my back.
___ Where in your back?	Between my shoulder blades.
Intensity	
___ On a **scale** of 1 to 10, where is it now?	An 8.

Exacerbation	
___ What makes it **worse**?	I don't know.
Remission	
___ Does anything make it **better**?	No.
Symptoms associated	
___ **Heartburn**?	No.
___ **Nausea or vomiting**?	Yes, I vomited a couple of times.
___ What did it look like?	Just mucous and food.
___ When was the last time?	After breakfast this morning.
___ **Changes** to your **bowel movements**?	The stools are kind of whitish.
___ **Changes** in your **urine**?	That's darker, looks like tea.
___ **Fever, chills**?	I get hot and cold.
___ **Eyes yellow**?	My wife said that they were.
___ When did she tell you that?	For about a week or so now.
___ **Pain with deep breathing**?	Maybe a little.
___ **SOB or cough**?	No.
SMASH FM	
Social History (FED TACOS)	
___ Does any type of **food** have an effect?	Maybe greasy stuff.
___ Have you ever used **tobacco**?	No.
___ Do you drink **alcohol**?	A beer or two a month.
___ Do you use any **drugs**?	No.
___ What's your **occupation**?	I work for a security company.
___ Have you **traveled** anywhere?	We were in Mexico last month.
___ Did you get sick then?	We got a little diarrhea for a few days.

___ Are you **sexually active**?	Yes.
___ How many partners in the last 6 months?	One for the last 20 years.
___ Do you have any **medical** conditions?	I just found out that I have high cholesterol.
___ Were you ever **immunized** for hepatitis?	Yes, for the military.
___ Do you have any **allergies**?	No.
___ Any prior **surgeries**?	I was shot in the leg when I was in the military.
___ When was that?	Couple of years ago.
___ Any prior **hospitalizations**?	No.
___ Medical conditions in the **family**?	Nothing much.
___ Any **contacts** with similar symptoms?	No.
___ Are you on any **medications**?	Only a cholesterol medication, a statin?
___ How many milligrams?	I'm sorry, I don't know.
___ How many pills a day?	One.
___ How long have you been on those?	About a month.

Case 16 Review

The patient presents with abdominal pain with some hint of chronicity, as it has occurred in the past on several occasions but self-resolved. An early differential might include gastritis, reflux, peptic ulcer disease, cholelithiasis, and even dissecting aneurysm. Very valuable is the location in the right upper quadrant with radiation to the back, not exactly to the right shoulder blade but more between the shoulder blades. Again, consider dissecting aneurysm and cholelithiasis, but expand the differential using anatomy.

This patient has pain in the right upper quadrant. If you pointed to the site and went straight through the body, what organ systems could be affected? First considerations are the skin and subcutaneous tissues, as herpetic zoster is a very painful condition easily confirmed on physical examination. Next the inferior anterior rib cage would be encountered; could this patient have a somatic rib dysfunction that could lead to musculoskeletal pain? Next, we hit the liver and gallbladder; consider any condition that would involve these organs, such as cholelithiasis and hepatitis. The transverse bowel and descending small bowel also lie in the area; could this be colitis or a duodenal ulcer? Even the inferior lobe of the right lung may be encountered with our straight line. Could pneumonia be possible? This demonstrates the anatomy-based approach to diagnosis.

Now with these possibilities ask the appropriate questions. Most likely is liver or gallbladder involvement, so focus on these areas first. Symptoms from gallstones are commonly associated with fatty food intake. Inquire about changes to the stools and urine. With obstruction of bile ducts from stones or tumor the stools become clay-colored and the urine darker from bilirubinuria. Does the lack of a report of green bile in his emesis correspond? The patient admits that his wife has noticed his eyes were yellow. Probe to see if he has ever had this before. Perhaps he has a metabolic disorder in the processing of bilirubin for elimination, such as Gilbert's disease. This seems unlikely in this case, so focus on acute causes of hyperbilirubinemia. Is he hemolyzing red blood cells, such as that which could occur with splenomegaly?

The importance of SMASH FM is seen here. We find out the gentleman has hyperlipidemia and that he was started on a cholesterol pill not long ago. Could this be drug-induced hepatotoxicity? We also discover a risk for infectious hepatitis by his recent travel to Mexico, or are both of these argued against by the previous occurrences, which self-resolved as would be more common with cholelithiasis? You have your work cut out for you trying to find out which is the real diagnosis.

Possible differential diagnosis:

1. Hyperbilirubinemia
2. Rule out choledocholithiasis
3. Rule out viral hepatitis
4. Rule out drug-induced hepatoxocity

CASE 17

Clinical Setting: Emergency Room
Cheryl R. Canton—65-year-old female
CC: Dizziness

Vital Signs

Blood pressure: 102/48

Respirations: 20 per minute

Pulse: 108 bpm

Temperature: 98.3 degrees F

Weight: 118 lbs

Height: 5′2″

CASE 17

Cheryl R. Canton
65-year-old female
CC: Dizziness

___ Addresses patient by name	
___ Introduces self and explains role	
___ Properly washes hands prior to touching patient	
___ What brings you in today?	I've been dizzy.
Chronology/Onset	
___ **When** did you first notice it?	It's been going on for about a month.
___ **What are you doing** when it occurs?	Mostly when I stand up.
___ Did you ever have this **before**?	No.
___ **How often** does it happen?	At first only once a week, but now it's daily.
Description/Duration	
___ **Describe** the dizziness.	It feels like the room is closing in on me and getting darker.
___ Does the **room spin**?	No.
___ **How long** does it last?	Maybe 5 to 10 minutes.
Intensity	
___ Have you **fallen or passed out**?	No.
Exacerbation	
___ What makes it **worse**?	Standing up too fast.
Remission	
___ What makes it **better**?	I just sit back down for a few minutes and try again slowly.
Symptoms associated	
___ Have you had **a cold** recently?	No.

___ Does your **heart beat fast**?	Yes, when I feel dizzy.
___ **Vomiting or diarrhea**?	No.
___ **Eating and drinking** well?	Yes.
___ **Heartburn or stomach pain**?	No.
___ **Abdominal distention**?	Yes, I'm all puffed up.
___ **Changes to your stools**?	It's embarrassing but my hemorrhoids have been bleeding quite a bit.
___ Change in **caliber or size** of your stools?	Yes, I'm constipated. It comes out like little ropes.
___ Have you **lost** any **weight**?	I think I've lost a little weight.
___ How much, over how long?	20 pounds in the last year or so.
___ **Fever or night sweats**?	No.
SMASH FM	
Social History (FED TACOS)	
___ What types of **food** do you eat?	I haven't had much of an appetite. I feel all backed up.
___ Have you ever used **tobacco**?	No.
___ Do you drink **alcohol**?	No.
___ Do you have any **medical** conditions?	High blood pressure.
___ Do you have any **allergies**?	No.
___ Any prior **surgeries**?	No.
___ Any prior **hospitalizations**?	Just to deliver my kids.
___ How many children did you have?	6, and I have 15 grandkids.
___ Any **family** history of colon polyps or cancer?	No.
___ Are you on any **medications**?	Hydrochlorothiazide.
___ How many milligrams?	Twenty-five.
___ How many pills a day?	Twice a day.

Case 17 Review

Ms. Canton presents with dizziness. Dizziness can mean many things, so a description should be explored early on. The room spinning around is vertigo, whereas the perception of the room getting darker and the patient's feeling as if he/she is going to pass out is near syncope. Often you will get a description of lightheadedness or imbalance.

The patient has had this going on for a month but the frequency is increasing, suggesting a somewhat chronic process. She denies a sensation of the room spinning, decreasing the likelihood of labyrinthitis, or inner ear dysfunction, which is often associated with recent colds, hence the symptom associated question.

The patient admits tachycardia or palpitations when the dizziness occurs. Is it because the heart is trying to increase output, or could it be an arrhythmia causing the dizziness?

Dizziness with standing suggests decreased cerebral perfusion such as with autonomic or carotid body dysfunction or hypovolemia. She has been eating and drinking well without nausea or vomiting, which suggests that dehydration is not likely the cause. Could she be anemic? To explore this question consider what the most common causes of blood loss are. GI bleeding comes to mind.

The patient is obviously embarrassed about her rectal bleeding and unfortunately has attributed it to hemorrhoids. Weight loss and change in caliber of stools are not consistent with hemorrhoids and along with abdominal distension points us to colon cancer as a source of blood loss. Notice the follow-up to a positive weight loss screen; ask how much and over what period of time.

When you learn of the patient's 6 children and she proudly tells you of her 15 grandchildren you have a great opportunity for humanistic interaction. Don't move on to the next question; spend a little time talking about how important that is to her.

The patient is likely faced with a serious diagnosis, but short-term measures should not be overlooked. She has a history of hypertension and at one time likely needed her blood pressure medications. With her anemia she is now relatively hypotensive and her medication should be adjusted as appropriate.

Possible differential diagnosis:

1. Hematochezia
2. Rule out colorectal cancer
3. Rule out anemia
4. Hypotension

CASE 18

Clinical Setting: Emergency Room
Diana Rhetta—38-year-old female
CC: Diarrhea

Vital Signs

Blood pressure: 112/62

Respirations: 14 per minute

Pulse: 72 bpm

Temperature: 98.4 degrees F

Weight: 120 lbs

Height: 5'4"

CASE 18	
Diana Rhetta **38-year-old female** **CC: Diarrhea**	
___ Addresses patient by name	
___ Introduces self and explains role	
___ Properly washes hands prior to touching patient	
___ What brings you in today?	I have diarrhea.
Chronology/Onset	
___ When did it **start**?	About 3 days ago.
___ How **many times** do you go a day?	About 6 or 7 times.
___ When was the **last time**?	About 10 minutes ago.
___ Did you ever **have this before**?	No.
___ Has it **changed** in any way?	No.
Description/Duration	
___ **Describe** what you mean by **diarrhea**.	My stools are all watery.
___ Is there any **blood or mucous** in it?	No.
Intensity	
___ Does it affect your **daily activities**?	I'm afraid to go anywhere.
Exacerbation	
___ What makes it **worse**?	Nothing that I know of.
Remission	
___ Does anything make it **better**?	That pink diarrhea stuff helped a little.
___ **How often** do you take it?	3 times a day.
___ **How much** at a time?	A tablespoon.

Symptoms associated	
____ Any **nausea or vomiting**?	No.
____ Any **fever or chills**?	No.
____ **Abdominal pain**?	Yes.
____ Can you **describe** the pain?	It's crampy.
____ **Level** of the pain on a scale of 1 to 10?	Oh, about a 3 or 4.
SMASH FM	
Social History (FED TACOS)	
____ How does your **diet** look?	I try to eat right.
____ Have you eaten food that was **left out** or **was undercooked**?	I was at a picnic last week but was fine.
____ Have you ever used **tobacco**?	Yes, I smoke.
____ **How much** a day?	About a half a pack.
____ **How long** have you been smoking?	About 10 years or so.
____ Do you drink **alcohol**?	No.
____ When was the **FDLNMP**?	I don't have one. I'm on the Depo shot.
____ Do you have any **medical** conditions?	I just got over a sinus infection.
____ Do you have any **allergies**?	Yes. Ibuprofen.
____ What reaction do you have?	It really messes up my stomach.
____ Any prior **surgeries**?	No.
____ Any prior **hospitalizations**?	No.
____ **Family or contacts** with the same symptoms?	No.
____ Recent **travel**?	No.
____ Are you on any **medications**?	Just the antibiotic for my sinuses.
____ Do you know the name of it?	Bactrim?

___ How many milligrams?	I'm not sure.
___ How many times a day?	Twice.

Case 18 Review

The definition of diarrhea will vary from patient to patient, so defining the condition with the patient is important. Some patients will present complaining of diarrhea and will only have one liquid stool a day. Others may not truly have any liquid stools but only stools that are softer than what the patient considers to be normal for them. Therefore identify first occurrence, frequency, and, equally important, when the last episode occurred. It is common for a patient to complain of diarrhea but to try to "weather the storm" and present when the clinical picture is actually improving. For example, if she had six liquid stools the day before, but none so far on the day that she sees you, your clinical decision-making is altered. Perhaps you will not treat this patient with aggressive antidiarrheals but rather let it run its course naturally with supportive care such as a bland diet and increased liquids only.

Acute diarrhea is often viral in nature and requires little diagnostic workup beyond the history and physical examination. Chronic diarrhea, however, may require an extensive evaluation including microscopic evaluation for infectious agents, allergy testing, and even a colonoscopy. The presence of excessive flatulence, explosive qualities, and the presence of blood or mucous in the stools should also be discerned. By clearly defining the past history of diarrhea, duration of episodes, and frequency of occurrence, the most appropriate evaluation can be undertaken.

Your differential diagnosis may be drawn more to an infectious etiology if you ascertain that the patient has recently been to a picnic where food may have been left out, has eaten undercooked foods, or has traveled to areas with unsanitary water supplies.

It is also important to ask about other family members or contacts with similar conditions. It should be noted if patients have recently dined out. If a community outbreak should occur, this information will be invaluable in helping to isolate the infectious cause.

Asking about medical conditions and medication is the key to this case, as we discover a recent course of antibiotics, which may suggest *Clostridium difficile* as the infectious agent. Recently eating fried rice is associated specifically with *Bacillus cereus*. Skipping the history of medical conditions is tempting in so young a patient, but the diagnosis would likely have been missed if you had done so.

Possible differential diagnosis:

1. Diarrhea
2. Rule out *C. difficile* enteritis
3. Consider side effect of medication

Congratulations! You have completed the history section and will start to learn the examination component of the patient visit when you begin the comprehensive flows.

SECTION III

Physical Examination

CHAPTER 5

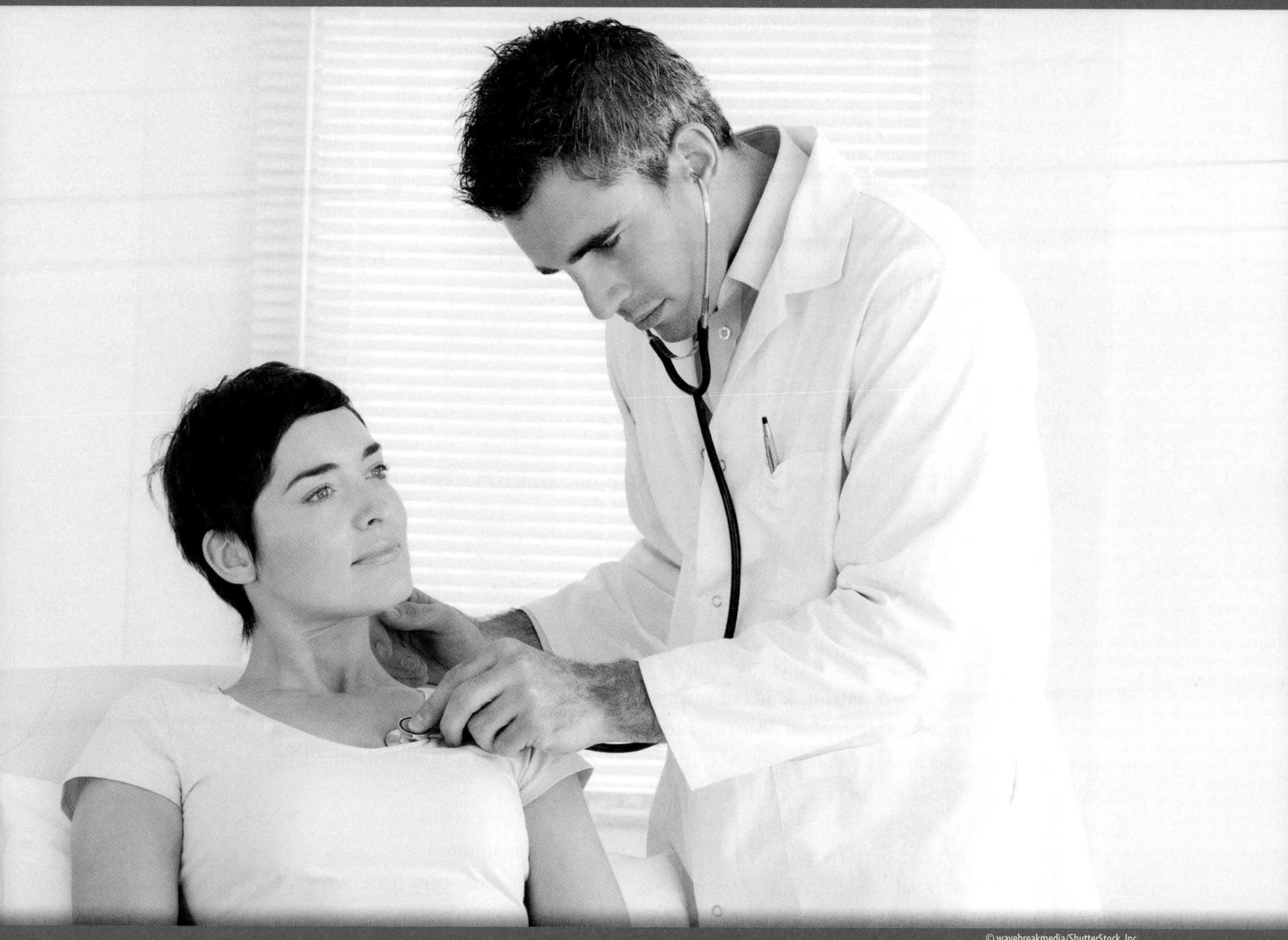

© wavebreakmedia/ShutterStock, Inc.

Introduction to Physical Examination

OBJECTIVES

At the conclusion of this chapter, the student will be able to

1. Organize physical examination in a head-to-toe, systems-based approach
2. Define the Target Method of examination through Absolute, Adjacent, and Associated areas
3. Employ the correct techniques when using a stethoscope, including the use of the bell and diaphragm in identification of low- and high-frequency sounds during physical examination
4. Recognize and avoid the drift toward complacency in physical examination

KEY TERMS

Sensitive examinations
Target Method
Problem-specific examinations
Absolute area of examination
Adjacent areas of examination
Associated areas of examination
Techniques of examination
Inspection
Auscultation
Palpation
Percussion

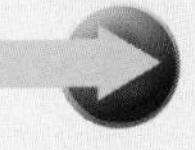

Where this icon appears, visit **go.jblearning.com/HPECWS** to view the video.

When students of medicine first begin studying history and physical examination, it is common to segment each step: Available patient information is reviewed first, the medical history is then obtained, a physical examination is performed, a differential diagnosis is offered, and a plan of care is devised. Once in clinical practice, providers frequently find themselves examining their patient while concurrently asking questions: Jill, a 23-year-old, complains of a rash on her right forearm. How convenient it is to have her push up her sleeve so that the rash can be observed as you ask questions about it.

Providers develop individual styles and approaches to patient evaluation based on their own experience, training, and logic. Yet early in the practice of physical examination, developing a system that follows a consistent, reproducible pattern assures the competence of the provider in observation and assessment of the patient, both in maintenance of health and in detection of disease states. A head-to-toe approach offers consistency, accuracy, and thoroughness.

Sensitive examinations: components of the physical examination requiring exposure of male and female genitalia and breasts

Head-to-Toe Approach

This approach breaks down the body in systems for examination and follows an order as such:

- General assessment
- Vital signs
- Integumentary (interwoven with other systems)
- HEENT
- Neck and lymphatics
- Respiratory
- Cardiovascular
- Abdominal
- Musculoskeletal
- Neurological
- Breast
- Female genitalia
- Male genitalia and rectum

Sensitive examinations are saved for last. This allows for performance of the examination followed by allowing the patient to redress or at least gown, and preservation of modesty.

General assessment of the patient is often completed through observation while eliciting the history. The systematic examination then begins with vital signs and generally follows a head-to-toe approach. Unless the patient presents with a dermatologic complaint, the examination of the integumentary system is typically interwoven throughout the system examinations. For example, examination of the skin of the lower thorax would be completed when beginning the abdominal examination instead of following vital signs with the integumentary system, having the patient disrobe, examining the skin, and then beginning again with a head-to-toe approach.

Variation is common. Some providers will examine the heart before the lungs. Some may do the upper extremities before the thorax, then the lower extremities after the abdominal exam. What is important is to follow an order of examination consistently.

FRONT TO BACK

Also include an order of front to back within the head-to-toe approach. For example, when examining the ear begin at the front, the area closest to you—the external ear—covering all surfaces. Next examine the conchal bowel and the visible external canal. Working toward the back, utilize the otoscope to see the remaining external canal, following it backward to the surface of the tympanic membrane. Visualize the boney prominence of the malleolus, seen through the tympanic member, and inner ear findings such as effusions. If a perforation of the tympanic membrane is present, inspection of the inner ear structures would then finish the exam.

The Target Method: Absolute, Adjacent, and Associated Areas of Examination

The **Target Method** approach to physical examination incorporates a targeted area examination technique. This method is more commonly used in **problem-specific examinations** where the physical examination is limited only to those areas directly related to the concern or complaint presented by the patient or potential diagnoses. The examination would again begin with the general assessment and vital signs; however, from this point a target would be imagined overlying the patient with the bullseye over the area of primary concern. The bullseye represents the "Absolute" area. The next ring in the target, which lies in close proximity, would be the "Adjacent" areas, and the distal areas or third ring requiring examination would be the "Associated" areas.

If the patient history leads you to believe the patient is in heart failure, the bullseye of the target would be over the heart. This is the **Absolute area**, or the area that "absolutely" needs to be examined: the heart in heart failure, the throat in a patient with a sore throat, or the shoulder in a patient with shoulder pain. From the bullseye (see **FIGURE 5-1**), you would then spread outward to adjacent organ systems, as would the rings of a target.

In the case of heart failure, you would then move laterally to the first ring of the target, the **Adjacent areas**. The Adjacent area would include the lungs and, moving upward, the neck, which is closely associated through vasculature to the heart.

Finally, you would examine the second ring of **Associated areas**, which are those areas that are related to the proposed diagnosis by system or disease. Thinking of the typical signs of heart failure, one could examine the abdomen for ascites and hepatomegaly and the extremities for edema and peripheral pulses.

A summary then of the Target Method would be:

- Absolute (Bullseye)—Cardiac exam
- Adjacent (First ring)
  - Respiratory exam
  - Neck exam

Target Method: technique of physical examination where the provider examines the primary area of concern or complaint first and then continues the examination by moving outward from the central focus

Problem-specific examination: physical examination that is limited only to those areas related to the concern or complaint presented by the patient or potential diagnoses

Absolute area: area of primary concern or complaint that must be included in the physical examination

Adjacent areas: areas in anatomic proximity to the primary area of concern or complaint requiring inclusion in the physical examination

Associated areas: areas outside of anatomic proximity to the primary area of concern or complaint but that are related to the proposed diagnosis by system or disease, prompting inclusion in the problem-specific physical examination

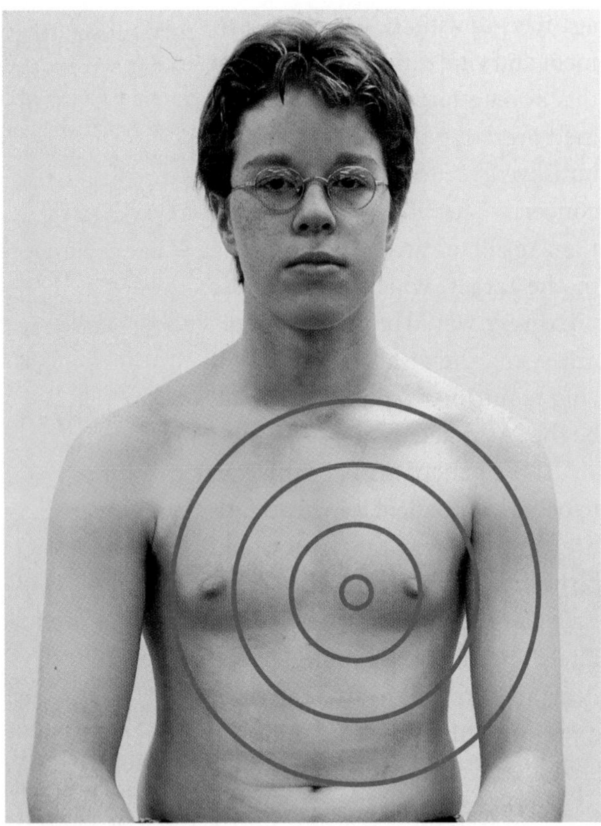

FIGURE 5-1 Target method of examination where the provider examines the primary area of concern or complaint, the bull's-eye, first and then continues the examination by moving outward from the central focus.

- Associated (Second ring)
  - Abdominal exam
  - Extremity exam

Beginning the Examination

When beginning the examination, keep in mind the humanistic domain, following these guidelines:

- Advise the patient that you are about to start the physical examination.
- Ask the patient's permission to do so.
- Rewash your hands if you have contaminated yourself in any way.
- Ask for permission to expose areas of examination.
- Recover the areas of examination as soon as possible.

Techniques of examination: standard methods of physical examination, which include assessment of function, inspection, auscultation, palpation, and percussion

- Assist the patient in position changes no matter what the age of the patient.
- Use a sheet to drape the patient from the waist down when exposing the abdomen.
- Slide the sheet upward to examine the lower extremities, keeping the pelvis covered at all times.

Techniques of Examination

Techniques of examination include assessment of Function, Inspection, Auscultation, Palpation, and Percussion. The order of applying these techniques is commonly described as Inspection, Percussion, Palpation, and then Auscultation. However, there were noted exceptions to the rule where the neck should be auscultated prior to palpation to avoid compressing stenotic carotid arteries, and auscultation prior to palpation of the abdomen to avoid changing the pattern of bowel sounds, which could occur if palpating the abdomen prior to auscultating it.

This argument was then presented by Merrine, a first-year medical student: Is there any system that would be adversely affected if you auscultated prior to palpating, and if not, why remember an order of examination that requires adjustments under certain conditions? Why not use an order that does not have exceptions? Not being able to find a contraindication to auscultating prior to palpating in all systems, we recommend the order as noted:

- Function
- Inspection
- Auscultation
- Palpation
- Percussion

Not all body systems will have each component of examination. For example, auscultation is not part of the neurologic exam, nor is percussion part of the neck and lymphatic exam.

FUNCTION

Common areas requiring assessment of function include the eyes for visual acuity, nose for smell, ears for auditory acuity, tongue for taste, and throat for swallow. Other areas of function are ingrained within the system, such as the sensory examination in the neurologic system and range of motion testing in the musculoskeletal system. Assessing function prior to inspection provides a baseline for comparison between before and after treatment.

A patient presents with blurred vision. Assessing function through visual acuity and peripheral fields should be performed first as a baseline prior to intervention. If light were shown into the eye either with pen light or ophthalmoscope prior to the visual acuity assessment, the acuity could be measured as falsely low. Following intervention, reassessment of acuity documents the outcome of treatment. Assessing baseline visual acuity at patient presentation documents preexisting loss of acuity should the outcome be adverse and the patient claim that the treatment intervention, rather than the condition itself, caused loss of vision.

INSPECTION

Inspection is next in the order of examination for each body system. Proper exposure is a rule that must be followed. If you cannot see the area being examined, then you cannot make a proper diagnosis. Consider the following case reported by Amanda, then a third-year medical student on clinical rotations:

> I'm on surgery rotation this month with the trauma service so I spend a lot of time in the ER. I happened to be in the ER two days ago and was reviewing a chart when I heard an ER doctor scolding a patient across the hall. It drew my attention but [I] couldn't really hear why he was yelling at her. She was a 70-year-old lady, had no one with her and was lying on the stretcher with a gown on. I didn't think anything of it so I went back to what I was doing.
>
> Ten hours later I got a consult in the ER for something else and when I came down, lo and behold there she still was, upset and agitated. I had no idea why she was there, but while I was doing my consult on another patient, a resident came over and said, "I'm about to teach you the most important thing you could ever learn in medicine. Come with me."
>
> Sure enough, I find myself standing outside of this lady's room. He tells me she presented to her family doctor 3–4 days ago with horrible pain in the right flank area that wrapped around to the front and was getting worse. He said nothing she did made it better or worse and she hadn't taken anything for it. Other than this new pain, she had a pretty benign history, lived alone, etc. The family doc sent her for a CT scan of the abdomen/pelvis, which she had that same day. It came back normal. The family doctor gave her "reassurance" and sent her home with a follow-up in two weeks.
>
> She came into our ER that morning because the pain woke her up from sleep and "was just unbearable." She gave the HPI to the ER doctor, who rescanned her. She's now had two CTs in four days and both are normal. I now found out that when I saw him talking to her in the AM, ten hours earlier, he was scolding her about being a frequent flyer and telling her there was nothing wrong with her. She was refusing to leave the ER because she knew that something was wrong, and the ER doctor was yelling at her for it.
>
> In frustration the ER doctor consults one of the residents on general surgery just to "make her happy" . . . which is how my resident and I find ourselves standing in front of her door. So with that history, he sends me in to see her and he follows. As I start my exam I lift up her gown and, clear as day, couldn't be any more textbook, this poor little old lady had shingles. Not one doctor in that whole 4 days lifted up her gown or checked on bare skin. If they had, they would have seen her rash and she wouldn't have been scanned twice, or accused of being a frequent flyer.
>
> It gave me the chills, I felt so bad for her. The ER doctor ended up coming in and apologizing and was highly embarrassed, and with good reason. He should have been.

In the simplest of terms, if you can't see the area, you can't examine it. Inspection is paramount.

When inspecting small body areas, a tendency to drift to cursory examination should be avoided. Consider examination of smaller body areas in a head-to-toe fashion as well. For example, looking at a fingernail, consider each component. Begin at the proximal nail fold representing the head, then moving distally, looking at the lunula, nail surface, nail bed, and free edge. Then examine the lateral nail folds as you would the extremities following examination

Inspection: technique of physical examination where the provider carefully observes an area of the body under conditions of proper exposure, comparing side to side when paired anatomy exists

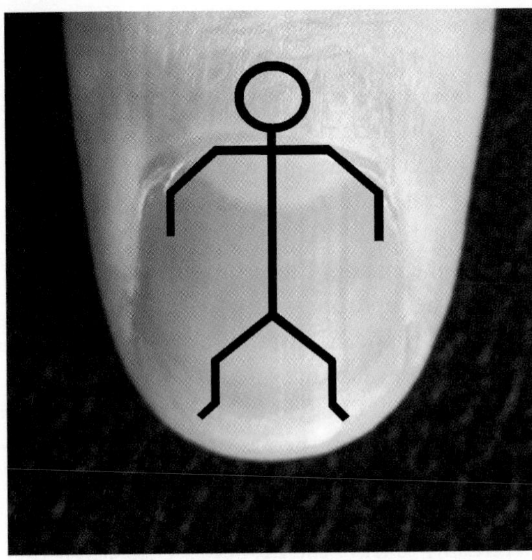

FIGURE 5-2 Concise examination of small body areas utilizing the head-to-toe approach.

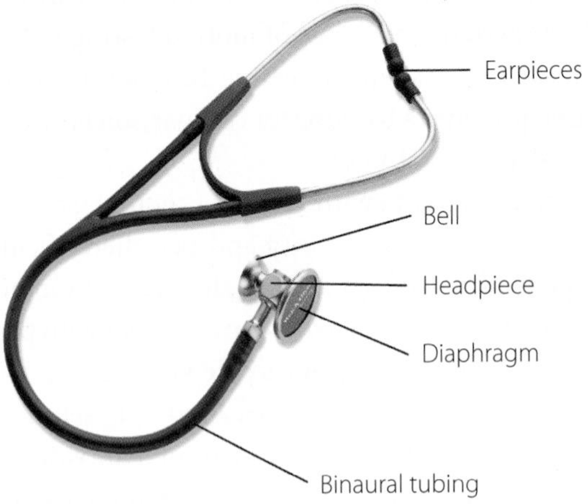

FIGURE 5-3 Labeled stethoscope.
Courtesy of: Welch Allyn.

of the thorax. This approach provides detailed examination (see **FIGURE 5-2**).

AUSCULTATION

Auscultation is completed through the use of a stethoscope.

Stethoscopes (see **FIGURE 5-3**) typically consist of a headset of two earpieces, binaural tubing, and a chestpiece. Chestpieces vary in construction but most commonly have two sides, one with a diaphragm that is best used for identifying higher-frequency sounds such as those found in diastolic murmurs, splitting of sounds, clicks, and ejection sounds.

The other side is the bell, used for identifying lower-frequency sounds such as bruits, S3, and S4. In older-model stethoscopes, the practitioner was advised to avoid placing the thumb on the chestpiece to hold it against the skin, as noise artifact could be experienced. Most chestpieces now rotate, allowing transmission of sound through only one side at a time. The thumb can be placed firmly on the other side without causing artifact.

A simple mistake can significantly reduce clarity of auscultation. The ear canals of adults angle forward between 10 and 20 degrees. When placing the earpieces into the ears, make sure the binaural tubes are adjusted so that they point slightly forward toward the tympanic membranes; otherwise the sound will be transmitted against the ear canal.

Other stethoscope models have tunable diaphragms. When the stethoscope chestpiece is laid lightly against the skin, it functions as a bell, better identifying low-pitched sounds. Applying pressure seals an inner ring, converting it to a diaphragm with better detection of high-pitched sounds.

Stethoscope chestpieces also typically have small (pediatric) and large (adult) sizes. The smaller-diameter chestpieces are also convenient to use over smaller areas of examination such as the carotid arteries.

Auscultation must always be performed on bare skin. As experience is gained, providers begin to take shortcuts, shaving a few seconds off the time taken for examination by auscultating through clothing. This decreases accuracy, introduces aberrant noises, and is poor technique.

Auscultation: technique of physical examination where the provider listens to the internal sounds of the body, which is amplified by the use of a stethoscope

Palpation: technique of physical examination where the provider touches the area being examined to assess such things as temperature, texture, mobility, size, shape, and consistency

PALPATION

Palpation should be performed with the pads of the fingers, where sensory preceptors are richest. The pads should be laid parallel to the surface being palpated. Angling above parallel lifts the pads from the surface, resulting in use of the firmer tips of the fingers, which are less sensitive and more likely to cause discomfort during the examination, especially in soft areas like the abdomen.

Palpation should be done in a circular fashion. Avoid a poking approach where the fingers are pressed in one area and then lifted to an adjacent one. This results in skipped areas, where even a centimeter missed can result in an undetected lesion, with potentially devastating effects such as those of a breast cancer.

Palpation should also be used in attempting to reproduce pain. Utilize the least amount of pressure to reproduce the pain while gradually increasing the force, but not to the point where the technique itself induces pain.

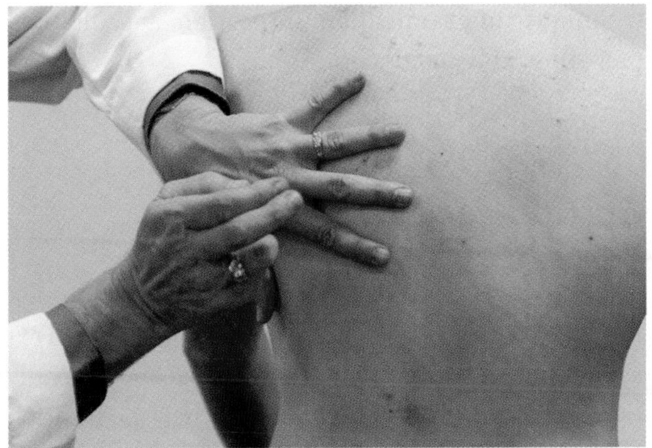

FIGURE 5-4A To perform percussion the provider first places one hand flatly against the area to be examined while hinging the wrist of the opposite hand in preparation of striking the first.

PERCUSSION

Percussion is perhaps the least-utilized technique in physical examination, though it lies hidden in the system examination where it may be overlooked. For example, with the HEENT exam, percussion is used for the detection of sinus tenderness associated with sinusitis. In the neurologic examination, a percussion technique is utilized to reproduce symptoms of cubital or carpal tunnel syndromes.

The percussion technique utilized for the respiratory and abdominal exams (see **FIGURES 5-4A** and **5-4B**) is to place one hand flatly against the chest or abdominal wall with the fingers spread apart. Then using the third digit or a combination of the second and third digit of the other hand the provider sharply strikes the third digit of the outstretched hand while assessing resonance of the area. The action of striking is from the hinged wrist, not the elbow.

5-1 The transmission of the force through the wall allows for detection of density through the resonance created. Gas-filled structures such as the lungs or large bowel resonate with drum-like tympany. Disease states are identified when tympany is increased, such as with a pneumothorax, where lung tissue is collapsed and replaced by air, or decreased, such as when the lungs fill with fluids.

Percussion is also used in the measurement of organs, such as the size of the liver, spleen, or bladder.

While advancing through the order of examination techniques, the provider must perform only those techniques that are necessary for that system.

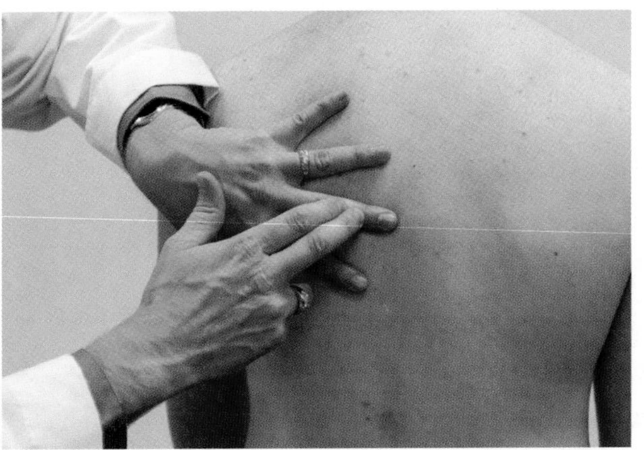

FIGURE 5-4B One digit of the flattened hand is struck sharply as the provider assesses resonance of the created sound.

For example, working in a head-to-toe fashion while examining a patient with abdominal discomfort, you would perform the respiratory system exam prior to reaching the abdomen. First you would inspect the chest. Moving to auscultation, you find that all areas have breath sounds that are full and clear, without adventitious sounds or diminished breath sounds in the bases. Palpation and percussion would not be indicated in this problem-specific case of abdominal pain.

However, if the patient had presented with a cough, a more detailed chest examination would have been appropriate, incorporating all

Percussion: technique of physical examination where the provider places one hand against the patient and uses the other hand to strike the first with a hinged wrist movement in order to assess resonance of the area

techniques of examination: inspection, auscultation, palpation, and percussion.

Complacency in Physical Examination

In addition to the avoidance of taking shortcuts in examination, such as placing the stethoscope centrally over the heart and listening only in that one position instead of over the four valvular areas of auscultation, providers must guard against the tendency to simply go through the motions without actually paying attention to what they are doing.

For example, you listen to the heart and then move on in the exam, only to find yourself thinking, "Wait a minute. I think I heard something." Returning to the area you find a low-grade murmur. If this occurs, you must reset yourself, recognizing the danger of complacency and moving forward with renewed attention to detail.

CHAPTER 6

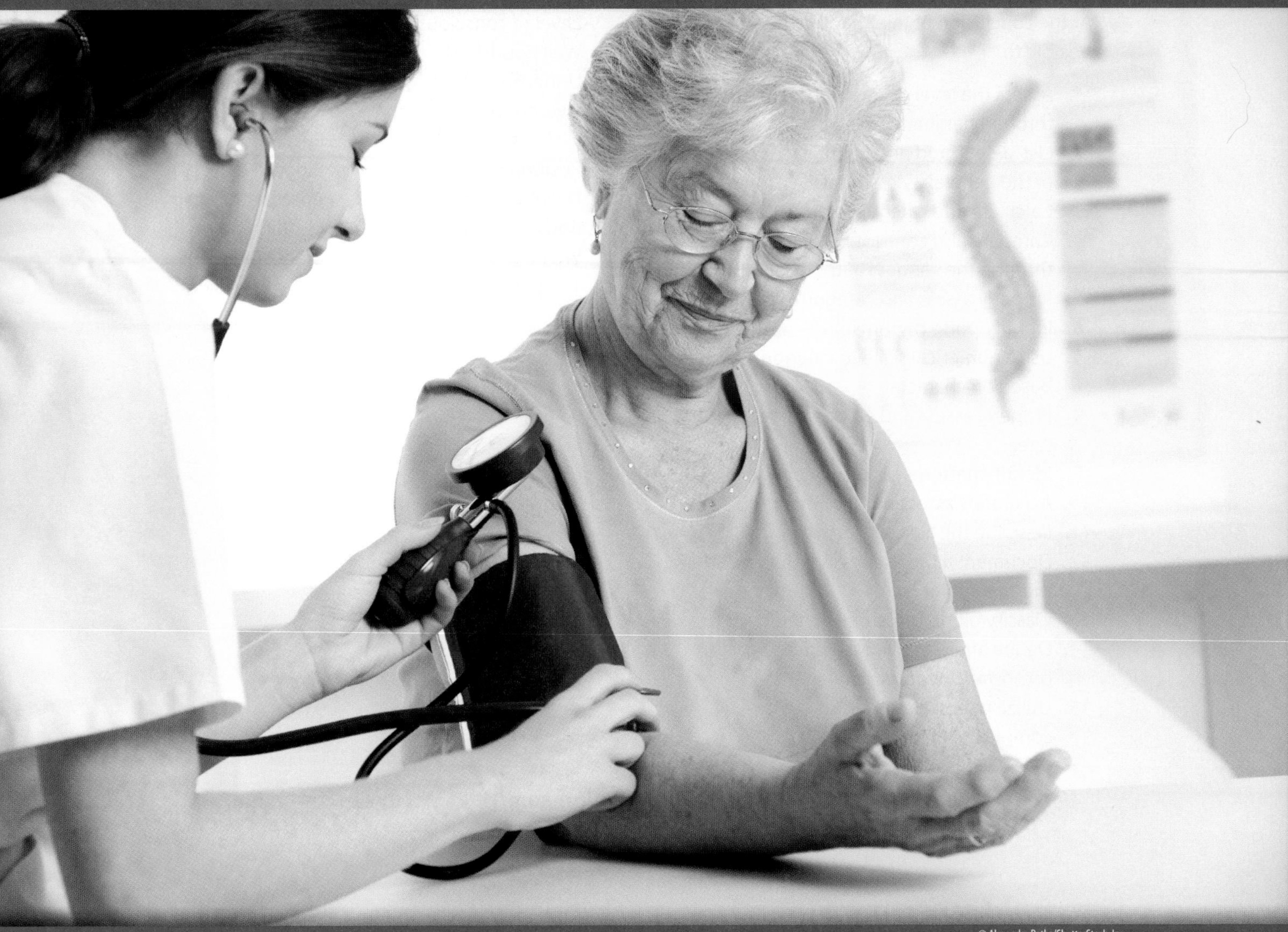

© Alexander Raths/ShutterStock, Inc.

General Assessment and Vital Signs

OBJECTIVES

At the conclusion of this chapter, the student will be able to

1. Assess the level of consciousness of a patient through heightening levels of stimuli
2. List, assess, and document each component of the general assessment
3. Calculate and categorize body mass index
4. Compare and contrast body temperature through the various methods of assessment
5. Properly assess and categorize pulse rates
6. Identify pulse rhythms
7. Use a numerical scale to categorize pulses based on character
8. Properly assess and categorize respiratory rates
9. Identify patterns of respiration
10. Accurately assess blood pressure
11. Describe the auscultatory gap
12. Document a blood pressure that includes a muffling point
13. Classify blood pressures by category
14. Define and perform assessments for orthostatic hypotension
15. Utilize pain scales in assessment of complaints of pain

KEY TERMS

Level of consciousness
Well nourished
Undernourished
Overnourished
Distress
Position of comfort
Development
Body mass index
Vital signs
Temperature
Pyrexia
Hyperthermia
Hypothermia
Pulse
Bradycardia
Tachycardia
Respiration
Respiratory rate
Blood pressure
Auscultatory gap
Muffling point
Orthostatic hypotension
Pain
Pain scale

Where this icon appears, visit **go.jblearning.com/HPECWS** to view the video.

General Assessment

General assessment is interwoven throughout the patient encounter from first observation of the patient through the history gathering and physical examination. It provides a brief assessment of the patient with detailed examination being completed within each system.

LEVEL OF CONSCIOUSNESS

Level of consciousness: the state of arousability, behavior, and response to stimuli

Much confusion has been caused by improper use of terms employed to describe **level of consciousness**. Providers should strive to describe a patient's behavior, arousability, and responses to stimuli rather than attempt to use terminology that often lacks universal acceptance in definition. When assessing level of consciousness, approach the patient with heightening levels of stimuli starting with verbal stimuli, then light touch, and finally painful or noxious stimuli such as the sternal rub, squeezing the trapezius, or pinching the patient's thumbnail between the provider's thumb and index finger.

As standard definitions are often used inappropriately, the provider should instead observe and document eye opening, verbal, and motor responses that occur. It is best to follow descriptives with responses to various stimuli such as, "drowsy but awakens to verbal stimulation, follows simple commands, and falls asleep within a few minutes." "Comatose" should be followed by "no response to verbal or noxious stimulation." Any rudimentary responses such as groaning should be documented.

Examples of documentation of level of stimuli would include:

- Alert to verbal stimuli, answers questions appropriately
- Opens eyes to light touch and follows commands
- Groans with sternal rub
- Unarousable to painful stimuli

NUTRITIONAL STATUS

Within a complete history and physical examination, nutritional status is an approximation of the level of nutrition of the patient. It is not a critical analysis of body mass index or percentile of body fat. Advanced evaluation techniques can be employed when appropriate, such as for the evaluation of nutritional status in hospitalized patients.

A patient's nutritional status affects a wide range of organ systems. Most easily recognized for this general assessment would include the amount of subcutaneous tissue and muscle mass. Edema and ascites may represent significant protein loss and are also easily assessed.

Common categories for documentation of the general nutritional status include:

- **Well nourished**: Appearance suggesting caloric intake over expenditure that allows for preservation of subcutaneous tissues and muscle mass.
- **Undernourished**: Appearance of having overall caloric expenditure greater than intake presented by a body habitus that is underweight and shows loss of subcutaneous tissues and muscle mass. Children and adolescents may also be short of stature. Edema and ascites hallmark severe undernourishment and protein deficiency.
- **Overnourished**: Appearance of having overall caloric intake greater than that of expenditure. Patients present with increase in subcutaneous tissues, visceral adipose, and body weight.

COMPARISON TO STATED AGE

Comparing a patient's stated age to his/her physical appearance allows for an approximation of the cumulative state of health. Though imprecise, it does afford the reader a general appreciation of patient morbidity.

- "Appears younger than the stated age": implies overall higher state of health than others in the same age group as the patient
- "Appears stated age": implies state of health equal to that of others in the same age group
- "Appears older than the stated age": implies a lower state of health than, and past or present morbidity greater than, those of others in the same age group

Again, this is imprecise as someone who has had a high cumulative sun exposure may appear quite advanced in age yet be cardiovascularly fit, running 10 miles a day, and in an excellent state of health.

DISTRESS

Distress in a patient can be on both a physical and an emotional basis.

- Physical pain
  - Somatic: Such as seen with musculoskeletal conditions or trauma. It is often described as sharp or stabbing. This pain is usually very well localized. Patients may demonstrate protective guarding or hesitancy in moving the area. Movement may appear stiff, slow, and purposeful in an attempt to avoid triggering the pain. Facial grimacing may be present that exaggerates urgently when the pain is triggered.
  - Cardiac: Such as seen with acute coronary syndrome. Parasympathetic innervation provides for the perception of more diffuse, vague pain often described as heaviness or pressure. Stimulation of the vagus nerve may result in nausea, vomiting, or sweating.
  - Acute visceral: Such as seen with perforated viscus. Perforation of abdominal

Well nourished: appearance suggesting caloric intake over expenditure that allows for preservation of subcutaneous tissues and muscle mass

Undernourished: appearance of having overall caloric expenditure greater than intake presented by a body habitus that is underweight and shows loss of subcutaneous tissues and muscle mass

Overnourished: appearance of having overall caloric intake greater than that of expenditure

Distress: state of mental or physical suffering

organs such as the gallbladder, appendix, or bowel results in diffuse peritonitis. Movement exacerbates the pain, resulting in the patient attempting to remain still. Respirations are shallow in avoidance of moving the diaphragm. The abdomen is often guarded by the upper extremities and there is hesitancy in allowing examination. Contracture of abdominal muscles results in rigidity. Patients appear in an extreme amount of pain.

- Respiratory Distress
  - Respiratory distress occurs with poor gas exchange. Breathing becomes labored, with increase in respiratory rate, open-mouth breathing, exaggerated chest wall motion, use of accessory muscles, and intercostal retractions. Facial expression may show the patient to be fearful. Cyanosis is more frequently central and is seen in the perioral area. Infants may demonstrate nasal flaring, while children may tripod, leaning forward on outstretched arms in the seated position. Position of comfort is often seated upright with intolerance to supine positioning even for brief examinations. "Abdominal breathing" may occur, with protrusion of the abdomen with each breath.
- Emotional Pain
  - Anxiety and depression are common causes of distress. Facial expressions range from sadness to anguish. Tearfulness, crying, nervousness, apprehension, muted responses, and even hysteria may be encountered.

POSITION OF COMFORT

Position of comfort: body position employed by the patient in an attempt to lessen discomfort

Development: within the general assessment, a comparison of musculoskeletal symmetry and proportion in relation to expected averages for the patient's age, sex, and race

Position of comfort most commonly accompanies pain. Patients favor contralateral sides when discomfort is encountered. This reflective mechanism attempts to avoid additional pressure, stress, or pain on the affected area.

Abdominal pain often results in flexion at the waist and rotation toward the side of pain, splinting around the area in avoidance of stretching it.

Restlessness also may be seen, such as with nephrolithiasis, wherein patients report an inability to find a position of comfort.

Patients in respiratory distress may show an exaggerated upright seated position with cervical lordosis and jaw thrust.

DEVELOPMENT

Under general assessment, notation of **development** is a brief observation of the musculoskeletal development of the patient. A general survey of head-to-body proportion, extremity length, muscle mass, and height is sufficient. Detailed examination is completed with the musculoskeletal assessment.

SKIN COLORATION

Assess the patient's generalized color. Particular attention should be made to note diffuse pallor, which may reflect anemia, cyanosis for hypooxygenation, jaundice for hyperbilirubinemia, erythema for polycythemia, infection, drug reaction, or carbon monoxide poisoning, all of which may require acute intervention.

The patient's skin type should be noted for likelihood of skin lesion prevalence, which will later guide the integumentary examination.

HYGIENE

Hygiene can be a reflection of the overall health of the patient. Poor hygiene may equate to self-neglect in more than grooming; poor preventive care and compliance are also suggested. Poor grooming, malodor, and halitosis may be signs of medical conditions or an inability to care for oneself.

Providers may find it difficult to discuss poor hygiene for fear of insulting the patient, as patients with malodor are often unaware that they have it.

- "Jim, I wanted to ask if you were having any difficulty taking care of yourself."
  - "No, I do okay."
- "I asked because our health can be affected by the way we take care of ourselves. I'm a little concerned because it doesn't appear you showered

or washed your clothes today. Do you find you're having difficulty doing those things?"

This concern was presented by relating health issues and grooming to an inquiry about the ability of the patient to care for himself.

DOCUMENTATION

- General Assessment: Alert, well developed and well nourished (wdwn), appropriately groomed with light tan complexion, seated on the examination table in no apparent distress.

Height and Weight

Height and weight measurements are required for calculation of body mass index and identification of ideal body weight as well as underweight and overweight conditions. In children these routine measurements document appropriate growth. Weight measurements are also important in the monitoring of disease conditions in which the status of fluid balance is imperative, such as heart and renal failure.

Conversion of typical U.S. measurements of pounds and inches to kilograms and centimeters (see **TABLE 6-1**) is essential for calculation of medication dosages.

- Height: measure in centimeters (cm) or convert inches to cm
  - Centimeters = inches × 2.54 centimeters/inch
  - Example: 6 feet 1 inches converted to centimeters
    - Convert feet to inches
      - (6 feet × 12 inches/foot) + 1 inches
      - 72 + 1 = 73 inches
    - Convert inches to centimeters
      - Centimeters = inches × 2.54 centimeters/inch
      - Centimeters = 73 inches × 2.54 cm/inch
      - Centimeters = 185.42 cm
- Weight: measure in kilograms (kg) or convert pounds (lbs) to kg
  - Pounds = kilograms × 2.2
    - Kilograms = pounds/2.2
  - Example: 180-pound male converted to kg
    - Kilograms = pounds/2.2
    - Kilograms = 180/2.2
    - Kilograms = 81.8 kg

BODY MASS INDEX

Body mass index (BMI): an approximation of the amount of body fat, used to categorize patients along a range from severely underweight to obese

Body mass index (BMI) is an approximation of the amount of body fat and is used to categorize patients along a range from severely underweight to obese, allowing providers to recognize these conditions and provide interventions where appropriate. (See **TABLE 6-2**.) Individual consideration must be given for BMI measurements in that certain characteristics may result in incorrectly categorizing patients as obese when they are not, such as individuals who have increased body weight due to muscle conditioning (for example, weightlifters).

BMI is calculated as follows:

$$\text{BMI} = \frac{\text{weight (kilograms)}}{(\text{height (m)})^2} = \text{kg/m}^2$$

For example, calculating the BMI for a 6′ 1″ male who weighs 180 pounds:

- BMI = weight in kg/(height (m))^2
  - Convert weight in pounds to kilograms
    - kg = 180 lbs/2.2 = 81.8
  - Convert height in inches to meters
    - m = 6′1″ × 2.54
    - m = 73″ × 2.54
    - m = 1.85
  - Calculate BMI
    - BMI = kg/m^2
    - BMI = 81.8/(1.85)^2
    - BMI = 81.8/3.43
    - BMI = 23.8

The calculated BMI for this patient would put him into the Healthy Weight category.

An alternative formula using pounds and inches without conversion may be used.

- BMI = weight in pounds/(height in inches)^2 × 703
- Using the same example:
  - BMI = 180 lbs/(73 inches)^2 × 703
  - BMI = 180 lbs/5329 × 703
  - BMI = 0.033 × 703
  - BMI = 23.8

TABLE 6-1 Height and Weight Conversion Table

Pound to Kilogram		Inch to Centimeter and Meter				
Pounds	**Kilograms**	**Feet (′) Inches (″)**		**Total Inches**	**Centimeters**	**Meters**
lbs	**kg**	**ft**	**in**	**in**	**cm**	**m**
80	36	3	7	43	109	1.09
85	39	3	8	44	112	1.12
90	41	3	9	45	114	1.14
95	43	3	10	46	117	1.17
100	45	3	11	47	119	1.19
105	48	4	0	48	122	1.22
110	50	4	1	49	124	1.24
115	52	4	2	50	127	1.27
120	55	4	3	51	130	1.30
125	57	4	4	52	132	1.32
130	59	4	5	53	135	1.35
135	61	4	6	54	137	1.37
140	64	4	7	55	140	1.40
145	66	4	8	56	142	1.42
150	68	4	9	57	145	1.45
155	70	4	10	58	147	1.47
160	73	4	11	59	150	1.50
165	75	5	0	60	152	1.52
170	77	5	1	61	155	1.55
175	80	5	2	62	157	1.57
180	82	5	3	63	160	1.60
185	84	5	4	64	163	1.63
190	86	5	5	65	165	1.65
195	89	5	6	66	168	1.68
200	91	5	7	67	170	1.70
205	93	5	8	68	173	1.73
210	95	5	9	69	175	1.75
215	98	5	10	70	178	1.78
220	100	5	11	71	180	1.80
225	102	6	0	72	183	1.83
230	105	6	1	73	185	1.85
235	107	6	2	74	188	1.88
240	109	6	3	75	191	1.91
245	111	6	4	76	193	1.93
250	114	6	5	77	196	1.96

TABLE 6-2 Body Mass Index[1]

Body Mass Index—kg/m²	
Underweight	Less than 18.5
Healthy weight	18.5 to 24.9
Overweight	25 to 29.9
Obese—Class 1	30 to 34.9
Obese—Class 2	35 to 39.9
Obese—Class 3	Over 40

Source: National Institutes of Health. National Heart, Lung, and Blood Institute. Clinical Guidelines on the Identification, Evaluation, and Treatment of Overweight and Obesity in Adults: The Evidence Report. http://www.nhlbi.nih.gov/guidelines/obesity/ob_gdlns.pdf. Published September 1998. Accessed January 20, 2012.

Vital Signs

Vital signs consist of measurements of temperature, pulse, respirations, blood pressure, and pain.

TEMPERATURE

Formulas for converting between Fahrenheit and Celsius (see **TABLE 6-3**) are:

$$°F = °C \times 9/5 + 32$$

$$°C = (°F - 32) \times 5/9$$

TABLE 6-3 Temperature Conversion Chart—Degrees Fahrenheit (F) to Celsius (C)

F	C	F	C	F	C
98.0	36.7	100.0	37.8	102.0	38.9
98.1	36.7	100.1	37.8	102.1	39.0
98.2	36.8	100.2	37.9	102.2	39.0
98.3	36.8	100.3	37.9	102.3	39.1
98.4	36.9	100.4	38.0	102.4	39.1
98.5	36.9	100.5	38.1	102.6	39.2
98.6	37.0	100.6	38.1	102.7	39.3
98.7	37.1	100.7	38.2	102.8	39.3
98.8	37.1	100.8	38.2	102.9	39.4
98.9	37.2	100.9	38.3	103.0	39.4
99.0	37.2	101.0	38.3	103.1	39.5
99.1	37.3	101.1	38.4	103.2	39.6
99.2	37.3	101.2	38.4	103.3	39.6
99.3	37.4	101.3	38.5	103.4	39.7
99.4	37.4	101.4	38.6	103.5	39.7
99.5	37.5	101.5	38.6	103.7	39.8
99.6	37.6	101.6	38.7	103.8	39.9
99.7	37.6	101.7	38.7	103.9	39.9
99.8	37.7	101.8	38.8	104.0	40.0
99.9	37.7	101.9	38.8	104.1	40.1

There are multiple, common methods for assessment of body temperature, including oral, rectal, axillary, tympanic, and temporal artery.

Oral temperatures have long been the most common method of body temperature measurement. A normal oral body temperature of 98.6 degrees Fahrenheit (F) or 37 degrees Celsius (C) was first proposed by German physician Carl Wunderlich in the nineteenth century. The normal value has since been adjusted to 98.2 degrees F and 36.8 degrees C.[2]

Taking an oral temperature requires the patient to be old enough to be able to understand and comply with the need to hold the probe under the tongue. Glass thermometers that require cleaning between uses have largely been replaced with electronic units with disposable probe covers (see **FIGURE 6-1**).

Rectal thermometry utilizes the insertion of the probe into the rectum and represents a more accurate reflection of core body temperature, measuring approximately 1 degree F higher than an oral temperature. Glass thermometers should be avoided due to the risk of breakage and patient injury.

Axillary temperature taking, wherein the probe is placed in the axilla, is a useful method in infants and

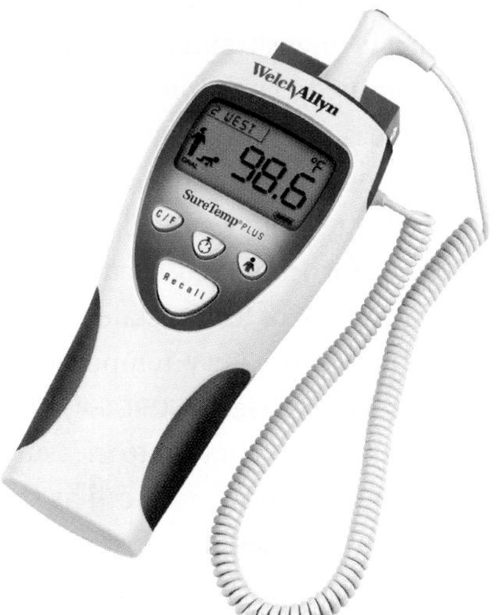

FIGURE 6-1 Electronic thermometer.

Vital signs: measurements of the patient's temperature, pulse, respirations, blood pressure, and pain in assessment of basic functioning and need for urgency in treatment intervention

Temperature: amount of heat maintained by the body, most frequently measured in Fahrenheit or Celsius

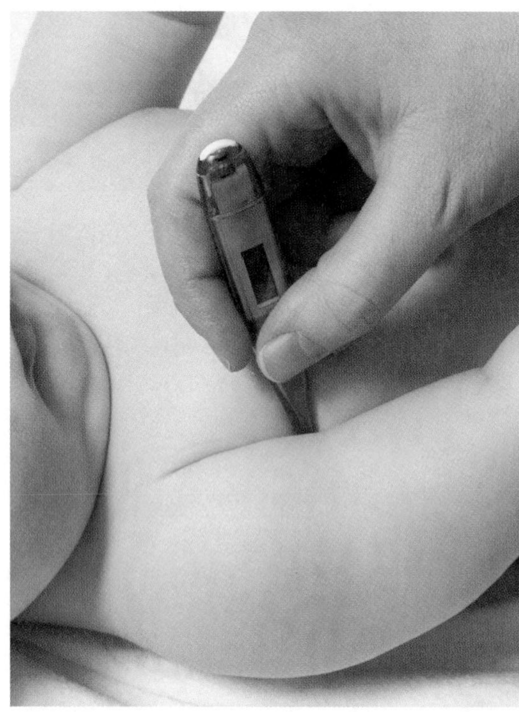

FIGURE 6-2 Taking an axillary temperature on an infant.
© fred goldstein/ShutterStock, Inc.

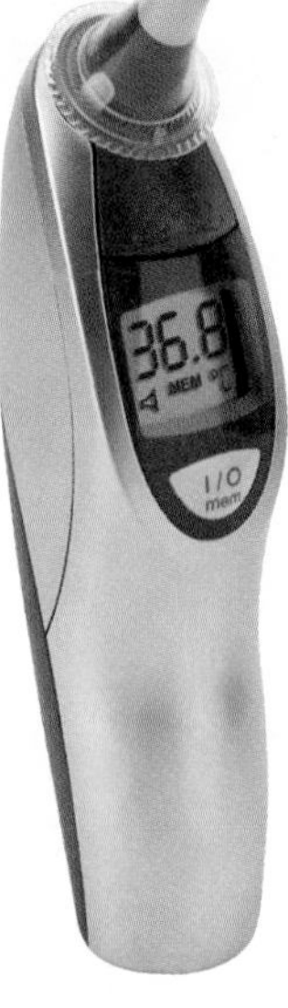

FIGURE 6-3A Tympanic thermometer.

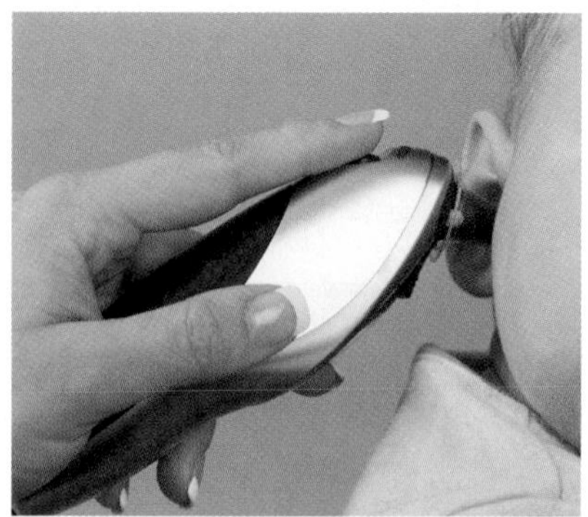

FIGURE 6-3B Taking a tympanic temperature on an infant.

children due to ease of use and better tolerance by the patient, but it offers a measurement that is approximately 1 degree F lower than the oral measurements (see **FIGURE 6-2**).

Tympanic membrane (TM) measurements utilize infrared technology to measure the amount of heat produced by the tympanic membrane and are close to core temperatures (see **FIGURE 6-3A** and **B**). This technique relies on operator competency. If the measurement is directed at the ear canal instead of the TM, accurate measurements will not be obtained. Therefore the use of TM measurements may be appropriate for experienced individuals, but other techniques should be considered for improved accuracy in management of febrile states.

Pyrexia: elevated body temperature, also referred to as fever, most commonly associated with inflammation and infection resulting in an elevation of the body's temperature set point

Hyperthermia: elevation of body temperature that is not caused by fever but rather the inability of the body to dissipate heat, commonly related to certain medications, drugs, and heatstroke

Temporal artery temperature measurements (see **FIGURE 6-4**) also use infrared technology to measure the amount of heat produced by the temporal arteries. The instrument head is run over the forehead along the temporal artery and takes only seconds to perform. The extreme ease and speed of use make these thermometers useful in standard screening, such as in immediate postoperative states. For improved precision, other techniques should again be utilized for febrile states.

Fever, **pyrexia**, is elevated body temperature most commonly associated with inflammation and infection resulting in an elevation of the body's temperature set point. **Hyperthermia** is elevation of body

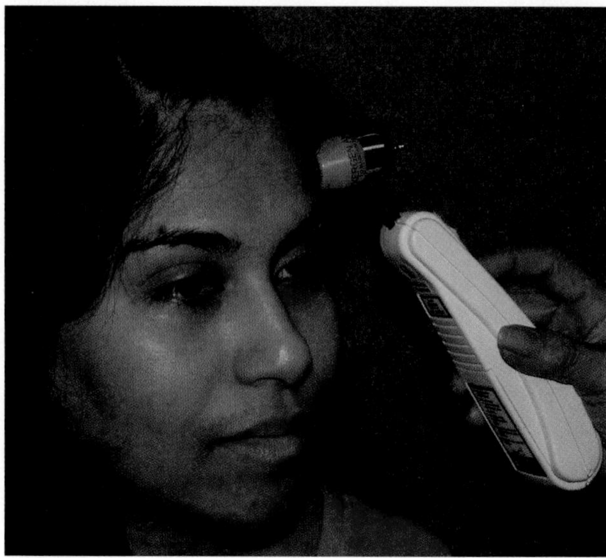

FIGURE 6-4 A temporal artery temperature uses infrared technology and is taken by dragging the thermometer over the temporal artery.

temperature that is not caused by fever but rather the inability of the body to dissipate heat, commonly related to certain medications, drugs, and heatstroke. Hyperpyrexia refers to an extremely elevated body temperature.

Hypothermia refers to lower than normal body temperature, most commonly as a result of environmental exposure.

PULSE

Pulse is typically palpated at the radial artery, laying the pads of the fingers parallel to the skin surface and avoiding use of the tips of the fingers in perpendicular positioning (see **FIGURE 6-5**). Also avoid using the thumb, since the provider's pulse may be mistaken for that of the patient. Extension of the wrist helps to bring the radial artery to a more superficial position. Palpate at the distal radius and metacarpal junction, avoiding positioning the finger pads too proximally where the radial artery is deeper.

Pulse in smaller children can be assessed at the brachial artery. Infant pulse can be checked at the femoral artery. Carotids may also be palpated for pulse assessment. This should be done lightly in aging patients after auscultation for bruits.

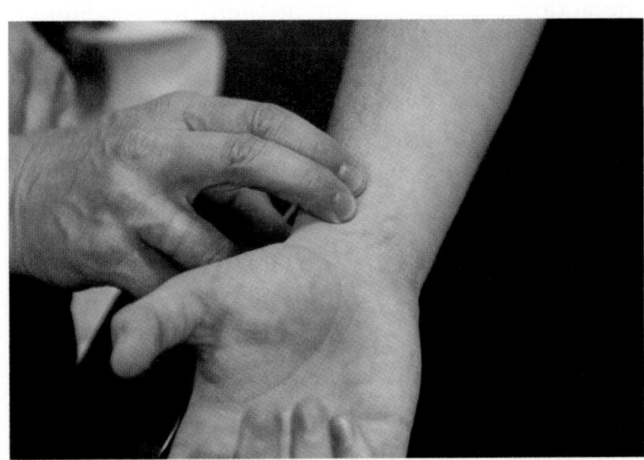

FIGURE 6-5 Radial artery palpation.

- Rate—Count number of pulses for 15 seconds and multiply by 4
  - Normal heart rate: between 60 and 100 beats per minute
  - **Bradycardia**: slow pulse—pulse rate < 60 per minute
    - Examples: athletic conditioning, sick sinus syndrome, increased intracranial pressure, hypothyroidism, hypothermia, medications that block sympathetic nerve conduction, such as beta blockers
  - **Tachycardia**: rapid pulse—pulse rate > 100 beats per minute
    - Examples: fever, hyperthyroidism, anxiety, anemia, exertion, pulmonary embolism, fear, acute coronary syndrome, stimulant medications or drugs
- Rhythm
  - Regular: each beat occurs at a regular interval from the previous beat
    - Examples: AV nodal or junctional rhythms
  - Regularly irregular: irregular beats occur with predicted regularity
    - Examples: bigeminy and trigeminy
  - Irregularly irregular: no pattern of beats is present
    - Classic for atrial fibrillation
- Character—refers to strength of pulse (see **TABLE 6-4**). These are documented on a scale from 0, absent pulse, to 4, bounding pulse. The character

Hypothermia: lower than normal body temperature, most commonly as a result of environmental exposure

Pulse: the palpable perception of throbbing as blood moves through the arterial system as a result of left ventricle contraction

Bradycardia: a pulse rate of less than 60 beats per minute

Tachycardia: a pulse rate greater than 100 beats per minute

TABLE 6-4 Pulse Character

Pulse Description	Scale	Examples
Absent: nonpalpable	0	Asystole, thrombosis, or occlusion
Weak: diminished amplitude, may have difficulty locating	1	Stenosis, left ventricular failure, hypovolemia, anemia, dehydration
Normal: readily palpable	2	Hemodynamic stability
Strong: increased amplitude, quickly palpable	3	Anxiety, mild exertion, caffeine
Bounding	4	Fever, strenuous exercise, fear, cocaine

Respiration: a breath consisting of two phases: inspiration and expiration

Respiratory rate: number of respirations per minute

of the pulse is an estimation of the amount of blood ejected into the arterial system through left ventricular contraction minus any obstruction of arterial flow. An abnormality that decreases the amount of blood or obstructs the flow of blood to the peripheral artery diminishes the pulse. Anything that increases ventricular contraction or the amount of blood ejected per contraction increases the pulse strength.

RESPIRATIONS

A normal breath or **respiration** in a healthy adult at rest is composed of an inspiratory and an expiratory phase that are equal in length (see **FIGURE 6-6**).

Technique

Respiratory breathing patterns and rates are controlled by both voluntary and involuntary musculature. If you announce to a patient that you intend to count his/her respirations, the patient may consciously or subconsciously alter the pattern or rate, not as an intentionally misleading gesture but because he/she knows you are focused on that area. For this reason, a distraction technique should be employed. Count respirations by combining the technique with that of checking his/her pulse. Advise the patient that you will be checking their pulse. Sit beside the patient, and raise your arm on which you wear your watch so that the watch rests in a line of vision between your eyes and the patient's chest. Palpate the radial artery with your opposite hand. Instead of counting the pulse, for the first 30 seconds count each rise of the chest seen in your peripheral vision just slightly above your watch. You may lightly rest your elevated forearm against the lateral shoulder of the patient to add tactile perception of the inspiration (see **FIGURE 6-7**).

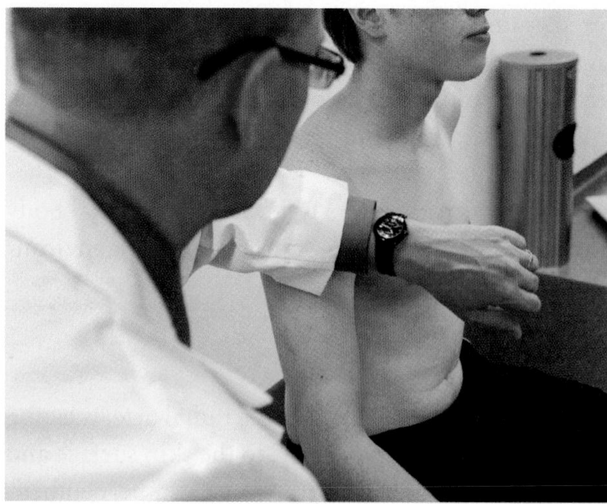

FIGURE 6-7 Distraction technique for assessing respiratory rate where the provider counts respirations by observing the rise of the chest wall and lightly placing a forearm against the patient's shoulder.

Avoid sitting directly in front of female patients using this technique as, should they see you intermittently glancing over your wrist, they might mistake the action as your looking at their breasts. Should this occur, simply explain that you are counting their respirations.

When examining the patient, take note of the rate, pattern, and depth of the respirations.

Rate

- **Respiratory Rate**—count the number of breaths for 30 seconds and multiply by 2 to get the rate of breaths per minute (bmp).
  - Eupnea (see **FIGURE 6-8**): normal respiratory rate of adults at rest—12 to 20 bpm
  - Bradypnea (see **FIGURE 6-9**): slow breathing—< 12 bpm—count for full 60 seconds

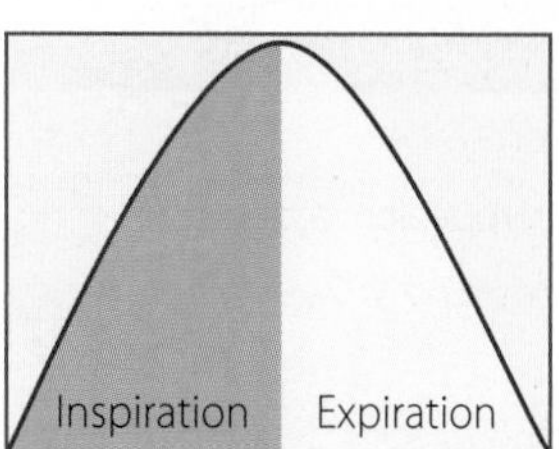

FIGURE 6-6 Respiratory phases.

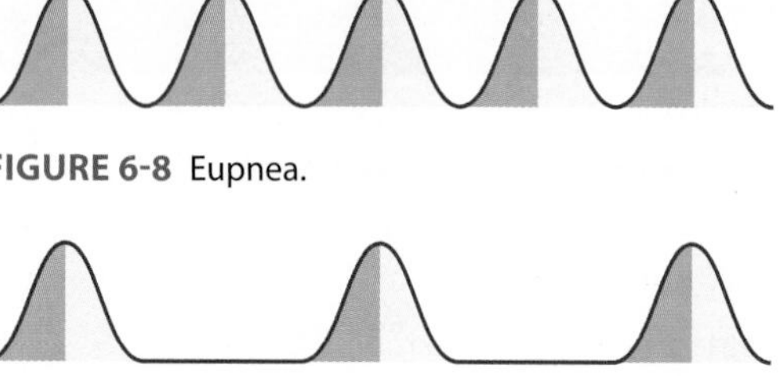

FIGURE 6-8 Eupnea.

FIGURE 6-9 Bradypnea.

- Examples: athletic conditioning, depressant medications or drugs, hypothermia
- Tachypnea (see **FIGURE 6-10**): rapid breathing—> 20 bpm—count for a full 60 seconds.
  - Examples: Acidosis, fever, exertion, anxiety, fear, carbon monoxide poisoning

Depth

- Depth—note abnormalities of depth of inspiration
  - Shallow
  - Deep

Pattern

- Pattern—observe the pattern of respirations
  - Apneustic (see **FIGURE 6-11**): inspiratory phase longer than expiratory phase
    - Example: Brainstem damage
  - Obstructive Pattern (see **FIGURE 6-12**): expiration phase longer than inspiratory phase
    - Examples: Asthma, COPD
  - Restrictive Pattern (see **FIGURE 6-13**): shallow inspirations that become rapid with exertion
    - Examples: restrictive lung diseases

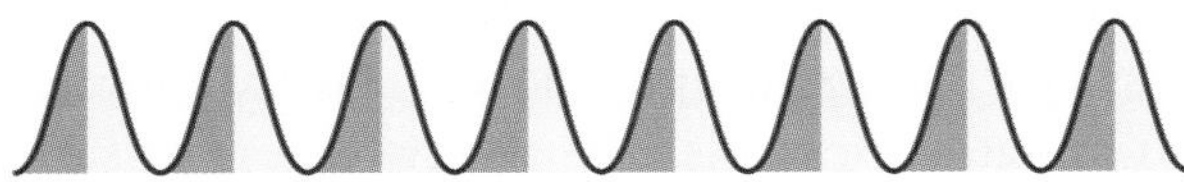

FIGURE 6-10 Tachypnea.

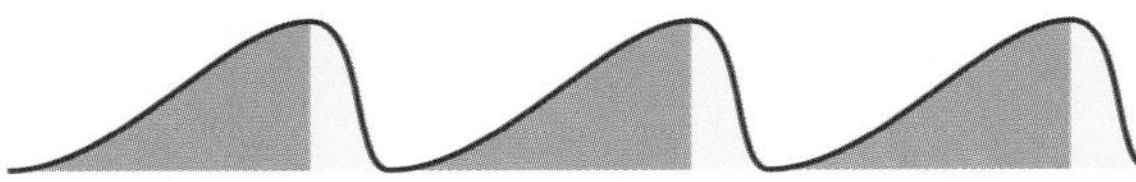

FIGURE 6-11 Apneustic.

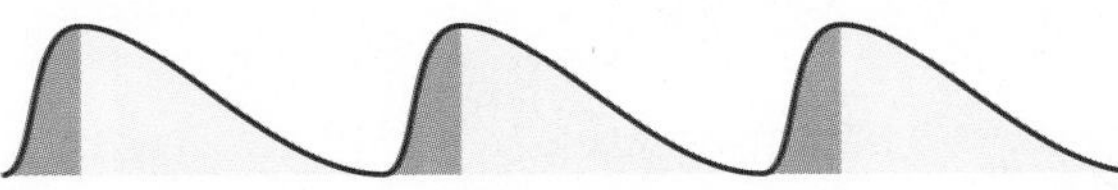

FIGURE 6-12 Obstructive pattern.

FIGURE 6-13 Restrictive pattern.

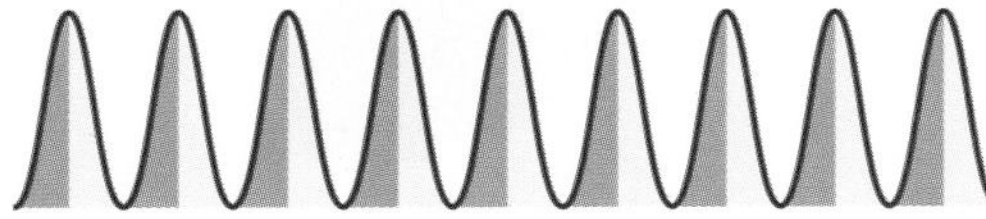

FIGURE 6-14 Hyperpnea.

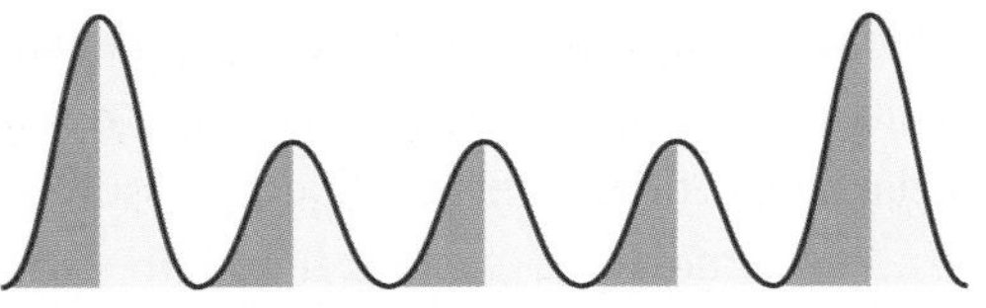

FIGURE 6-15 Sighing.

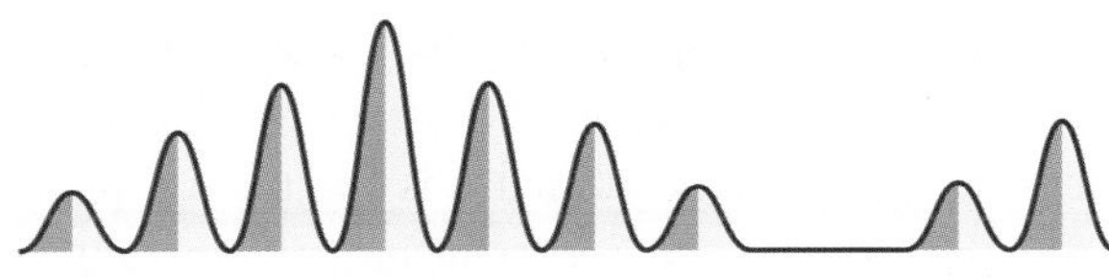

FIGURE 6-16 Cheyne-Stokes.

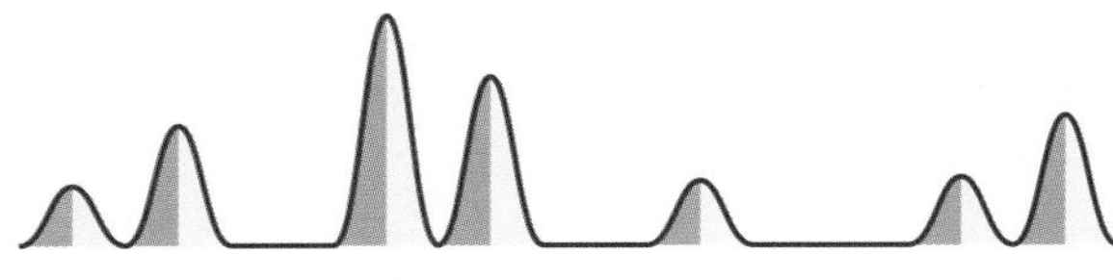

FIGURE 6-17 Ataxic.

- Hyperpnea (see **FIGURE 6-14**)—rapid, deep inspirations
  - Examples: pain, respiratory distress, acidosis, hysteria
  - Kussmaul: deep gasping respirations such as found in diabetic acidosis
- Sighing (see **FIGURE 6-15**): deep inspirations with the breathing pattern
  - Examples: normal variant if occasional
- Cheyne-Stokes (see **FIGURE 6-16**): increasing then decreasing amplitude of respiration with periods of apnea
  - Examples: depression of the frontal lobe
- Ataxic (see **FIGURE 6-17**)—irregular, unpredictable pattern with periods of apnea
  - Examples: meningitis, increased intracranial pressure

BLOOD PRESSURE

Competency in measuring **blood pressure** is more than obtaining a measurement to document in the chart. The consequences of untreated high blood pressure (hypertension) can be devastating: heart attack, stroke, and renal failure.

The measurement of arterial blood pressure is an estimation of

Blood pressure: the pressure of blood against the arterial vascular system consisting of two components: systolic, the measure of pressure at the peak of left ventricular contraction, and diastolic, the measure of pressure during left ventricular relaxation

the force of blood on the wall of the artery. It is affected by contractility of the heart, peripheral vascular resistance, and elasticity of the arteries. Blood pressure is measured and documented as systolic blood pressure over diastolic blood pressure: for example, 130/72.

The systolic measurement is the pressure of the blood on the arterial wall at the peak of left ventricular contraction as perfusion of the peripheral arteries occurs. Diastolic blood pressure is the resting pressure on the arterial wall, occurring during ventricular relaxation.

Equipment needed:

- Stethoscope
- Sphygmomanometer

Sphygmomanometer

Sphygmomanometers (see **FIGURE 6-18**) are instruments used in the measurement of blood pressure. There are two types: mercury manometers, which are larger units that maintain the accuracy of their calibration, and aneroid manometers, which are commonly smaller, handheld units that require intermittent recalibration. These manometers attach via a valve and bulb to an inflatable bladder inside a cuff that wraps around the extremity.

The manometer is a gauge that is marked in millimeters of mercury (mmHg). The needle points to the corresponding mmHg of pressure being exerted when the cuff is inflated. The valve allows for inflation of the bladder when closed and deflation when opened.

The cuff containing the bladder is labeled with an artery marker that is to be placed over the artery. This marker is at the midpoint of the bladder, allowing for appropriate compression of the vessel. If the bladder is misaligned so that the artery is not centered but is toward the edge, the cuff must be overinflated to compress the artery, resulting in a falsely elevated reading.

Cuffs are also marked with ranges to assure the use of proper-size cuffs. The bladder must encircle 80% of the arm. When wrapping the cuff around the arm, the artery marker must fall within the range markers. If the artery marker falls short of the markers, the cuff is too small and a larger cuff should be chosen. Using a cuff that is too small again results in a falsely elevated blood pressure. If the artery marker wraps beyond the range, the cuff is too large and a small cuff should be chosen to avoid a falsely low blood pressure.

Mechanism of Action

Auscultation of a peripheral artery is normally silent. Heartbeats are typically heard only when turbulence from a partial obstruction is present, such as with significant atherosclerosis. The ability to hear a heartbeat while auscultating a peripheral artery during

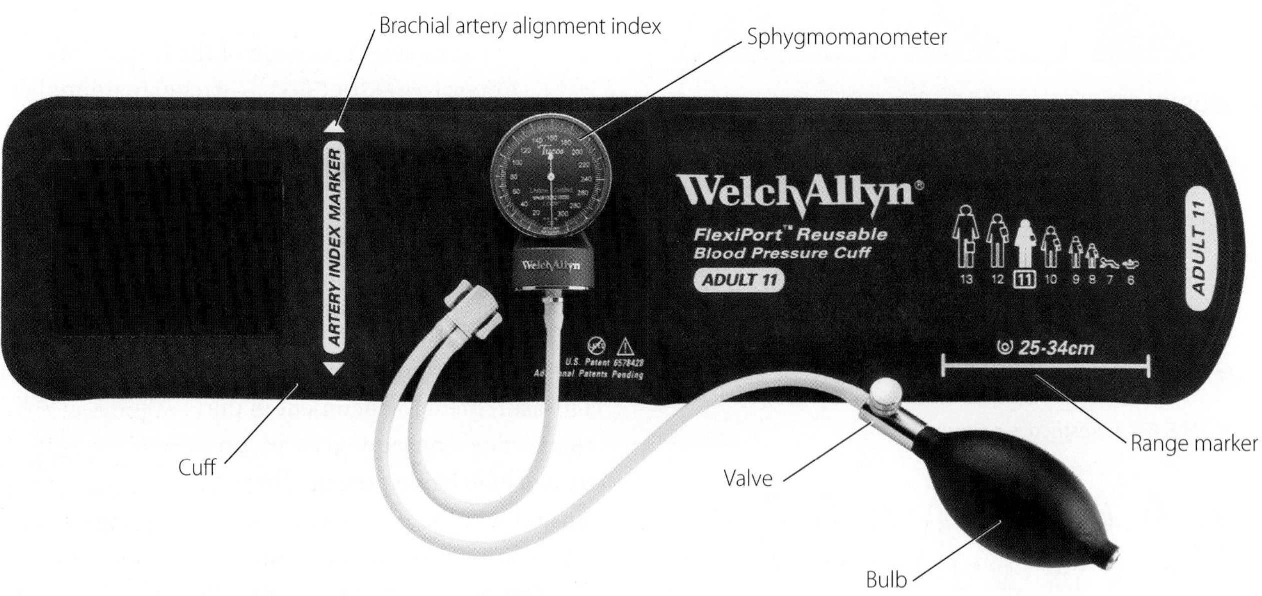

FIGURE 6-18 Sphygmomanometer and blood pressure cuff.
Courtesy of: Welch Allyn

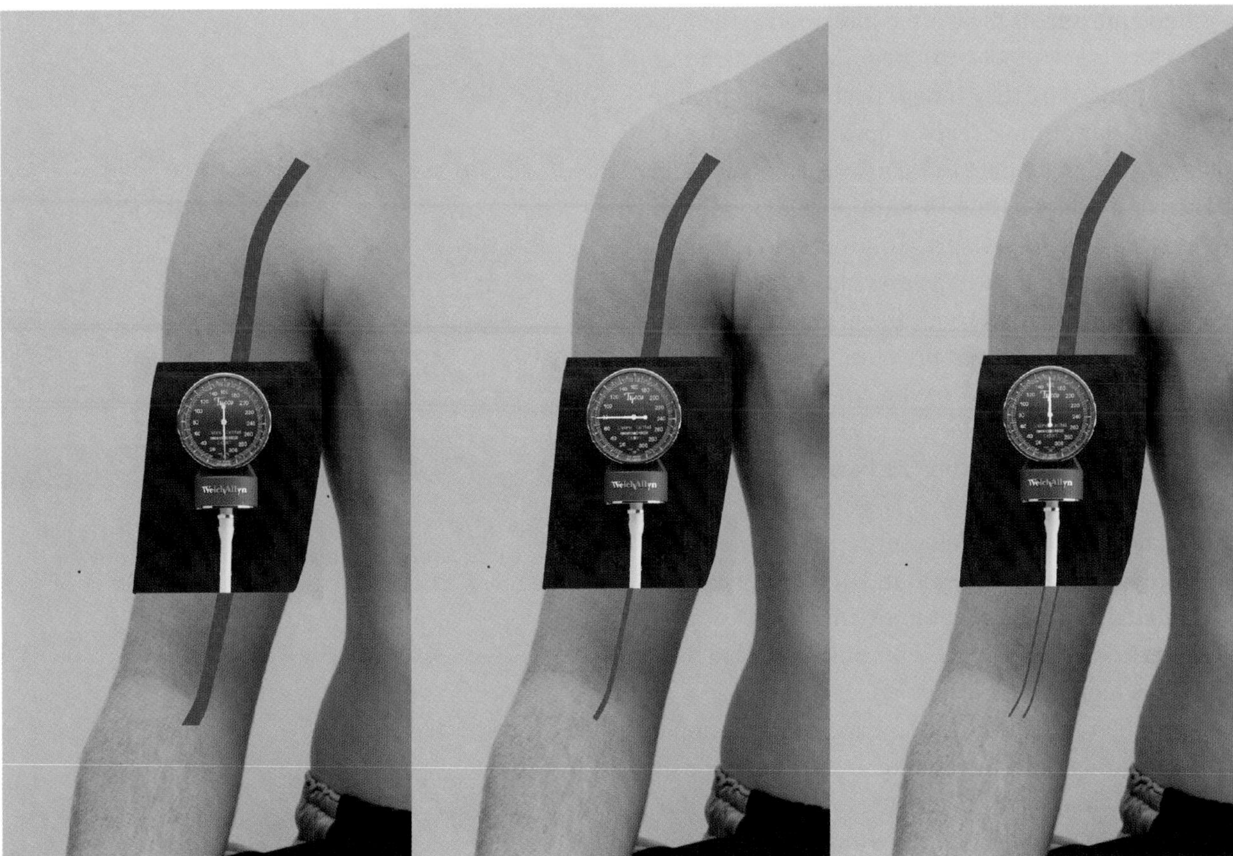

No occlusion of arterial flow. Pulse is readily felt but cannot be ausculatated.

Cuff is being inflated. Partial occlusion of arterial flow. Pulse becomes weak and partial occlusion allows for auscultation of pulse.

Cuff is inflated higher than maximum left ventricular pressure. Artery is collapsed. Pulse cannot be palpated or auscultated.

FIGURE 6-19 Blood pressure mechanism of action.

measurements of blood pressure is a result of creating partial obstruction of the flow of blood as it pulses through the artery during ventricular contraction (see **FIGURE 6-19**). This partial obstruction is generated by the external pressure of the blood pressure cuff as it is inflated. For this reason, prior to taking a blood pressure, you must locate a brachial artery by palpation rather than by auscultation. Once located, the blood pressure cuff is applied to the arm and the head of the stethoscope placed over the artery in the antecubital fossa.

Technique

Vital signs are often completed by ancillary office staff such as medical assistants prior to the provider's seeing the patient. Common practice is to escort the patient to the examining room and immediately assess the vital signs, including the blood pressure. Blood pressures, however, should be taken only after the patient has been seated for five minutes, and office staff performing the screens should be instructed to refrain from taking the blood pressure until five minutes of rest has been assured. It behooves the provider to repeat blood pressures when elevated screens have been documented to assure compliance with this guideline.

Patients should also be asked about nicotine or caffeine use within the prior 30 minutes, as elevations of blood pressure can occur. If the blood pressure cuff about to be used contains latex, patients must also be asked about latex allergies. Finally, before taking the blood pressure, ask patients if there are any restrictions to taking a blood pressure in either arm, such as their having had mastectomies or arteriovenous shunts for dialysis.

Blood pressure is most often measured at the brachial artery (see FIGURE 6-20). Begin with an arm free of restrictions. Bare the arm, preferably by having the arm taken out of the sleeve or gown. Sleeves should not be pushed up to bare the arm as them may cause constriction of blood flow. In addition, it is poor practice to place a blood pressure cuff over any clothing.

Have patients sit with their wrists on their thighs. Palpate the brachial artery in the arm on which you are about to take the blood pressure. The brachial artery is most commonly located medially to the biceps tendon. To palpate the artery, first lay the pads of your index and middle finger on the biceps tendon, then slide medially over the tendon, pressing more deeply toward the humerus. Search gently around the area if the pulse is not immediately found. If difficulty is still encountered, ask the patient to extend his/her arm at the elbow while you palpate. This pushes the brachial artery to a more superficial position.

The blood pressure cuff is now applied to the upper arm by aligning the artery marker over the previously palpated brachial artery, being sure to keep the edge of the cuff approximately 5 cm proximal to the antecubital fossa. This allows placement of the stethoscope head away from the cuff edge so that sound distortion from the cuff rubbing against the head is avoided.

Ensure that the appropriate cuff size is being used by confirming that the artery marker falls within the range markers on the cuff (see FIGURES 6-21A, 6-21B, and 6-21C).

It is important to apply the cuff snugly. Ask the patient for assistance in applying the cuff by having

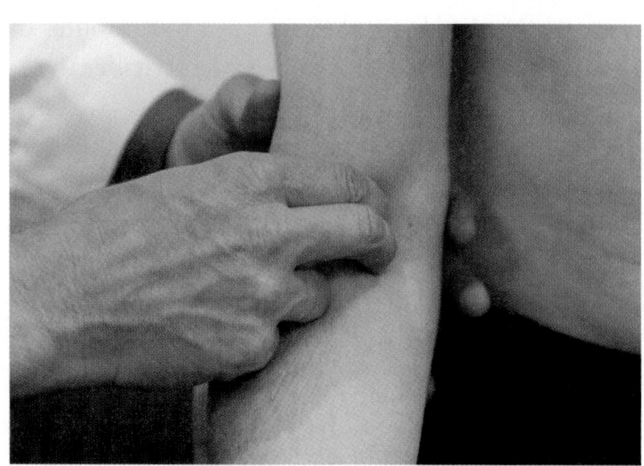

FIGURE 6-20 Deep brachial artery palpation.

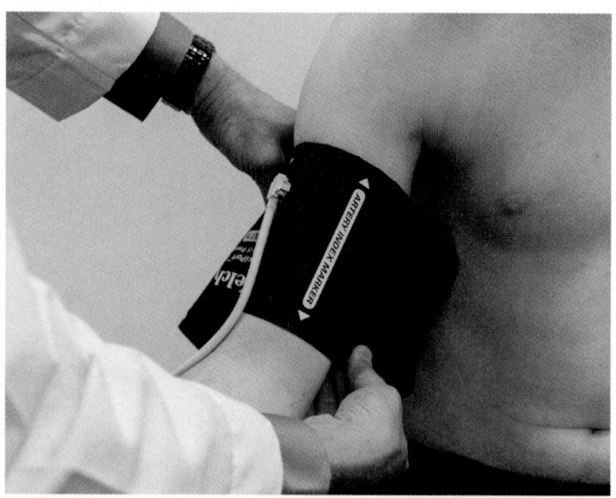

FIGURE 6-21A To ensure that the appropriately sized blood pressure cuff is used, the artery index is first aligned over the brachial artery.

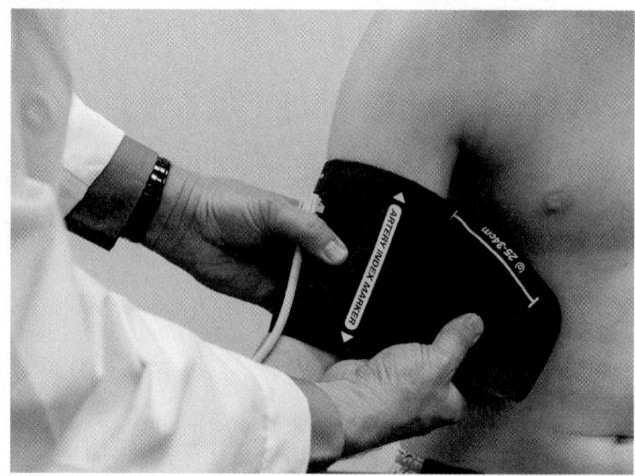

FIGURE 6-21B The provider wraps the cuff around the arm so that the range marker comes into view.

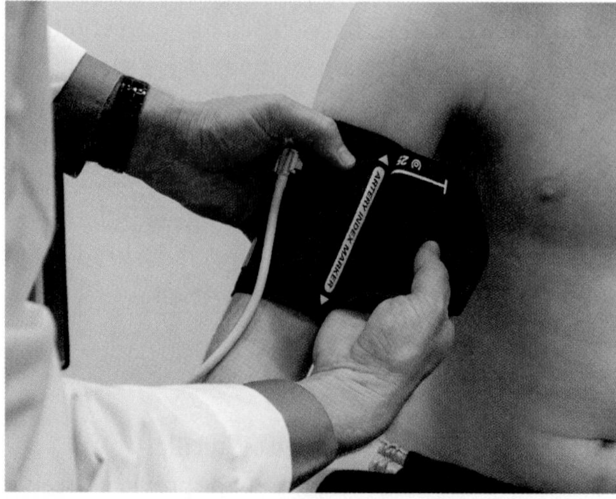

FIGURE 6-21C The correct cuff size is ensured when the artery index falls within the range marker.

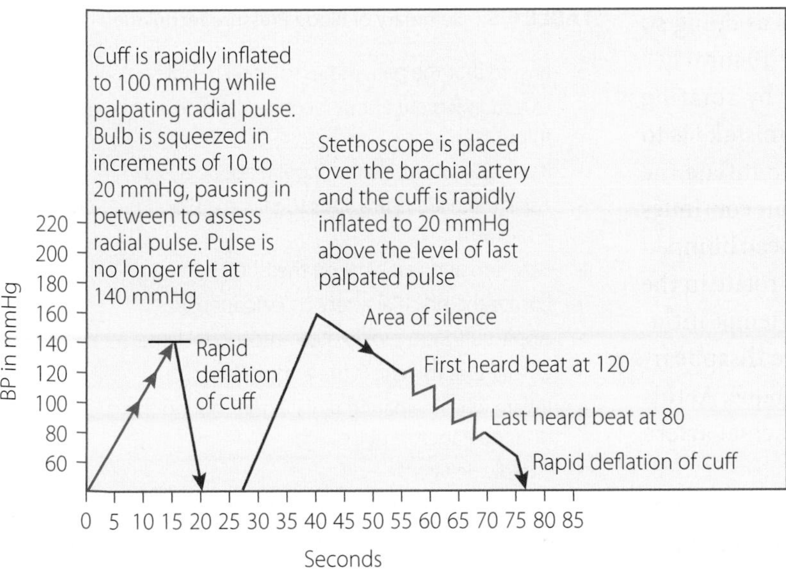

FIGURE 6-22 Assessment of blood pressure using palpatory followed by auscultatory techniques.

the patient elevate his/her arm to a position parallel to the floor and supinating his/her hand. This maneuver rotates the brachial artery laterally and supports the cuff as you wrap and secure it around the arm. Then have the patient rest the wrist back on his/her thigh.

Without using the stethoscope, locate the radial artery. Inflate the cuff so that the needle points to approximately 100 mmHg while palpating radial artery. If the pulse has disappeared, deflate the cuff quickly; however, in the vast majority the pulse will still be palpable. If it is, squeeze the bulb only enough to raise the manometer by about 10 more mmHg, to 110 mmHg. Again, feel for a pulse. If present, advance another 10 mmHg. Continue this pattern until no pulse is palpable with a 10 mmHg advancement. When an advancement results in a significant reduction in pulse strength, it should be anticipated that the next advancement will result in complete absence of a palpable pulse. Once the pulse is nondetectable with an advancement, note the reading and then rapidly and immediately deflate the cuff. This is the systolic blood pressure by palpation (see **FIGURE 6-22**). In an environment where the level of noise is too great for auscultation, such as transporting a patient by ambulance, the provider should minimally be able to report the systolic blood pressure as a sign of hemodynamic stability via this method.

Position the stethoscope earpieces into the ears with the binaural tubes adjusted so that they point slightly forward. Elevate the patient's arm to heart level utilizing a cross-arm technique wherein the provider is supporting the patient's right arm with his/her arm, or left arm with his/her left arm. Support the arm with a hand under the elbow while the thumb wraps around to secure the head of the stethoscope firmly in place, flat against the antecubital fossa over the brachial artery but below the edge of the cuff (see **FIGURE 6-23**).

If the provider fails to support the arm, resulting in the patient's elevating his or her own, the blood pressure can be raised by 10%. In addition, the elbow

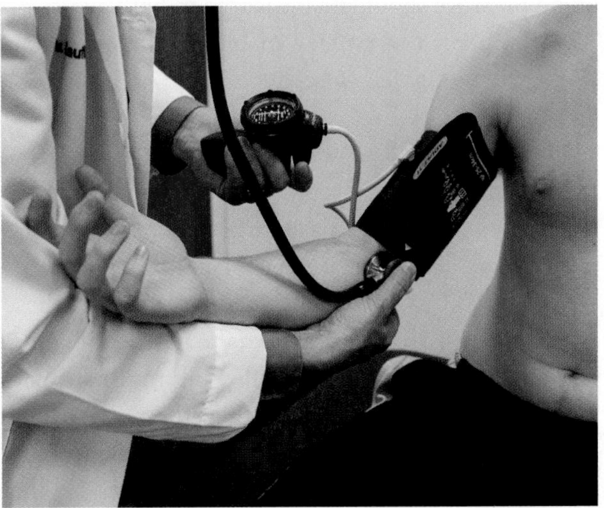

FIGURE 6-23 The bell of the stethoscope is placed over the brachial artery in the antecubital space below the edge of the cuff.

should not be bent more than 45 degrees as doing so can elevate the diastolic measurement by 10 mmHg.[3]

Close the valve on the manometer by rotating the knob only until it stops. A common mistake is to torque the knob too tightly. Now begin to inflate the cuff. If you attempt to inflate the cuff but air continues to escape, confirm that the valve has not been bumped open. If it is at the end of rotation, simply rotate in the opposite direction until it stops, and reattempt inflation. Inflate the cuff to 20 mmHg above disappearance of pulse noted by the palpatory technique. At this level no pulse should be heard, as the brachial artery is completely compressed by the cuff.

Slowly open the valve to allow the cuff to deflate at a rate of 2–3 mm per second. If the valve has been closed too tightly, extra torque is required to open it, resulting in a sudden, significant drop. Close the valve and pump the cuff back up to the desired level, then release more slowly. Note the measurement when the first pulse is audible. This is the point where the pressure from the external cuff has dropped just below the pressure of the ventricle at contraction: the systolic blood pressure. Continue watching the manometer while auscultating. When the pulse disappears, note the measurement at the point where the last pulse was heard. This is the point where the pressure from the external cuff has dropped below the resting ventricular pressure during its resting phase: the diastolic blood pressure. Open the valve to rapidly deflate the cuff. For every new patient and at least once a year, the blood pressure should be measured in both arms.

For a summary of blood pressure technique, see **TABLE 6-5**.

TABLE 6-5 Summary of Blood Pressure Technique

- Ensure that the patient has sat for 5 minutes
- Question patient about nicotine/caffeine in the prior 30 minutes
- If using a cuff with latex, inquire about allergy
- Ask if there are restrictions to taking a blood pressure in either arm
- Bare arm and rest wrist on the thigh
- Locate the brachial artery by palpation
- Apply cuff 5 cm proximal to antecubital fossa
- Ensure that the cuff is the appropriate size
- Inflate while palpating radial artery, noting the disappearance of pulse
- Rapidly deflate the cuff
- Elevate the arm with cross-arm technique
- Reinflate to 20 mmHg above disappearance
- Auscultate the brachial artery
- Deflate cuff at a rate of 2–3 mm per second
- Note first pulse to return, reflecting the systolic blood pressure
- Note any muffling point
- Note the disappearance point, reflecting diastolic pressure
- Repeat in other arm

Auscultatory Gap

Infrequently during auscultation there is a period between the systolic and diastolic blood pressure where the pulse is not audible but returns with continued deflation. In these cases there is a period of audible pulse following the first heart sound, and then the pulse disappears, but it reappears later and finally disappears once again. This phenomenon is called an **auscultatory gap** and may reflect arthrosclerosis, or hardening of the arteries (see **FIGURE 6-24**). The result of this may be the documentation of an artificially low blood pressure when hypertension actually exists.

Auscultatory gap: period of silence during auscultation of the blood pressure where the first beat is heard representing systole, a period of silence occurs followed by a return of audible pulse and a second disappearance representing diastole

As providers become comfortable with routine, it is tempting to save a few seconds by skipping the palpatory technique for estimating the systolic blood pressure before auscultating. For example, the cuff is placed and inflated to around 160 mmHg assuming most patients will have a systolic blood pressure lower than this level. Doing so and finding no audible pulse falsely reassures the provider that the brachial artery is completely occluded and they are therefore above the systolic pressure. While deflating, a first pulse is noted at 120 mmHg and the disappearance of pulse at 80 mmHg, which is documented as systolic/diastolic blood pressure of 120/80. The patient is advised that he/she has pre-hypertension, should follow behavioral modification such as weight loss and exercise, and should be seen again in several months.

In fact had the radial artery been palpated during inflation, it would have remained palpable until a level just over 200 mmHg. The cuff would have required inflation to 220 mmHg before deflation began. Now while auscultating, the first pulse is heard at 210

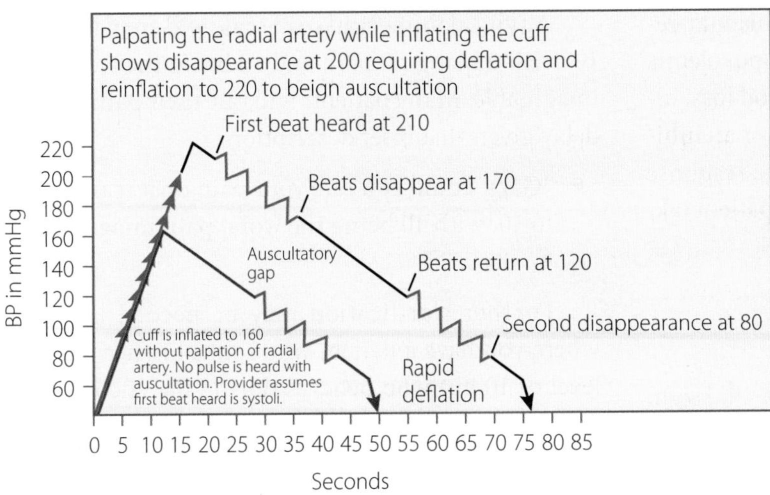

FIGURE 6-24 Auscultatory gap.

mmHg, and then it disappears at 170 mmHg, reappears at 120 mmHg, and disappears for the second time at 80 mmHg. This is documented as 210/80 with an auscultatory gap of 170/120. This patient requires urgent treatment instead of being sent home. Investing the 5 to 20 seconds required to do a palpatory technique with every blood pressure prior to auscultation simply saves lives.

Muffling Point

Another observation during auscultation of blood pressure is a point where the strength of the pulse is heard to muffle but continues and disappears at a lower measurement. There is a longstanding debate as to whether the diastolic blood pressure is more accurately portrayed by the point at which the sound muffles or by the point of disappearance. It is noted, however, that detecting the point of disappearance is more reproducible in early practitioners. If a **muffling point** is encountered, the blood pressure should be documented by systolic/muffling point/diastolic, such as 152/84/68.[3]

Peripheral Pulse Palpation and Estimating Blood Pressure

In acute emergency or trauma situations it has long been taught that if the provider is able to detect a radial, femoral, or carotid pulse by palpation, the corresponding systolic blood pressure was at a range of above 80 mmHg, 70 to 80 mmHg, and 60 to 70 mmHg, respectively.[4]

This theory has since been shown to overestimate systolic blood pressure. In these emergent situations, however, it is still valuable to note that as blood pressure drops, the pulse is no longer palpable, losing the radial first, then the femoral, and finally the carotid. During acute triage or assessment of the patient, noting the lack of peripheral pulse helps to direct urgency of intervention.

Blood Pressure Goals

The Seventh Report of the Joint National Committee on Prevention, Detection, Evaluation, and Treatment of High Blood Pressure (JNC 7) recognizes the categories of blood pressure described in **TABLE 6-6**.

Orthostatic Hypotension

If a patient presents with complaints that suggest hypovolemia, blood loss, or anemia, such as tachycardia, dizziness upon rising, shortness of breath with exertion, presyncope, or syncope, the provider should rule out **orthostatic hypotension**.

To assess a patient, first take the blood pressure and pulse in the supine position. Then assist the patient to the seated position and repeat, and then assist the patient to standing, guarding against a fall should the patient become lightheaded, and take a final blood pressure and pulse.

Orthostatic hypotension is defined as a drop in blood pressure of 20 mmHg or the rise of pulse by 20 beats per minute from the supine

Muffling point: observation during auscultation of blood pressure where the strength of the pulse is heard to significantly muffle but continues and disappears at a lower measurement; this is debated as representing true diastolic blood pressure

Orthostatic hypotension: a drop in blood pressure of 20 mmHg or the rise of pulse by 20 beats per minute as the patient changes from supine to standing position

TABLE 6-6 Classification of Blood Pressure

Category	SBP mmHg	DBP mmHg
Normal	< 120 and	< 80
Prehypertension	120–139 or	80–89
Hypertension—Stage 1	140–159 or	90–99
Hypertension—Stage 2	≥ 160 or	≥ 100

Pain: the perception of physical discomfort, the intensity of which can be represented by scale; this is now considered a vital sign

Pain scale: a numerical or graphical display utilized by providers to help patients decrease subjectivity in assigning intensity to the amount of pain being experienced

to standing position.[5] This may reflect disorders such as hypovolemia from dehydration or blood loss, inadequate venous return, or an inhibition of the sympathetic response to standing, such as in a patient taking beta blockers.

PAIN

Pain is now considered a vital sign, with assessment to occur at each encounter where blood pressure, pulse, or respirations would be assessed. Blood pressure and pulse are strictly objective. They are measured and documented with a scale that is used across all patient populations. Pain, however, is subjective. It is a historical inquiry that defines the patient's perception of the severity of the symptom. It is a scale that is not shared from patient to patient, in that one person's definition of moderate pain may be considered mild or severe by others. Therefore, the **pain scale** is most accurate in the monitoring of pain over a series of visits or encounters.

Many pain scales exist, including visual pain scales depicting facial expressions (such as Wong-Baker FACES), colored analogue, descriptive pain, and numerical scales, each with some variation. The Wong-Baker FACES scale (see **FIGURE 6-25**) is commonly used for pediatric patients, ages 3 years and older. When using the Wong-Baker FACES rating scale, physicians should instruct patients to point to each face using the words to describe the pain intensity and ask the child to choose the face that best describes his/her pain. The physician should then record the appropriate number associated with the face that the child chooses.

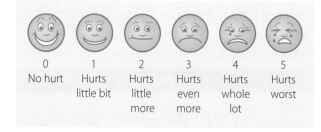

FIGURE 6-25 Wong-Baker FACES pain rating scale.

Source: Hockenberry MJ, Wilson D. *Wong's Essentials of Pediatric Nursing*. 8th ed. St. Louis, MO: Mosby; 2009. Used with permission. Copyright Mosby.

A typical numerical pain scale will span from 0 to 10, with 0 being no pain and 10 being the worst pain imaginable. Many patients will rate their pain without delay given that brief description.

- "Gary, could you rate your pain on a scale from 0 to 10, with 10 being the worst pain imaginable?"
  - "It's a 3."

Further clarification may be needed in a case where you have a patient who ranks his/her pain at a level of 10 but who behaves during the encounter by smiling, joking, moving freely, and lacking a facial grimace, suggesting exaggeration of the level. You might first clarify that a 10 is the worst imaginable pain, for which the patient would seek hospitalization to help treat the pain.

In cases of chronic or severe pain, the use of printed numerical and facial grimace scales help patients more accurately assign the level of pain intensity they are experiencing. An example of a pain scale is given in **FIGURE 6-26**.

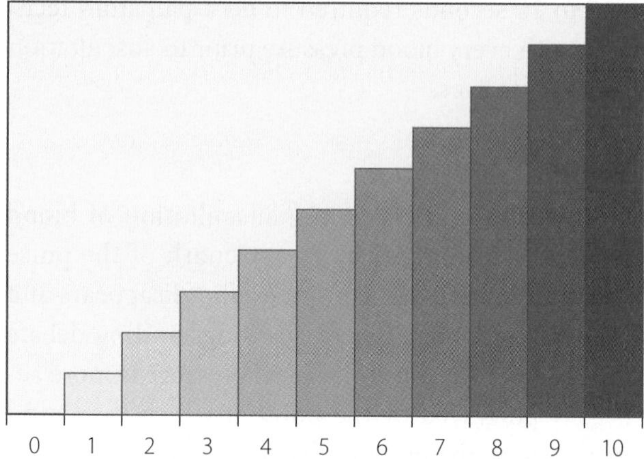

0	You have no pain at all.
1	You have mild pain but sometimes you actually have to think about it to notice it.
2	You have mild pain that is always noticeable.
3	You have mild pain that is always noticeable but occasionally jumps in intensity.
4	You have a moderate amount of pain.
5	You have a moderate amount of pain that occasionally jumps in intensity.
6	You have a moderate amount of pain that frequently jumps in intensity.
7	You have severe pain.
8	You have severe pain that occasionally jumps in intensity.
9	You have severe pain that frequently jumps in intensity.
10	You have the worst possible pain imaginable, so bad you would seek admission to the hospital.

FIGURE 6-26 Sample pain scale.

TABLE 6-7 General Assessment and Vital Signs Flow

Introduces self and explains that physical exam will now be performed
Washes hands for 15 seconds, turning off water with towel
General Assessment
Level of consciousness: alert, drowsy, stuporous, comatose
Distress: pain, respiratory/cardiac, emotional
Nutritional status: well nourished, malnourished, overnourished, increased BMI
Development
Skin coloration: describe general skin tone
Hygiene: describe overall hygiene
Posture/position of comfort: describe posture/position
Vitals
TEMPERATURE—Facilitator: prompt student to discuss
Rectal—one degree above oral
Oral
Axillary—one degree below oral
RESPIRATIONS
Places fingers on radial pulse as distractive technique
Observe respirations through peripheral vision
Calculate rate for 30 seconds and multiply by 2
Student must state, noting:
Rhythm: describe the rhythm
Character: inspiration = expiration, shallow, deep
PULSE
Calculate rate—measure for 15 seconds and multiply by 4
Student must state, noting:
Rhythm: regular, regularly irregular, irregularly irregular
Character: weak (small), normal, bounding (large)
BLOOD PRESSURE
Student must ask patient if he/she has been sitting for 5 minutes
Student must question patient about nicotine/caffeine in the prior 30 minutes
Student must ask patient if there is a restriction to taking blood pressure in either arm
Bare arm
Locate the brachial artery by palpation
Apply cuff with artery marker overlying brachial artery
Apply cuff at least 2.5 cm proximal to antecubital fossa with correct side down
Demonstrate appropriate size cuff use by evaluating range markers
Inflate while palpating radial artery, note disappearance
Deflate quickly
Place earpieces in ears facing forward
Elevate arm placing stethoscope head over brachial artery
Reinflate to 20 mmHg above disappearance
Deflate cuff at a rate of 2–3 mm per second
Note first sounds to return—systolic
Note disappearance point—diastolic pressure
Repeat in other arm
SPECIAL CONSIDERATIONS—Facilitator: prompt student to discuss:
Ask student to describe auscultatory gap
Ask student to describe test to be used if suspected blood volume loss or syncope
Take in supine, seated, and then standing positions
Define orthostatic hypotension: 20 mmHg fall systolic or 10 mmHg diastolic

DOCUMENTATION

- Vital Signs: Pulse reg 78 bpm, Resp 14 bpm, BP 112/62 R arm, Temp 98.5 F, Ht 5′6″, Wt 132 lb, Pain 0/10

References

1. National Institutes of Health. National Heart, Lung, and Blood Institute. Clinical Guidelines on the Identification, Evaluation, and Treatment of Overweight and Obesity in Adults: The Evidence Report. http://www.nhlbi.nih.gov/guidelines/obesity/ob_gdlns.pdf. Published September 1998. Accessed January 20, 2012.
2. Mackowiak, PA, Wasserman SS, Levine MM. A critical appraisal of 98.6°F (37.0°C), the upper limit of the normal body temperature, and other legacies of Carl Reinhold August Wunderlich. *JAMA*. 1992;268(12):1578–1580.
3. National Institutes of Health. Session 1. Measurement of Blood Pressure. http://www.ncbi.nlm.nih.gov/pmc/articles/PMC2573776/pdf/rcgpoccpaper00052-0009b.pdf. Accessed January 28, 2012.
4. Deakin CD, Low JL. Accuracy of the advanced trauma life support guidelines for predicting systolic blood pressure using carotid, femoral, and radial pulses: observational study. *BMJ*. 2000 Sep 16;321:673–674.
5. Venes D, ed. *Taber's Encyclopedic Medical Dictionary*. 20th ed. Philadelphia, PA: F.A. Davis; 2005:1536.

CHAPTER 7

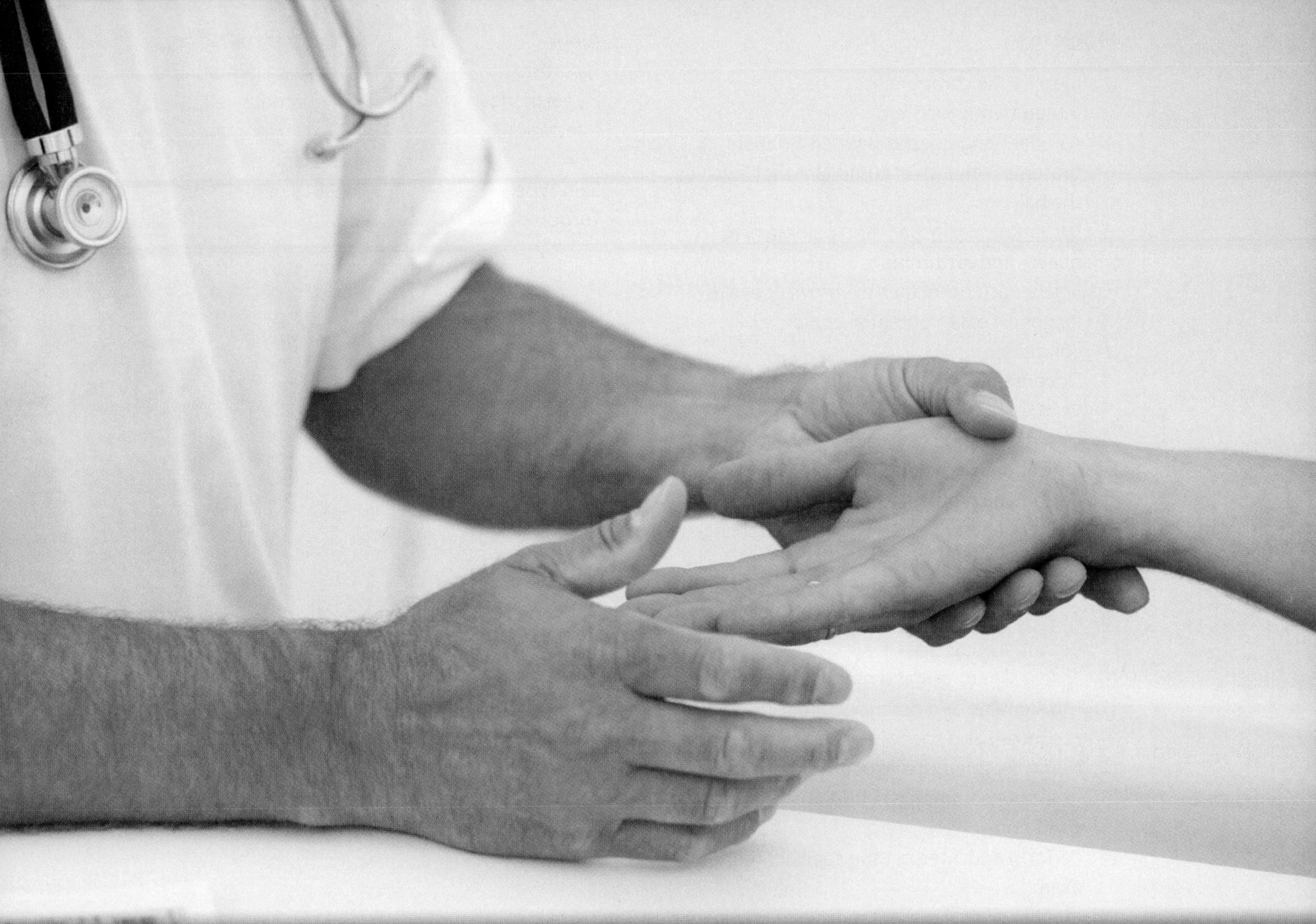

© Yuri Arcurs/ShutterStock, Inc.

Integumentary System

Scott J. M. Lim, DO, FAOCD
Mark Kauffman, DO, MS (Med Ed), PA

OBJECTIVES

At the conclusion of this chapter, the student will be able to

1. Identify the components of the integumentary system
2. Ask clarifying questions when a patient presents with a chief complaint that involves the hair
3. Systematically inspect and palpate hair quality and distribution
4. Relate patterns of hair, eyebrow, or eyelash loss or excess to potential etiologic conditions
5. Document findings of the integumentary examination
6. Describe hair pull and pluck tests and indications of the findings
7. Perform a complete examination of the integumentary system with limited changes of position
8. Categorize patients by skin types
9. Associate color variation of the skin with potential etiologies
10. Assess skin turgor and mobility
11. Differentiate and describe primary, secondary and special skin lesions
12. Name the anatomic structures of the nail
13. Associate common nail findings with medical conditions
14. Perform and interpret the capillary refill exam
15. Identify clinical presentations and prevalence of the three most common types of skin cancer
16. Provide patient education on melanoma recognition

KEY TERMS

Hair
Alopecia
Hirsutism
Hypertrichosis
Infestations
Skin
Skin type
Turgor
Nail
Capillary refill
Cell carcinoma
Squamous cell carcinoma
Melanoma
ABCs of melanoma

Where this icon appears, visit **go.jblearning.com/HPECWS** to view the video.

The integumentary system consists of three major components: the hair, skin, and nails. Each component can reflect specific localized conditions, nonspecific reaction patterns, or features that implicate a systemic disease. At times, pathology of the integumentary system can be related to other organ systems in seemingly random but well-documented and predictable ways as part of a syndrome. When encountering a patient, consider that the patient may not appreciate the scope of his/her disease when presenting with a specific skin complaint. For example, a patient may complain only of a scaly scalp rash, but in addition to seeing a silvery, scaly, papulosquamous plaque in the scalp, you may also look for and note a pink nonscaly patch in the gluteal cleft, a small plaque evolving on the knee, and pitting of the nail plate. The collective findings strengthen your clinical diagnosis for psoriasis, yet the patient may not have thought to tell you about these findings or have even been aware of these manifestations. It requires that you not only perform a complete exam, but also have some knowledge of how and where psoriasis may present.

Experience will help you know what to look for and when to look, making you more efficient. When the patient doesn't present with a specific dermatologic complaint, the examination of the integumentary system is typically interwoven throughout the system examinations as the provider progresses from head to toe. Findings during the course of your integument exam may be common or benign in nature, important but *incidental* to the primary complaint, or important and clinically *relevant* to the presenting complaint. A complete head-to-toe general exam can be illuminating. With this approach, following a brief survey of the skin during the general assessment, we encounter the first component of the integumentary system: the hair.

Hair

If a condition of the **hair** (see **FIGURE 7-1**) is the chief complaint or concern, then some of the questions to clarify are:

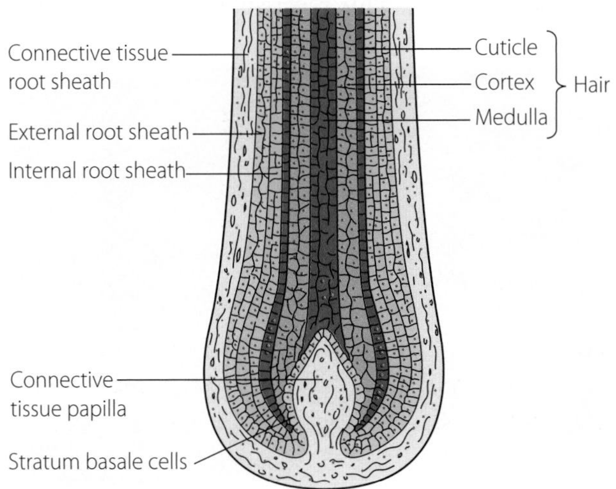

FIGURE 7-1 Anatomy of hair structure.

- What is the hair problem?
- Where is the hair problem (e.g., scalp, eyebrows, body)?
- Is the problem acute or chronic?
- Could there be a temporal association with medications (e.g., vitamin A supplementation)?
- Could there be a temporal association with diet?
- Could there be systemic disease symptoms (e.g., thyroid disease)?
- Are there any other associated events?

Hair: in humans, keratinous filaments growing from the skin of two types: fine, light-colored Vellus hair found at birth and distributed across the body and Terminal or androgenic hair, which develops under hormonal influence

Inspection of the hair begins with general observation of the quality and distribution of hair. Two types of hair are found on the body. Vellus hair is the fine, light-colored hair found at birth and distributed across the body, such as that found on the arms and legs. Terminal or androgenic hair is hair that develops under the hormonal influence of androgens, arising on the face in men, as well as in the axilla and pubic areas.[1]

Reviewing the techniques of examination for the integumentary system, we would perform only inspection and palpation of this system with no areas for auscultation or percussion.

INSPECTION

Quality

When evaluating the hair, consider the general appearance:

- Is it well kempt or is there poor hygiene?
- Are the hair shafts oily or dry?
- What is the condition of the hair shafts? Intact? Broken or brittle? Damaged?

Distribution

When inspecting for distribution of hair, two conditions should be considered:

1. Is there loss of hair from where it would typically be found?
2. Is there abnormal growth of hair where it should not be?

Areas for examination would include the scalp, eyebrows, eyelashes, face, thorax, pubic areas, and extremities.

HAIR LOSS

When evaluating hair loss, **alopecia**, determine:

- Is the hair loss localized or generalized?
- Is it scarring or nonscarring?
- Is it inflammatory or noninflammatory?
- Is there any follicular plugging?
- Are there other areas of the body with skin diseases that may be related to this?

Beginning at the top, hair distribution on the head focuses on patterns of hair loss. One approach of classification would be to categorize alopecia as localized or diffuse. If the hair loss on the scalp is localized, then your clinical differential diagnosis may include disorders such as alopecia areata, hair loss associated with underlying skin disorders like psoriasis, or hair loss from mechanical damage (e.g., trichotillomania or traction alopecia). If the hair loss is diffuse or generalized, then your clinical differential diagnosis might consider androgenic alopecia, hormonal-related causes like thyroid disease, medications (e.g., anticoagulants, anticonvulsants, and beta blockers), or systemic disease (e.g., nutritional disorders, chronic diseases, and infectious diseases).[2]

Alopecia may also be classified as either scarring or nonscarring. As the name suggests, scarring alopecia is associated with a scar and destruction of the hair follicle. Scarring alopecia may be associated with a localized cutaneous disease such as lichen planopilaris or part of a systemic disorder such as lupus. Nonscarring alopecia is more common where hair loss occurs without destruction of the hair follicle. The most common nonscarring form of alopecia is genetic or androgenic alopecia. In men there is the characteristic "horseshoe" pattern of hair loss also known as male pattern baldness (see **FIGURE 7-2**). Women who are genetically prone to lose their hair, referred to as female pattern hair loss, tend to have more diffuse loss on the vertex rather than on the sides of the head but are never bald like men. This common pattern of loss is incremental with a progressively receding hairline.

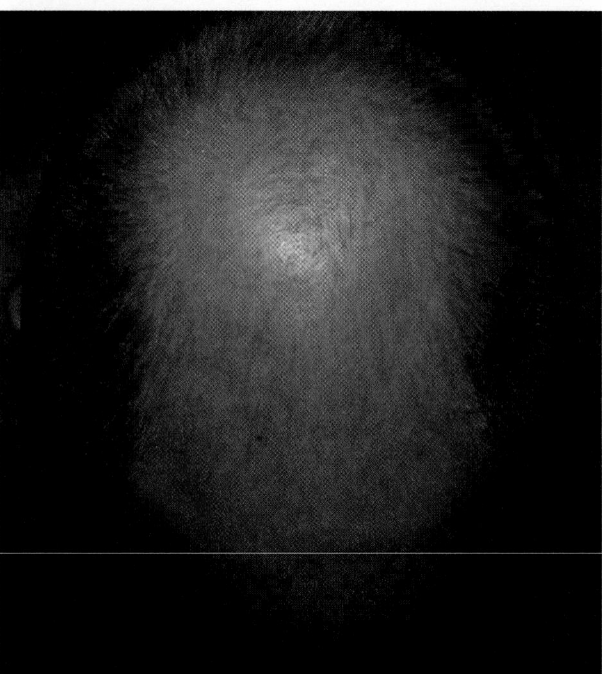

FIGURE 7-2 Male alopecia.

An example of localized nonscarring hair loss would be alopecia areata (see **FIGURE 7-3**). In addition to being nonscarring, it also characteristically presents with sharply defined circular patches. Alopecia totalis would be loss of nearly all hair from the scalp, where alopecia universalis would refer to loss of hair from the entire body. This extensive form of alopecia is rare and also associated with a poor prognosis. Recognizing that alopecia is an autoimmune phenomenon and that it can be associated with other autoimmune disorders (such as lupus, thyroid, and/or vitiligo) helps you to consider these diagnoses when taking a history and examining the patient.[2]

Alopecia: localized or diffuse hair loss classified as scarring or nonscarring

Diffuse, nonscarring hair loss is also seen in telogen effluvium. This reversible condition usually

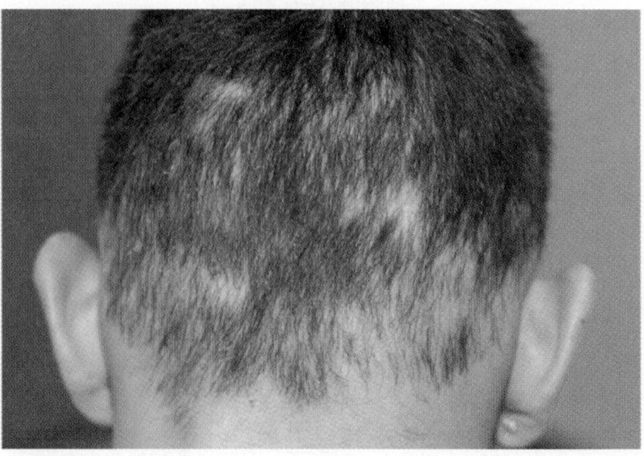

FIGURE 7-3 Localized alopecia.

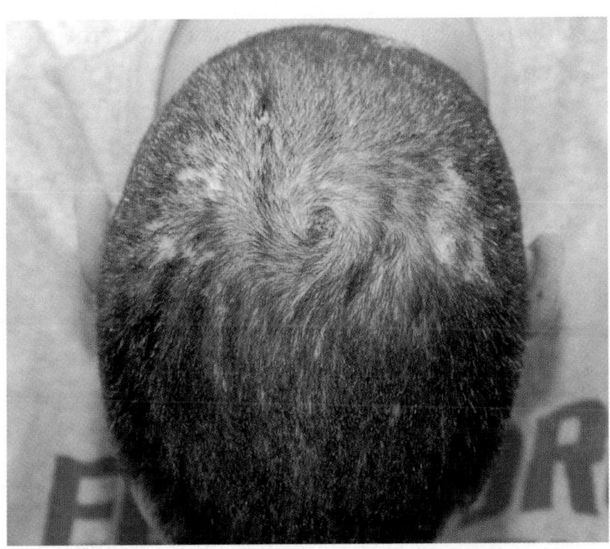

FIGURE 7-4 Scarring alopecia from lichen planopilaris.

occurs about three months following a major stress such as illness, surgery, psychological trauma, severe weight loss, or pregnancy. Therefore, reviewing history again can be important when confronting this physical finding.

Scarring alopecia is more commonly associated with localized patterns of loss. This patchy loss is due to destruction of the hair follicle and results in permanent loss of hairs. Trauma (e.g., chemical and thermal burns, surgery, radiation, and injury), infections (e.g., chronic untreated dermatophyte infections), tumors (e.g., basal cell carcinoma), and dermatologic diseases such as discoid lupus and lichen planopilaris can cause scarring alopecia (see **FIGURE 7-4**).

Poor oxygen delivery through compromised blood flow also results in hair loss. This is commonly seen in peripheral arterial disease (see **FIGURE 7-5**). The finding of lack of hair on the lower extremities should prompt consideration of this disorder. Patients who shave their legs should be questioned about hair loss of the lower extremities by inquiry into the frequency of the need for shaving.

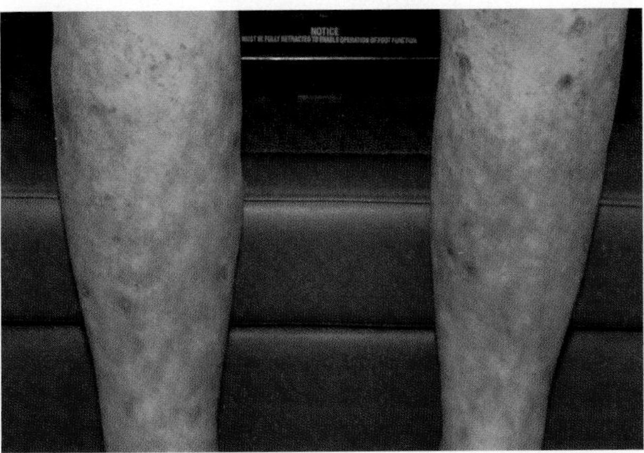

FIGURE 7-5 Hair loss due to peripheral arterial disease.

Hirsutism: a condition of excessive terminal hair growth or growth of hair in unusual places

DOCUMENTATION

- Male pattern alopecia without patchy loss

HAIR EXCESS

Hirsutism is defined as a condition of excessive terminal hair growth or growth of hair in unusual places (see **FIGURE 7-6**).[3] In women, increased terminal hair growth may be more noticeable on the face, but examination will also reveal occurrence on the chest, abdomen, and back. On exam, hirsutism may not be obvious as the woman may be using depilatories or have already pursued electrolysis or laser hair removal. Therefore, when encountering other body parts with abnormal coarse terminal hairs, one should review the history of facial hair and depilatory use.

Hirsutism may be the result of abnormal androgen production such as found with polycystic ovary syndrome, adrenal hyperplasia, and ovarian and adrenal tumors. Severe insulin resistance and certain medications such as hormonal therapies may also result in hirsutism.

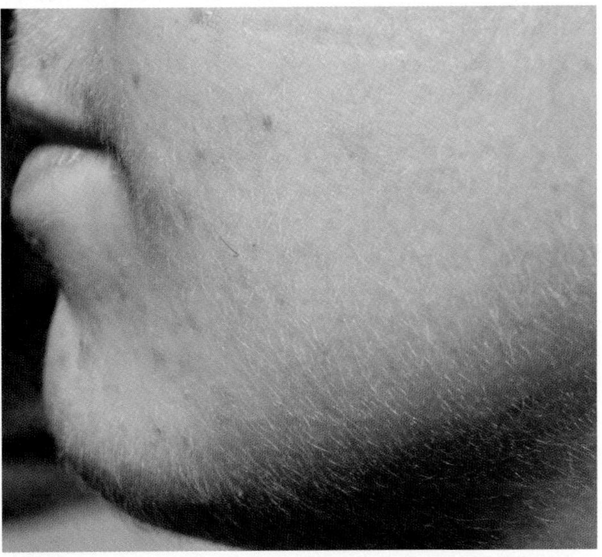

FIGURE 7-6 Hirsutism.

Hypertrichosis: a diffuse increase in body hair commonly associated with medications such as phenytoin, glucocorticoids, minoxidil, and cyclosporin.

Infestations: parasitic infections commonly involving areas of hair growth

When hirsutism is suspected, the patient should be questioned about chronological presentation and ethnic and/or genetic tendencies. A report of changes in hair growth, including distribution or acceleration of growth, would heighten suspicion and investigation for a medical cause of the disorder. Women of certain ethnic backgrounds may report familial tendency for excessive hair growth, especially above the lip, and be entirely normal.

In contrast, **hypertrichosis** is a diffuse increase in body hair commonly associated with medications such as phenytoin, glucocorticoids, minoxidil, and cyclosporin.

DOCUMENTATION

- Hirsute appearance with facial hair growth above the lip and below the chin

INFESTATIONS

The hair, eyebrows, eyelashes, and pubic hair areas are frequent sites for **infestations** by parasites. Look for evidence of nits or lice (see **FIGURES 7-7A** and **7-7B**). For pediculosis corporus (head lice), visualization of live lice can be best achieved by using a fine-toothed comb technique, sequentially searching all areas intently. Wetting the hair with a conditioner aids in detection. Nits—eggs of lice attached to hair follicles—are more easily detected, but the detection of nits does not guarantee active infection. Following eradication of an infection, nits that were not removed will progress distally as the hair grows, which may clue in the provider to the likelihood of active infection.

Pediculosis pubis (pubic area) and ciliaris (eyelashes) involve the crab louse, which is typically spread through sexual contact. These infestations may also be found in the axilla.

EYEBROWS AND EYELASHES

Eyebrow and eyelash distribution should also be considered. Patients with apparent loss of eyebrows or eyelashes should be questioned about grooming habits. Patchy areas of hair loss in these areas might suggest alopecia areata. Damaged, irregular hair shafts of different lengths may suggest mechanical damage from grooming techniques, or neuroses such as trichotillomania. Other causes for hair loss in these areas could be telogen effluvium, hypothyroidism, infections, eczema, and certain medications. Advancing age can contribute to thinning of the eyebrows as well as cause longer hairs.

Hypertrichosis of eyelashes is often iatrogenic in nature with patients on bimatoprost ophthalmic (Lumigan) for glaucoma. Topical bimatoprost (Latisse) is also FDA-approved for cosmetic treatment of hypotrichosis, in order to achieve a more aesthetically pleasing "hypertrichosis" of the eyelashes (see **FIGURE 7-8**).

PALPATION

Palpate the hair for texture. Note whether it is smooth, silky, oily, fine, coarse, or brittle. Thyroid disorders are commonly associated with hair texture changes. Hypothyroidism is characterized by the hair becoming coarse. Conversely, hyperthyroidism is associated with thinning of the hair. Anorexia nervosa and nutritional

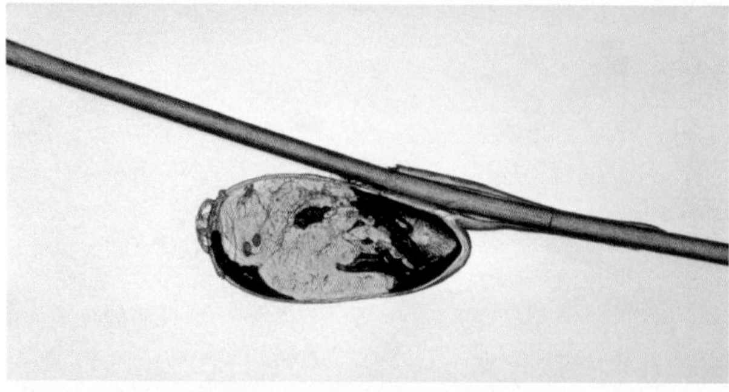

FIGURE 7-7A Nits/lice.
Courtesy of: CDC/ Dr. Dennis D. Juranek.

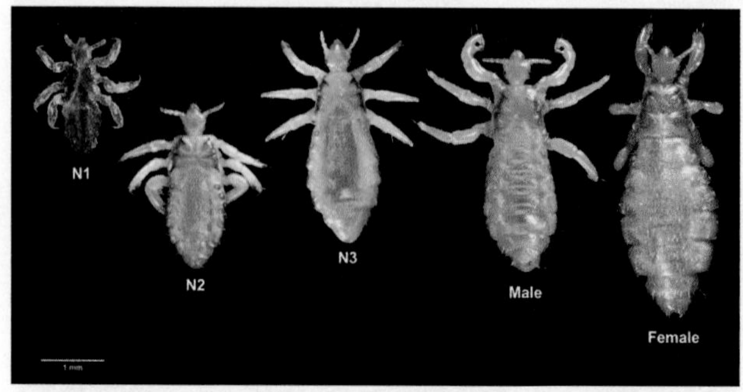

FIGURE 7-7B Nits/lice.
Courtesy of: CDC/Joseph Strycharz, PhD; Kyong Sup Yoon, PhD; Frank Collins, PhD

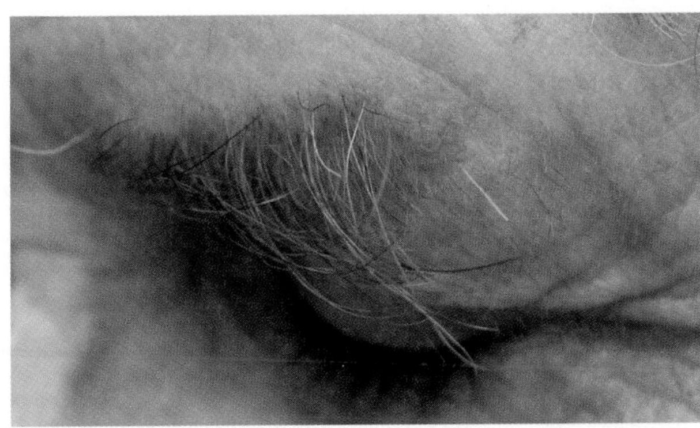

FIGURE 7-8 Localized hypertrichosis of eyelashes and eyebrow from use of bimatoprost.

deficiencies can be associated with brittleness and loss of hair.

SPECIAL TESTING IN ALOPECIA

Hair Pull Test

Firmly grasp about 50–60 hairs from the sides of the scalp above the ear and exert slow, constant traction to slightly tent the scalp skin while slowly sliding the fingers up the hair shaft. Anagen growing hairs should remain rooted in place while telogen hairs should easily come out. There should be fewer than six club hairs extracted. If more than six hairs are extracted, then there is active shedding. A potential pitfall in interpretation, however, can occur if the patient shampoos just prior to the test, as many of the telogen hairs may have already come out. Repeat the process on the opposite side of the scalp and two or three other areas. Evaluate the hair bulbs as well. If the percentage of hairs in telogen phase is up to 10%, this is excellent; up to 25%, typical; over 30%, a problem. An excessive number of telogen hairs, an event referred to as telogen effluvium, can occur following childbirth, crash diets, high fever, and physical and psychological stresses.

Hair Pluck Test—Trichogram

Using a rubber-tipped needle nose hemostat or holder, abruptly extract approximately 50 hairs from the scalp. Trim the excess hairs about 1 cm from the roots. Examine the hairs on a wet microscope slide with a hand lens. Telogen hairs will have a small unpigmented ovoid bulb without internal root sheath. Anagen hairs have larger elongated pigmented bulbs surrounded by a gelatinous internal root sheath. Some diseases like alopecia areata and drugs with antimetabolite therapy may interrupt the mitotic activity in cells normally involved in hair growth. This can result in hair shafts that break under tension and fragment during the hair pluck test.

DOCUMENTATION

- Hair—Inspection: female pattern distribution, well kempt with mildly oily appearance. No evidence of shaft damage, alopecia, or hirsutism. Eyebrows with evidence of manual thinning laterally. Eyelashes intact. No infestations. Palpation: smooth and slightly oily. Negative hair pull test.

Skin

STRUCTURE

The **skin** is the largest organ system in the body, with many functions including the production of vitamin E, temperature regulation, and the prevention of dehydration and infection. It is composed of three layers: the epidermis, the dermis, and the subcutaneous tissues. The epidermis is the thinnest, most superficial layer, under which lies the thicker dermis and then the subcutaneous tissues at the deepest level (see FIGURE 7-9).

INSPECTION

In order to perform a thorough dermatologic exam, the following conditions should be in place:

- The patient adequately disrobed
- Adequate lighting
- Ancillary tools
  - Wood's lamp
  - Magnifying lens

Although a complete exam of the skin will provide the most information and certainly could screen for life-threatening melanomas, not everyone will be receptive to such thorough inspection. The practice of routine "full-body examination" of the skin on new patients is

Skin: the largest organ system in the body, composed of three layers: the epidermis, the dermis, and the subcutaneous tissues. It has many functions, including the production of vitamin E, temperature regulation, and the prevention of dehydration and infection

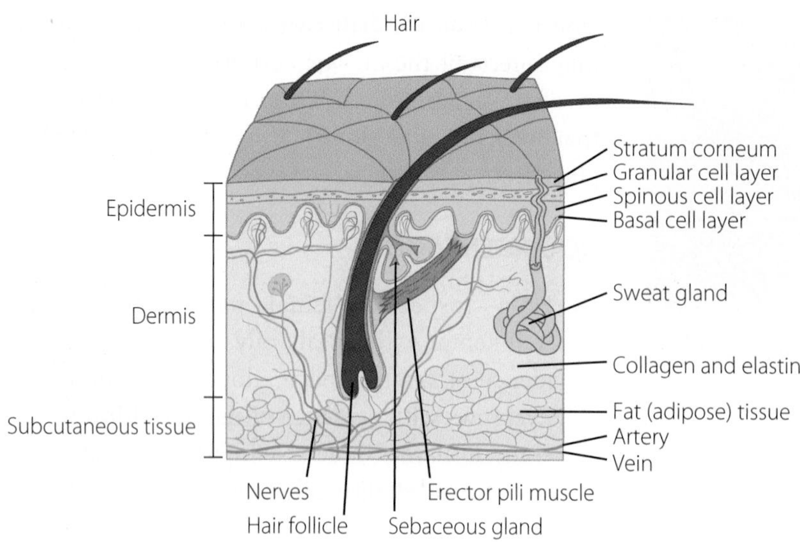

FIGURE 7-9 Anatomy of human skin.

In physically compromised patients, there may be limitations to what areas can be physically examined. Every effort should be made, however, to accommodate such patients. For example, in wheelchair patients, exam tables are available that are compliant with the Americans with Disabilities Act (ADA)—that is, mechanically able to be lowered to the height of the wheelchair, enabling easier transfer to the exam table. Once the patient is on the exam table, the examiner can better see his/her back and can then recline the patient to examine the ventral surfaces of the body.

controversial. Some would argue that such practice would not only help in the assessment of the patient's chief complaint but would also screen for skin cancers, which, although incidental to the chief complaint, could save lives. Others argue that it is inappropriate in situations where, for example, the patient is modest or an adolescent, or a when a complete exam is not relevant to the chief complaint (e.g., a patient presents for a wart on the hand). Consideration should be given to the nature of the complaint, the potential scope of the disease process, the willingness of the patient to comply with an exam, the physical capability of the patient to comply with the exam, and the time constraints on pursuing a good exam. When a full exam is declined or refused despite the indication and/or benefits of such a complete exam, documentation of such refusal and/or inability to perform the exam may be helpful for medicolegal purposes.

When performing a complete exam, consider the most efficient approach to accomplishing your goals. For example, much of the skin can be examined while the patient is in the seated position provided there is ample illumination and you can position yourself properly. Begin by looking at the easily visualized areas first. Then assist the patient to the supine position for inspection of the inguinal and abdominal fold areas. Finally, assist the patient to standing in order to observe the posterior legs and buttock regions. In this example, only three position changes would be needed.

Scalp

7-1 Inspection of the scalp is best achieved by utilizing a tongue blade to part the hair at consistent intervals (see **FIGURE 7-10**). Again, the rule applies that if the area cannot be seen, the disorder cannot be detected. If a general screen is being completed, 1-cm intervals are sufficient. Systematically work front to back from the frontal to the temporal, parietal, crown, and occipital areas, first one side and then the other. If the patient has a specific complaint, smaller parts should be made. Note the condition and integrity of the scalp and the presence of lesions.

Once inspection is complete, you should search for missed lesions by palpating the scalp with the same meticulous approach.

Face and Neck

The face is a frequent site for skin lesions as it generally has more sun exposure than any other body area. Pay close attention to the nose, a common site of basal cell carcinoma, and lips, a common site for squamous cell carcinoma, especially in smokers. Also be sure to fold the ear forward to inspect behind it. Many lesions are missed in this area.

Thorax

Appropriate exposure requires that the patient be disrobed. If a breast examination is to be performed on

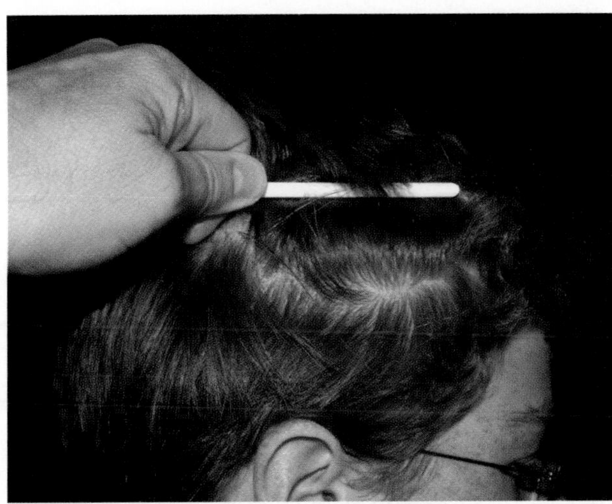

FIGURE 7-10 Detailed inspection of the scalp.

a female patient, this should be reserved for a time closer to the end of the exam, where all sensitive examinations can be completed together and the patient can be allowed to dress immediately following. Immediately re-cover the thorax when the examination is completed. Be sure to inspect all skin fold areas and the axilla. Ask both men and women to lift pendulous breasts. Areas such as these have increased warmth and moisture, increasing the likelihood of fungal and yeast infections.

Extremities

Some providers may elect to examine the upper extremities after the neck and before the thorax, then follow the thorax with the lower extremities. Others choose to move cephalad to caudad: head, neck, thorax, lower extremities, and then back to the upper extremities. In either case, break the surface area of the extremities into four sections: dorsal, ventral, medial, and lateral. Drape the pelvis with a sheet while examining the lower extremities, sliding the sheet up the thighs for proper exposure. You may have the patient rest his/her hands between the upper thighs to anchor the sheet as appropriate. Palpate each section while inspecting to aid in detection of small or skin-colored lesions.

Sensitive Examinations

When examination of sensitive areas is appropriate, you should save these areas until near the end of the examination. Explain the necessity for including the exam and ask for permission before exposing the area. For instance, psoriasis is commonly seen in the intergluteal folds. This should be explained to patients so that they understand the need for this component of the exam as well as to heighten their awareness so that they can include it during self-assessments. Allow the patient to dress or gown immediately after the exam is concluded.

Skin type: categorization by reaction of the skin based on what occurs after 30–45 minutes of sun exposure after at least several months of exposure to the sun

Generalized Scanning

Start the skin examination with a generalized scanning for symmetry of color, areas of exposure, and tendency toward lesions. Note areas of thickening or thinning.

Color.

Color variation can be seen with either generalized distribution or localized discoloration. **Skin type** should be documented as an assessment of the level of risk for developing skin cancer and to facilitate education of the patient in frequency of skin cancer surveillance (see **TABLE 7-1**).

These characteristics are based on what the patient would experience in the 30–45 minutes of sun exposure after the winter season or no prior sun exposure. When assessing skin type, be aware that this reflects the color of unexposed buttock skin. Types I to III are white, type IV is white or brown, type V is brown, and type VI has dark brown or black buttock skin.

When considering etiologies associated with color variation, group colors with associated diagnoses.

TABLE 7-1 Skin Types

Skin Types[4]	
Type I	Always burns easily, never tans
Type II	Burns easily, tans slightly
Type III	Sometimes burns, then tans gradually and moderately
Type IV	Burns minimally, always tans well
Type V	Burns rarely, tans deeply
Type VI	Almost never burns, deeply pigmented

Adapted from: Lowe, NJ. An overview of ultraviolet radiation, sunscreens, and photo-induced dermatoses. *Dermatol Clin*. 2006;24(1):9–17.

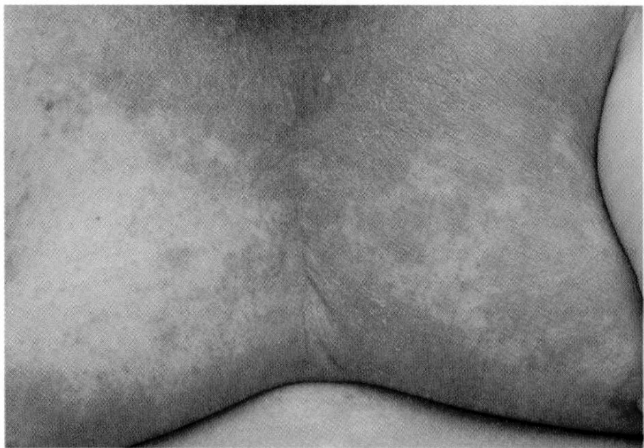

FIGURE 7-11 Diffuse erythema.

Generalized Distribution.

- Red (Erythema) (see **FIGURE 7-11**): exertion, flushing, viral exanthem, medication reaction, thermal injury including solar injury or radiation therapy, polycythemia, trauma, allergy, carbon monoxide poisoning.
- White:
  - Pallor: Reduced oxyhemoglobin: anemia, vasovagal effect from fear or embarrassment, hypovolemia, acute blood loss, lead poisoning
  - Hypopigmentation (see **FIGURE 7-12**): lack of sun exposure, ethnic tendency
  - Amelanosis: albinism
- Blue (Cyanosis) (see **FIGURE 7-13**): hypoventilation, chronic lung disease, congenital heart disease, hemoglobin abnormalities.
- Yellow (Jaundice) (see **FIGURE 7-14**): hyperbilirubinemia, hemolysis, protein deficiency, enzyme deficiency, liver disease, bile duct obstruction.

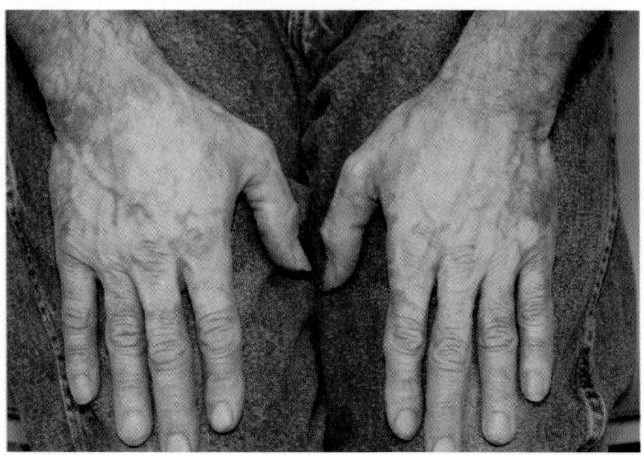

FIGURE 7-12 Diffuse hypopigmentation.

- Orange: carotenemia, dietary intake.
- Brown: pituitary disorder, adrenal disorder, hemochromatosis, tetracycline or minocycline hyperpigmentation (see **FIGURE 7-15**).

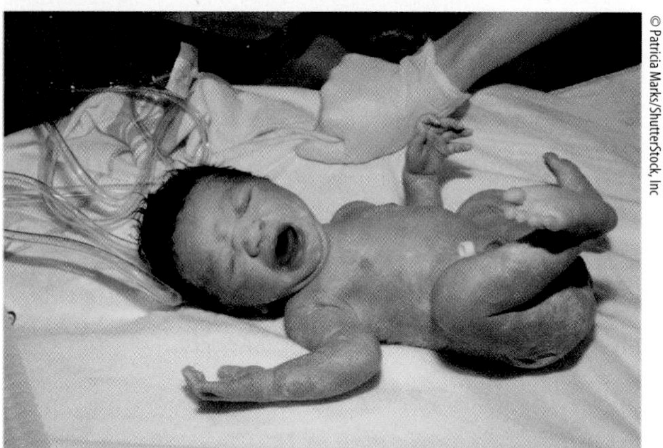

© Patricia Marks/ShutterStock, Inc

FIGURE 7-13 Cyanosis of the hands, feet, and scalp in a newborn.

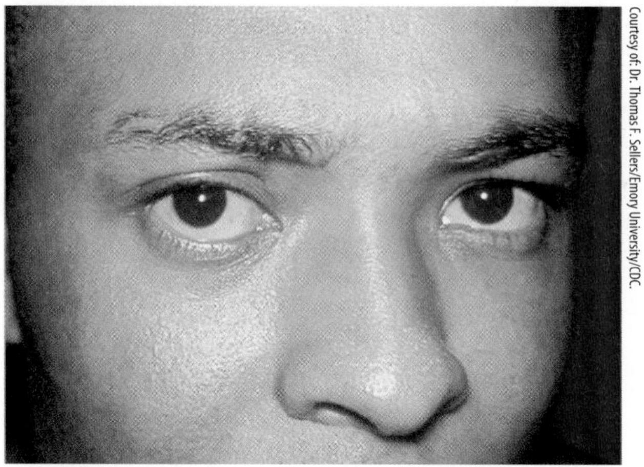

Courtesy of: Dr. Thomas F. Sellers/Emory University/CDC.

FIGURE 7-14 Jaundice.

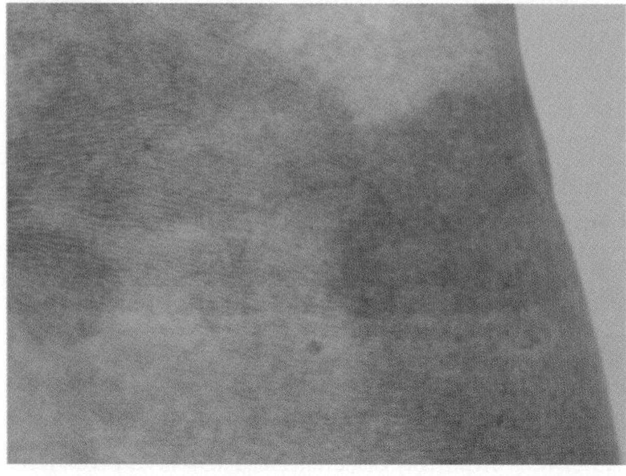

FIGURE 7-15 Diffuse minocycline hyperpigmentation of torso.

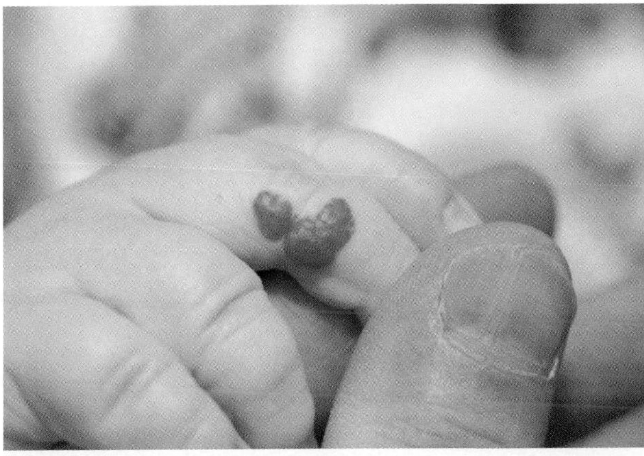

FIGURE 7-16 Localized erythema: hemangioma of the finger.

Localized Discoloration.

- Red (see **FIGURE 7-16**): cellulitis, inflammation, hemangioma, venous obstruction, viral infection.
- White (see **FIGURE 7-17**): amelanotic vs. hypopigmentation: vitiligo, scar, peripheral arterial occlusion, Raynaud's phenomenon (vasospasm), tinea versicolor.
- Blue (see **FIGURE 7-18**): venous pulling, nevi, Raynaud's phenomenon.
- Brown/black (see **FIGURE 7-19** and **FIGURE 7-20**): nevi, café au lait, melanoma, melasma, acanthosis nigrans, drug reaction.

DOCUMENTATION

- Skin—Inspection: general scanning with even tan coloration, low tendency toward lesions, without thickening or thinning. No evidence of localized or diffuse discoloration, hyper- or hypopigmentation. No suspicious lesions.

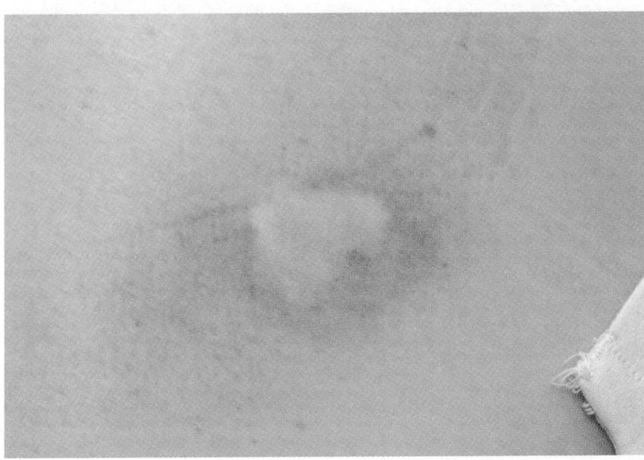

FIGURE 7-17 Localized white: hypopigmentation.

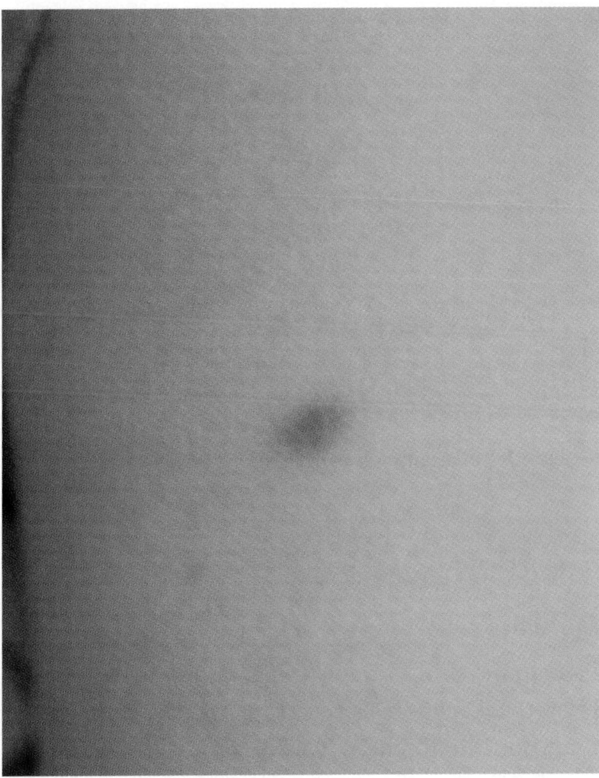

FIGURE 7-18 Localized blue: blue nevus.

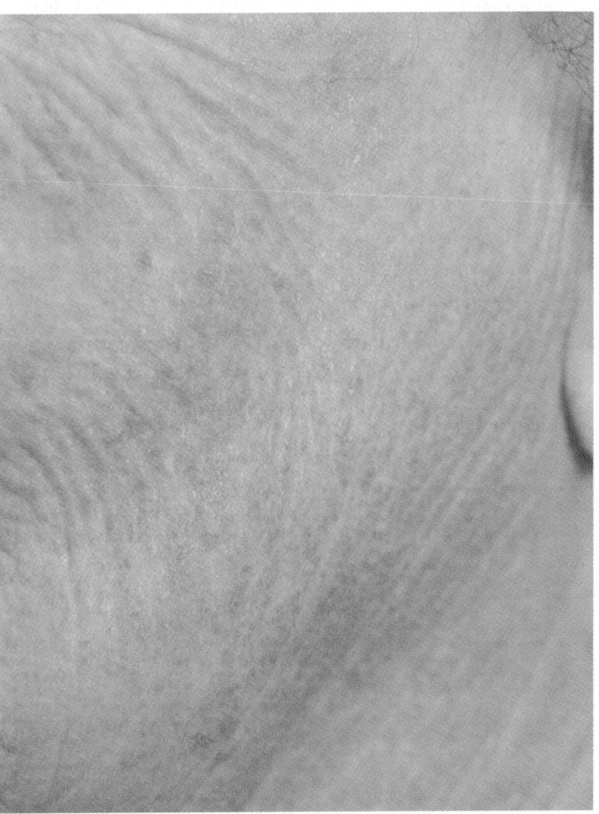

FIGURE 7-19 Localized minocycline hyperpigmentation of the face.

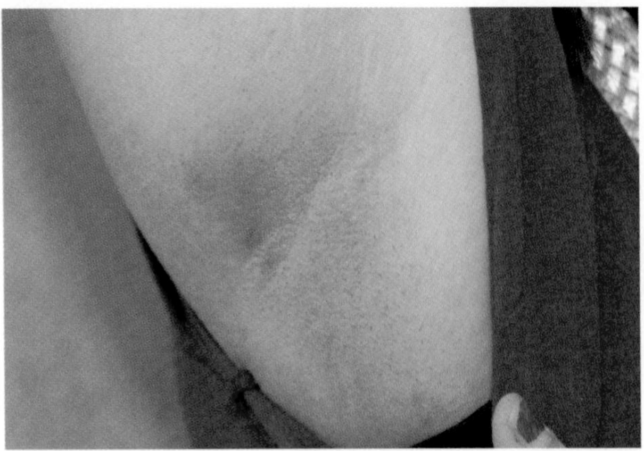

FIGURE 7-20 Acanthosis nigricans of the axilla.

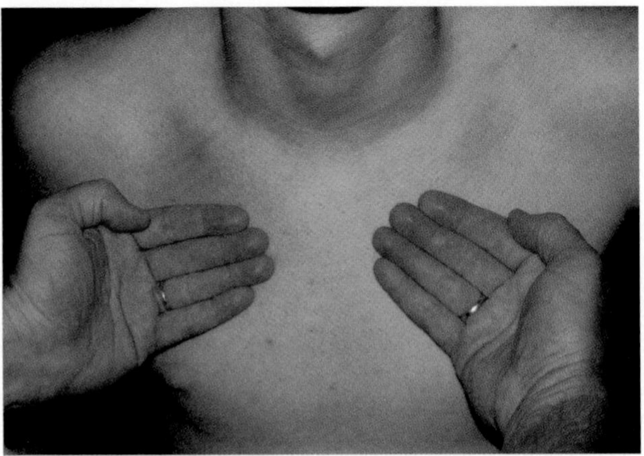

FIGURE 7-21 Temperature variation is better appreciated through palpation using the back of the hands.

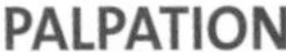

PALPATION

Moisture

Palpate the skin for moisture. Is it dry, moist, or diaphoretic? Diaphoresis is easily noted and commonly found on the forehead. Vasovagal diaphoresis commonly involves the thorax. The palms of the hands, soles of the feet, and axillary regions have the greatest concentration of eccrine glands and if excessively sweaty they may demonstrate hyperhidrosis. Examine the intertriginous areas such as between the fingers, toes, and skin folds and under the breasts, where moisture aids fungal or yeast growth.

Temperature

Palpate temperature with the back of the hands using a bilateral comparison approach (see **FIGURE 7-21**). This is especially useful in comparison of extremities for discernible temperature variation and aids in diagnosis of arterial occlusion with coolness and venous obstruction with increased warmth. Localized areas of erythema should be assessed for increased warmth, which may reflect inflammation or infection.

Texture/Thickness

Palpate for texture and thickness, noting if the skin is soft, rough, smooth, thinned, or thickened.

Turgor: an assessment of the state of hydration wherein the provider gently pinches the skin of the patient's forearm, causing it to tent, and assesses the speed of retraction

Turgor

Turgor is an assessment of the state of hydration. In this technique, the provider gently pinches the skin of the patient's forearm, causing it to tent (see **FIGURE 7-22**). In normal states of hydration, the skin quickly retracts back to its resting position. When a state of dehydration occurs, the skin will remain tented longer, slowly returning to the resting position. This is documented as a delay in turgor.

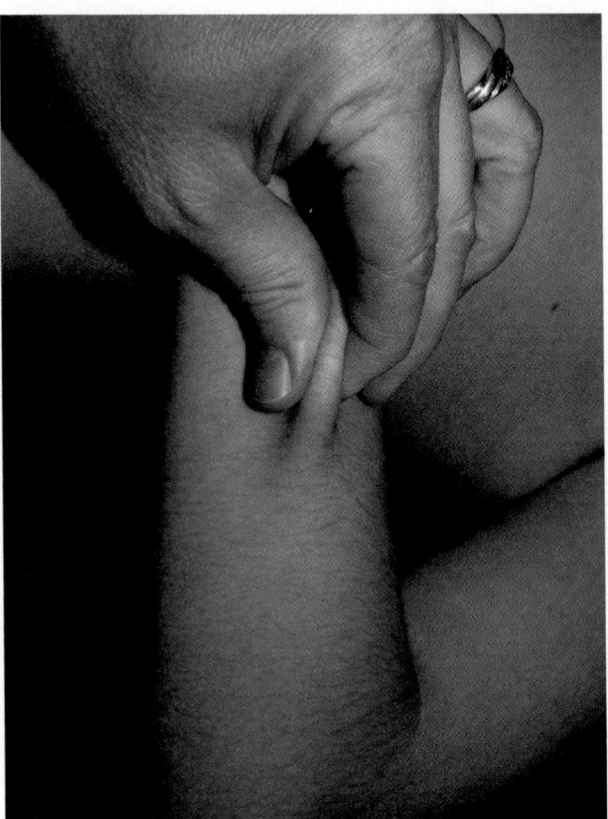

FIGURE 7-22 Assessment of turgor through tenting of the forearm skin.

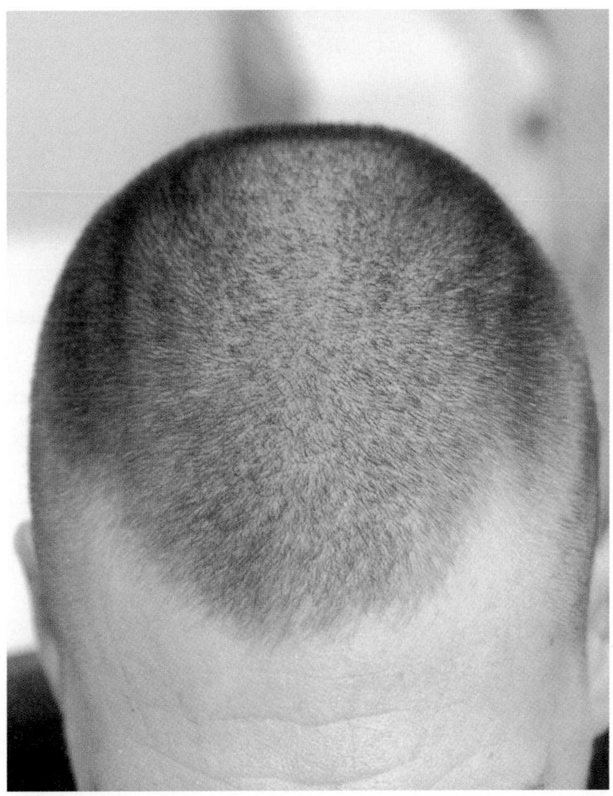

FIGURE 7-23 Static inspection of the scalp in the assessment of mobility prior to excision of a lesion.

This test had commonly been described as being performed on the dorsum of the hand; however, in the elderly population, loss of elasticity and subcutaneous tissues result in falsely positive testing. Testing on the forearm is a more accurate assessment.

Mobility

General mobility may also be assessed using the pads of the fingers in circular motion and is typically performed on the extremities with bilateral comparison. Diminished subcutaneous tissues such as that seen with aging increases mobility. If one observes excessive stretch of the skin as well as hypermobile joint flexibility, then consideration of a syndrome such as Ehlers-Danlos might be made.

Firm, "bound down" skin of the face and taut skin of the hands causing contractures and progression to a "claw like" deformity should prompt for consideration of systemic scleroderma.

Assessment of mobility has clinical importance with surgical planning as well. When confronted with neoplasms that will need surgical excision, one will need to consider the resulting surgical defect size, the anticipated repair needed, and the limitations of certain repairs based on peripheral skin mobility. Some anatomic locations such as the scalp and pretibial areas will be more challenging to close surgical defects than the cheek or neck, which are more mobile.

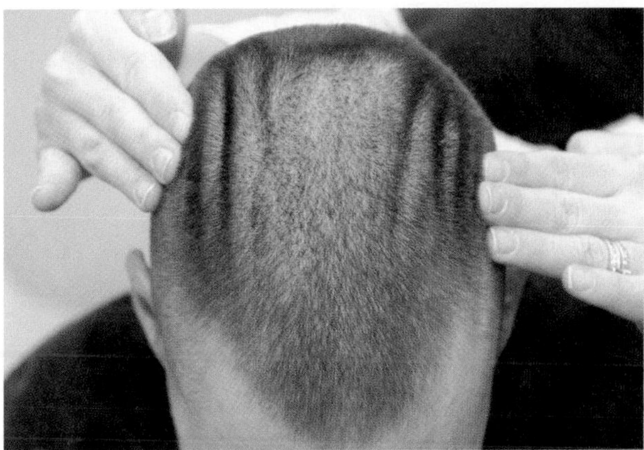

FIGURE 7-24 Direction of greatest mobility of the scalp.

Furthermore, aging skin may have more laxity and be more forgiving in repairing a large facial defect than the same defect in a 20-year-old. When planning a flap repair, one needs to consider the mobility of the skin peripheral to the surgical defect in order to know the direction from which to recruit skin for the repair while minimizing functional impairment or undesired cosmetic appearance (see **FIGURES 7-23** and **7-24**).

Consider a basal cell carcinoma of the forehead (see **FIGURE 7-25**). Excision requires consideration of the anticipated defect, the mobility of the surrounding tissue, and anticipation of how and where peripheral

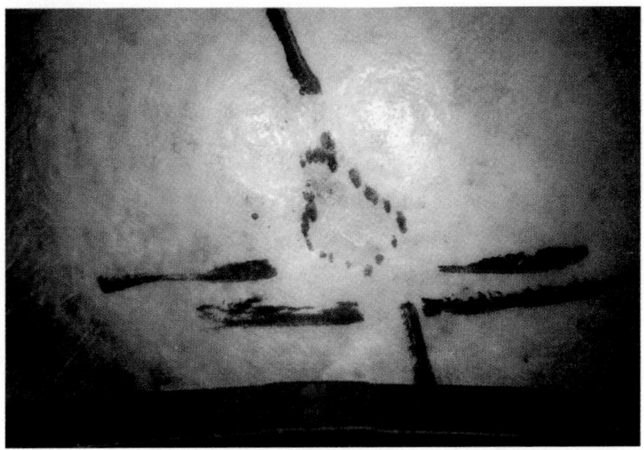

FIGURE 7-25 Marking of a basal cell carcinoma of the forehead prior to excision.

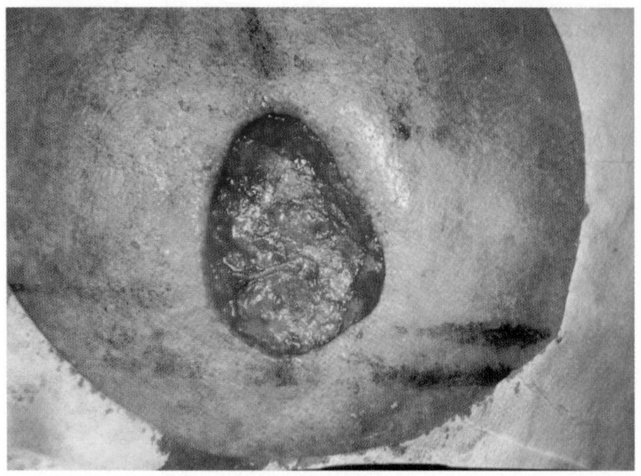

FIGURE 7-26 Surgical defect after removing basal cell carcinoma from glabella area of forehead.

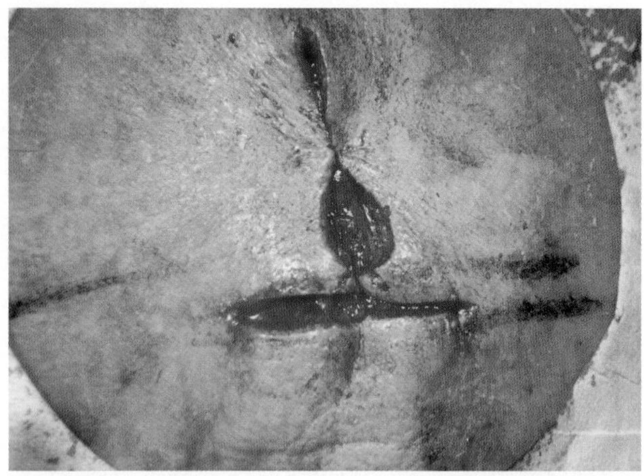

FIGURE 7-27 Beginning of "O to T" flap with key sutures in place.

skin will be recruited to repair the wound without functional impairment and yield the best cosmetic result. Excision requires a large surgical resection (see **FIGURE 7-26**).

To avoid elevation of the brow, the flap must come from the lateral directions of the defect. An "O to T" flap is created and the key sutures are in place (see **FIGURE 7-27**). All subcutaneous sutures are in place and superficial sutures ready to be placed.

The final repair will not create any unnatural pulling on the eyebrow and the subcutaneous sutures are approximating tissue without tension, allowing superficial cutaneous sutures to repair the wound with excellent cosmetic results (see **FIGURE 7-28**).

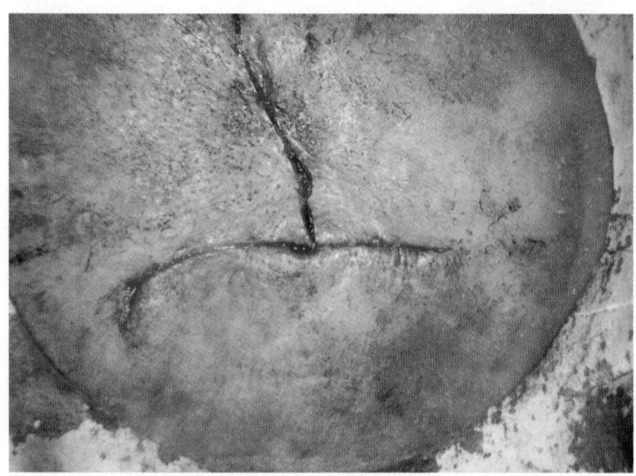

FIGURE 7-28 "O to T" flap with subcutaneous sutures completed.

DOCUMENTATION

- Skin—Palpation: soft, dry, symmetrically warm throughout. Slightly delayed turgor b/l forearms and increased mobility.

SKIN LESIONS

When a skin lesion is encountered, it is important to accurately document the lesion. Proper documentation and proper use of nomenclature will enable you and other readers of your records to accurately visualize the lesion. This is critical for proper communication with other health professionals. For example, if you need to call your local dermatologist for advice on a lesion, improper nomenclature and description will mislead the dermatologist's visualization of the lesion and hence the possible diagnoses.

Type of Lesion

Begin with the type of lesion. As the provider gains experience in identification of skin lesions, being able to correctly describe the lesion by its type significantly narrows the differential diagnosis. Dermatological texts frequently categorize skin lesions by type. You may not readily know what the lesion is, but being able to describe it as "papular" allows you to reference that section of the text, aiding in your diagnosis.

Skin lesions can be broken down into three categories:

1. Primary skin lesions
2. Secondary skin lesions
3. Special lesions

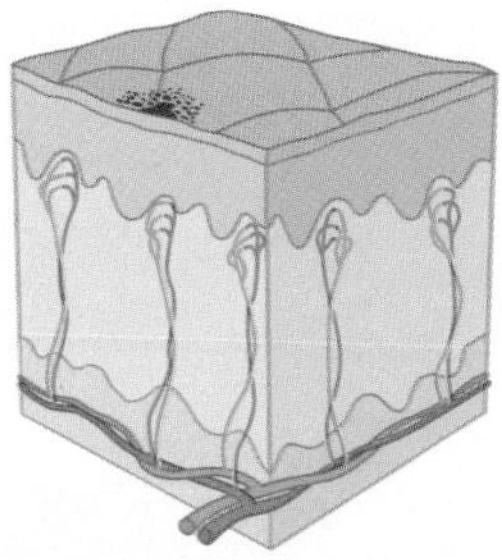

FIGURE 7-29 Diagram of macule.

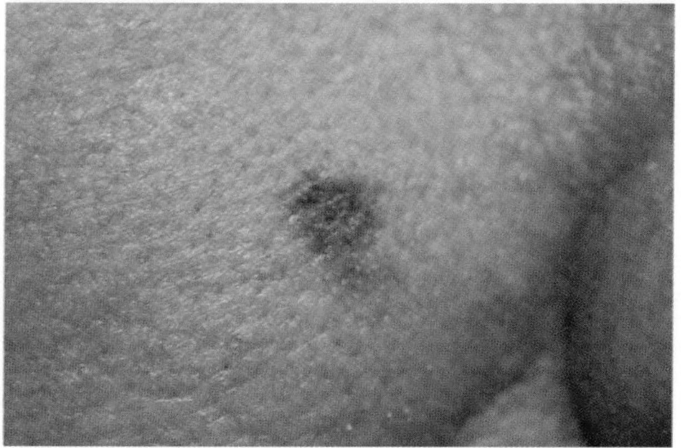

FIGURE 7-30 Macule.

Primary Lesions.

- Macule (see **FIGURES 7-29** and **7-30**): a flat skin lesion less than 10 mm in diameter that varies from the surrounding skin by color, but not by texture or thickness. If the provider closes his/her eyes and rubs a finger over the area, he/she cannot discern the location of the lesion.
- Patch (see **FIGURE 7-31**): a macule that is larger than 10 mm in size. Consider a patch of blue paint on a green wall. If you rub your hand over it with your eyes closed, you cannot tell where the patch of blue paint starts.

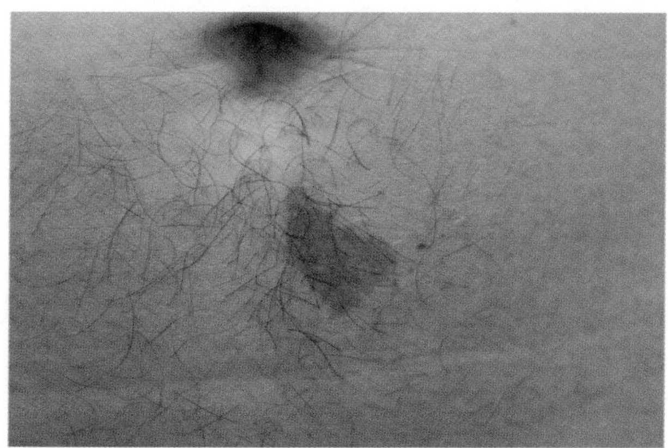

FIGURE 7-31 Patch.

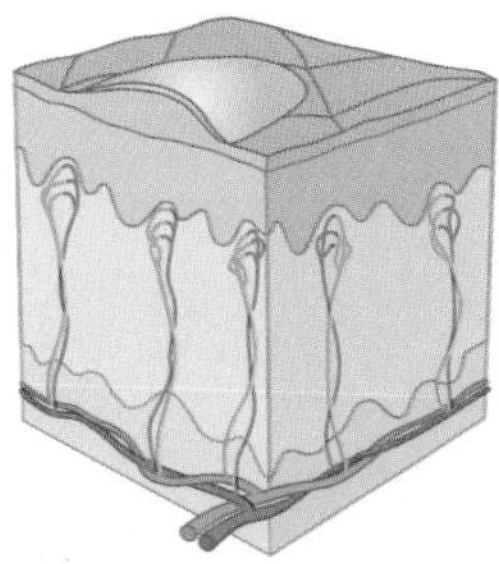

FIGURE 7-32 Diagram of papule.

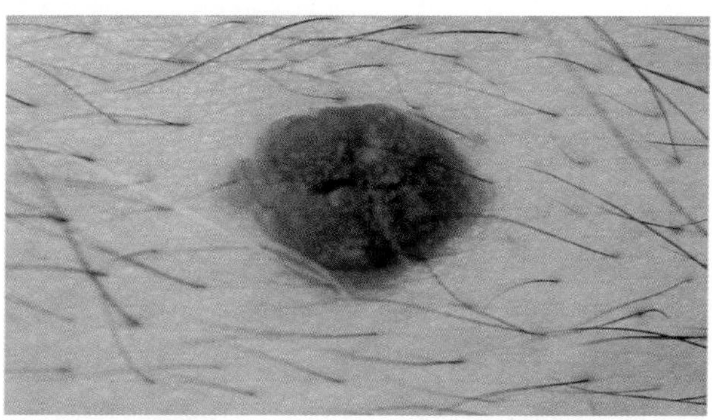

FIGURE 7-33 Papule.

- Papule (see **FIGURES 7-32** and **7-33**): an elevated, solid skin lesion that is less than 1.0 cm in diameter. Papules often arise in the epidermis or epidermal/dermal junction. These lesions are detectible by touch when rubbing your finger over the area. Utilizing the technique of lightly palpating a region of skin while inspecting for lesions increases detection of smaller, skin-colored lesions that may otherwise have been missed by inspection alone, especially in areas such as the scalp.
- Plaque: a circumscribed, elevated, superficial, solid lesion greater than 1.0 cm in diameter. Often it is formed by a confluence of papules.
- Nodule (see **FIGURES 7-34** and **7-35**): a circumscribed, elevated, solid lesion greater than 1.0 cm in diameter. Large nodules are referred to as tumors.
- Vesicle (see **FIGURES 7-36** and **7-37**): a circumscribed collection of free fluid that is less than 0.5 cm in diameter. This fluid collection lifts the epithelium from the dermal skin layer.

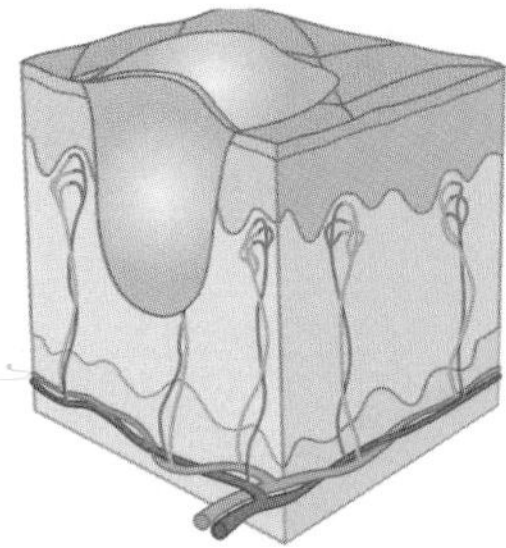

FIGURE 7-34 Diagram of nodule.

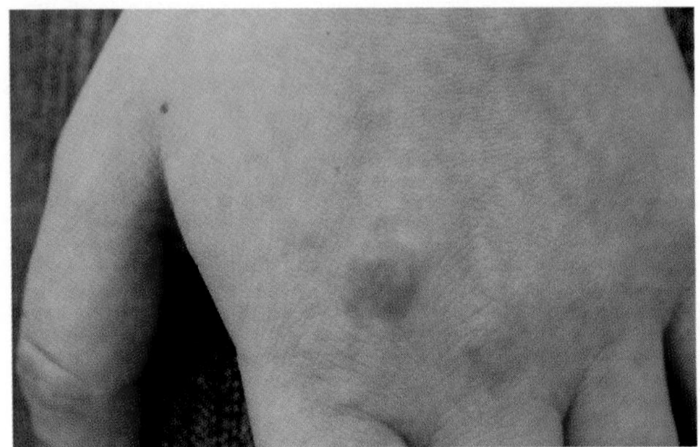

FIGURE 7-35 Nodule.

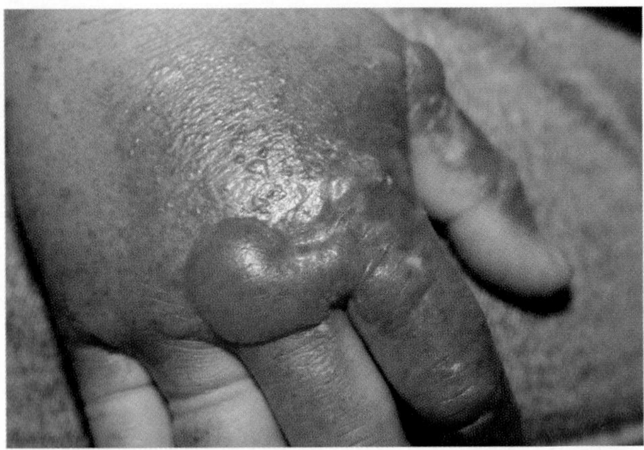

FIGURE 7-38 Bulla.

- Bulla (see FIGURE 7-38): a circumscribed collection of free fluid greater than 0.5 cm in diameter.
- Pustule (see FIGURES 7-39 and 7-40): a vesicle that contains inflammatory cells or, as the name implies, "pus," causing the fluid to appear cloudy or purulent. A common example would be an acne pustule. Some vesicles progress to pustules, such as with herpes virus lesions.

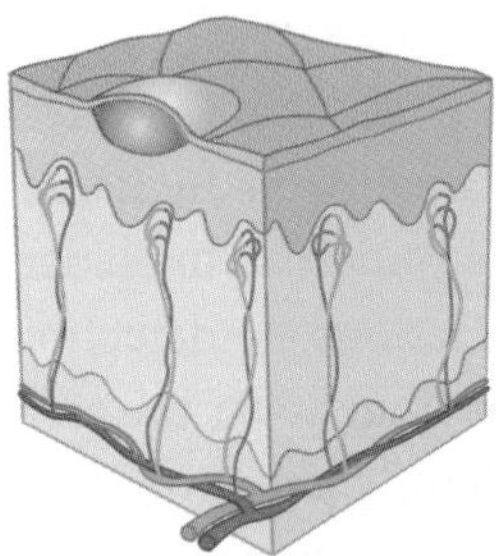

FIGURE 7-36 Diagram of vesicle.

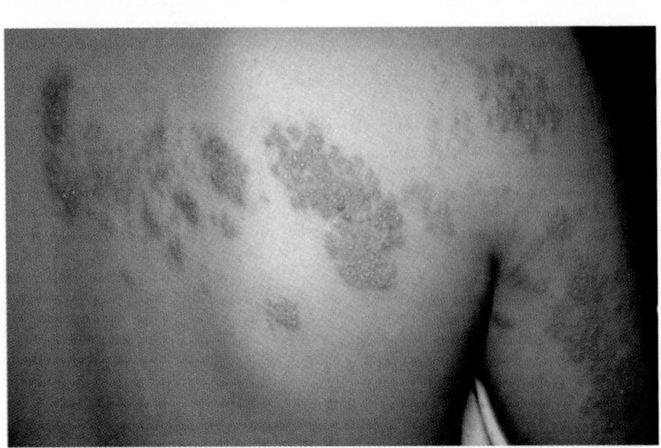

FIGURE 7-37 Vesicle.

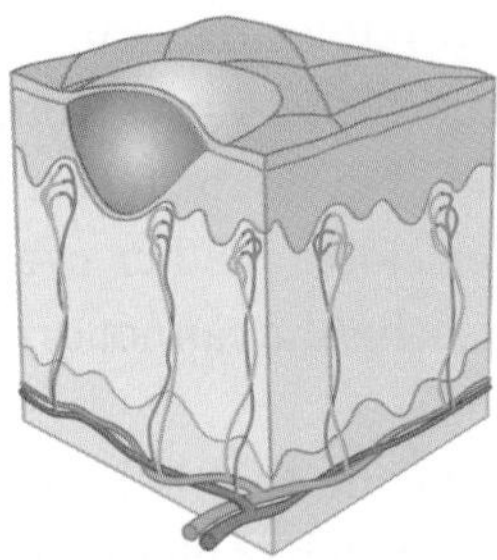

FIGURE 7-39 Diagram of pustule.

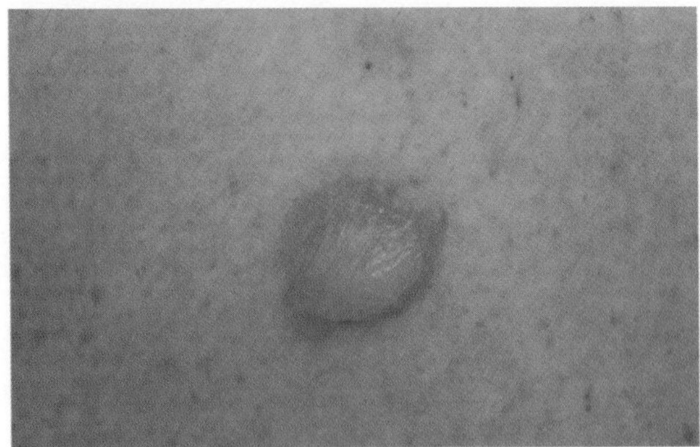

FIGURE 7-40 Pustule.

Secondary Lesions.

- Erosion (see **FIGURES 7-41** and **7-42**): an erosion is a focal loss of part of the epidermal layer of skin, leaving the dermis intact. Acutely it appears moist and slightly depressed. Because the loss of tissue does not penetrate the dermoepidermal junction, it typically heals without scarring. A denuded blister is an example of an erosion.
- Ulcer (see **FIGURES 7-43** and **7-44**): an erosion that involves the epidermis and dermis. Ulcers typically heal with scarring. Common examples would include pressure ulcerations, venous stasis, and basal cell carcinoma.
- Fissure (see **FIGURES 7-45** and **7-46**): a split in the skin that extends through the epidermis and dermis. The split is linear and sharply defined, with near-vertical walls. Chapped hands from wind and cold exposure that crack and bleed are an example.

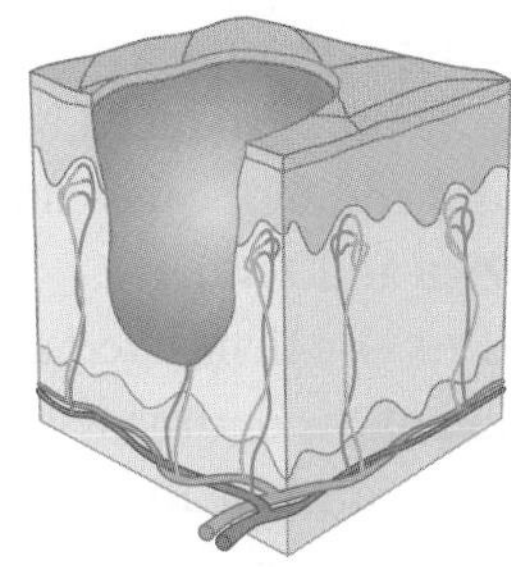

FIGURE 7-43 Diagram of ulcer.

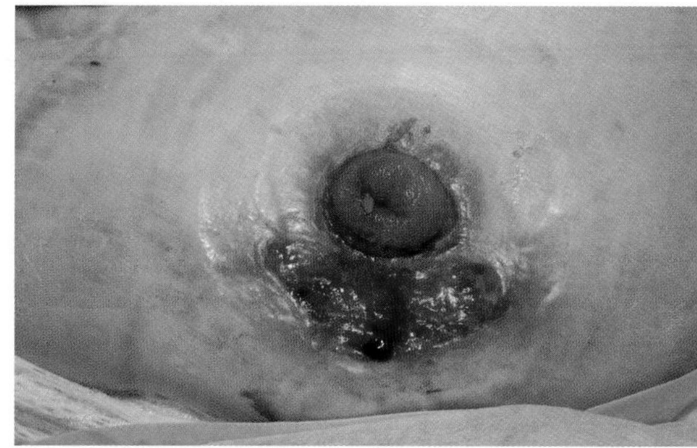

FIGURE 7-44 Ulcer.

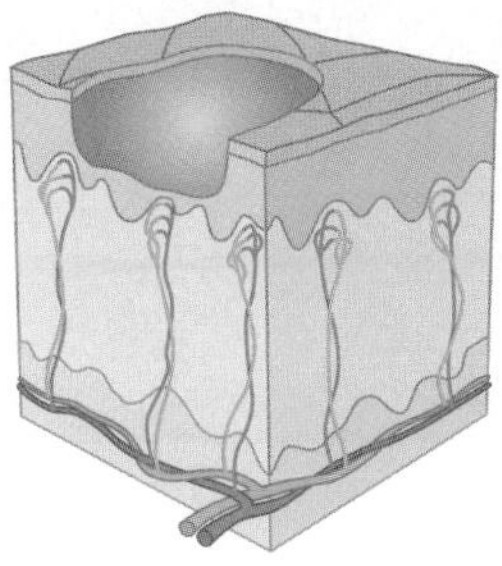

FIGURE 7-41 Diagram of erosion.

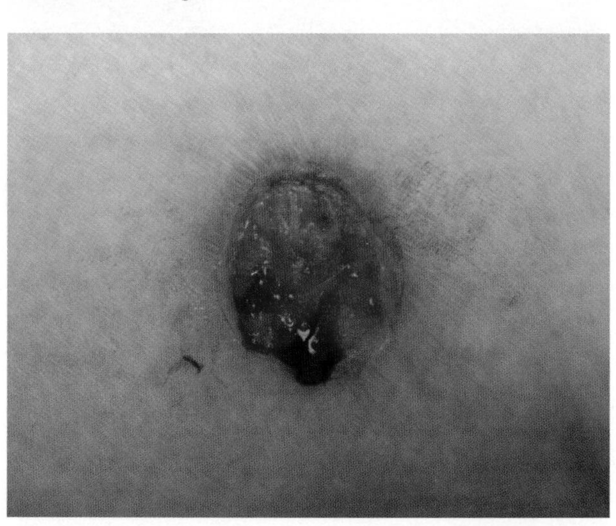

FIGURE 7-42 Denuded bullous lesion with a moist erosion.

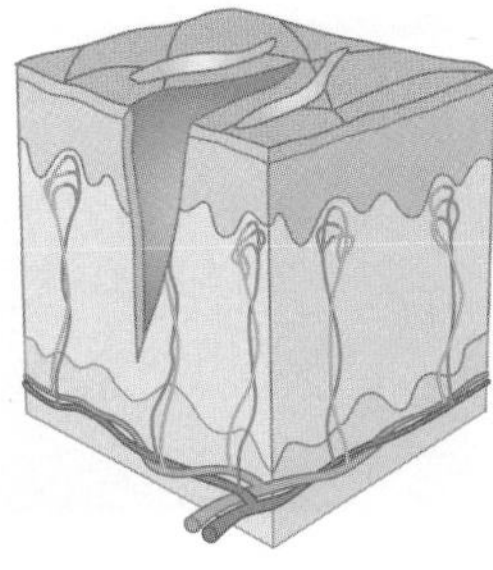

FIGURE 7-45 Diagram of fissure.

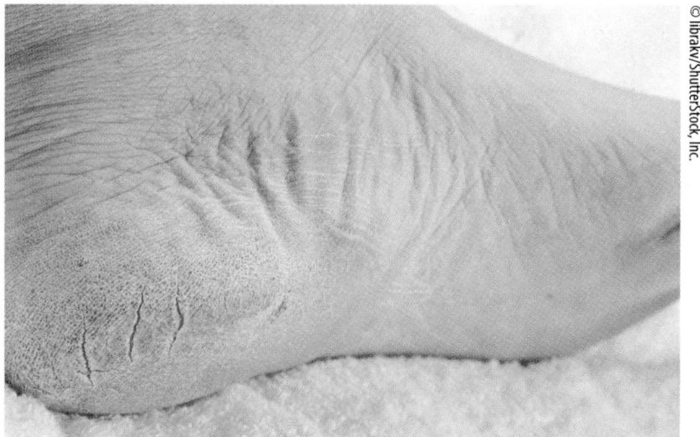

© librakv/ShutterStock, Inc.

FIGURE 7-46 Fissure.

- Scale (see **FIGURE 7-47**): a flaking of the uppermost layer of skin, the stratum corneum. Produced by abnormal keratinization and shedding. Scales can be dry or oily (see **FIGURES 7-48** and **7-49**).
- Wheal (see **FIGURES 7-50** and **7-51**): a firm, edematous plaque due to infiltration of the dermis with fluid. These lesions are usually transient and may last for only a few hours. They are often associated with an allergic reaction, making them pruritic. Common terminology includes a welt or hive. More severe deep-tissue edema with more diffuse swelling is referred to as angioedema.

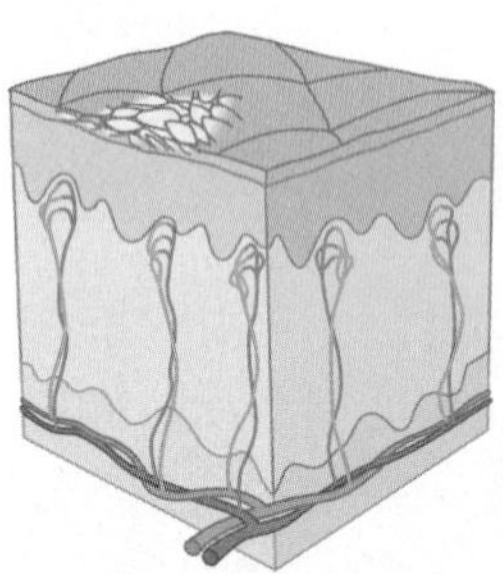

FIGURE 7-47 Diagram of scale.

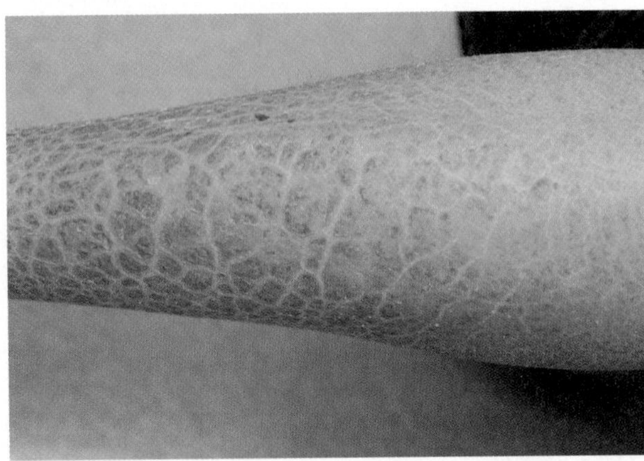

FIGURE 7-48 Icthyosis.

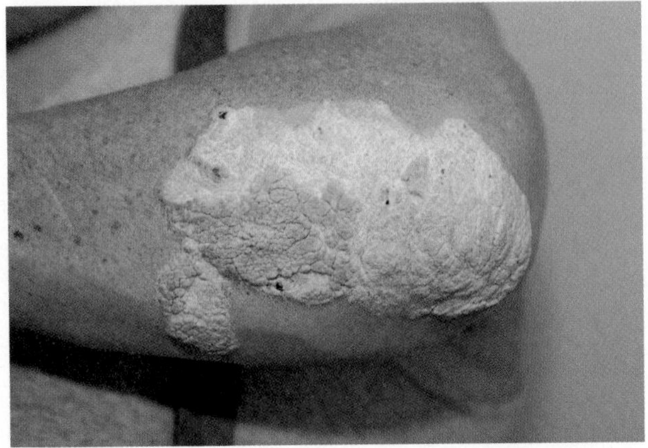

FIGURE 7-49 Psoriasis.

Special Skin Lesions.

- Comedone (see **FIGURE 7-52**): a plug of sebaceous and keratinous material in the opening of the hair follicle. When the orifice is dilated (open

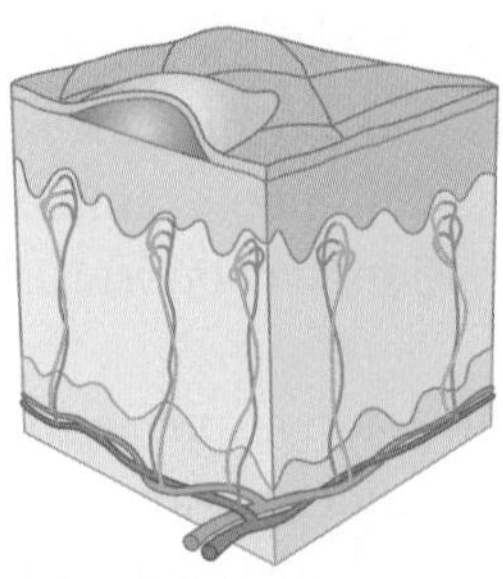

FIGURE 7-50 Diagram of wheal.

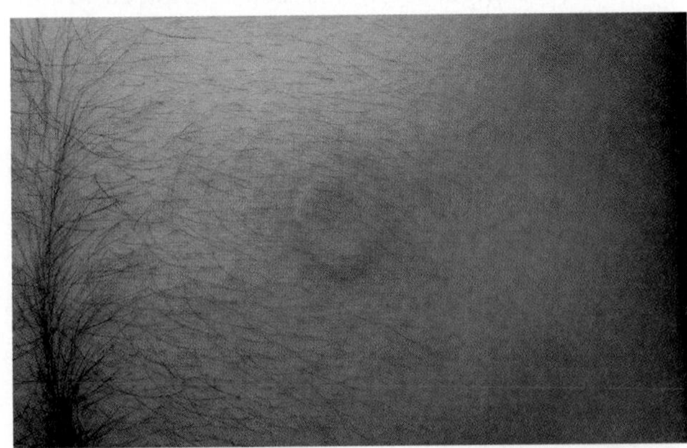

FIGURE 7-51 Wheal.

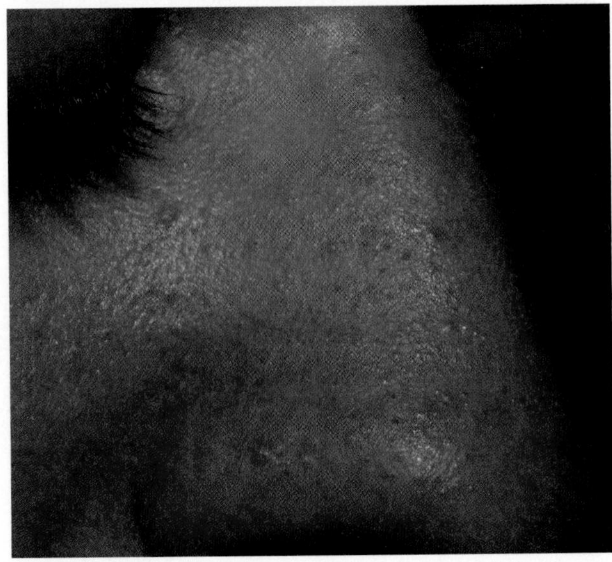

FIGURE 7-52 Comedone.

comedone), it is commonly referred to as a "blackhead." When the orifice is narrowed (closed comedone), it is commonly referred to as a "whitehead." Comedones are the primary lesion of acne and their absence is helpful when entertaining a diagnosis for rosacea.

- Milia (see **FIGURE 7-53**): small, circumscribed, superficial keratin cysts with no visible opening.
- Cyst (see **FIGURE 7-54**): a closed saclike structure that may be filled with liquid or solid material. It has a distinct wall often composed of epithelial cells. There are many different types of cysts: chalazion, ganglion, pilar, pilonidal, sebaceous.
- Lichenification (see **FIGURE 7-55**): a thickening of the skin with exaggeration of skin lines, often due to chronic irritation such as rubbing or scratching the area.
- Atrophy (see **FIGURE 7-56**): a thinning of skin that may include the subcutaneous layer. The skin may appear shiny, translucent, tight, or depressed.

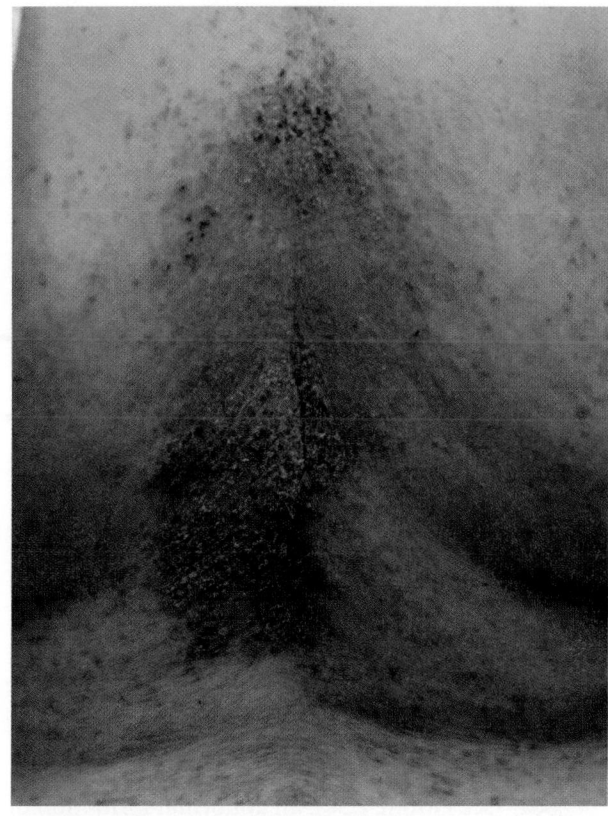

FIGURE 7-55 Lichenification of the back.

FIGURE 7-53 Milium.

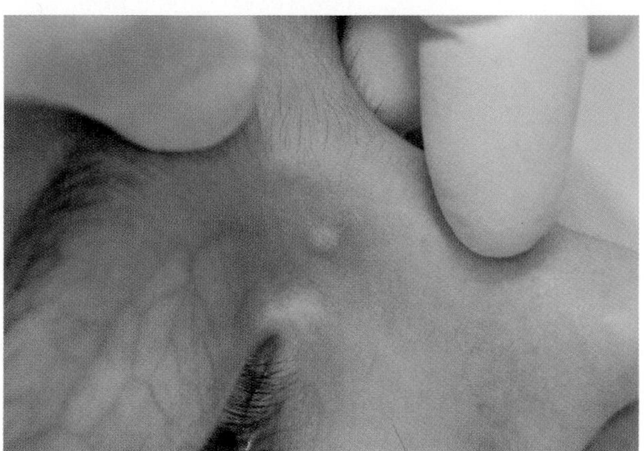

FIGURE 7-54 Epidermal cyst of the nose.

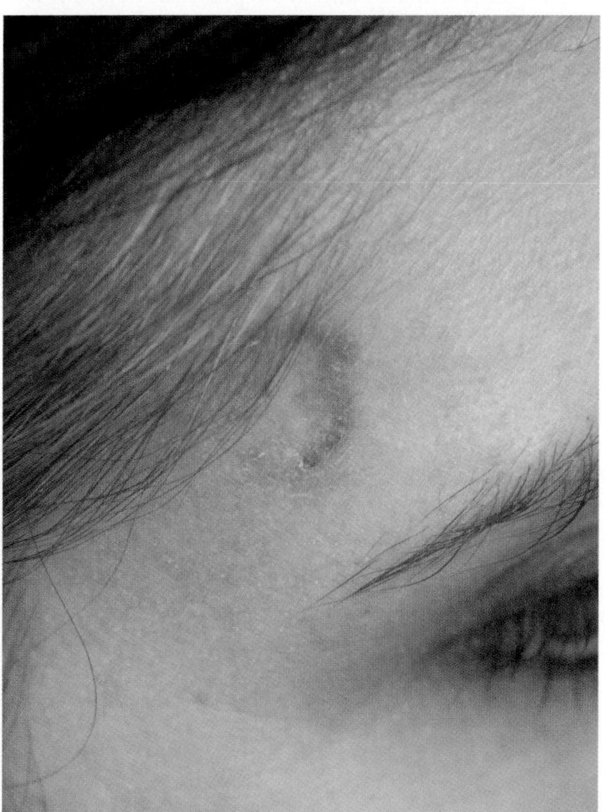

FIGURE 7-56 Atrophy.

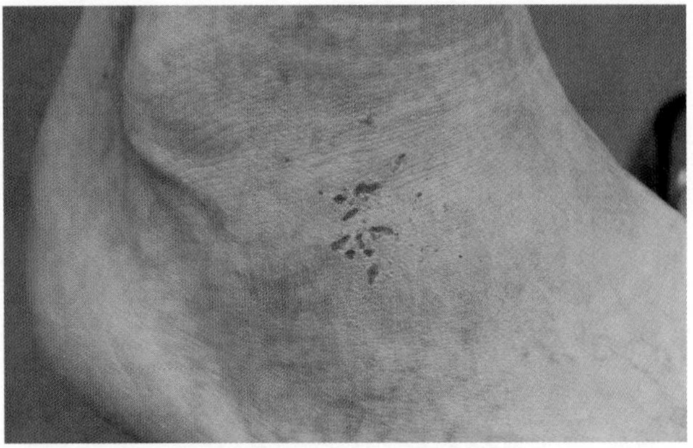

FIGURE 7-57 Excoriation.

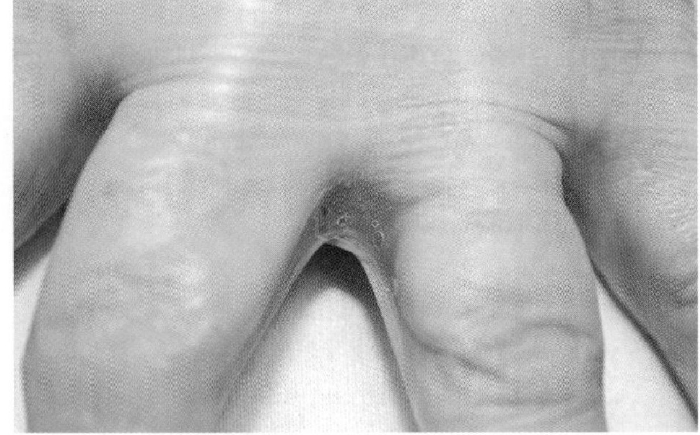

FIGURE 7-59 Maceration.

- Excoriation (see **FIGURE 7-57**): an abrasion of the skin, often caused by scratching of the area, resulting in a linear pattern. Excoriation often destroys the characteristics of primary lesions, making diagnosis difficult. Search the patient for undisturbed primary lesions, such as in the middle of the back, where the patient cannot reach to scratch the lesions. Also look for newly forming lesions.
- Scar (see **FIGURE 7-58**): an abnormal formation of connective tissue that suggests a previous damage to the dermis by injury or previous surgery. Initially scars can be pink and thick, but they often mature into white and atrophic lesions.
- Maceration (see **FIGURE 7-59**): a condition caused by chronic moisture, which softens and makes the tissues opaque. Maceration is commonly seen in the corners of the mouth, between skin folds such as under the breasts, and between the toes.
- Telangiectasia (see **FIGURE 7-60**): dilated blood vessels appearing within a lesion or on the surface of the skin. Commonly seen as a component of basal cell carcinoma and rosacea.
- Petechiae (see **FIGURE 7-61**): a circumscribed deposit of blood less than 0.5 cm in diameter.

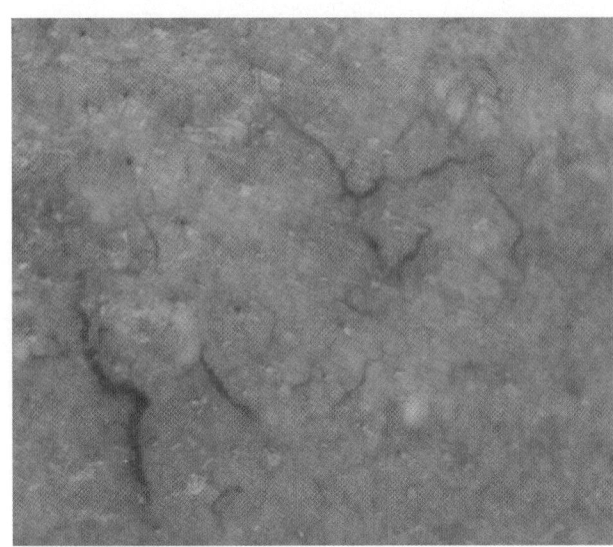

FIGURE 7-60 Telangiectasia.

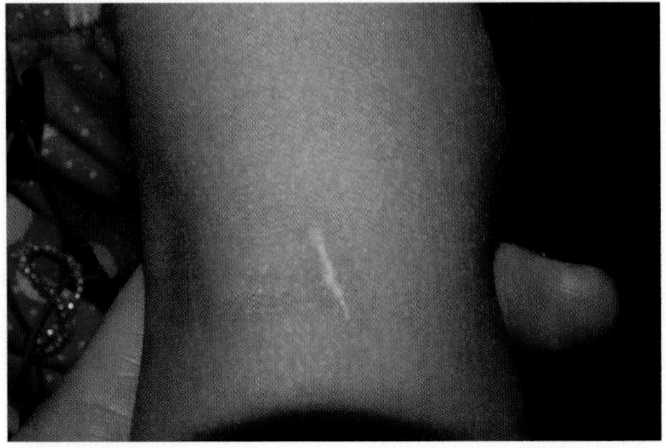

FIGURE 7-58 Scar.

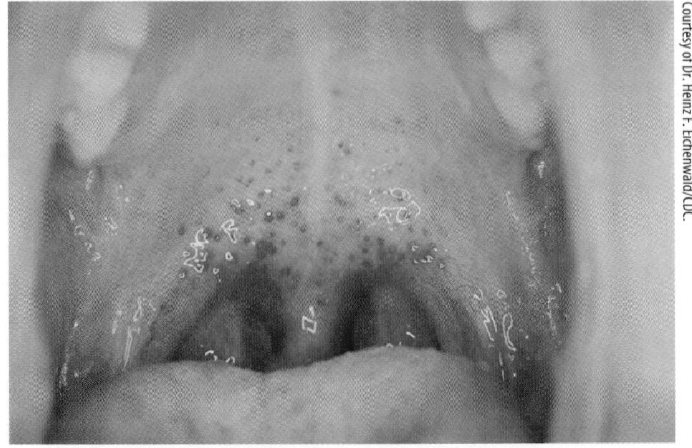

Courtesy of Dr. Heinz F. Eichenwald/CDC.

FIGURE 7-61 Petechiae.

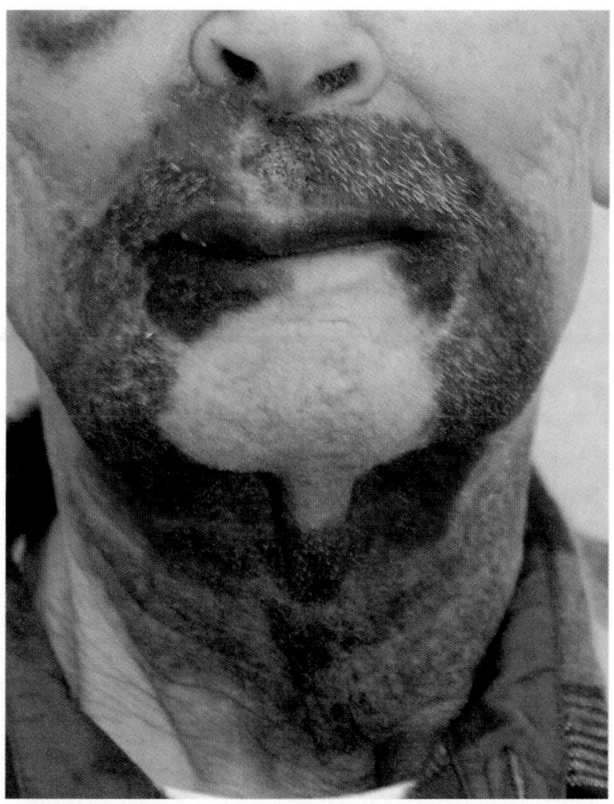

FIGURE 7-62 Purpura secondary to surgical trauma.

- Purpura (see FIGURE 7-62): a circumscribed deposit of blood greater than 0.5 cm in diameter.
- Burrow (see FIGURE 7-63): a thin, elevated tortuous channel produced by a parasite. Scabies burrows are typically found in webspaces or hypothenar eminence of the hand, wrists, elbows, and ankles. Scabies scrapings should be done of these areas to have the best chance of confirming the diagnosis.
- Crust (see FIGURE 7-64): Dried exudate, commonly called a scab.

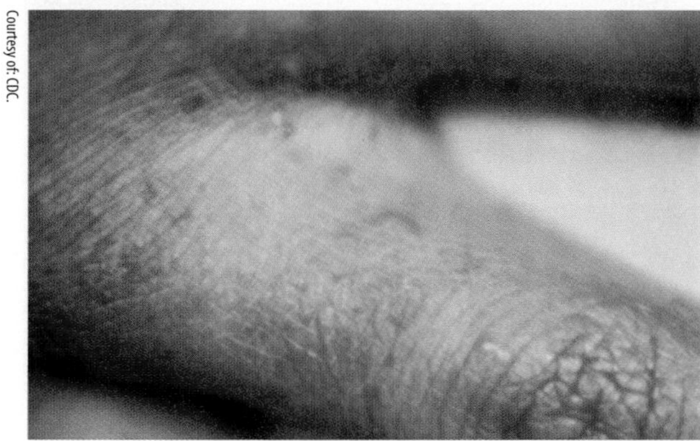

Courtesy of: CDC.

FIGURE 7-63 Burrow.

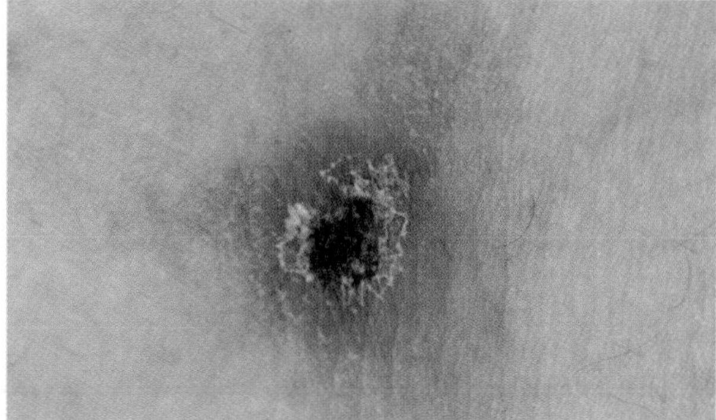

FIGURE 7-64 Cutaneous calciphylaxis related to secondary hyperparathyroidism.

Shape and Configuration

What is the shape of the individual lesion? Is it oval, annular (round), arciform (archlike), angulated? Are the lesions symmetrical or asymmetrical? Are the borders well circumscribed or are they blurred or jagged? Look for any configuration of the lesions and document this, as it may help to support or not support certain diagnoses. For example, are the lesions individual and scattered or do they form patterns, becoming linear, clustered, serpiginous, or coalesced? Could the lesions be associated with sites of trauma (Koebner phenomenon)?

Consider the following lesion for description:

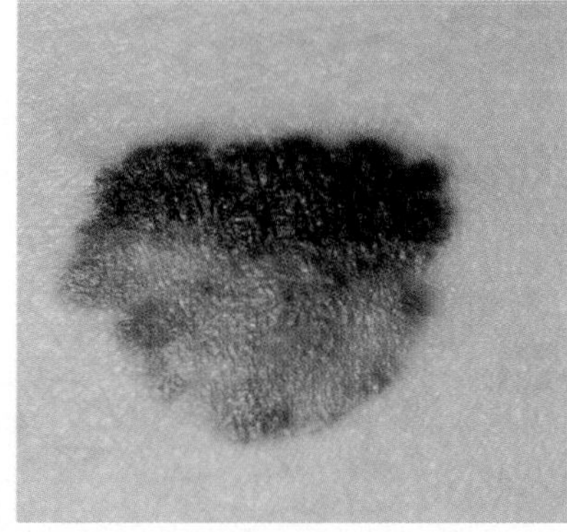

- The lesion depicted is somewhat annular.

Border.

Look closely at the border. Is it regular and easily discernible? Or is it irregular, even to the point that you cannot discern where the actual edge of the border merges with normal skin?

- It has an irregular border

Nail: horny plates of the distal, ventral surfaces of the fingers and toes, produced by the nail matrix

Color Variation.

Is the lesion monotone, consisting of only one color? Describe the color: brown, black, red, blue, white, tan, pink, etc. Or, is it composed of several colors in combination?

- The lesion is two-tone brown and black.

Size.

Measure the lesion. If composed of multiple colors or a combination of shapes, describe each.

- The lesion is two-tone brown and black measuring 13 × 9 mm at its greatest width and length—the approximate lower two-thirds being brown and the upper 10- × 3-mm section of the lesion being black.

Location.

Certain lesions have a predilection for different locations on the body, such as squamous cell carcinomas on the dorsum of the hand and basal cell carcinomas on the face. Observe for patterns of distribution, such as areas limited to sun exposure. Lesions caused by contact with offending agents often take on the shape of the object, such as jewelry or footwear (see **FIGURE 7-65**).

- The lesion is on his back above the left scapula.

Combining the findings, you give your report:

- A 26-year-old male presents with an isolated, somewhat circular, but irregular bordered, two-tone brown and black plaque above his left scapula with the lower two-thirds of the lesion being brown and the upper 10- × 3-mm section of the lesion being black.

This detailed description allows the lesion to be visualized as much as possible.

DOCUMENTATION

- Isolated, somewhat circular, irregular bordered, two-tone brown and black plaque above the left scapula with the lower two-thirds of the lesion being brown and the upper 10- × 3-mm section of the lesion being black.

Nails

The fingernails and toenails should be examined for both local pathology and evidence of systemic disease. **Nail** changes may be associated with skin and hair disorders and may be supportive evidence for a clinical diagnosis. Some nail changes are "reaction patterns" that are not necessarily pathognomonic of any specific condition but can be associated with a variety of diseases. For example, "pitting" of the nail plate is often associated with psoriasis, but it can also be seen with other conditions. When inspecting small body areas, do so with purposeful attention to detail. Looking at a nail, consider each component (see **FIGURE 7-65**). Begin at the proximal nail fold, then move distally, looking at the lunula, nail surface, nail bed, and free edge. Then examine the lateral nail folds as you would the extremities following examination of the thorax. This approach provides a detailed examination.

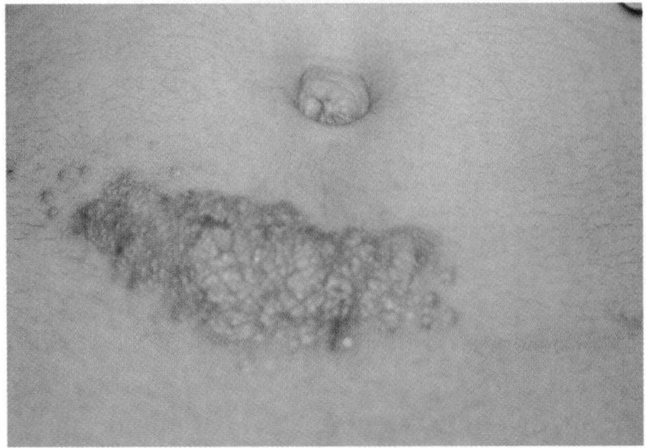

FIGURE 7-65 Contact dermatitis from belt buckle.

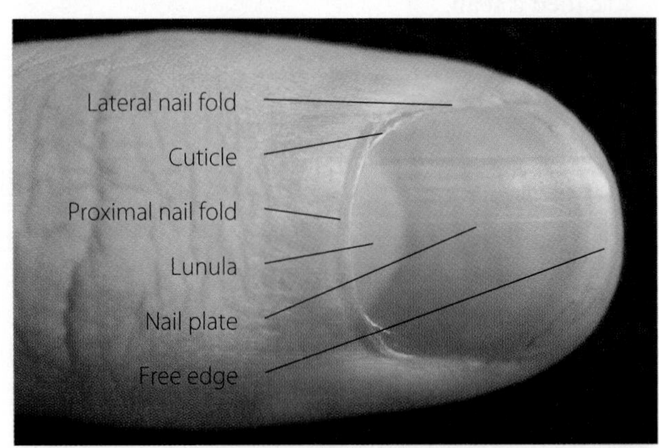

FIGURE 7-66 Labeled nail.

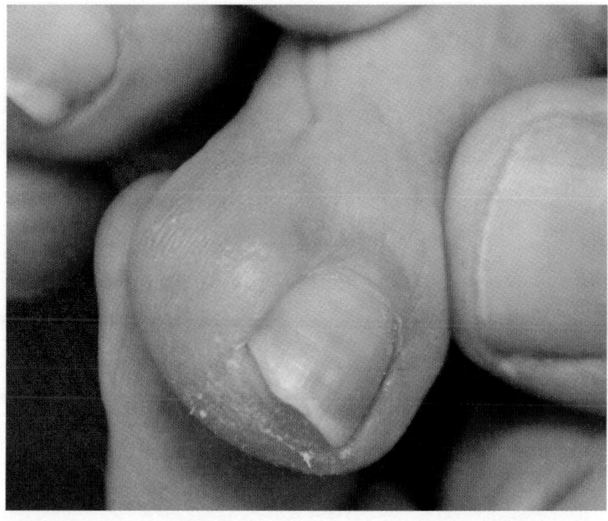

FIGURE 7-67 Paronychia.

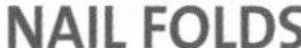

NAIL FOLDS

The nail folds serve as a barrier to infection. Observe the folds for signs of inflammation: erythema, swelling, tenderness, and abscess formation associated with paronychia (see **FIGURE 7-67**).

NAIL

Moving distally, look at the nail itself. Work from front to back, first observing the surface of the nail.

- Surface: Is it smooth or does it have deformity? Pits represent small foci or "footprints" of nail plate shedding that occurred previously under the cuticle and will grow out with the nail (see **FIGURE 7-68**). Pits can represent conditions such as psoriasis, lichen planus, contact dermatitis, or alopecia areata. Vertical splits that extend to the proximal nail fold represent damage to the matrix where nail growth occurs (see **FIGURE 7-69**). This can be associated with a number of conditions or can be a reaction pattern seen in contact dermatitis, trauma, or the aging process. Beau's lines are transverse depressions that may be related to acute illness (see **FIGURE 7-70**).
- Color: Is the surface translucent or discolored? Leukonychia, whitening, and opacification of the nail is the most common color change (see **FIGURE 7-71**). Onset with progression from the distal

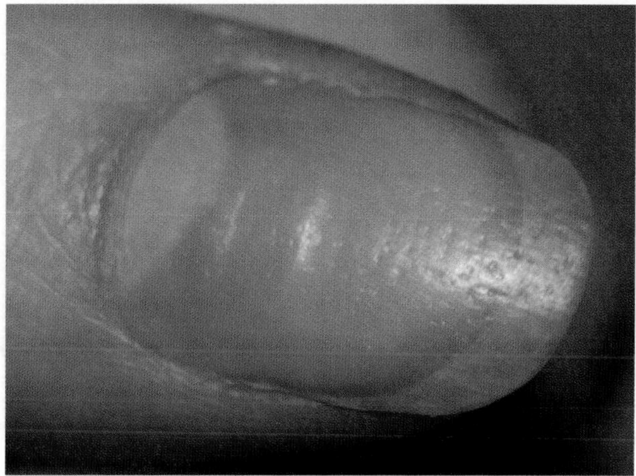

FIGURE 7-68 Nail pitting.

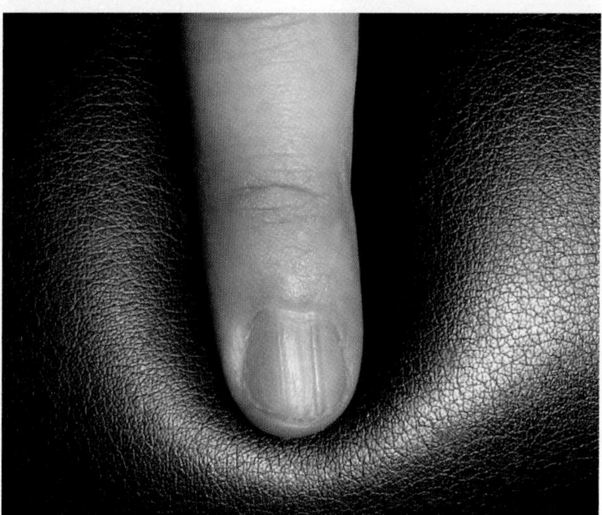

FIGURE 7-69 Linear nail defect.

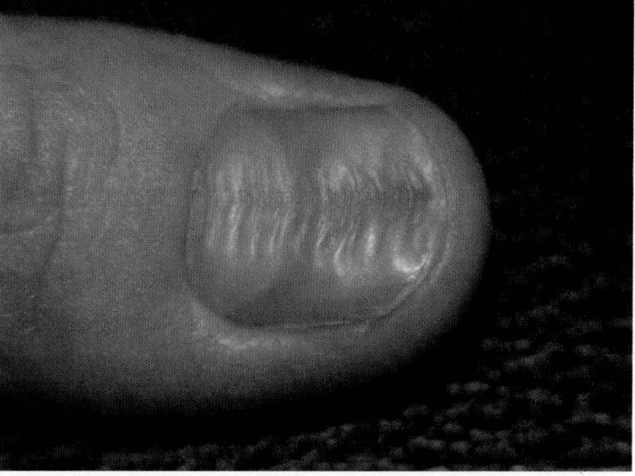

FIGURE 7-70 Beau's lines appear as transverse depressions of the nail however these are from repeated trauma caused by the patient pushing down the proximal nail fold with the adjacent finger.

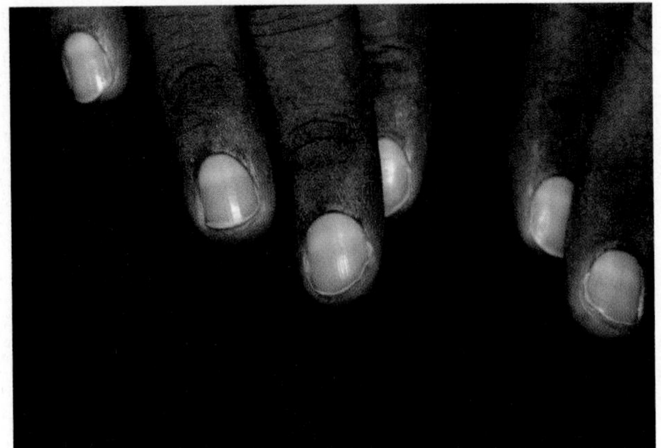

FIGURE 7-71 Leukonychia.

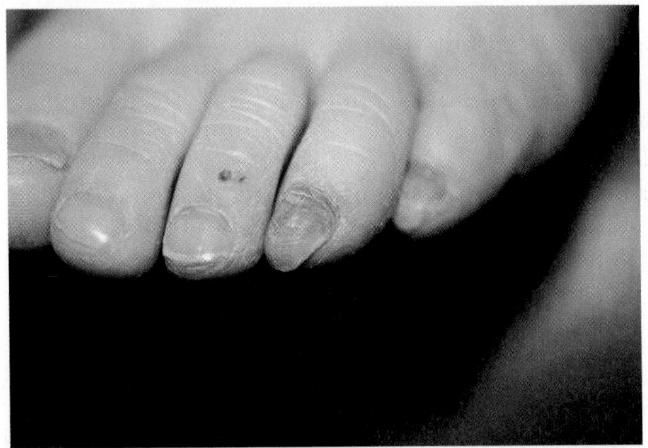

FIGURE 7-72 Onychomycosis.

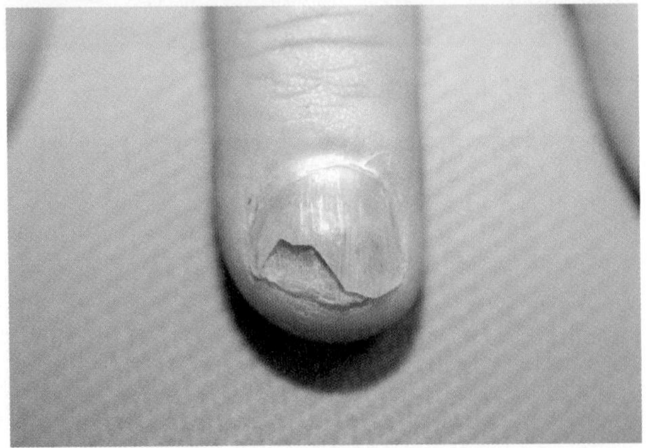

FIGURE 7-73 Onycholysis.

nail edge, especially with subungual debris, may represent fungal infection or onychomycosis (see FIGURE 7-72). Separation of the nail from the bed is called onycholysis (see FIGURE 7-73). Terry's nails are mostly white with a distal band and may be

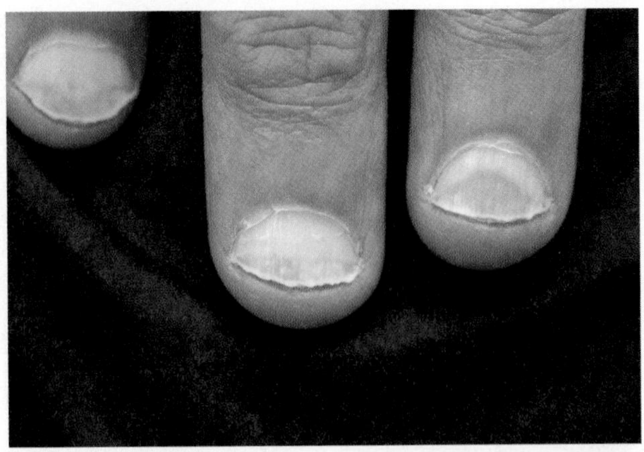

FIGURE 7-74 Terry's nails.

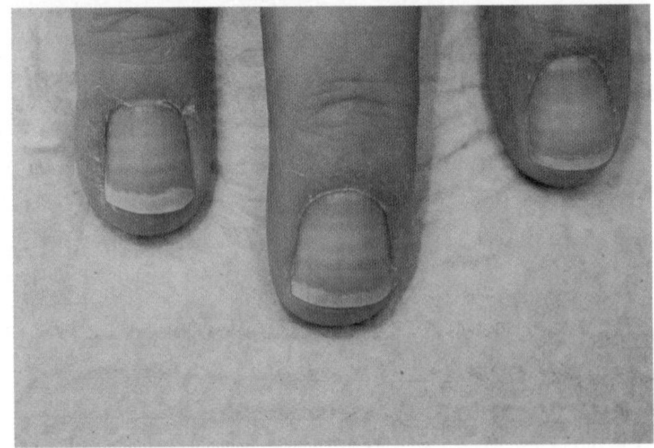

FIGURE 7-75 Mees' lines.

related to aging, end-stage liver disease, diabetes mellitus, or heart failure (see FIGURE 7-74). Mees' lines follow the curve of lunula and may occur after acute or severe illness (see FIGURE 7-75).

- Thickness: Increased thickness may represent fungal infection, psoriasis, lichen planus, contact dermatitis, onychogryphosis, or response to repeated trauma.
- Length and Hygiene: Observe for hygienic care of the nails. Are the nails trimmed or neglected? Elongated nails may simply reflect lack of self-care or may mark dementia. In care-dependent patients, they may also show a level of neglect from the caregiver. Elongation of a single nail may have the connotation of drug abuse. Overly shortened nails with evidence of biting may be habit or evidence of a more severe anxiety disorder (see FIGURE 7-76).

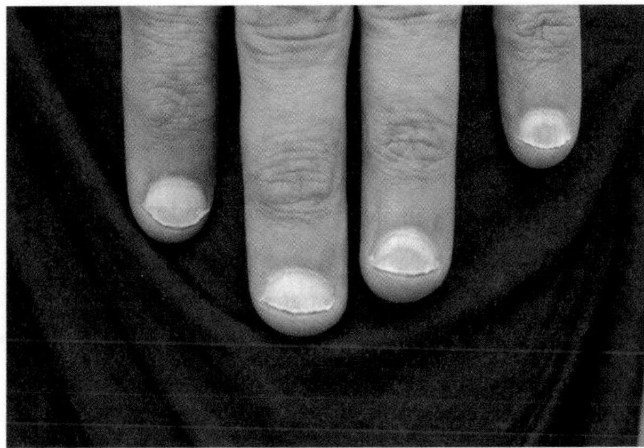

FIGURE 7-76 Bitten nails.

NAIL BED

- Color: Observe the whiteness of the lunula at the proximal edge of the nail, then the pinkness of the nail bed itself. Look for pallor and cyanosis.
- Observe for lesions within the nail bed. As the name suggests, splinter hemorrhages appear as thin linear brownish-red or brown splinters and are caused by microinfarcts from endocarditis or vasculitis (see **FIGURE 7-77**). The splinter configuration is due to the longitudinal "tongue and groove" interface of the nail bed and underside of the nail plate that "channels" the subungual blood in a linear fashion. Subungual or acral lentiginous melanomas appear as darkening of the nail bed, most commonly of the great toe and thumb. Periungual extension of brown-black pigmentation to the proximal or lateral nail folds is an important indicator of subungual melanoma and is referred to as Hutchinson's sign (see **FIGURE 7-78**). They are

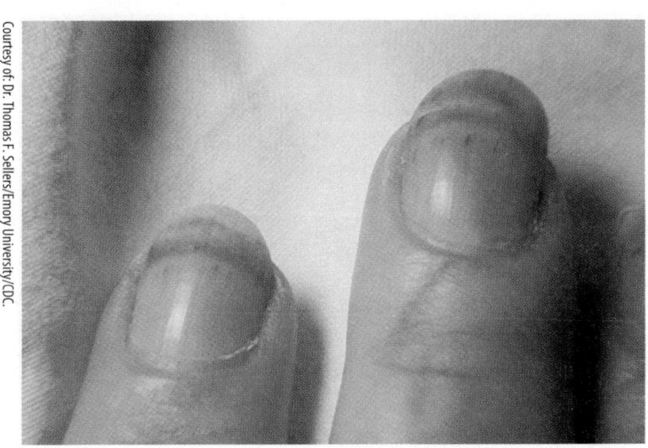

Courtesy of: Dr. Thomas F. Sellers/Emory University/CDC.

FIGURE 7-77 Splinter hemorrhages.

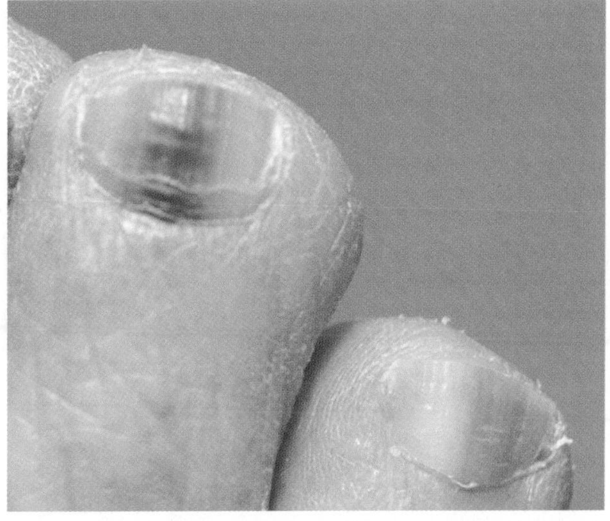

FIGURE 7-78 Nail melanoma.

more common in dark-skinned ethnic groups, where they comprise 15–35% of melanoma occurrences, as compared to only 3% of cases of melanoma in Caucasians.[5]

7-2

- **Capillary Refill** (see **FIGURE 7-79**): assessment of peripheral perfusion can be made by performing a capillary refill test. The nail is compressed between the provider's thumb and index finger, blanching the nail bed. When released, reperfusion, evidenced by pinking of the nail, should occur in less than two seconds. Systemic perfusion can be assessed by performing

Capillary refill: assessment of peripheral perfusion performed by compressing the nail between the provider's thumb and index finger, blanching the nail bed, and assessing reperfusion when released

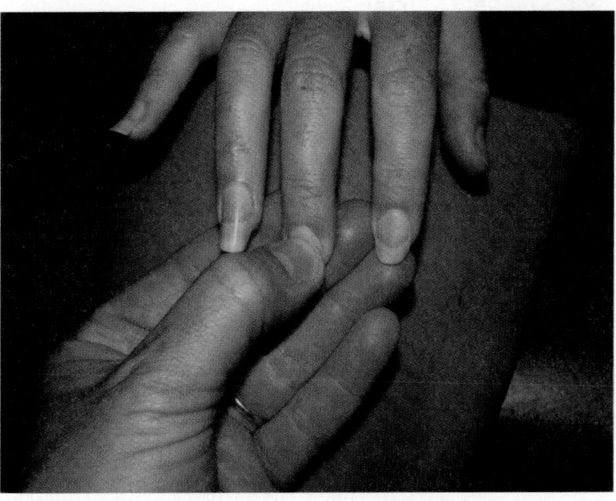

FIGURE 7-79 Assessment of capillary refill.

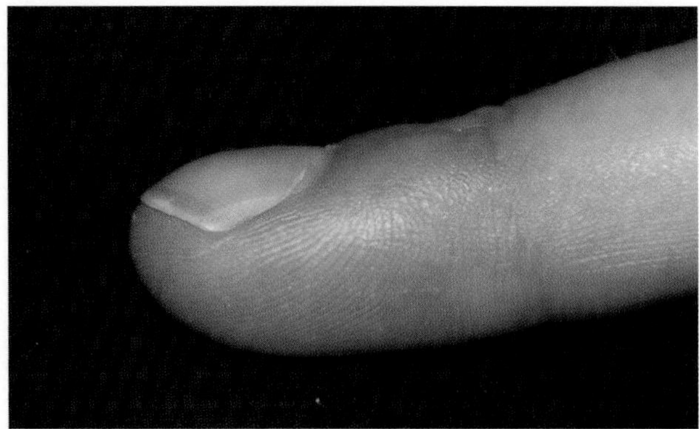

FIGURE 7-80 Clubbing in a patient with a congenital heart defect.

the exam on a few digits of each extremity. Each digit of an individual extremity should be examined when assessing localized perfusion, such as after cast placement, trauma, or cold injury.

SHAPE

Clubbing

Clubbing consists of excessive growth of tissues beneath the cuticles, which causes enlargement and sponginess of the surrounding nail folds, resulting in a "drumstick" appearance (see **FIGURE 7-80**). Nail deformity occurs with spoonlike curvature. Clubbing is most commonly associated with hypo-oxygenation, such as with chronic lung or heart disease, but may also be associated with liver disease such as cirrhosis with hepatopulmonary syndrome, gastrointestinal disorders such as Crohn's disease, and malabsorptions, lung cancer, and infection.

DOCUMENTATION

- Nails—Inspection: well kempt with nail folds intact. Surface smooth, translucent without pits. Bed pink without lesions. No clubbing.

Basal cell carcinoma: the most common type of skin cancer, arising from the epidermis, classically described as a dome-shaped lesion with translucent, pearly white borders and telangiectasias that frequently ulcerate, forming a central depression

Skin Cancer

According to the American Academy of Dermatology and the Skin Cancer Foundation, skin cancer is the most common form of cancer in the United States. More than 3.5 million skin cancers in over two million people are diagnosed annually.[6] That is more than the combined incidence of cancers of the breast, prostate, lung, and colon. Almost one out of every two people in the United States who live to age 65 years will be diagnosed with skin cancer.[7] Patient education on the signs and symptoms of skin cancer and the need for and methods of self-assessment is vital in prevention of the disease, early detection, and management.

BASAL CELL CARCINOMA

Basal cell carcinoma (BCC) (see **FIGURE 7-81**) is the most common type of skin cancer, with estimates approaching nearly three million diagnosed cases annually in the United States.[7] Although rarely fatal, these carcinomas can be highly disfiguring if allowed to grow.

BCC arises from the epidermis. There are variable histologic types including nodular, superficial, and morpheaform. Nodular is the most common form, classically being described as a dome-shaped lesion with translucent, pearly white borders and telangiectasias that frequently ulcerate, forming a central depression.

These lesions are directly related to ultraviolet exposure and are most commonly found on sun-exposed areas such as the face, head, and neck. It is more common in men and with advancing age.

SQUAMOUS CELL CARCINOMA

Squamous cell carcinoma (SCC) (see **FIGURE 7-82**) is the second-most-common form of skin cancer, with an estimated 700,000 new cases being diagnosed annually in the United States.[8] Although when caught

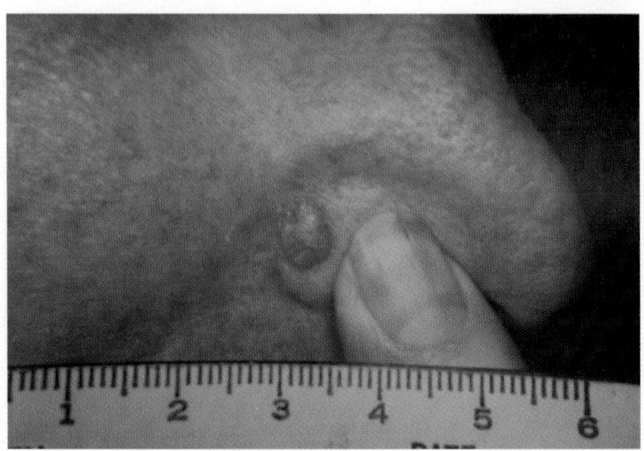

FIGURE 7-81 Basal cell carcinoma.

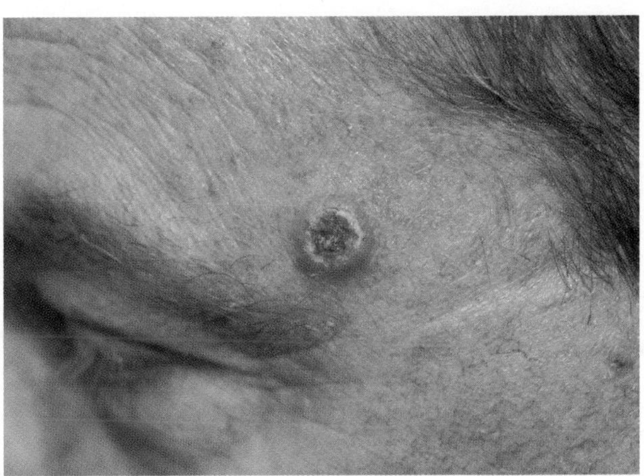

FIGURE 7-82 Squamous cell carcinoma.

early it can be cured, SCC can metastasize and be fatal. The greatest contributing factor to the occurrence of nonmelanoma skin cancers is exposure to ultraviolet (UV) radiation from the sun, resulting in occurrence most commonly on sun-exposed areas.

These lesions occur more commonly in men of advancing age. They commonly present as scaly, red papules, or plaques.

MELANOMA

Melanoma is not as common as the nonmelanoma skin cancers, but incidence continues to rise and it can quickly metastasize and become fatal when not caught early. It accounts for less than 5% of the skin cancer cases but causes more than 75% of skin cancer deaths. In fact, statistically, one person dies from melanoma every hour.[9] According to the American Cancer Society's journal *CA*, the lifetime risk for female whites to get melanoma is now 1 in 55 and the lifetime risk for male whites to get melanoma is now 1 in 36.[10] Melanoma is the most common form of cancer for young adults 25–29 years old and the second-most-common form of cancer for young people 15–29 years old.[11] The survival rate for patients whose melanoma has not spread to the lymph nodes is approximately 98%, but it falls to 15% for those with distant node involvement.[9] An estimated 130,000 new cases of melanoma are expected to be diagnosed in the United States in 2012.[9]

The greatest risk factor for melanoma is exposure to ultraviolet light from the sun, especially when the patient has a history of recurrent or blistering sunburns. Another disturbing trend is increased incidence of melanoma with tanning bed use, often unrecognized as an equally dangerous source of ultraviolet radiation. For these reasons prevention education, which includes avoidance of ultraviolet radiation and the use of protective clothing and sunscreen, should begin with parental guidance and persist throughout the lifetime.

Squamous cell carcinoma: the second-most-common form of skin cancer, arising from epithelial cells and commonly presenting as scaly, red papules or plaques on sun-exposed areas

Melanoma: a highly malignant form of skin cancer, arising from melanocytes and causing the majority of skin cancer related deaths

ABCs of melanoma: a common educational tool useful in instructing patients on the signs and symptoms of possible melanoma

SELF-ASSESSMENT

Patients should be instructed in monthly self–skin assessment. Partnered examinations help in the assessment of hard-to-examine areas such as the back. The **ABCs of melanoma** is a common educational tool useful in instructing patients on the signs and symptoms of possible melanoma. This tool, where each letter from A to E represents a lesion characteristic to look for, is designed to heighten awareness of abnormalities in lesions, which may suggest the lesion is a melanoma (see **FIGURE 7-83**).

A—Asymmetry

The ability to draw an imaginary line down the center of a lesion and create two equal sides where one flipped on top of the other would match is called symmetry.

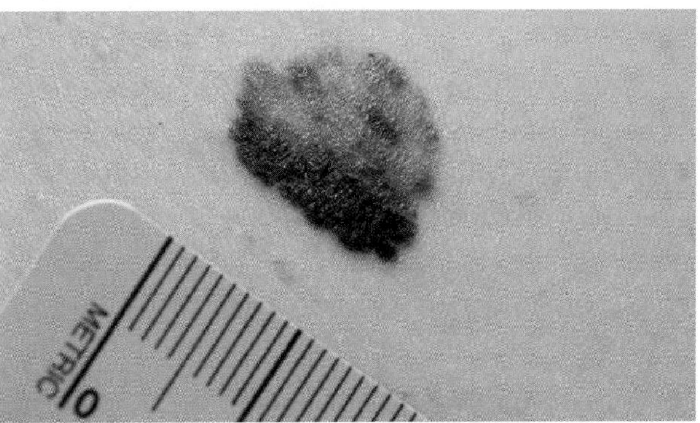

FIGURE 7-83 Lesion meeting all of the characteristics of ABCs of melanoma: asymmetry, border irregularity, color variation, diameter greater than 6 mm, and evolution with a history of growth.

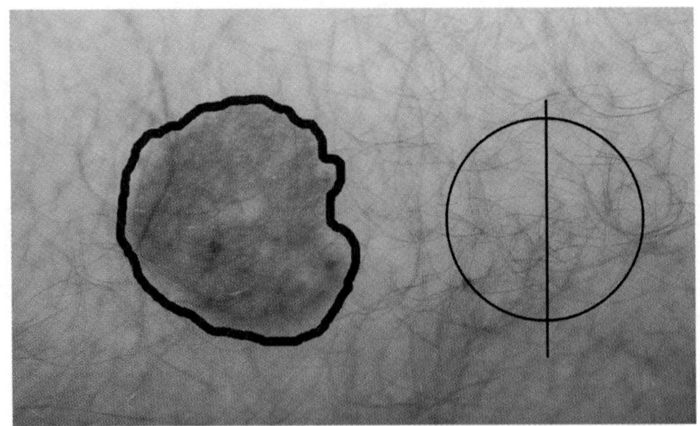

FIGURE 7-84 Diagram of asymmetry.

Asymmetry of a lesion, where one side doesn't match the appearance of the other half, increases concern (see FIGURE 7-84).

B—Border Irregularity

The edges are ragged, notched, blurred, indistinct, or otherwise poorly defined.

C—Color Variation

Lesions of multiple color arouse more suspicion than monotoned lesions. However, patients should be educated to observe lesions for changes in color and darker pigmentation. Patients will often state that they have had a lesion since childhood. It should be confirmed that no color change has occurred and that they should be attuned to watch for color changes from the baseline.

D—Diameter

Lesions greater than 6 mm, the size of an average pencil eraser, are of greater concern.

E—Evolution

7-3 If the lesion is changing in any way, for example elevating or doubling in size, this could be a warning sign of melanoma. Although the American Academy of Dermatology recently added the "E" to broaden the screening tool for melanoma, one should understand that there are pitfalls in specificity with this addition. For example, in children moles are typically evolving, which would cause false alarms. In elderly patients, many benign age-related lesions are evolving, such as seborrheic keratoses and lentigines, that may cause false alarms.

TABLE 7-2 Integumentary Flow

Introduces self by name and title
Asks for permission to begin the physical examination
Washes hands for 15 seconds before touching patient, turning off water with towel
HAIR
Inspection: uses tongue blade to separate hair if needed
Distribution: patterns of loss or excess
Scalp: lesions, flaking
Infestations
Eyebrows: distribution, infestations
Eyelashes: infestations
Palpation: Texture—Smooth, silky, dry, brittle
SKIN
Inspection
Areas
Face
Neck
Thorax
Provides appropriate exposure
Covers lower extremities and pelvis with sheet
Asks patient to lower gown for thorax exam
Immediately covers thorax when exam is completed
Upper extremities
Lower extremities: asks permission to lift sheet to expose legs
Intertriginous areas: between skin folds and digits, under breasts
Findings
Generalized scanning: symmetry, exposure, tendency toward lesions
Thickness: areas of thickening or thinning
Color
Skin Type
Generalized: tan, erythematous, pale, cyanotic, jaundiced
Localized discoloration
Lesions: educate the patient on the ABCs of melanoma
Asymmetry (shape and configuration)
Border irregularity
Color variation
Diameter greater than 6 mm (size)
Elevation (type)
Feeling
Growth

TABLE 7-2 Integumentary Flow *(Continued)*

Palpation
Moisture: dry, moist, diaphoretic, oily
Temperature: palpation with the back of the hand
Texture: soft, rough, smooth
Turgor/mobility: pinch skin on forearm and release
NAILS
Inspection
Nail folds: disruption, paronychia
Nail
Surface: deformity
Color
Separation
Thickness
Length
Hygiene
Nail Bed
Color
Lesions
Shape
Clubbing
Palpation: capillary refill—compress nail and release. Count speed of refill.

References

1. Wolff K, Johnson RA. Disorders of hair follicles and related disorders. In: *Fitzpatrick's Color Atlas and Synopsis of Clinical Dermatology.* 6th ed. New York, NY: McGraw-Hill Professional; 2009.
2. Goldstein BG, Goldstein AO. Androgenetic alopecia. In: Dellavalle RP, ed. *UpToDate.* Waltham, MA: UpToDate; 2012.
3. Venes D, ed. *Taber's Encyclopedic Medical Dictionary.* 20th ed. Philadelphia, PA: F.A. Davis; 2005:1000.
4. Lowe NJ. An overview of ultraviolet radiation, sunscreens, and photo-induced dermatoses. *Dermatol Clin.* 1996;24(1):9–17.
5. NYU Langone Medical Center. Subungual (Nail Bed) Melanoma. http://surgery.med.nyu.edu/oncology/patient-care/melanoma/special-situations/subungual-nail-bed. Accessed February 12, 2012.
6. Rogers HW, Weinstock MA, Harris AR, et al. Incidence estimate of nonmelanoma skin cancer in the United States, 2006. *Arch Dermatol.* 2010;146(3):283–287.
7. National Cancer Institute. Cancer Trends Progress Report—2009/2010 Update. Sun Protection. http://progressreport.cancer.gov/doc_detail.asp?pid=1&did=2007&chid=71&coid=711&mid+=. Accessed February 24, 2012.
8. Skin Cancer Foundation. Skin Cancer Facts. http://www.skincancer.org/skin-cancer-information/skin-cancer-facts. Accessed February 24, 2012.
9. American Cancer Society. Cancer Facts and Figures 2012. Atlanta: American Cancer Society; 2012. http://www.cancer.org/Research/CancerFactsFigures/ACSPC-031941. Accessed April 21, 2012.
10. Kushi L, Doyle C, McCullough M. American Cancer Society guidelines on nutrition and physical activity for cancer prevention. *CA.* 2012;62(1):30–67.
11. Howlader N, Noone AM, Krapcho M, et al., eds. National Cancer Institute. SEER Cancer Statistics Review, 1975–2009 (Vintage 2009 Populations). http://seer.cancer.gov/csr/1975_2009_pops09/. Updated August 20, 2012. Accessed October 10, 2012.

CHAPTER 8

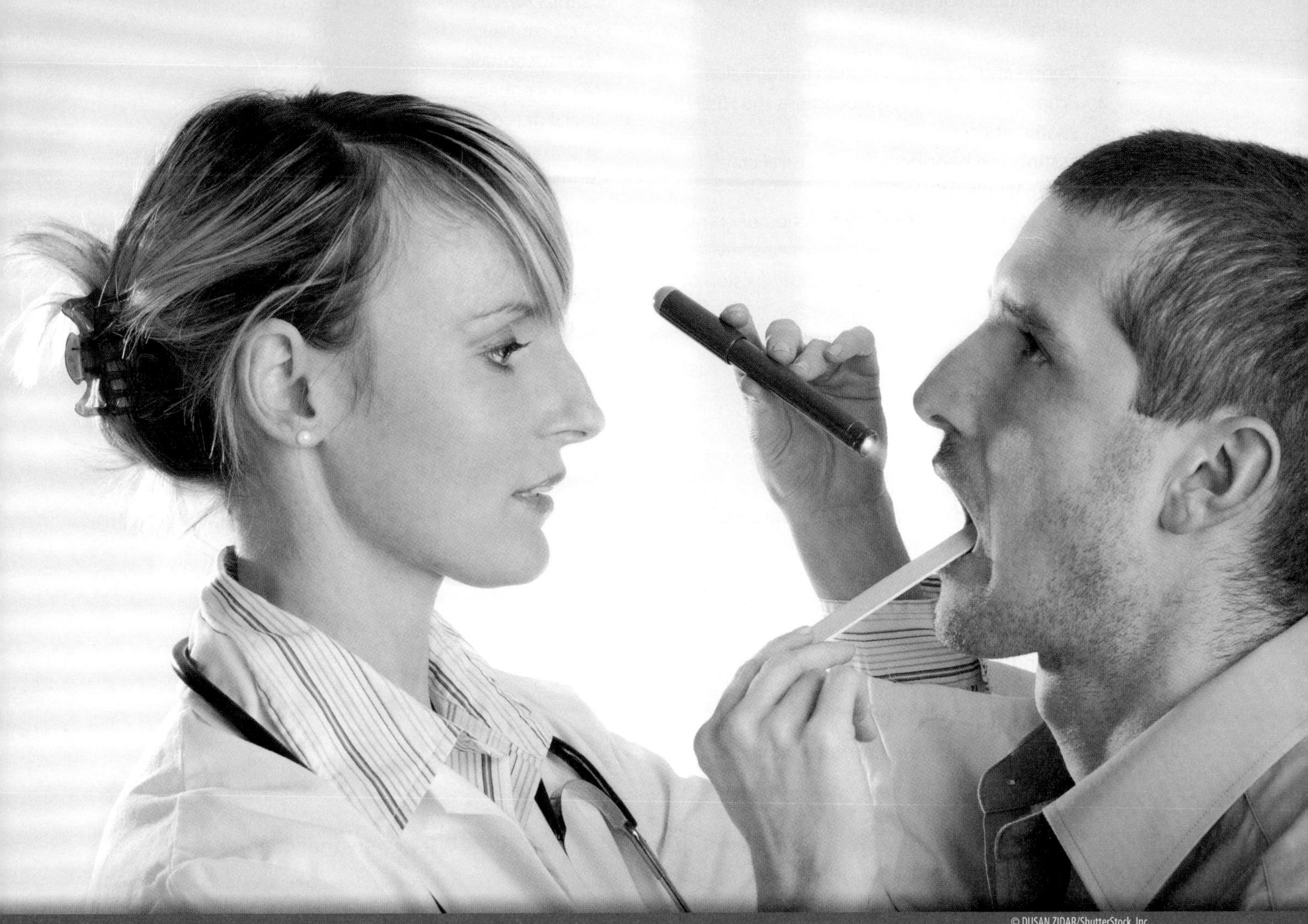

© DUSAN ZIDAR/ShutterStock, Inc.

Head, Eyes, Ears, Nose, and Throat Examination

Mark Kauffman, DO, MS (Med Ed), PA
Rizwan Aslam, DO, MS, FACS
Frank Fatica, DO

OBJECTIVES

At the conclusion of this chapter, the student will be able to

1. Define and contrast variation in head size
2. Properly and concisely document the HEENT examination
3. Distinguish peripheral from central cranial nerve VII disruption
4. Assess motor and sensory function of cranial nerve V
5. Perform transillumination and percussion of the sinuses
6. Describe and perform a complete eye examination, including assessment of visual acuity and peripheral fields
7. Understand the mechanisms and demonstrate proper use of ophthalmoscopes and otoscopes
8. Compare and contrast normal anatomic structures of the eye to common pathologic conditions
9. Perform complete examinations of the nose, mouth, and throat
10. Diagnose and document hearing loss through general screening, Weber testing, and Rinne testing
11. Recognize common disorders of the ear seen during otoscopy

KEY TERMS

Cranial nerves
Microcephalic
Normocephalic
Macrocephalic
Facial nerve
Trigeminal nerve
Sinuses
Transillumination
Visual acuity
Peripheral fields
Extraocular movements
Cornea
Pupillary reaction
Ophthalmoscopy
Retina
Papilledema
Fundus
Macula
Optic disc
Retinopathy
Exudate
Drusen
Hypoglossal nerve
Tympanic membrane
Conductive hearing loss
Sensorineural hearing loss
Weber test
Rinne test
Otoscopy
Insufflation
Otitis

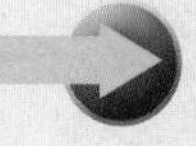
Where this icon appears, visit **go.jblearning.com/HPECWS** to view the video.

The head, eyes, ears, nose, and throat (HEENT) system comes early in the head-to-toe approach to completing a full physical examination. Examination of one body area often involves the overlapping of multiple organ systems. The HEENT system significantly overlaps with the neurologic system in many ways. The testing of **cranial nerves**, for example, can be performed initially in the HEENT examination or later in the neurologic examination. A thorough examination in conjunction with an adequate history is critical in the identification of diseases of the head and neck.

Cranial nerves: nerves that arise directly from the brain as opposed to the spinal column

Head

INSPECTION

Inspection of the head usually begins with incorporation of the integumentary system by examining the hair and scalp and then the head itself.

Size

Inspection of the head begins with the observation of the size of the head in comparison to others of the same sex and age. Mean head circumference for the adult increases with height. If the head size appears large or small on general observation, measurement of circumference should be made. The measurement should then be compared against the mean through the following formulas:[1]

- Male: 42.4 + (0.08673 × height)
- Female: 41.02 + (0.08673 × height)

For example, a 5′ 11″ male patient has a head circumference measuring 55.88 cm:

- 5′ 11″ = 71 inches × 2.54 cm/inch = 180.34 cm
- Male: 42.4 + (0.08673 × 180.34)
- 42.4 + 15.64
- 58.04
- Comparison: 55.88 cm (patient measurement) – 58.04 cm (mean) = -2.16 cm

One standard deviation = +/– 1.41 cm[1]
Two standard deviations = +/– 2.82 cm

- This patient's measurement would fall between the first and second standard deviation.

The nomenclature used to describe head size for documentation is:

- **Microcephalic** (small head): head circumference measures more than two standard deviations below the average
- **Normocephalic** (normal head): head circumference measures within two standard deviations
- **Macrocephalic** (large head): head circumference measures more than two standard deviations above the average

Symmetry

Note symmetry, comparing each section of the head bilaterally: frontal, temporal, parietal, crown, and occipital.

Trauma

Inspection for trauma is prompted by history or symptoms such as fall, loss of consciousness, confusion, head or neck pain, cephalgia, visual changes, loss of coordination or balance, dizziness, otalgia, bloody otorrhea, or confusion.

PALPATION

Palpate the head for tenderness, lesions, and deformity.

DOCUMENTATION

- Head: Normocephalic, atraumatic. Palpation without tenderness, masses, lesions, or deformity.

Microcephalic: "small head," referring to head circumference measuring more than two standard deviations below the average for others of the same age and sex

Normocephalic: "normal head," referring to head circumference measuring within two standard deviations of the average for others of the same age and sex

Macrocephalic: "large head," referring to head circumference measuring more than two standard deviations above the average for others of the same age and sex

Facial nerve: cranial nerve VII, responsible for innervation of the musculature of facial expression and the ability to close the eyes

Face

INSPECTION

Lesions

Inspect the skin of the face for lesions. Sun exposure increases rate of incidence of skin cancer in this area.

Symmetry

Observe for facial symmetry. The motor component of the **facial nerve**, cranial nerve VII (CNVII), is responsible for muscle movements that occur with facial expressions. Ask the patient to complete a series of facial expression motions:

- Please raise your eyebrows.
- Puff out your cheeks.
- Show me your teeth.
- Frown.

Compare symmetry. Disruption of the innervation to the facial nerve can result in weakness of facial muscles and can be seen as flattening of the forehead wrinkles, loss of the nasolabial fold, drooping of the mouth, and inability to close the eye fully. If the disruption to the facial nerve is peripheral, deficits will be found throughout the entire side of the face, with loss of both forehead wrinkling and lower facial droop (see **FIGURES 8-1** and

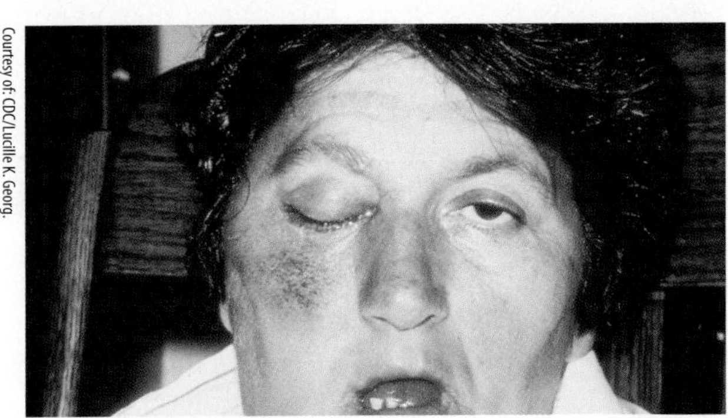

Courtesy of: CDC/Lucille K. Georg.

FIGURE 8-1 Facial droop from cranial nerve VII dysfunction.

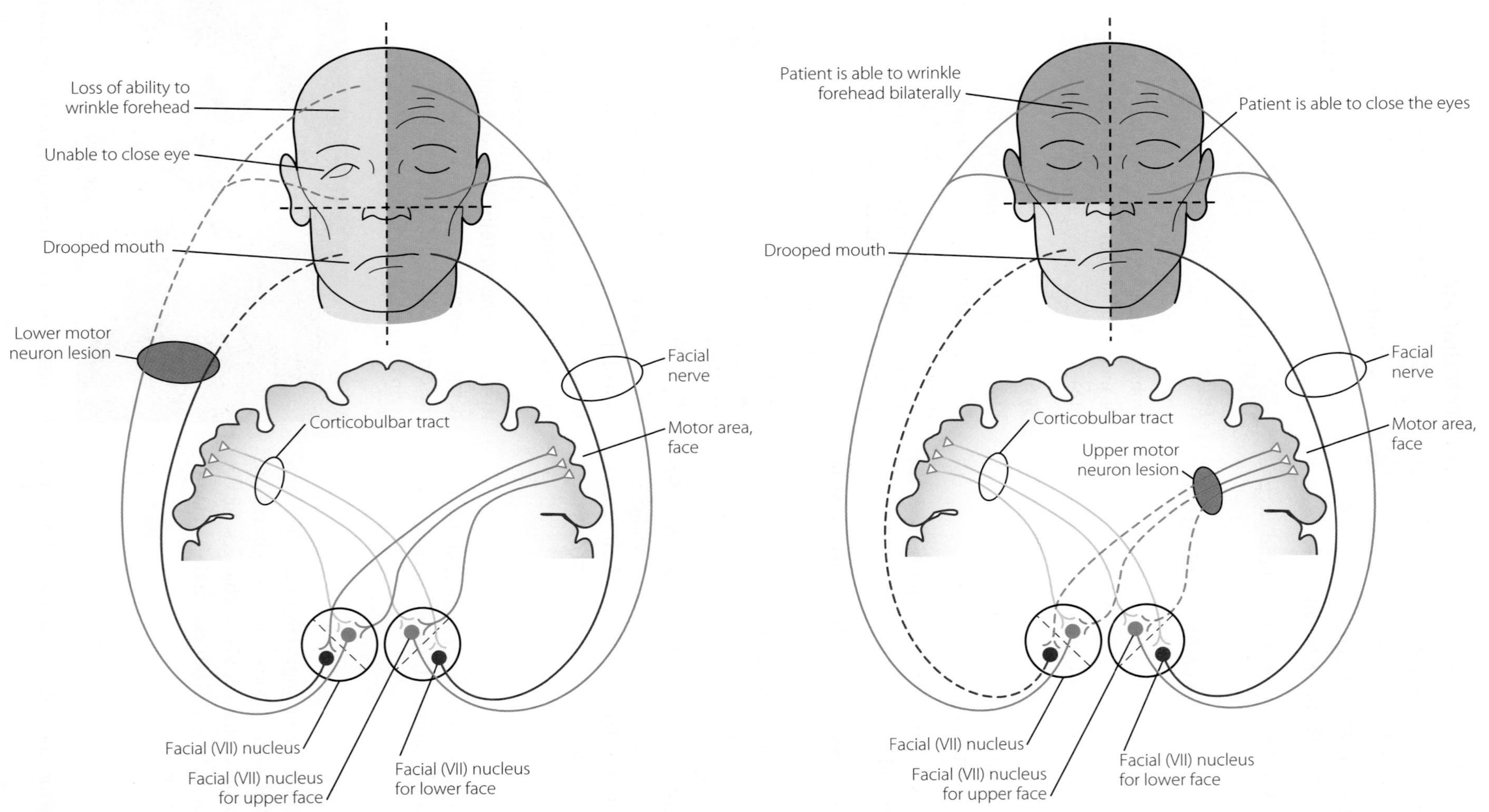

FIGURE 8-2A Lower motor neuron lesion.

FIGURE 8-2B Upper motor neuron lesion.

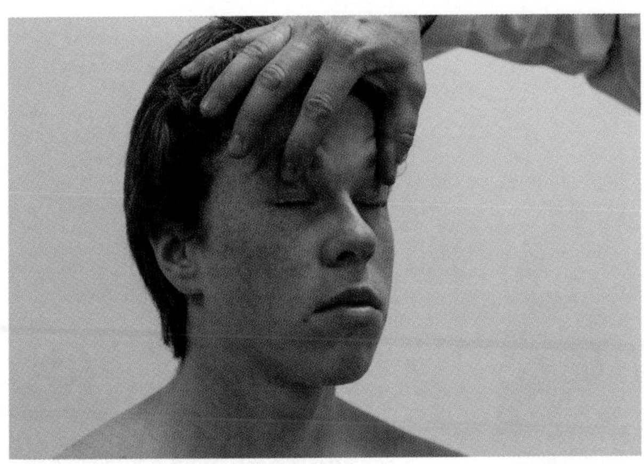

FIGURE 8-3 Testing the ability to close the eyes tightly as a function of the motor component of cranial never VII.

8-2A). If the disruption occurs centrally, the forehead wrinkling is preserved through cross-innervation from CNVII on the opposite side (see FIGURES 8-2B).

CNVII innervates the orbicularis oculi muscle, which allows the eyes to be forceably closed, a memory tool being the hook-like shape of a "7," pulling the eyelid down. To test, the patient is asked to hold his/her eyes closed tightly while the provider places a thumb and finger between the upper lids and eyebrows and tries to raise the lids against resistance (see FIGURE 8-3).

PALPATION

The sensory branch of CNV, the **trigeminal nerve**, supplies sensation to the face via three branches to the forehead, cheek, and jaw. Use soft touch or a sharp object to test both sides of the face (see FIGURES 8-4A–C). This can be done simultaneously, side to side, looking for symmetry, or it can be tested separately on all three areas. Do not test at the angle of jaw, as this is innervated by the great auricular nerve.

Advise the patient that you will be lightly touching him face, asking him to identify which side is being touched. Then ask him to close his eyes and randomly assess each area—the forehead, the cheek, and the jaw—on both sides using a cotton ball or the extended tip of a cotton-tipped applicator.

The motor component of CNV innervates the muscles of mastication. To examine these, have the patient clench his/her teeth while palpating the muscles of mastication.

DOCUMENTATION

- Face: Symmetrical without lesions. CNV and CNVII intact.

Sinuses

INSPECTION

After examining the face, begin working downward from the top of the head. We first encounter the **sinuses**. Hollow organs located within the bone of the skull, the major sinuses include the frontal, maxillary, and ethmoids (see FIGURE 8-5). Sinuses are normally

Trigeminal nerve: cranial nerve V, responsible for sensory perception of the face and the motor function of the muscles of mastication

Sinuses: paired, hollow organs located within the bone of the anterior skull that are normally air-filled

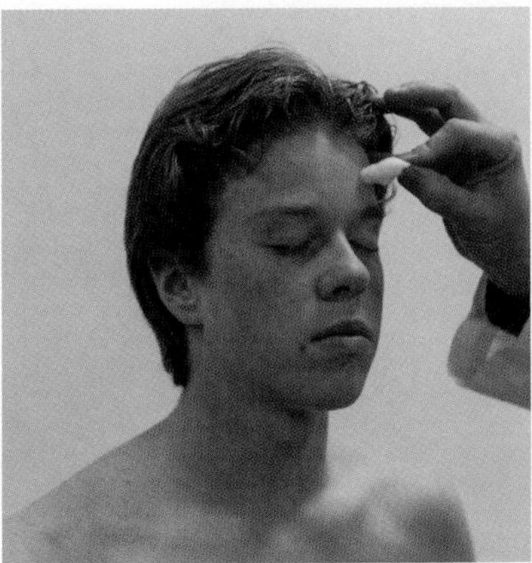

FIGURE 8-4A Testing sensation of soft touch of the trigeminal nerve—forehead.

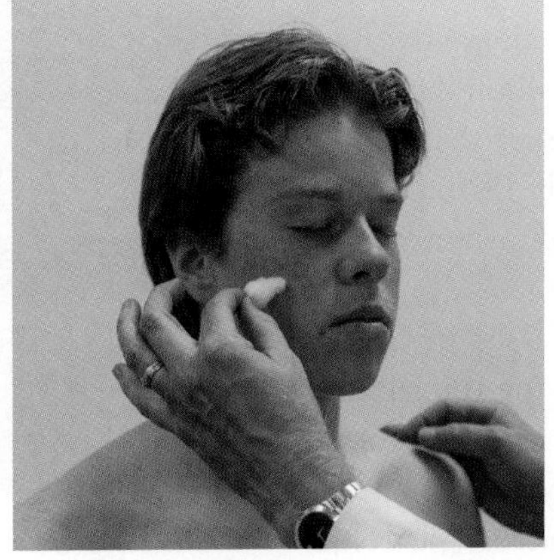

FIGURE 8-4B Testing sensation of soft touch of the trigeminal nerve—cheek.

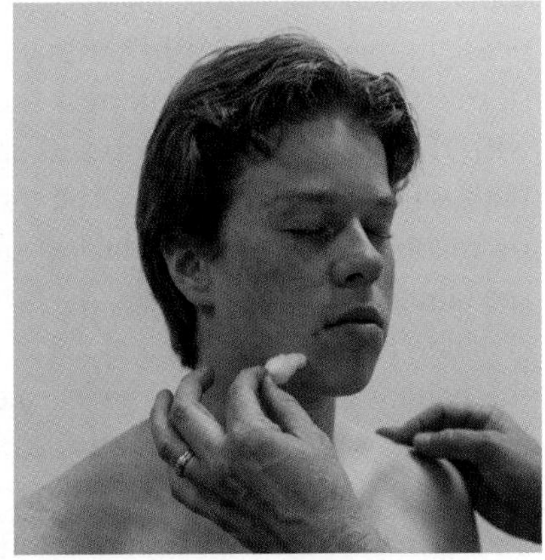

FIGURE 8-4C Testing sensation of soft touch of the trigeminal nerve—jaw.

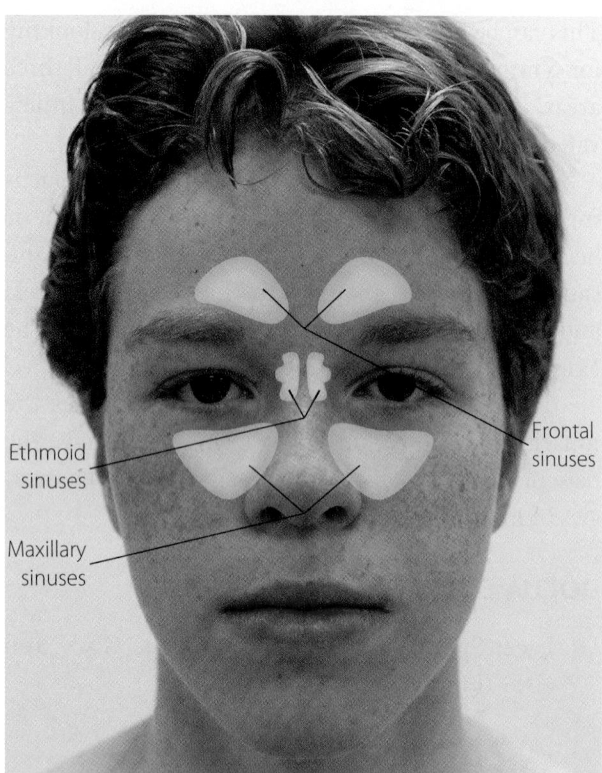

FIGURE 8-5 Sinus locations.

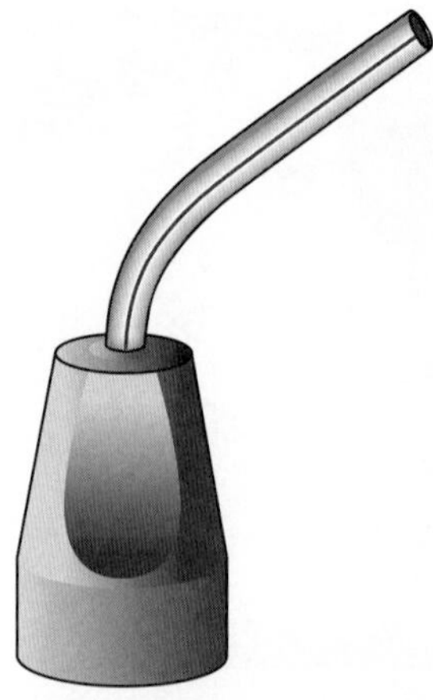

FIGURE 8-6 Sinus transilluminator.

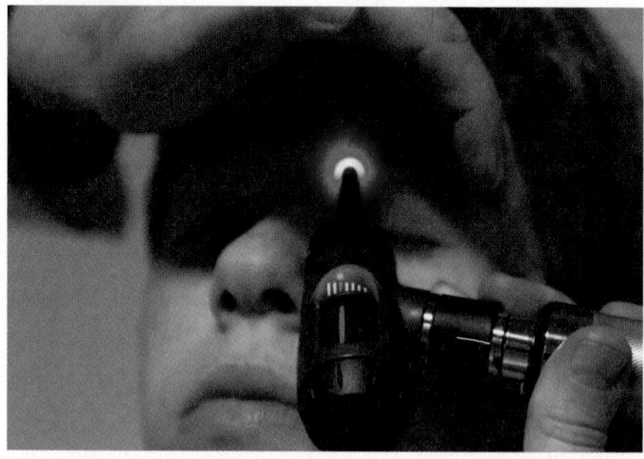

FIGURE 8-7 Frontal sinus transillumination.

Transillumination: the technique of passing a light through a body structure to aid in inspection such as in the detection of fluids

air-filled (pneumatized). When viral or bacterial infection of the sinuses occurs, the associated inflammation obstructs drainage of the sinuses. Fluid may accumulate within the cavities, causing the sensation of pressure, pain, and fullness.

To assess fluid accumulation through inspection, **transillumination** is required. This requires a light source. A sinus transilluminator is most efficient (see FIGURE 8-6). If one is not available, alternative light sources such as an otoscopic head with speculum or a penlight may suffice. When using an alternative light source the provider should test the illuminated end with the pad of his/her finger to ensure that the patient will not be burned by the bulb. If in an exam room, open the door a few inches and turn off or dim the lights.

The frontal sinuses may be accessed by having the patient close his/her eyes. Place the transilluminator under the ridge of the eyebrow in a line projecting vertically through the frontal bone (see FIGURE 8-7). Compare the transillumination across the frontal bones bilaterally.

8-1 To assess the maxillary sinuses, ask the patient to tilt his/her head backward with the mouth open. Place the transilluminator on the maxillary bone at an angle to project the light toward the roof of the mouth (see FIGURE 8-8). Observe the pattern

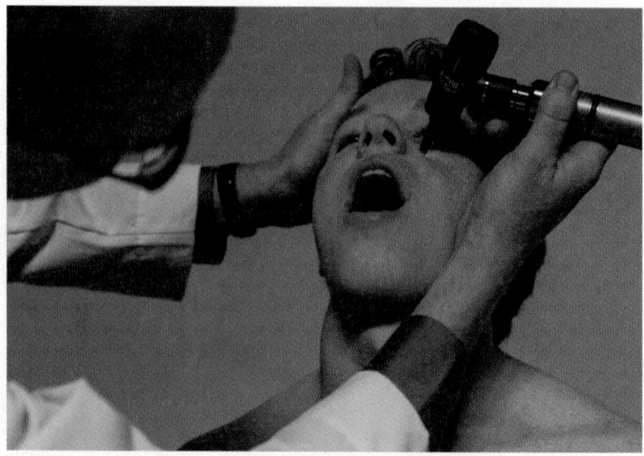

FIGURE 8-8 Maxillary sinus transillumination.

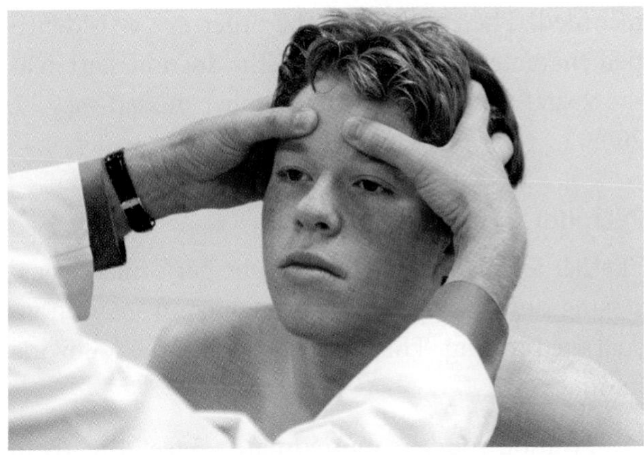

FIGURE 8-9 Frontal sinus palpation for tenderness.

of transillumination by looking through the open mouth to the palate. Sinusitis may be suspected with dullness to transillumination on one side compared to the other.

PALPATION

Now assess the sinuses for tenderness to palpation. Lightly place your hands along the patient's temples. Press firmly with the thumbs over the frontal sinuses simultaneously (see **FIGURE 8-9**). Ask the patient if tenderness is felt and, if so, which side is greater. Unilateral tenderness may correlate with sinusitis on that side.

8-2 Now slide the thumbs inferiorly and repeat the examination over the maxillary sinuses (see **FIGURE 8-10**).

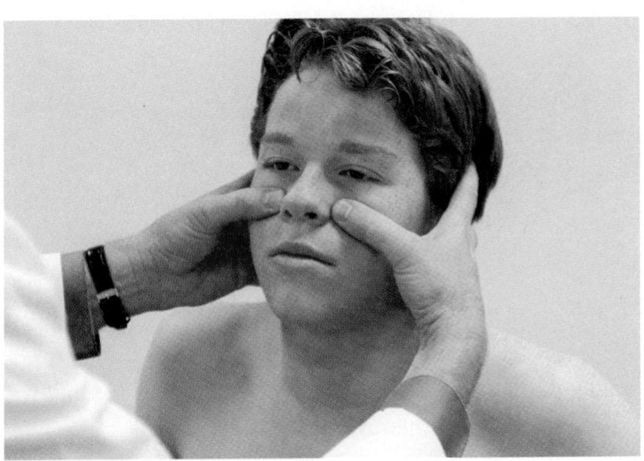

FIGURE 8-10 Maxillary sinus palpation for tenderness.

PERCUSSION

8-3 Percussion of the sinuses is performed by striking the tip of the finger bent at 90 degrees against the frontal and maxillary bones over the sinuses (see **FIGURES 8-11A** and **8-11B**). Ask the patient to close his/her eyes, then percuss each sinus area, one at a time, asking the patient if it causes discomfort. Sinusitis is suspected with pain isolated over the sinuses.

DOCUMENTATION

- Sinuses: Transillumination of frontal and maxillary sinuses symmetrical without dullness. Nontender to palpation and percussion.

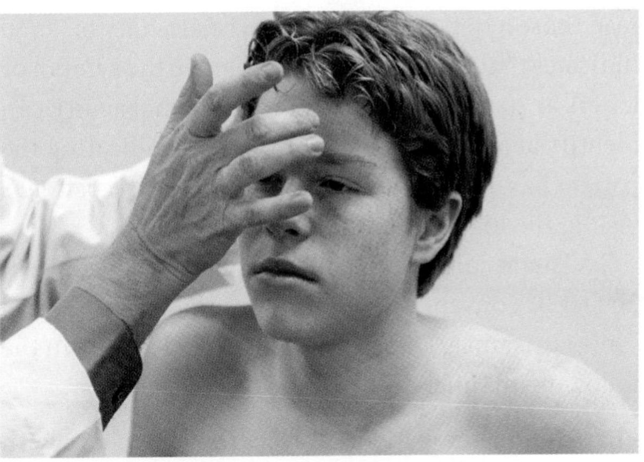

FIGURE 8-11A Hand cocked at hinged wrist preparing to strike over the sinus during percussion.

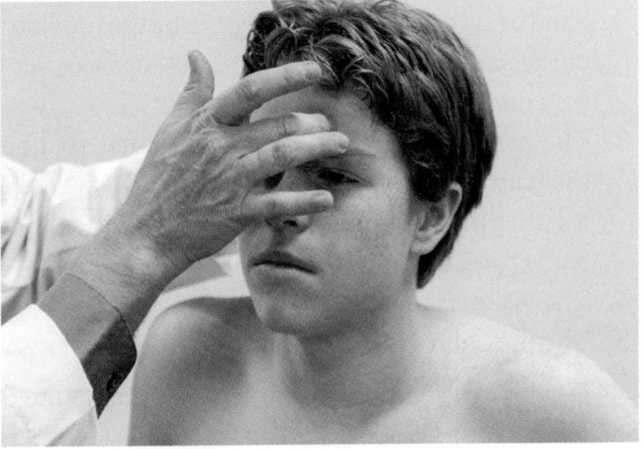

FIGURE 8-11B Striking the sinus during percussion to assess tenderness.

Eyes

BASIC OPHTHALMOLOGY EXAM

Visual Acuity

Visual acuity: the ability to see clearly

Peripheral fields: the area seen outwardly from the center of vision

Assessment of **visual acuity** (optic nerve, CNII) is the initial step in the ophthalmologic examination. It should be performed before shining any light in the eye. Each eye should be assessed separately and each assessment should be performed with the patient's glasses or contact lenses in place. Visual acuity can be measured either at distance or closely. The acuity measurement is denoted as a ratio comparing the patient's vision with an agreed-upon standard where the first number denotes the distance the patient is from the chart and the second number corresponds to the distance at which a person with normal acuity can read those letters. For example, a visual acuity of 20/60 indicates that this patient can recognize the symbol or letters at 20 feet that a person with normal acuity can identify at a farther distance of 60 feet, indicating the patient has diminished vision. The worse the patient's vision, the higher the denominator becomes.

Visual acuity is typically tested from a distance of 20 feet. A conventional Snellen eye chart is calibrated for this distance. Distance visual acuity is tested in the following manner:

1. Position the patient 20 feet from the chart with distance glasses or contact lenses in place.
2. By convention, the right eye is tested first. The patient's left eye is completely covered with a cupped hand or an occluding device either by the provider or the patient, with instructions not to place pressure on the eye.
3. The patient is directed to read the smallest line that can be distinguished. The patient gets credit for that line if more than half of the letters are read correctly.
4. The vision is recorded accordingly (e.g., 20/20).
5. The procedure is then repeated for the other eye.

Near visual acuity can be tested using a handheld Snellen chart or a Rosenbaum pocket vision screener. The screening card should be held at the specified distance indicated on the card, which is typically about 14 inches. One eye should be occluded and the findings recorded. Then repeat for the other eye. Misidentified characters can be noted in the documentation as the visual acuity minus the number missed—e.g., L 20/20 (– 1).

Peripheral Fields

Further assessment of CNII can be performed by assessing **peripheral fields** through confrontation visual field testing. This is performed in the following manner:

1. Position yourself approximately 3 feet directly in front of the patient, making sure that you are on the same eye level (see **FIGURE 8-12**).
2. Have the patient cover his/her *left* eye with his/her left hand while you close your *right* eye. This allows you to use your own field of view as a reference, as you should be able to see your own fingers with your peripheral vision when placed for patient identification.
3. Ask the patient to fixate on your left eye.
4. Position your hands equidistant between you and the patient, and test each quadrant by holding up either 1 or 2 or 5 fingers. Be sure that the patient does not look directly at your fingers. 8-4
5. Repeat the procedure for the other eye by having the patient cover his/her *right* eye while you close your *left* eye.

DOCUMENTATION

- Visual acuity by handheld Snellen L 20/20 (–1), R 20/25. Peripheral fields intact.

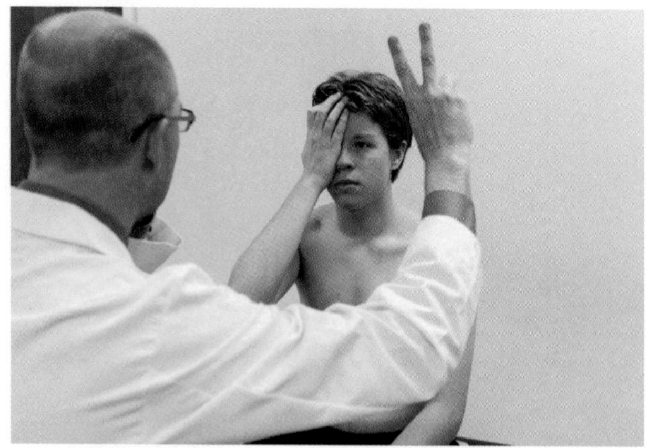

FIGURE 8-12 Peripheral field examination with provider at the same eye level as patient and hand placement halfway between the provider and the patient.

EXTERNAL EXAMINATION

The Distant Exam

It is also important to evaluate the patient for symmetry. From 3 or 4 feet away, evaluate the position of the upper eyelids for ptosis (CNIII). With an open eye, lid margins typically touch the top and bottom edges of the iris. An upper lid droop indicates the presence of ptosis with possible CNIII deficiency. Sclera visible above and below the iris may be caused by exophthalmus, protrusion of the eye that may be found with hyperthyroidism or space-occupying lesions.

8-5 Also check for symmetry of brow creases and facial droop. To check for eye misalignment or strabismus, shine a light directly in the eyes. Assess the symmetry of the position of the light reflex within the pupil. Any asymmetry of the reflex within the pupil could indicate strabismus.

Cranial nerves III, IV, and VI are assessed by evaluating extraocular muscle motility, termed **extraocular movements** (EOMs). This is performed by holding a fixation target such as a pen or your finger 12 to 14 inches away and having the patient follow it with his/her eyes through all nine positions of gaze. Be sure to hold the upper eyelids if necessary to evaluate inferior ocular movements. Have the patient fixate on the target and check for nystagmus, which can indicate a cranial nerve VIII dysfunction.

The Close Exam

Evaluation of the anterior anatomic structures of the eye is performed from approximately 1 foot in front of the patient. The conjunctiva can be inspected for hyperemia, pallor, exudate, or hemorrhage. Hyperemia of the conjunctival vasculature may be caused by an allergy, virus, or bacterium. An exudative discharge is often associated with a bacterial infection. The sclera should be evaluated for signs of dilated vasculature, lesions, or icterus, yellowing of the sclera as a result of hyperbilirubinemia often associated with bile duct obstruction or liver disease. The iris should be inspected for lesions and excessive heterochromia.

The **cornea** should be evaluated for signs of opacity, edema, or foreign body. A pterygium is an abnormal growth of conjunctival tissue that may progress to involve the cornea. It is usually triangular-shaped and inflamed, typically occurs on the nasal aspect of the eye, and is found most commonly in tropical climates. Metal foreign bodies in the cornea may cause corneal edema, anterior chamber inflammation, and a rust ring. Rust rings must be removed completely and carefully to minimize the potential for scarring.

Sudden opacification of the cornea can be a sign of increased intraocular pressure. This dulling of the otherwise crystal-clear cornea may indicate an acute angle-closure attack. Acute angle-closure glaucoma is a true ophthalmic emergency and requires immediate treatment. To assess the depth of the anterior chamber, shine a light from the temporal side of the head parallel to the plane of the iris (see **FIGURE 8-13**). Determine how much of the nasal iris is in shadow. If greater than two-thirds of the nasal iris is in shadow, then a shallow anterior chamber should be suspected (see **FIGURE 8-14**). Further evaluation of the cornea can include evaluating the sensory component as supplied by cranial nerve V (trigeminal). This is done by dragging a wisp of cotton, from either a cotton ball or the tip of cotton-tipped applicator formed into a point, gently across the corneal surface.

8-6 Pupillary evaluation should include inspection of the pupil for both the direct and consensual response as well as symmetry of size and shape. The direct **pupillary reaction** is performed by

Extraocular movements: movement of the eyes through nine positions of gaze as an assessment of cranial nerves III, VI, and VI

Cornea: the most ventral surface of the eye, appearing as a transparent mound lying directly over the pupil, iris, and anterior chamber

Pupillary reaction: reaction of the pupils when a light is shown into the eyes as an assessment of cranial nerves II and III

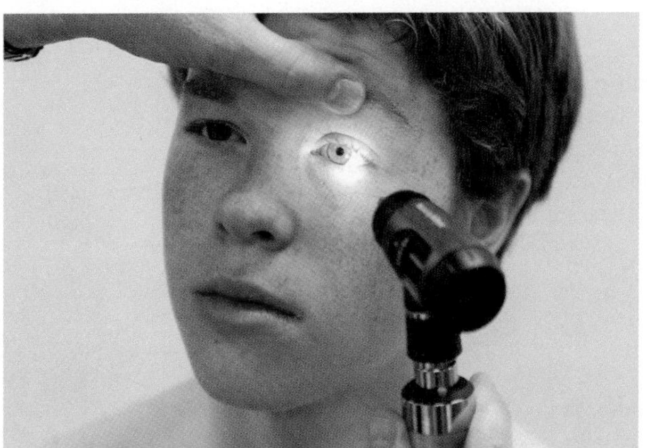

FIGURE 8-13 Assessment of the depth of the anterior chamber with the light source projected tangentially over the iris.

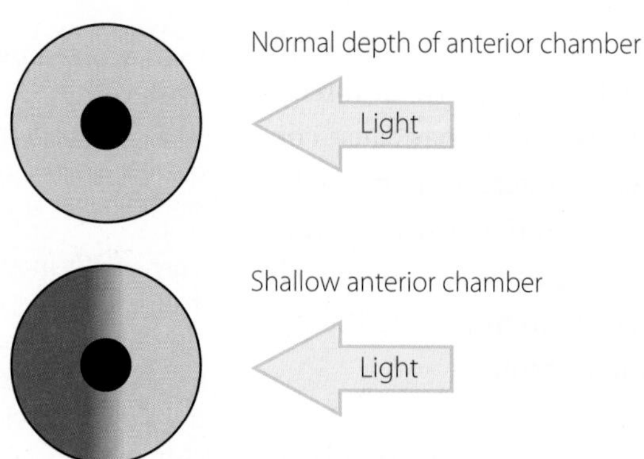

FIGURE 8-14 A shallow anterior chamber can be detected by evidence of a shadow following over the nasal iris under temporal tangential lighting.

having the patient look at a distant object and then shining the light in the right eye to see if it constricts, which is a normal response. This is repeated in the left eye. The consensual response is performed by shining the light in the right eye and watching to see if the left pupil constricts along with the right pupil. Again repeat in the left eye. The constriction of both pupils equally is a normal response.

8-7 An important neurologic assessment is the swinging flashlight test. This tests for an afferent pupillary defect, also known as a Marcus-Gunn pupil. The swinging flashlight test is performed in a room with dim ambient light while the patient fixates on a distant object. A bright light is then shined directly into one eye for three to five seconds, then moved quickly to the other eye for three to five seconds, and then shifted back to the other eye. This should be repeated several times. The important finding to observe is the reaction of the pupil when the light is first swung it into it. In a normal response, pupillary constriction occurs. An abnormal response is pupillary dilation without any initial constriction. This indicates an afferent pupillary defect of the optic nerve.

DOCUMENTATION

- Eye: Inspection—External examination without ptosis, strabismus, or exophthalmus. EOM intact. Conjunctiva pink without exudate. Sclera without injection or icterus. Cornea clear. Iris without lesions or shallow anterior chamber. PERRLA. Corneal reflex intact b/l.

OPHTHALMOSCOPY

Transparency of the cornea, lens, and vitreous humor permits the provider to directly view the optic nerve, arteries, veins, and **retina** (see **FIGURE 8-15**). Direct observation of these structures through an effective ophthalmoscope may show disease of the eye itself or may reveal abnormalities indicative of disease elsewhere in the body. Among the most important of these are vascular changes due to diabetes or hypertension, and **papilledema**, swelling of the optic nerve head due to increased intracranial pressure.

When a preliminary diagnosis of an imminently dangerous eye condition such as acute glaucoma or

Ophthalmoscopy: direct visualization of the posterior structures of the eye through the use of an ophthalmoscope

Retina: the inner surface of the posterior eye responsible for sensing light

Papilledema: edema of the optic nerve seen as blurring of the disc on examination

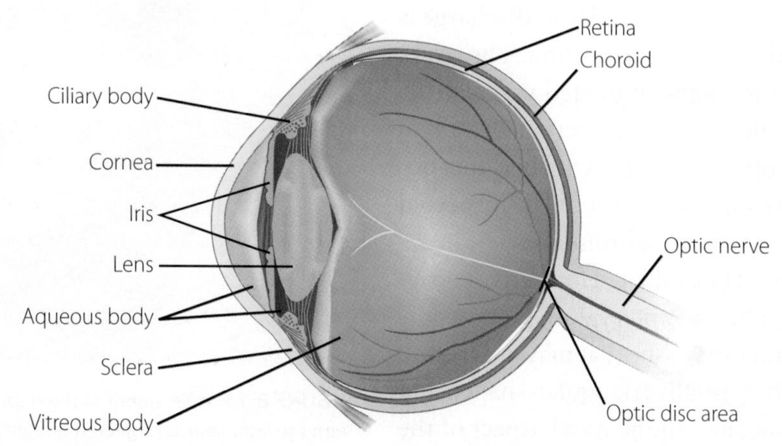

FIGURE 8-15 Eye anatomy.
© kovacevic/ShutterStock, Inc.

retinal detachment is made by the provider, urgent referral to an ophthalmologist may prevent irreversible damage. When distressing but less urgent conditions such as visual impairment due to cataract or vitreous floaters are recognized, the patient can be reassured and referred.

Because the ophthalmic examination can give so much information about a patient's well-being, correct use of the ophthalmoscope makes it one of the most valuable tools available for diagnostic use.

Ophthalmoscopy is best performed on a pharmacologically dilated pupil. This is typically done by using tropicamide 0.5% or 1%, or phenylephrine hydrochloride 2.5%. Dilation should not be performed if a shallow chamber or a narrow angle is suspected. If the patient has a history of narrow angle glaucoma or a family history of narrow angle glaucoma and you suspect that the patient's anterior chamber is shallow, or if there is sudden vision loss in the setting of a painful, red eye, the patient should not be dilated and the examination should be performed by an ophthalmologist. This may precipitate an angle-closure attack.

Coaxial Ophthalmoscopes

Coaxial optical systems achieve visualization of the retina by allowing the axis of illumination to coincide with the axis of vision into the retina for observation of the **fundus** and interior anatomy of the eye. Coaxial ophthalmoscopes (see **FIGURE 8-16**) offer wider ranges of diopters, from –25 to +40, which adjust to allow for focusing on structures.

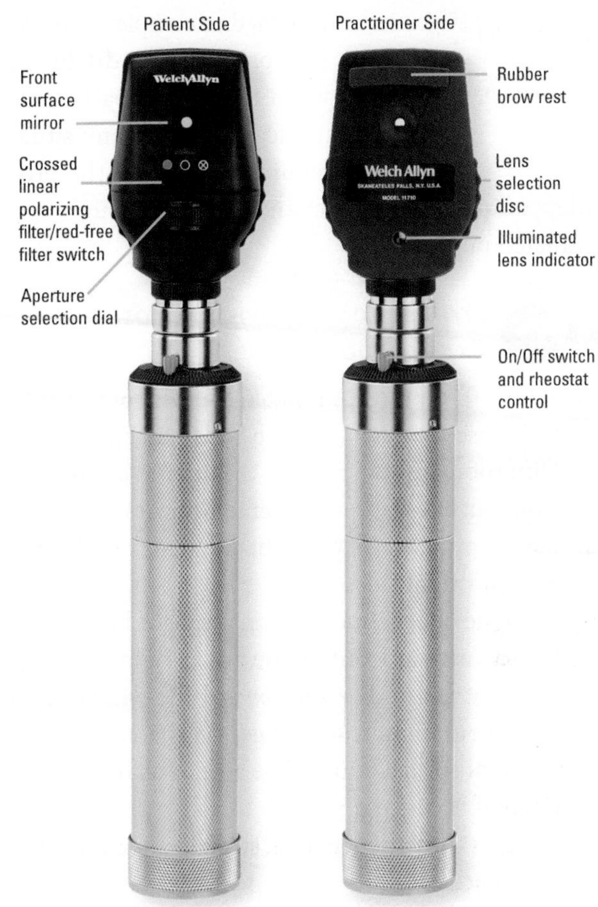

FIGURE 8-16 Coaxial ophthalmoscope.
Courtesy of: Welch Allyn.

Aperture and Filters.

A wide range of apertures and filters are typically available: small spot, large spot, micro spot, slit aperture, red-free filter, cobalt blue filter, half-moon, and fixation aperture.

- Micro Spot Aperture: Allows easy entry into very small, undilated pupils.
- Slit Aperture: Helpful in determining various elevations of lesions, particularly tumors and edematous discs.
- Small Aperture: Provides easy view of the fundus through an undilated pupil. Always start the examination with this aperture and proceed to micro spot aperture if the pupil is particularly small and/or sensitive to light.
- Large Aperture: Standard aperture for dilated pupil and general examination of the eye.
- Half-Moon Aperture: Provides a combination of depth perception and field of view.
- Fixation Aperture: The pattern of an open center and thin lines permits easy observation of eccentric fixation without masking the **macula**.
- Cobalt Blue Filter: Blue filter used with fluorescein dye permits easy viewing of small lesions, abrasions, and foreign objects.
- Red-Free Filter: Excludes red rays from examination field for easy identification of veins, arteries, and nerve fibers.

Fundus: posterior anatomic structures of the eye including the retina, optic nerve, macula and fovea, requiring ophthalmoscopy to be inspected

Macula: yellow area in the posterior retina responsible for central vision

Conducting the Examination

In order to conduct a successful examination of the fundus, the examining room should be either

Optic disc: head of the optic nerve which can be seen on ophthalmoscopic examination

semi-darkened or completely darkened. It is preferable to dilate the pupil when there is no pathologic contraindication, but many situations require the skill of the provider to perform the examination through the undilated pupil.

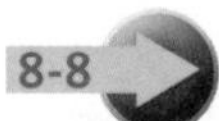

Steps in Coaxial Ophthalmoscopic Examination.

1. Select "0" on the illuminated lens disc of the ophthalmoscope and start with the small aperture.
2. Dim room lights, cracking the door to allow light from outside the room to enter if necessary.
3. For examination of the right eye, sit or stand at the patient's right side.
4. Take the ophthalmoscope in the right hand, hold it vertically in front of your own right eye with the light beam directed toward the patient, and place your right index finger on the edge of the lens dial so that you will be able to change lenses easily if necessary.
5. Instruct the patient to look straight ahead at a distant object.
6. Advise the patient that you may get in the way of his/her line of sight but that he/she should attempt to avoid moving the eyes.
7. Position the ophthalmoscope about 6 inches (15 cm) in front of and slightly (25 degrees) lateral of the patient. Look through the ophthalmoscope and direct the light beam into the pupil (see **FIGURES 8-17A** and **8-17B**). A red "reflex" should appear as you look at the pupil.
8. Rest your left hand on the patient's forehead and hold the upper lid of the eye near the eyelashes with the thumb. While the patient is fixating on the specified object, keep the "reflex" in view and slowly move toward the patient. The **optic disc** should come into view when you are about 1 to 2 inches (3 to 5 cm) from the patient. If it is not focused clearly, rotate lenses with your index finger until the optic disc is as clearly visible as possible.
   a. The hyperopic, or farsighted, eye requires more "plus" lenses (green numbers) for clear focus of the fundus.
   b. The myopic, or nearsighted, eye requires "minus" lenses (red numbers) for clear focus.
9. Examine the disc for clarity of outline, color, elevation, and condition of the vessels. Follow each vessel as far to the periphery as you can. Ask the patient to look at the light of the ophthalmoscope, which will automatically place the macula in full view, to inspect for abnormalities in the macula area. The red-free filter facilitates viewing of the center of the macula.

The PanOptic Ophthalmoscope

The PanOptic ophthalmoscope by Welch Allyn (see **FIGURE 8-18**) represents advancement in ophthalmoscopic design that improves the ability to see the fundus through constricted pupils by converging light to a point at the cornea. The light then diverges to the retina, illuminating the widest field of view of the fundus attainable in undilated ophthalmoscopy. A focusing range from –20 to +20 diopters is achievable by adjusting the focus wheel.

FIGURE 8-17A Distance alignment for ophthalmoscopic exam.

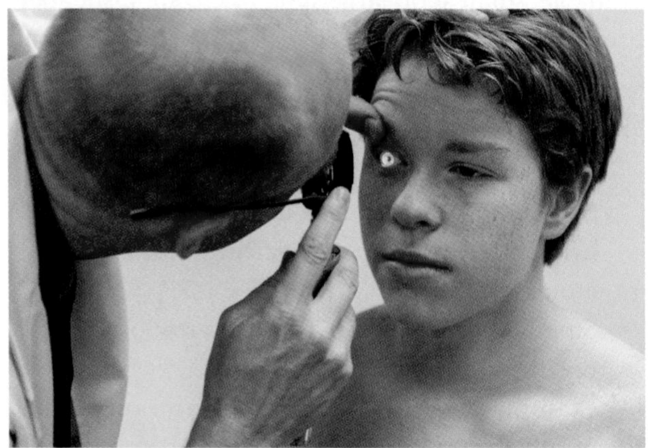

FIGURE 8-17B Near alignment for ophthalmoscopic exam.

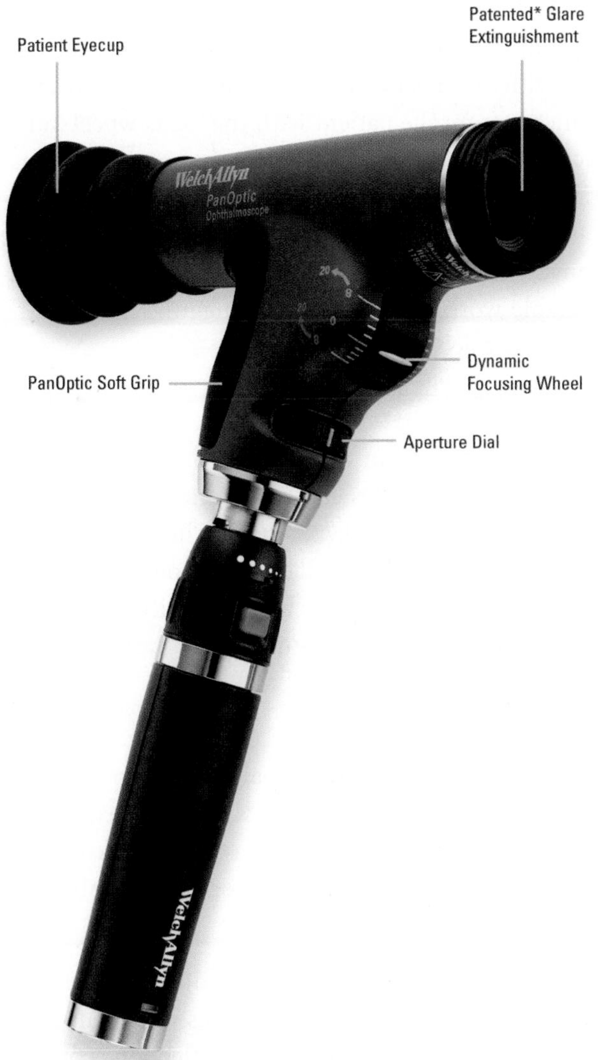

FIGURE 8-18 PanOptic ophthalmoscope.
Courtesy of: Welch Allyn.

Placing the eyecup on the patient side of the ophthalmoscope against the periorbital area of the eye helps the provider establish and maintain the proper viewing distance, provides stabilization for the view during the exam, and helps to eliminate interference from other light sources.

Conducting the Examination.

1. Use your right eye to examine the right eye of the patient and your left eye to examine the patient's left eye.
2. To examine the right eye, take the ophthalmoscope in your right hand with the eyepiece facing the patient and place your thumb on the focusing wheel. Hold the instrument up to your right eye and look through the eyepiece at an object approximately 20 feet away. Rotate the focusing wheel with your thumb to bring the object into focus.
3. Set the aperture/filter dial to the small spot.
4. Dim the room lights.
5. Instruct the patient to look straight ahead at a distant object. Advise the patient that you may get in the way of his/her line of sight but that he/she should attempt to avoid moving the eyes.
6. Hold the PanOptic up to your eye and position the ophthalmoscope about 6 inches (15 cm) in front of and at a slight angle (15 to 20 degrees) from midline on the temporal side of the patient. Direct the light beam into the pupil. A red "reflex" should appear as you look through the pupil
7. Adjust your height so that you are at the same eye level as the patient. The combination of being on eye level and being angled at 15 to 20 degrees from midline should allow illumination very close to or on the optic nerve. Being at a higher or lower eye level than the patient will result in observation of the periphery of the retina instead of the major structures.
8. Rest your left hand on the patient's forehead and hold the upper lid of the eye near the eyelashes with your thumb. This technique aids in the perception of depth while approaching the eye. While the patient is fixating on the specified object, keep the red "reflex" in view and move toward the patient in a slow, deliberate, and steady fashion until the eyecup rests on the orbit of the patient's eye (see **FIGURE 8-19**). The optic disc should come into

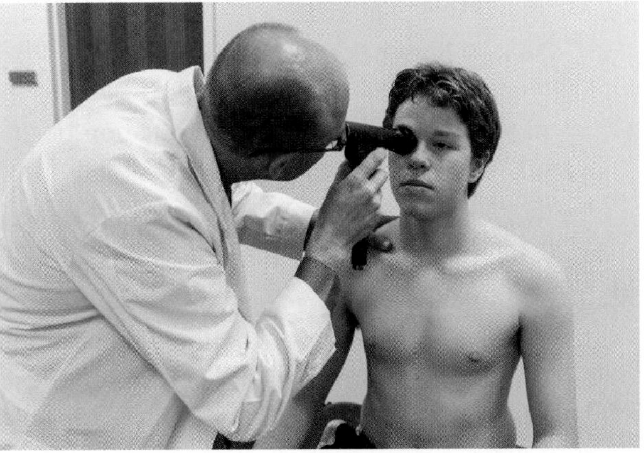

FIGURE 8-19 PanOptic exam with eyecup resting periorbitally.

view when you are about 1 to 2 inches (3 to 5 cm) from the patient. Gentle compression of the eyecup will maximize the field of view.

If the optic disc is not focused clearly, rotate the focusing wheel with your thumb until the optic disc is as clearly visible as possible. The hyperopic, or farsighted, eye requires more "plus" focus (rotation toward green) for clear focus of the fundus; the myopic, or nearsighted, eye requires "minus" focus (rotation toward red) for clear focus. If you lose the view of the optic disc while approaching the patient's eye, pull back slowly, relocate the red reflex, and try again.

9. Examine the disc for clarity of outline, color, elevation, and condition of the vessels. Follow each vessel as far to the periphery as you can.
10. To view the macula, instruct your patient to look directly into the light of the ophthalmoscope. This will automatically place the macula in full view. The red-free filter facilitates viewing of the center of the macula.
11. There are two methods of examining the extreme periphery:
    a. Instruct the patient to fixate straight ahead while performing the examination. Pivot around the eye by leveraging the eyecup against the orbit of the patient's eye to achieve the desired view. It is important to compress the eyecup to maximize this technique. Without full compression, the chances of losing your view increase significantly.
    b. As the lens of the eye inverts the image, instruct the patient to:
        i. Look up for examination of the superior retina
        ii. Look down for examination of the inferior retina
        iii. Look temporally for examination of the temporal retina
        iv. Look nasally for examination of the nasal retina
12. To examine the left eye, repeat the procedure outlined above but hold the ophthalmoscope in your left hand, stand at the patient's left side, and use your left eye.

Additional Examinations

To look for abrasions and foreign bodies on the cornea with a corneal viewing lens, begin the exam about 6 inches from the patient with the focus wheel in the neutral position. Look through the scope at the patient's cornea to direct the light at the target area. Adjust the focus wheel into the green (plus) diopters while moving slightly in (closer) or out (farther) until a comfortable working distance and magnification of the cornea are achieved.

Lens opacities can be detected by looking at the pupil through the +6 lens setting at a distance of 6 inches (15 cm) from the patient. In the same manner, vitreous opacities can be detected by having the patient look up and down, to the right and to the left. Any vitreous opacities will be seen moving across the pupillary area as the eye changes position or comes back to the primary position.

Corneal Reflection

One of the most troublesome barriers to a good view of the retina is the light reflected back into the examiner's eye from the patient's cornea—a condition known as corneal reflection. There are three ways to minimize this nuisance:

- A crossed linear polarizing filter may be used if the ophthalmoscope features one. This filter should be used when corneal reflection is present as it reduces corneal reflection by 99%.
- Use the small aperture. However, this reduces the area of the retina illuminated.
- Direct the light beam toward the edge of the pupil rather than directly through its center.

PATHOLOGIES OF THE EYE

Normal Fundus (see FIGURE 8-20)

Disc: Outline clear; central physiological cup is pale

Retina: Normal red/orange color, macula is dark; avascular area temporally

Vessels: Arterial/venous ratio 2 to 3; the arteries appear a bright red, the veins a slightly purplish color

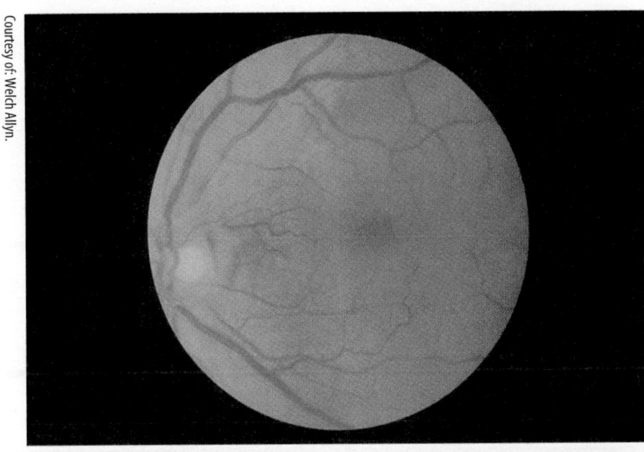
Courtesy of: Welch Allyn.

FIGURE 8-20 Normal fundus on ophthalmoscopic examination.

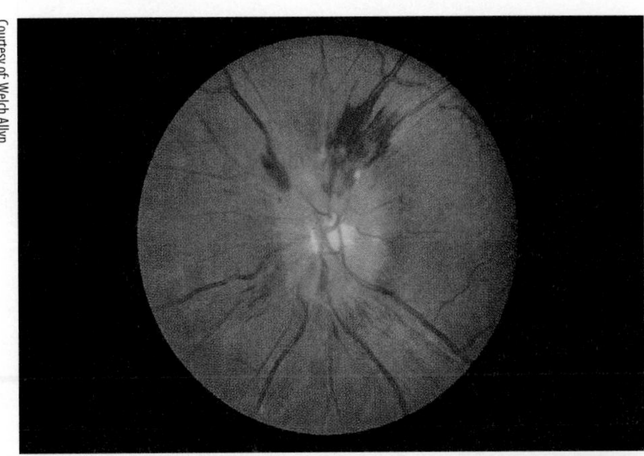
Courtesy of: Welch Allyn.

FIGURE 8-22 Hypertensive retinopathy, advanced malignancy.

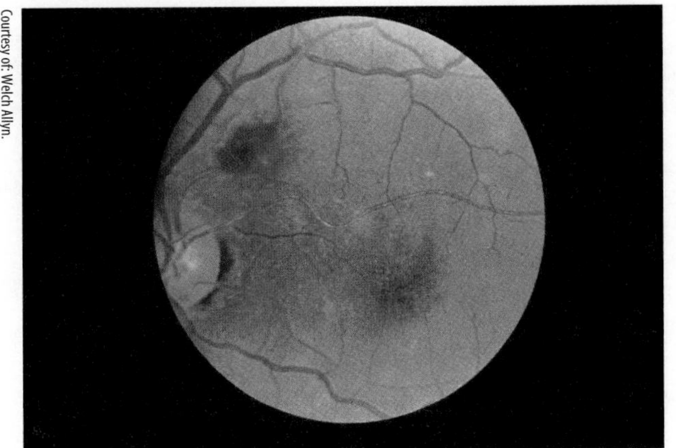
Courtesy of: Welch Allyn.

FIGURE 8-21 Hypertensive retinopathy.

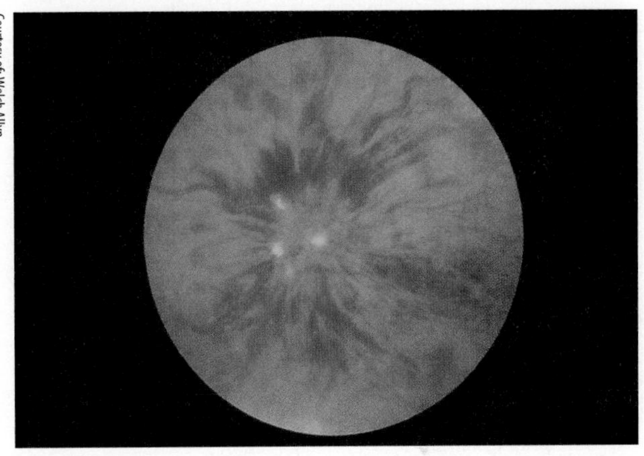
Courtesy of: Welch Allyn.

FIGURE 8-23 Central retinal vein occlusion.

Hypertensive Retinopathy (see FIGURE 8-21)

Disc: Outline clear

Retina: **Exudates** and flame hemorrhages

Vessels: Attenuated arterial reflex

Hypertensive Retinopathy, Advanced Malignancy (see FIGURE 8-22)

Disc: Elevated, edematous disc; blurred disc margins

Retina: Prominent flame hemorrhages surrounding vessels near disc border

Vessels: Attenuated retinal arterioles

Central Retinal Vein Occlusion (see FIGURE 8-23)

Disc: Virtually obscured by edema and hemorrhages

Retina: Extensive blot retinal hemorrhages in all quadrants to periphery

Vessels: Dilated tortuous veins; vessels partially obscured by hemorrhages

Inferior Branch Retinal Artery Occlusion Due to Embolus (see FIGURE 8-24)

Disc: Prominent embolus at retinal artery bifurcation

Retina: Inferior retina shows pale, milky edema; superior retina is normal

Vessels: Inferior arteriole tree greatly attenuated and irregular; superior vessel is normal

Retinopathy: non-inflammatory pathology of the retina

Exudates: fluid collections in the retina resulting from damaged blood vessels

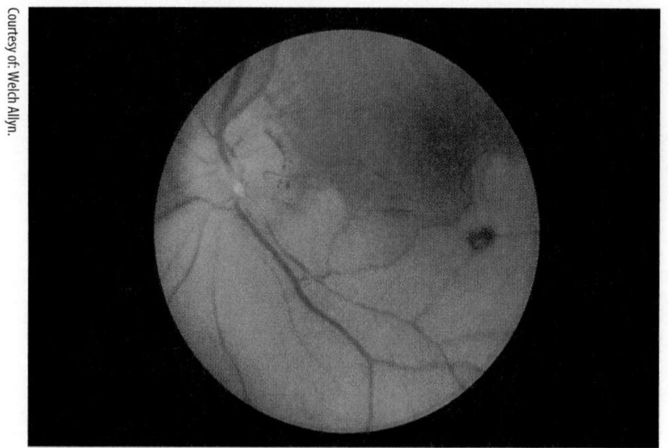

FIGURE 8-24 Inferior branch retinal artery occlusion.

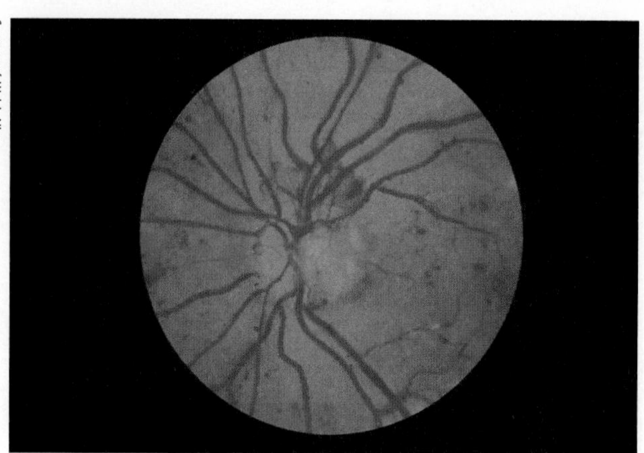

FIGURE 8-26 Proliferative diabetic retinopathy.

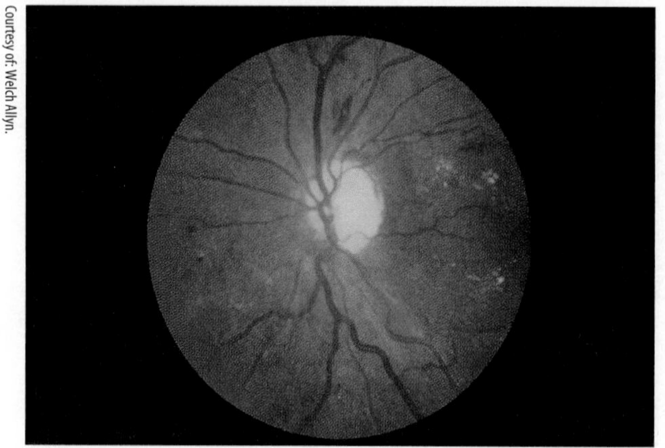

FIGURE 8-25 Nonproliferative diabetic retinopathy.

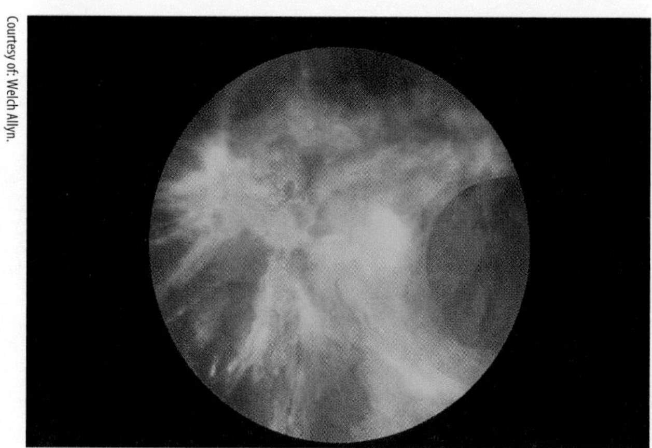

FIGURE 8-27 End-stage diabetic retinopathy.

Nonproliferative Diabetic Retinopathy (see FIGURE 8-25)

Disc: Normal

Retina: Numerous scattered exudates and hemorrhages

Vessels: Mild dilation of retinal veins

Proliferative Diabetic Retinopathy (see FIGURE 8-26)

Disc: Net of new vessels growing on disc surface

Retina: Numerous hemorrhages, new vessels at superior disc margin

Vessels: Dilated retinal veins

Drusen: small collections found on the retina and optic nerve often occurring with macular degeneration and aging

End-Stage Diabetic Retinopathy (see FIGURE 8-27)

Disc: Partially obscured by fibrovascular proliferation

Retina: Obscured by proliferating tissue; small area of retina with hemorrhage seen through "window" of fibrovascular membrane

Vessels: Abnormal new vessels in fibrous tissue

Vitreous: Prominent fibrovascular tissue

Advanced Hemorrhagic Macular Degeneration (see FIGURE 8-28)

Disc: Normal

Retina: Large macular scar with **drusen**; prominent macular hemorrhage

Vessels: Normal

Macular Drusen (Colloid Bodies) (see FIGURE 8-29)

Disc: Normal

Retina: Extensive white drusen of the retina

Vessels: Normal

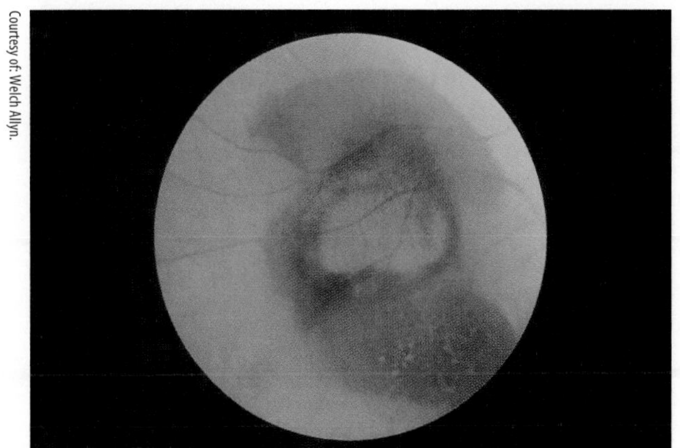
Courtesy of: Welch Allyn.

FIGURE 8-28 Advanced hemorrhagic macular degeneration.

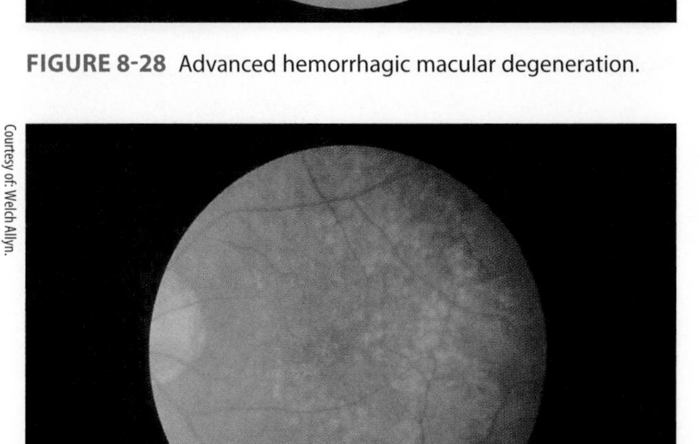
Courtesy of: Welch Allyn.

FIGURE 8-29 Macular drusen.

Inactive Chorioretinitis (Toxoplasmas) (see FIGURE 8-30)

Disc: Normal

Retina: Well-circumscribed lesion with areas of hyperpigmentation and atrophy of retina; white sclera showing through

Vessels: Normal

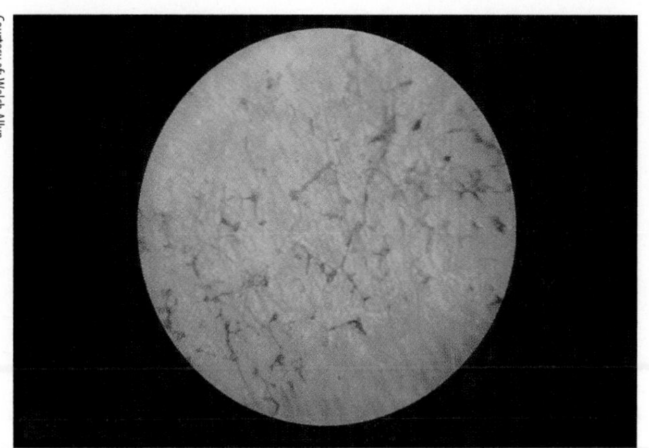
Courtesy of: Welch Allyn.

FIGURE 8-31 Advanced retinitis pigmentosa.

Advanced Retinitis Pigmentosa (see FIGURE 8-31)

Disc: Normal

Retina: Scattered retinal pigmentation in classic bone spicule pattern

Vessels: Greatly attenuated

Retinal Detachment (see FIGURE 8-32)

Disc: Normal

Retina: Gray elevation in temporal area with folds in detached section

Vessels: Tortuous and elevated over detached retina

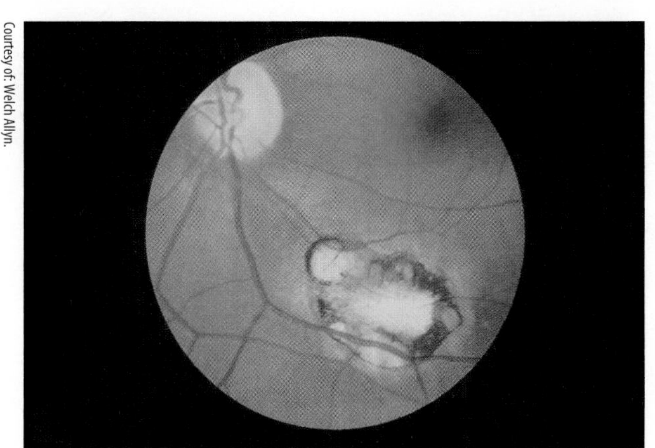
Courtesy of: Welch Allyn.

FIGURE 8-30 Inactive chorioretinitis.

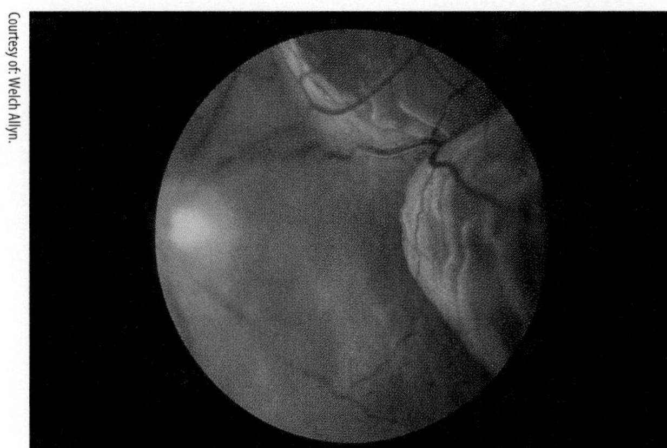
Courtesy of: Welch Allyn.

FIGURE 8-32 Retinal detachment.

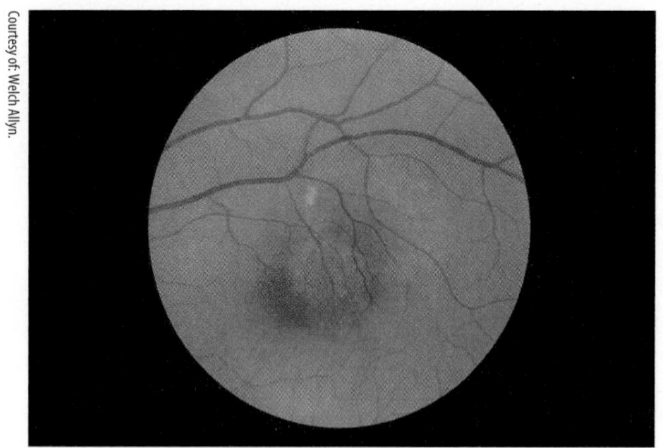
Courtesy of: Welch Allyn.

FIGURE 8-33 Benign choroidal nevus.

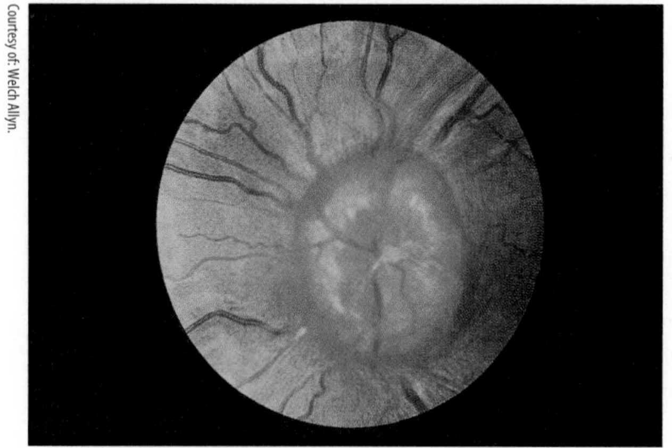
Courtesy of: Welch Allyn.

FIGURE 8-34 Papilledema.

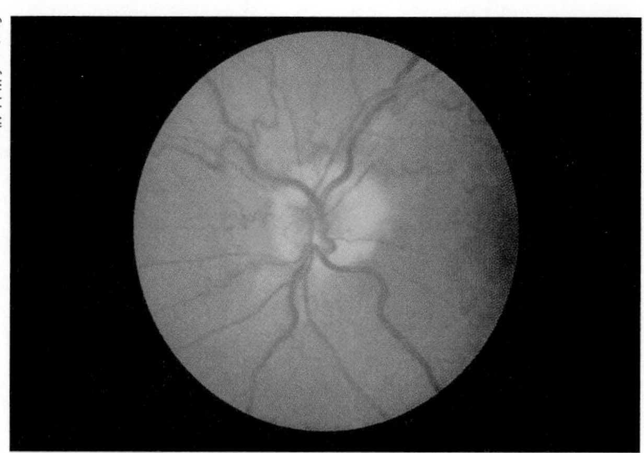
Courtesy of: Welch Allyn.

FIGURE 8-35 Optic neuritis.

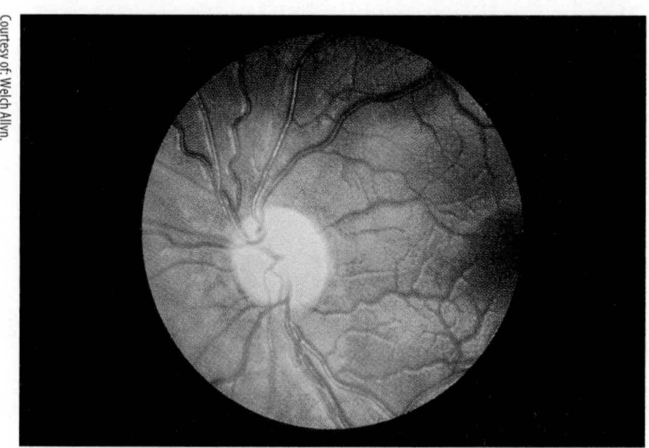
Courtesy of: Welch Allyn.

FIGURE 8-36 Optic atrophy.

Benign Choroidal Nevus (see FIGURE 8-33)

Disc: Normal
Retina: Slate gray, flat lesion under retina; several drusen overlying nevus
Vessels: Normal

Papilledema (see FIGURE 8-34)

Disc: Elevated, edematous disc; blurred disc margins; vessels engorged
Retina: Flame retinal hemorrhage close to disc
Vessels: Engorged tortuous veins

Optic Neuritis (see FIGURE 8-35)

Disc: Elevated with blurred margins
Retina: Mild peripapillary edema
Vessels: Mild dilation of vessels on disc

Optic Atrophy (see FIGURE 8-36)

Disc: Margins sharp and clear; pale white color
Retina: Normal
Vessels: Arteries attenuated; veins normal

Glaucomatous Cupping of the Disc (see FIGURE 8-37)

Disc: Large cup, disc vessels displaced peripherally; pale white color; pigment ring surrounding disc
Retina: Normal
Vessels: Normal

DOCUMENTATION

- Bilateral red reflex intact and symmetrical. No cataracts. Cup: disc ratio 2:1. No papilledema, exudate,

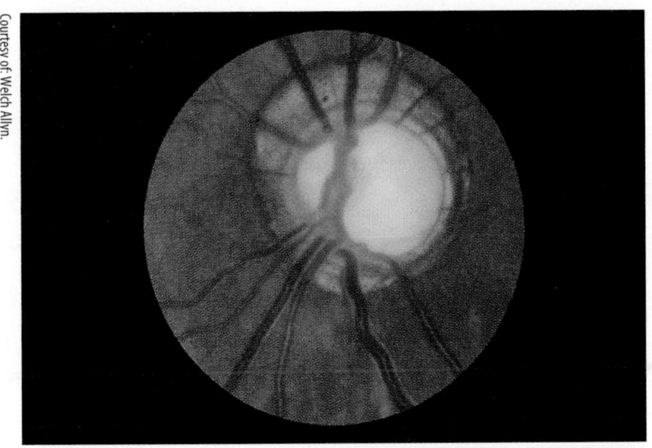

FIGURE 8-37 Glaucomatous cupping of the disc.

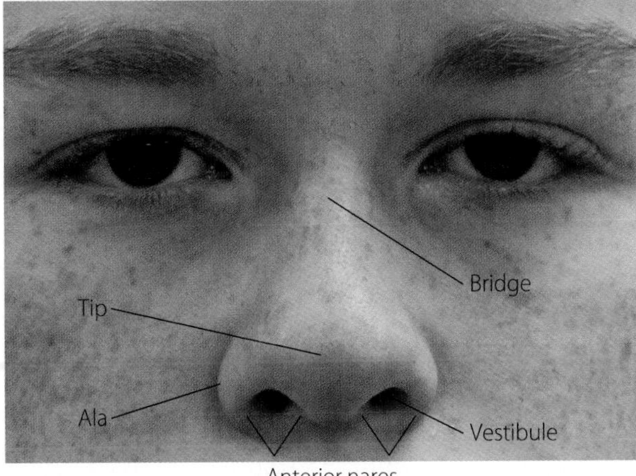

FIGURE 8-38 External nose anatomy.

hemorrhages, av nicking, copper or silver wiring, edema, detachments, or neovascularization.

Nose

INSPECTION

External Nose

Inspect the external nose for lesions and deformity (see **FIGURE 8-38**). Observe for symmetry of the nares.

Internal Nose

The patient is asked to tilt his/her head backward (see **FIGURE 8-39**). The provider places the fingers of the nondominant hand on the patient's forehead and lifts the tip of the nose with the thumb, which opens the nares for optimal inspection. Using a nasal speculum or light source, inspect the turbinates and septum. Also look for abnormalities such as exudate, polyps, bleeding, septal deviation, or foreign bodies.

PALPATION

Confirm patency of the nasal passages by having the patient breathe through one nare while occluding the other.

FUNCTION

The sensory function of the nose, smell, is governed by the olfactory nerve, CNI. This is the least frequently assessed of the cranial nerves due to lack of availability of samples. When smell is assessed, the provider should have two distinctly separate, easily identifiable samples, such as coffee and orange, preferably

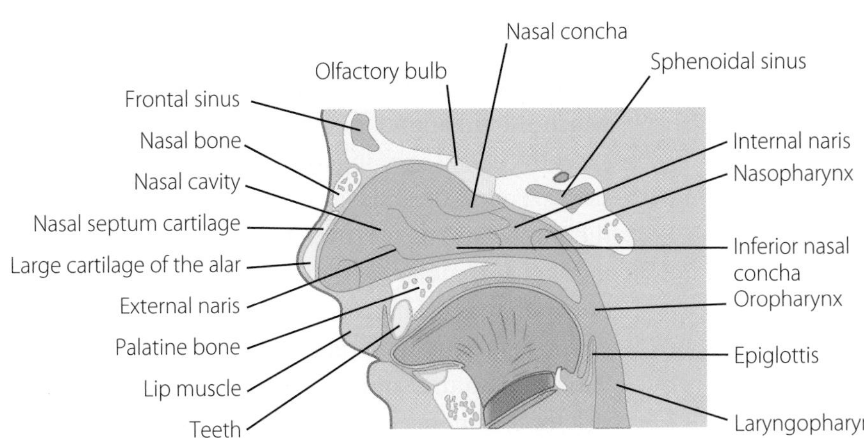

FIGURE 8-39 Internal nose anatomy.

Adapted from: Hess D, MacIntyre NR, Mishoe SC, Galvin WF, and Adams AB. *Respiratory Care: Principles and Practice.* 2nd ed. Burlington, MA: Jones and Bartlett Learning; 2012.

in identically capped containers that cannot be seen through. Avoid noxious samples such as ammonia.

Advise the patient that you will be testing his/her sense of smell. Ask the patient to close the eyes and occlude one side of the nose. Uncap one sample, place it several centimeters below the open nares, and ask the patient to identify the smell. Repeat on the other side with the second sample.

DOCUMENTATION

- Nose: External inspection without lesion or deformity. Septum midline. No exudate, edema, lesions, polyp, or foreign body. Nares patent bilaterally. CNI intact b/l.

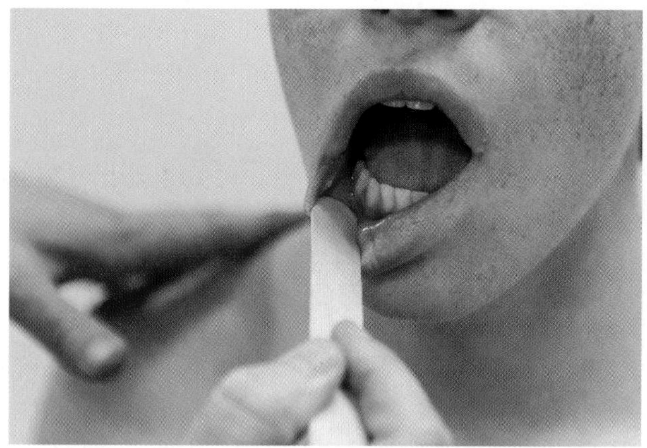

FIGURE 8-41 Appropriate inspection of the structures of the mouth requires the use of a tongue blade and light source.

Throat

INSPECTION

Traditionally the throat examination includes all of the structures of the mouth and throat (see **FIGURE 8-40**). The provider must use a light source and tongue blade for adequate inspection (see **FIGURE 8-41**). Working front to back, first examine the lips. The thin epithelium of the lips allows for improved detection of cyanosis and pallor. Inspect for lesions. A patient with a history of smoking is at increased risk for squamous cell carcinoma of the lips. Vesicular lesions are commonly caused by the herpes simplex virus. Pay particular attention to the corners of the lips (the labial commissures), where inflammation, cheilitis, may occur. This condition may be secondary to moisture-trapping and maceration as facial tone is lost with aging, but may also reflect other medical conditions such as deficiencies of riboflavin (vitamin B_3), iron, or zinc. It may also be caused by fungal or bacterial infection.

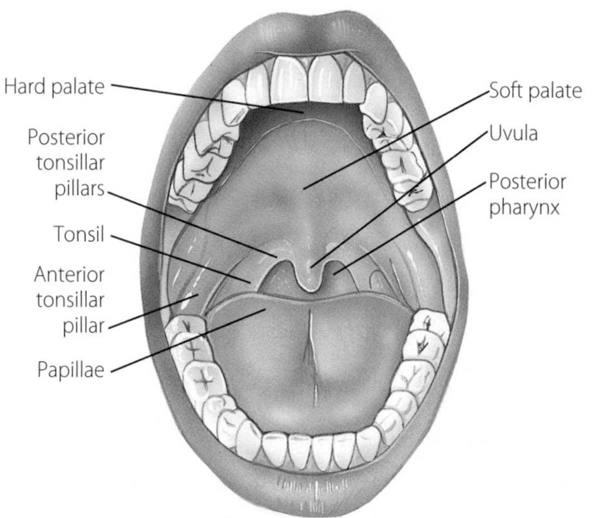

FIGURE 8-40 Anatomy of the mouth.

Use the tongue blade to evert the lips, inspecting the inner mucosal surface of the upper lip to the labial frenulum, then follow the anterior superior gingiva to the central and lateral incisors. Inspect for mucosal lesions and gingival hypertrophy, bleeding, retraction, or inflammation. Repeat the process with the lower lip, gingiva, and incisors. Now move the systematic examination laterally to inspect the buccal mucosa. Mentally divide the buccal mucosa into four sections: right superior, right inferior, left superior, and left inferior. Begin with the superior section of buccal mucosa, identifying the opening to the parotid duct, which should align laterally to the second molar. Inspect the ductal opening for inflammation, lesions, or stones. Follow the mucosa superiorly to the junction of the gingiva and then to the lateral surfaces of the upper incisors and molars. Continue with the inferior section of the buccal mucosa to the lower teeth, completing that side and then repeating on the opposite side. Patients who use smokeless tobacco are at increased risk for carcinoma of the buccal mucosa and gingiva, which can present in many forms from ulceration to plaque. White plaques may represent leukoplakia, hyperplasia of the epithelium that may be a precursor to carcinoma. Mucous-filled cysts (mucoceles) are a result of trauma to the salivary duct, resulting in obstruction and collection of the fluid. The warmth and moisture of the mouth provide a favorable environment for candidiasis, or thrush.

You are now ready to move centrally. Examine the top and inner surfaces of the teeth, looking for carries, accretions, cavitation, state of repair, or loss. To aid examination of the lower inner surface of the teeth, ask the patient to lift the tongue and try to touch the roof of the mouth while keeping the mouth open. Examine the floor of the mouth, moving front to back. Locate the openings of the ducts of the submandibular gland lateral to the frenulum and then the inferior surface of the tongue. Bony, mucosa-covered growths are called torus mandibularis and are a benign condition.

Ask the patient to stick the tongue out toward the right side, and examine the left lateral side and then move toward the left. Finally, have the patient stick the tongue out toward you. Note any deviation that occurs that would indicate a lesion of the **hypoglossal nerve**, CNXII, with the deviation of the tongue going toward the same side of the lesion. Sticking the tongue out midline involves equal muscle effort from each side of the tongue acting in conjunction. Envision the right side of your tongue being paralyzed. As you attempt to stick out your tongue, the right side remains flaccid with the only muscular effort coming from the left side. The lack of counterbalance results in the left side of the tongue pushing the flaccid right side farther toward the right.

Examine the top of the tongue, again looking for lesions. Some common conditions that are quite disturbing to patients are black hairy tongue and geographic tongue. Black hairy tongue may be associated with poor oral hygiene but may also be related to thrush and antibiotic use. The geographic tongue is so named due to a pattern papillae loss that makes the tongue look like a map. Though the etiology is unclear and usually benign, systemic conditions should also be considered should resolution not occur. Posterior papillae may occasionally be seen by the provider. Being of larger size than those on the anterior surface of the tongue, these papillae are sometimes confused with lesions by the inexperienced provider.

Next inspect the roof of the mouth, moving from hard to soft palate. Look for the mucosal-covered bony growth of torus palatinus along the midline on the hard palate. Follow the soft palate back to the anterior and posterior tonsillar pillars, noting the presence or absence of tonsils. Observe for tonsillar hypertrophy, exudate, or lesions. Ask the patient to say "Ahhhh." Observe the uvula as it rises with phonation. The uvula should rise in midline. Deviation to one side suggests a lesion of the vagus nerve, CNX, on the opposite side of the lesion. Note also the sound of phonation during this technique as well as during conversation, which may also indicate CNX dysfunction through the recurrent laryngeal branch of the vagus.

Inspect the posterior wall of the pharynx. If good visualization is not achieved, an alterative technique is to ask the patient to pant like a dog. This works especially well in children, asking them to pretend they are a dog and demonstrating how to pant. If an extended period of observation is required, a tongue blade may be used to depress the tongue. Attempt to avoid gagging the patient by placing the blade only midway back on the tongue and advising patients that you are attempting to avoid gagging them. Even with this instruction, some patients are hypersensitive to use of the tongue blade and may gag just by visualizing it even before placing it in the mouth.

Finally, to assess cranial nerves IX and X, the glossopharyngeal and vagal nerve, advise the patient that you will be checking the gag reflex, then depress the blade on the posterior tongue surface. Sensory stimulation occurs through CNIX with motor response through CNX.

PALPATION

Palpation of the mouth is primarily for lesions. When palpation is indicated, the provider should don latex-free gloves, washing the gloves to remove any residue prior to palpation. Palpate the lips and buccal mucosa, gently compressing each area between the thumb externally

Hypoglossal nerve: CNXII, responsible for motor function of the tongue

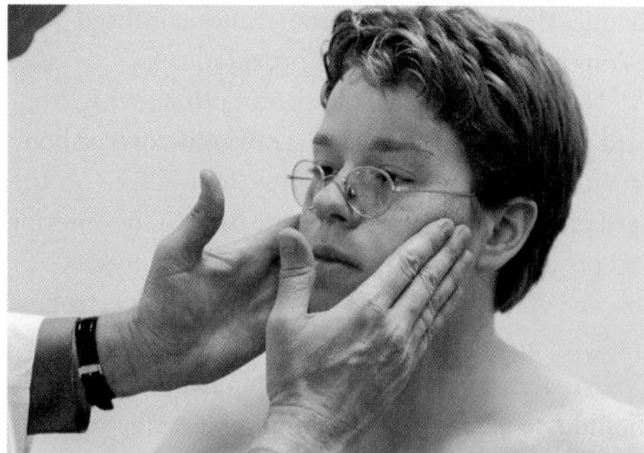

FIGURE 8-42 External palpation of the parotid glands.

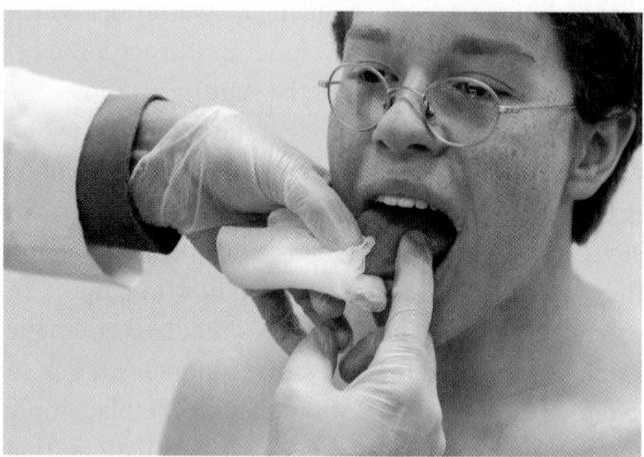

FIGURE 8-43 Palpation of the tongue utilizing a gauze pad.

and a finger inside the mouth. Gently sliding from one area to another helps to identify small lesions that may have no surface indication of presence. Assess the parotid gland for enlargement or stones (see **FIGURE 8-42**). Palpate the gingiva, under the tongue, and the hard palate. Finally, to palpate the tongue, ask the patient to stick the tongue out and use a dry piece of gauze to gently hold the tip, palpating for lesions with the other hand (see **FIGURE 8-43**).

DOCUMENTATION

- Mouth/Throat: Lips symmetrical, pink without cracking, lesions, or maceration. Buccal mucosa, palate, tonsillar pillars pink, moist without lesions. Gingiva without hypertrophy, retraction, or bleeding. Teeth in good repair. Tongue pink, smooth without lesions. Distends in midline CNXII intact. Tonsils without hypertrophy, exudate, or erythema. Uvula elevates midline with phonation. Posterior pharynx without erythema, exudate, postnasal drainage, or lesions.

Ears

FUNCTION

Hearing loss becomes intrusive as it enters the voice frequency range of conversation, which lies between 500 and 3000 Hz. Loss most commonly occurs at the higher-frequency ranges, with patients complaining of difficulty hearing the speech of women and children.

Begin examination of the ears through assessment of function (see **FIGURES 8-44** and **8-45**). Generalized screening can be completed through multiple techniques.

Whispered Word

With this technique the provider asks the patient to occlude one ear while the provider stands on the opposite side. The provider asks the patient to repeat a word, then whispers at a distance approximately 24 inches from the patient's ear (see **FIGURE 8-46**). If the patient cannot correctly identify the word, it is repeated at consecutively closer distances until correctly identified. The technique is then repeated in the opposite ear. For example, a patient is able to identify the whispered word at 24 inches in the left ear but is not able to identify the word in the right ear until the provider is 12 inches away.

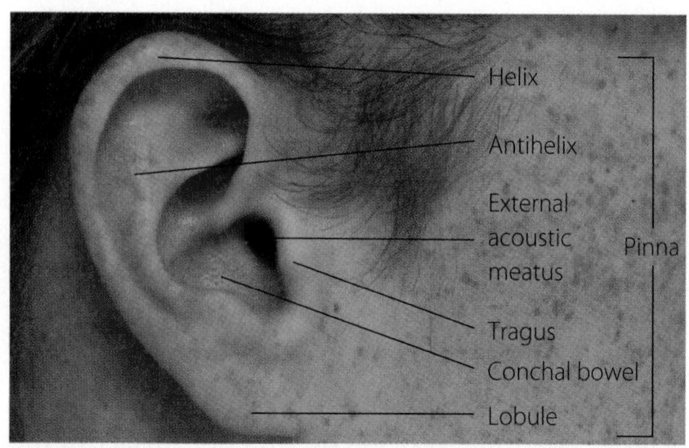

FIGURE 8-44 External ear anatomy.

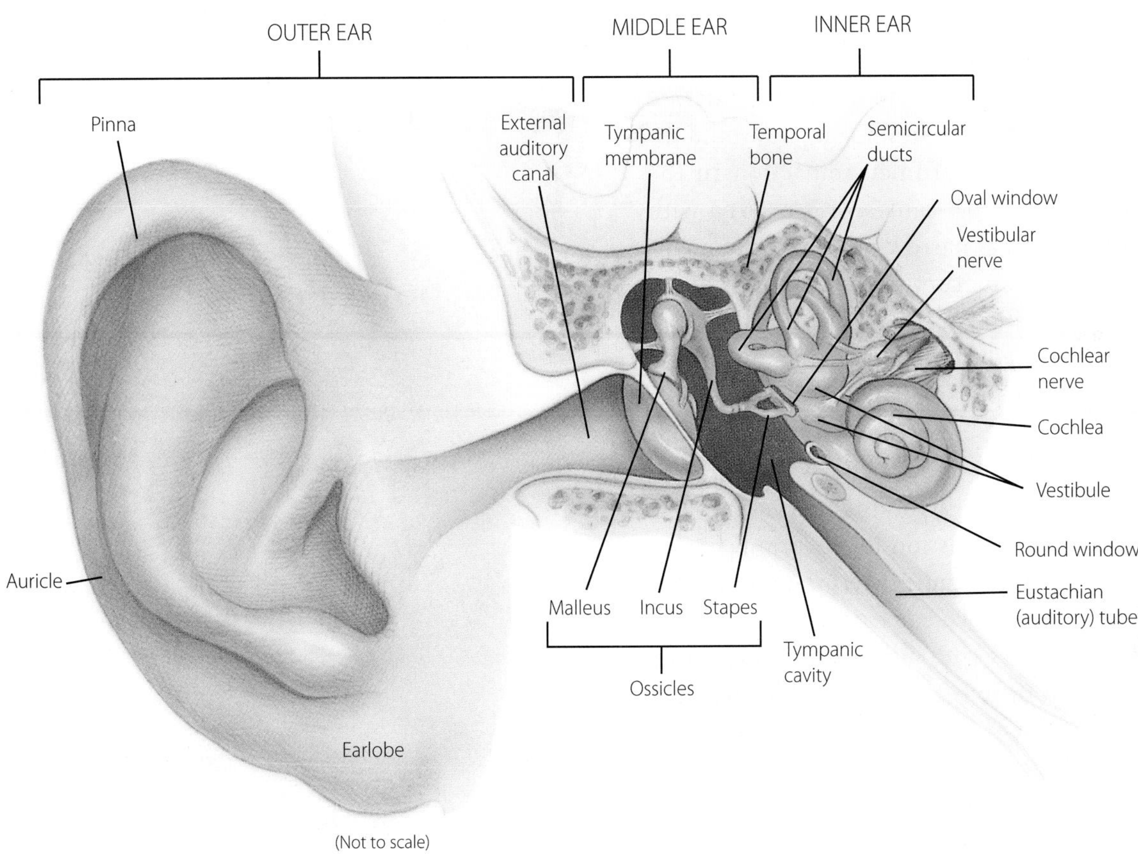

FIGURE 8-45 Internal ear anatomy.

DOCUMENTATION

- Hearing screen: Whispered word at 24 inches L, 12 inches R.

Finger Rub

With this general hearing screen, the provider asks the patient to close his/her eyes; the provider then rubs his/her thumb against the index and middle fingers approximately 3 to 4 inches from the patient's ear. The provider asks the patient to identify which ear he/she hears the rubbing in and alternates randomly between the right, left, or both ears.

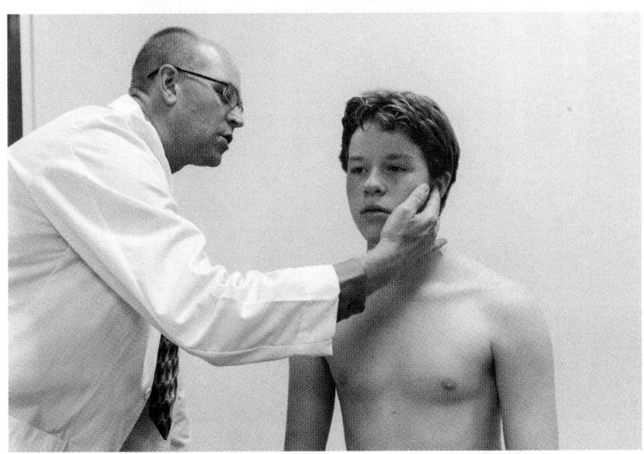

FIGURE 8-46 Whispered word testing.

DOCUMENTATION

- Hearing intact to finger rub b/l.

Specialized Testing

If the generalized screening tests show hearing deficit in one or both ears, two specialized tests are implemented to determine if the hearing loss is conductive or sensorineural.

Conductive hearing involves the passage of sound waves through the external auditory canal, against the **tympanic membrane** (TM), through the ossicles—the malleolus, incus, and stapes. Hearing

> **Tympanic membrane:** membrane within the ear that separates the external ear from the middle ear, collecting sound waves and transmitting them to the ossicles in the process of hearing

Conductive hearing loss: hearing loss caused by disruption of the transmission of sound waves through any component of the passages from external auditory canal, through the tympanic membrane and through the ossicles

Sensorineural hearing loss: hearing loss due to a deficiency within the cochlea, involving nerve impulse transmission to the brain

Weber test: hearing test performed with a 256-Hz vibratory tuning fork and used in conjunction with Rinne test to help distinguish between conductive and sensorineural hearing loss

loss caused by disruption of sound wave passage through any of these components results in **conductive hearing loss**. Examples would include cerumen impaction in the external canal, otitis externa with canal narrowing, tympanic membrane rupture or scarring, dislocation of the ossicular chain, otitis media, or ankylosing inhibiting mobility of the ossicles.

Sensorineural hearing loss is due to deficiency within the cochlea, involving nerve impulse transmission to the brain. Examples include deterioration of inner ear cochlear hair cells (which occurs with aging), noise exposure, and ototoxic drugs, which result in high-frequency hearing loss.

Mixed hearing loss occurs when there is a combination of conductive and sensorineural loss.

To distinguish between conductive and sensorineural hearing loss, two additional hearing tests must be utilized: the Weber and the Rinne.

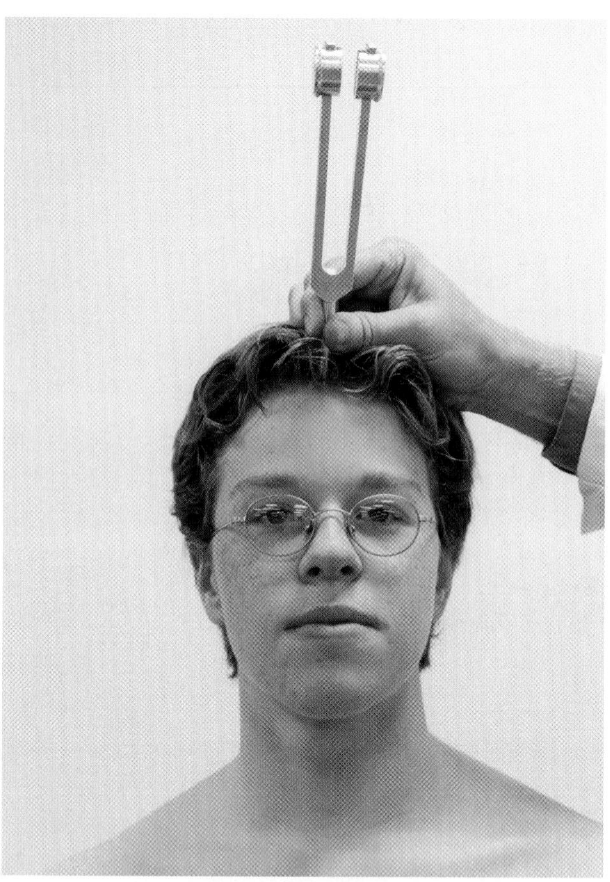

FIGURE 8-47 Placement of the tuning fork for the Weber test.

Weber.

8-10 The **Weber test** helps to distinguish conductive hearing loss from sensorineural loss when used in combination with the Rinne test. This test utilizes a 128- or 256-Hz vibratory tuning fork, which is struck and placed on the forehead equidistant between the ears to determine which ear the patient better hears the sound in (see **FIGURE 8-47**).

Technique (see **TABLE 8-1**). Instruct the patient that you will be striking a tuning fork (see **FIGURE 8-48**) and placing it on the top of his/her head to ascertain if the patient can hear it louder in one ear than in the other, or if it seems of equal volume in both. Then strike a vibratory tuning fork and place it in the middle of the patient's forehead, and ask the patient, "Do you hear the sound louder in your right ear or left ear, or is it equal in both?"

If lateralization occurs, there are two possibilities: conductive hearing loss and sensorineural hearing loss.

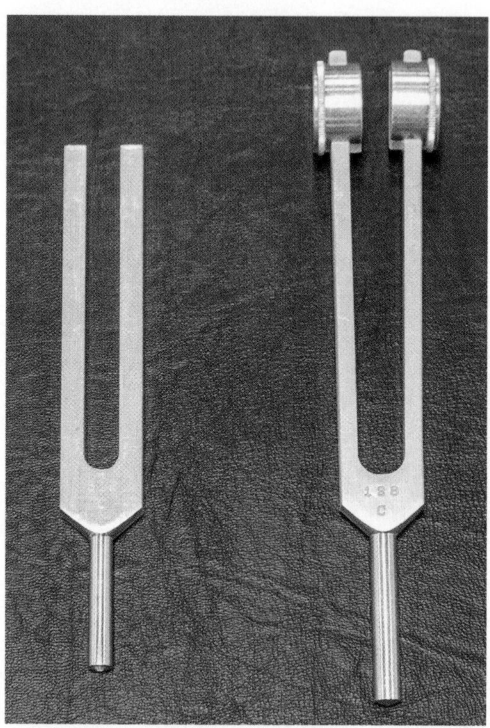

FIGURE 8-48 Common tuning forks used in the detection of conductive and sensorineural hearing loss.

TABLE 8-1 Performing the Weber Test

1. Instruct the patient that you will be striking a tuning fork and placing it on the top of his/her head.
2. Ask the patient to close his/her eyes.
3. Strike a 256-Hz vibratory tuning fork and place it on the forehead equidistant between the two ears.
4. Ask the patient, "Do you hear the sound louder in the right ear or left ear, or is it equal in both?"

Conductive loss. The patient perceives the sound to be louder in an ear with conductive hearing loss (CHL), as the defect of the transmission of sound to the cochlea is bypassed by providing an alternative direct pathway for sound transmission through the bones of the skull. The sound is perceived to be louder because the only sound reaching the nerve is provided through vibration, meaning there is no background noise to dampen it.

Sensorineural loss. With sensorineural loss (SNHL) the patient perceives the sound to be louder in the opposite ear. Even though a conduction pathway is being provided through the bone, once the sound reaches the cochlea of the ear with sensorineural loss, the deficit within the nerve itself diminishes perception of sound in that ear, resulting in a higher perception of sound in the opposite ear.

Case example. On general screening, a patient states that the sound is louder in the left ear, prompting the Weber and Rinne exams. When the Weber is performed, the patient states that the sound is heard loudest in the right ear. This indicates that there is either:

1. Conductive hearing loss in the *right* ear. The sound is perceived louder in the *right* ear because the conduction pathway being provided by the test is the only sound reaching the cochlea and it is not diminished by environmental background noise.
   or
2. Sensorineural hearing loss in the *left* ear. The sound is perceived louder in the *right* ear because even though a conduction pathway is being provided, once the sound reaches the cochlea of the left ear, deficit within the nerve itself diminishes perception of the noise.

To determine which it is, the provider must now perform the Rinne test.

Rinne.

To perform the **Rinne test**, a 528-Hz tuning fork is used to determine how the conduction of sound through the air compares to the conduction of sound through bone. With normal hearing, sound conducts through air better than through bone.

Rinne test: a hearing test commonly performed with a 528-Hz tuning fork used to determine how the conduction of sound through the air compares to the conduction of sound through bone

Technique. The tuning fork is struck and the handle is placed on the mastoid process with the tines directed posteriorly (see **FIGURE 8-49**). The ability to hear the tuning fork while on the mastoid process is assessing bone conduction (BC). An effective technique is to grasp the fork firmly by the handle, squeeze the tines between the thumb and index finger of the opposite hand, and drag the fork out from the thumb and finger. This results in a level of noise that is not overly loud and that will diminish at an appropriate rate. After positioning on the mastoid process, ask the patient if the sound can be heard; if it cannot, restrike the tuning fork with greater force. Leaving the fork in place, ask the patient to tell you when the sound can no longer be heard. When the patient indicates that the sound can no longer be heard, remove the handle from the malleolus and place the tines approximately 3 cm beside the patient's ear, being careful not to touch the tines while doing so. Placing the tines in front of the ear is assessing air conduction (AC). Now ask if the sound can be heard again. Repeat the process in the other ear.

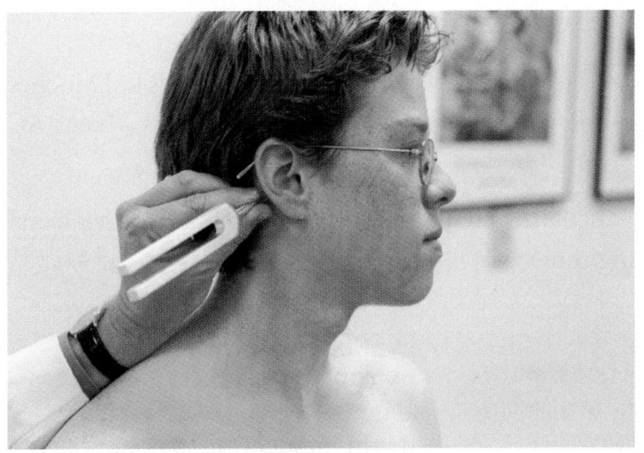

FIGURE 8-49 Placement of the tuning fork for the Rinne test.

Conductive loss. If the patient is unable to hear the tuning fork once it is removed from the malleolus and placed beside the ear, bone conduction is greater than air conduction and indicates conductive loss.

- Documentation
  - AC > BC or
  - BC > AC

Sensorineural loss. The patient's being able to hear the sound again when the tines are placed beside the ear indicates that two possibilities exist: (1) there is no hearing loss present, or (2) sensorineural hearing loss exists.

Case example continued. When performing the Rinne, the right ear demonstrates BC > AC. The left ear shows AC > BC. Combining the Weber and Rinne allows for differentiation of the type of hearing loss.

1. General screen—Whispered word: 24 inches L, 12 inches right prompting Weber/Rinne
2. Weber—Lateralizes right ear. This indicates that there is either:
   a. Conductive hearing loss in the *right* ear *or*
   b. Sensorineural hearing loss in the *left* ear
3. Rinne
   a. Right ear BC > AC—Indicates conductive loss in the *right*
   b. Left ear AC > BC—Indicates normal hearing or sensorineural loss in the *left*
4. Combining the results
   a. Lateralization to the right combined with BC > AC confirms conductive loss in the right
   b. General screen intact at 24 inches L, AC > BC indicates normal hearing

DOCUMENTATION

- Hearing: Whispered word at 24 inches L, 12 inches R. Weber lateralizes R. R ear BC > AC. L ear AC > BC.

TABLE 8-2 may be utilized following a positive hearing screen.

TABLE 8-2 Screening Deficit Follow-up Testing

	Step 1: Perform the Weber Test		
Step 2: Perform Rinne Result in ear of lateralization	**Lateralizes Right**	**Midline**	**Lateralizes Left**
AC > BC	SNHL L	SNHL B/L	SNHL R
BC > AC	CHL R	CHL B/L	CHL L

Otoscopy: examination of the ear using an otoscope, a medical device that provides amplification

INSPECTION OF THE EXTERNAL EAR

Begin inspection of the ear by working from outside to inside. Observe the external ear, looking for shape, lesions, or deformity. Be sure to fold the ear forward to inspect for lesions behind the ear, a common place for basal cell carcinoma to hide. Examine the meatus of the external auditory canal, looking for caliber of the canal, exudate, or lesions. The rest of the examination will require the use of the otoscope.

PALPATION OF THE EXTERNAL EAR

Prior to inspecting the external auditory canal and ear structures, palpate the external ear for lesions and tenderness. When a patient presents with ear pain, differentiation between an external ear infection (otitis external), and an inner ear infection (otitis media), can be aided through palpation. Tell the patient you will be touching the ear and ask the patient to tell you if he/she experiences any pain, then (1) depress the tragus against the conchal bowl, and (2) retract the pinna upward. If pain is elicited or intensified, otitis externa is anticipated. In this case, expect the auditory canal to be narrowed and inflamed, and use extra caution when attempting to perform the otoscopic exam.

DOCUMENTATION

- Ear: Inspection without lesions, erythema, edema, or deformity. Palpation without tenderness.

OTOSCOPY

Otoscopic examination is indicated both as routine screening and when a patient presents with ear pain.

The Otoscope

The otoscope consists of a power source, typically an AC-powered wall unit or a battery handle, and

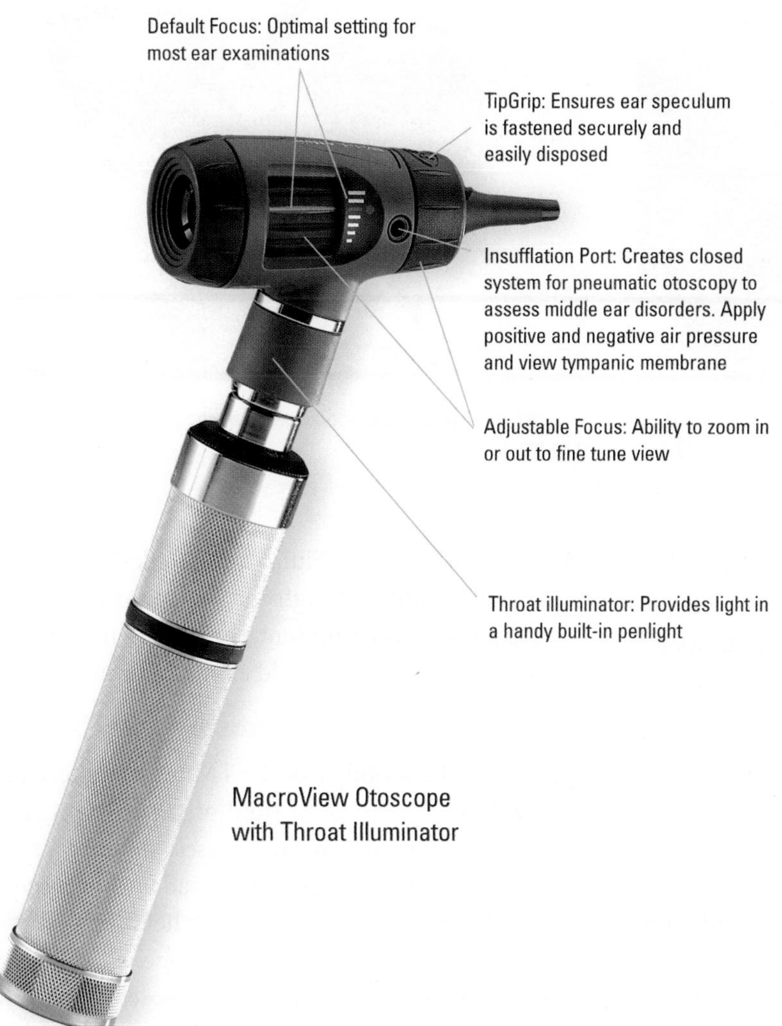
Default Focus: Optimal setting for most ear examinations
TipGrip: Ensures ear speculum is fastened securely and easily disposed
Insufflation Port: Creates closed system for pneumatic otoscopy to assess middle ear disorders. Apply positive and negative air pressure and view tympanic membrane
Adjustable Focus: Ability to zoom in or out to fine tune view
Throat illuminator: Provides light in a handy built-in penlight
MacroView Otoscope with Throat Illuminator

FIGURE 8-50 Otoscope.
Courtesy of Welch Allyn.

the otoscopic head (see **FIGURE 8-50**). The head of the otoscope has a posterior magnifier enlarging the field of view. Providers should choose an otoscope with maximal field of view and magnification to improve imaging of the tympanic membrane.[1] A light source is within the head. Light sources that avoid obstruction of the field of view are preferable. Advanced otoscopes produce optimal illumination through fiber-optic and halogen technologies. Fiber-optic light transmission provides a 360-degree ring of light without visual obstruction or specular reflection.[1] A speculum is placed on the conical tip. Disposable tips are preferred over reusable tips, which must be cleaned and disinfected between patients. The head should have a port for the attachment of an insufflation bulb, which is used to assess mobility of the tympanic membrane. Some advanced otoscopic heads have focus control, allowing for sharper visualization of the ear structures.

Technique.

- Inspect the meatus of the auditory canal for exudate or lesions.
- Depress the tragus and retract the pinnae to assess for tenderness.
- Observe the size of the auditory canal and select a speculum that most closely approximates the size of the canal.
- Turn on the light of the otoscope.
- Hold the inverted otoscope with the fifth finger extended and resting against the side of the patient's head (see **FIGURE 8-51A**). This is a precaution against the patient, especially a child, rapidly turning his/her head into the otoscope, resulting in the speculum tip being jammed into the ear canal and possibly rupturing the tympanic membrane.
- Grasp the pinnae with the opposite hand and straighten the ear canal by
  - Lifting up, back, and out for an adult.
  - Pulling down, back, and out for a child.
- Without looking through the magnifier, place the edge of the speculum against the tragus and push it anteriorly. This technique often allows the provider to observe the direction of the auditory canal, which is typically angled anteriorly, and often the tympanic membrane, even without magnification.
- Now look through the magnifier and adjust the angle of observation and depth of insertion until the tympanic membrane comes into clear view (see **FIGURE 8-51B**).

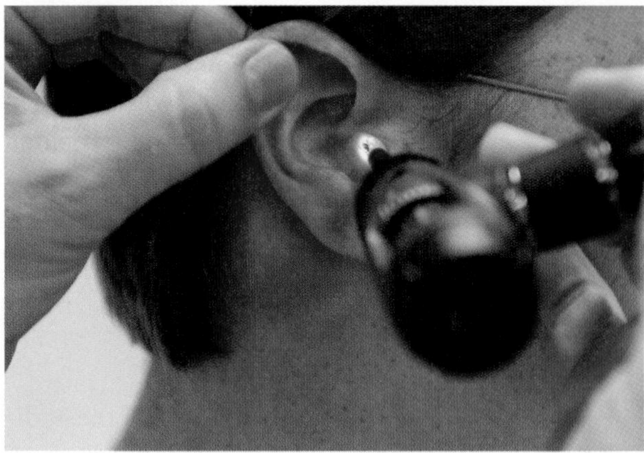

FIGURE 8-51A Early otoscopic exam as the provider places the tip of the otoscope against the posterior tragus while retracting the ear.

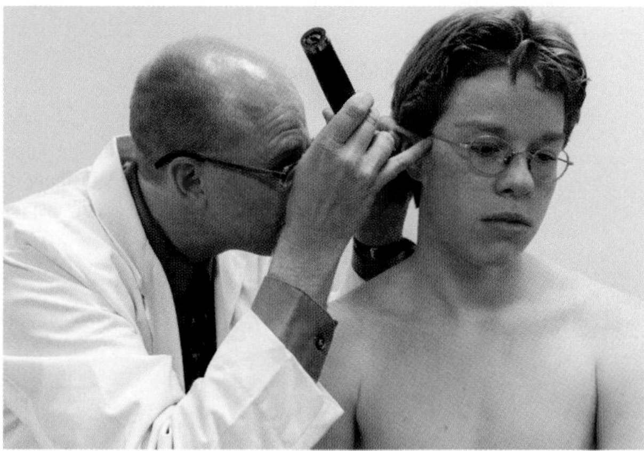

FIGURE 8-51B Late otoscopic exam as the provider looks through the magnifier.

Insufflation: the assessment of the mobility of the tympanic membrane in the evaluation of fluid and middle ear pressures by forcing air against it through the use of an insufflation bulb attached to an otoscope

Inspection.

Following the same sequential outside-to-inside approach allows for concise examination.

- Auditory Canal: Inspect the canal for lesions, foreign bodies, trauma, and signs of infection or inflammation such as erythema, edema, or exudate.
- Tympanic Membrane: Identify the normal landmarks of the TM, particularly the pars tensa, pars flaccida, malleolus with umbo, and cone of light (see FIGURE 8-52). Inspect for bulge associated with otitis media, retraction with negative inner ear pressure or serous otitis media, scars (tympanosclerotic plaques), perforation, or masses.
- Tympanic cavity: Fluid, air bubbles, or masses may be visible through the semitranslucent TM. If a perforation is present, the ossicles may be able to be visualized as would exudates or masses.

Insufflation *(Pneumatic Otoscopy).*

8-12 The mobility of the TM may be altered by the presence of fluid or negative pressure within the tympanic cavity. To assess mobility an insufflation bulb is attached to the head of the otoscope (see FIGURE 8-53). The bulb may be held between the thumb and the handle of the otoscope, allowing the provider to insufflate and hold the otoscope with the same hand while straightening the canal by positioning the ear with the other (see FIGURE 8-54). When fluid is present in the middle ear, for example, movement of the tympanic membrane is generally diminished or absent.[1] Eustachian tube dysfunction may lead

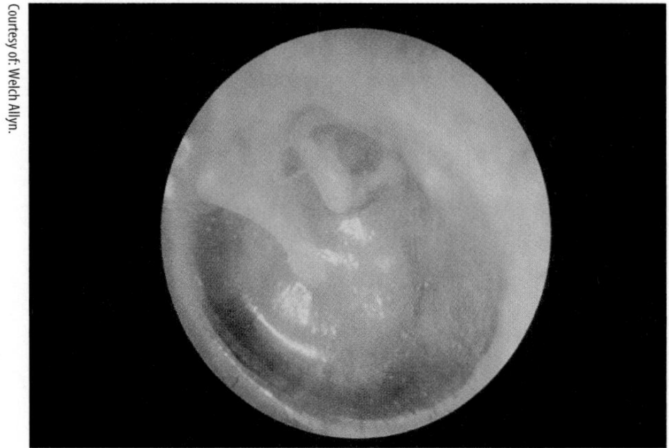

Courtesy of: Welch Allyn.

FIGURE 8-52 Normal tympanic membrane.

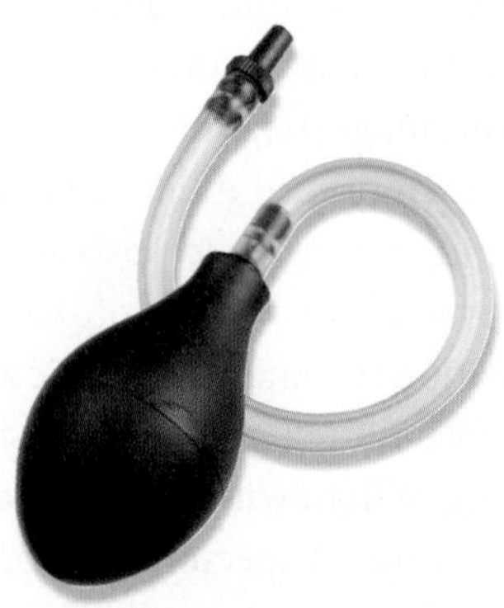

FIGURE 8-53 Insufflation bulb.

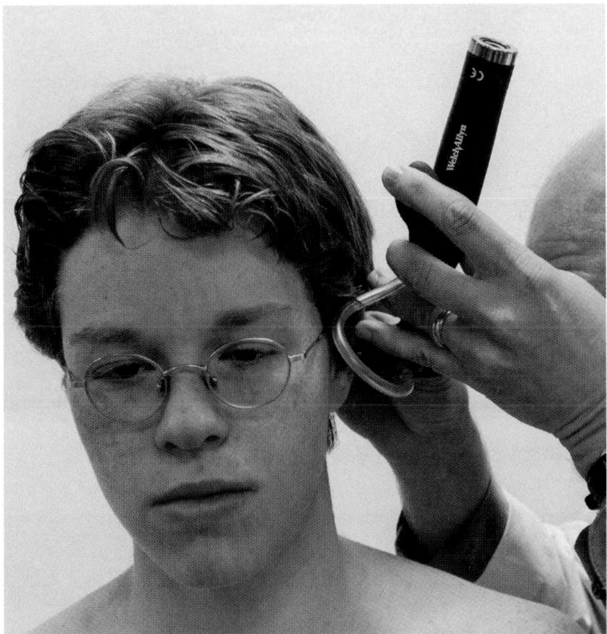

FIGURE 8-54 Proper positioning for the performance of insufflation during the otoscopic exam.

to negative inner ear pressure with retracted TM and immobility on insufflation. Insufflation in patients with complaints of dizziness related to barotrauma may induce further dizziness. This phenomenon is seen in patients with perilymphatic fistulae.

DOCUMENTATION

- Otoscopic exam: Auditory canal with edema, exudate, or lesions. TM intact with good light reflex free motion with insufflation. No bulge, retraction, or perforation.

COMMON PATHOLOGIES OF THE EAR

Red Reflex (see FIGURE 8-55)

On otoscopy, dilatation of the blood vessels supplying the tympanic membrane may result in an erythematous appearance in the crying child. This should not be confused with otitis media.

Exostosis (see FIGURE 8-56)

Exostoses appear as well-defined, hard nodules in the auditory canal. They are typically benign, requiring no intervention other than observation, and are common in swimmers. Occlusion of the meatus and the external auditory canal may lead to conductive hearing loss.

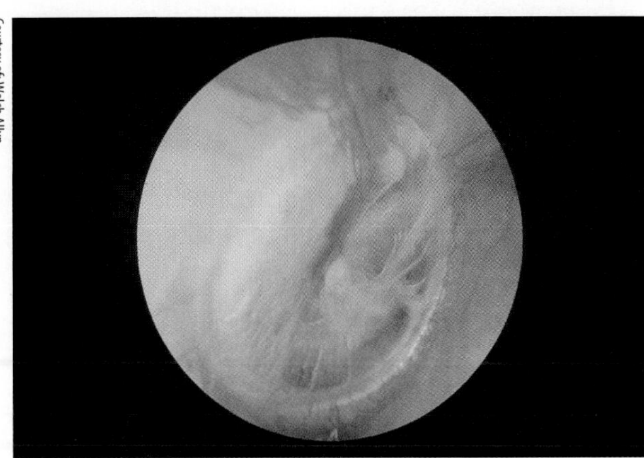

Courtesy of: Welch Allyn

FIGURE 8-55 Red reflex.

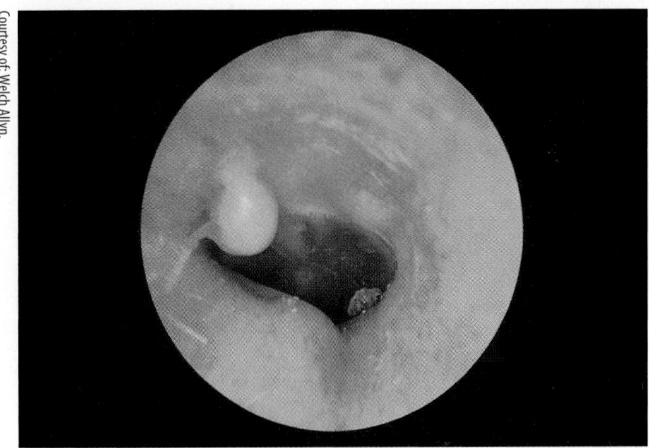

Courtesy of: Welch Allyn.

FIGURE 8-56 Exostosis.

Foreign Body (see FIGURE 8-57)

The auditory canal is a common place for foreign body insertion, especially in children. It is also common to encounter insects, with patients relating the sounds of their movements to be quite harsh against the TM.

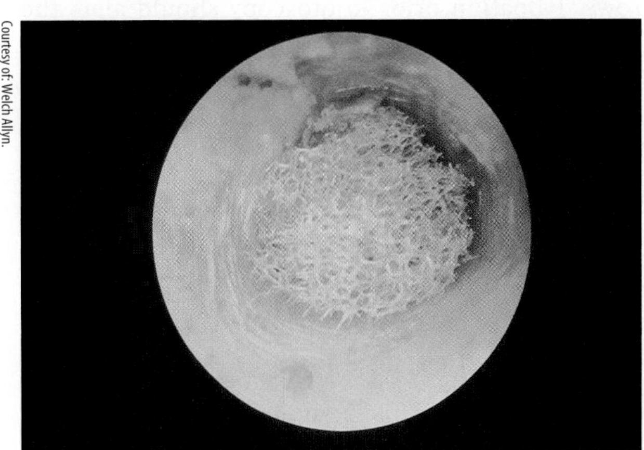

Courtesy of: Welch Allyn.

FIGURE 8-57 Foreign body.

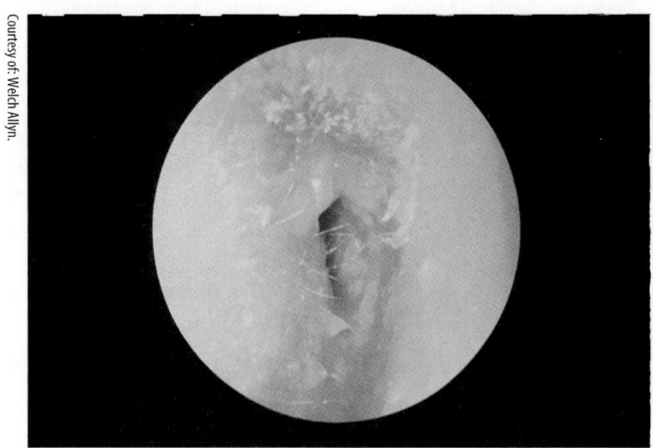
Courtesy of: Welch Allyn.

FIGURE 8-58 Acute otitis externa.

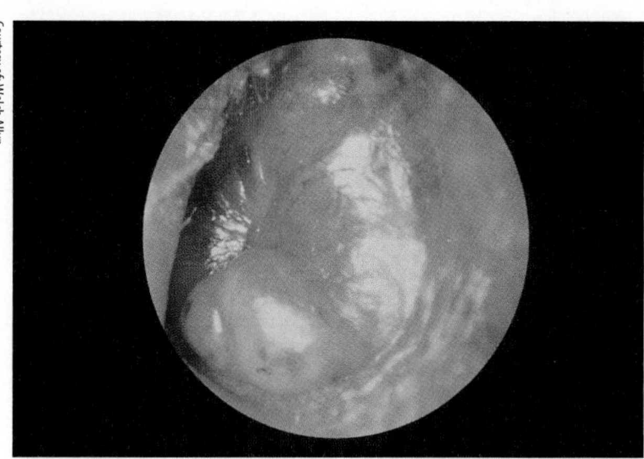
Courtesy of: Welch Allyn.

FIGURE 8-60 Acute otitis media.

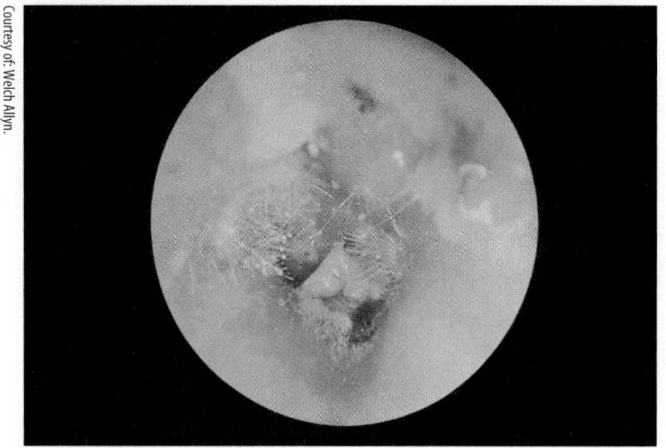
Courtesy of: Welch Allyn.

FIGURE 8-59 Otomycosis.

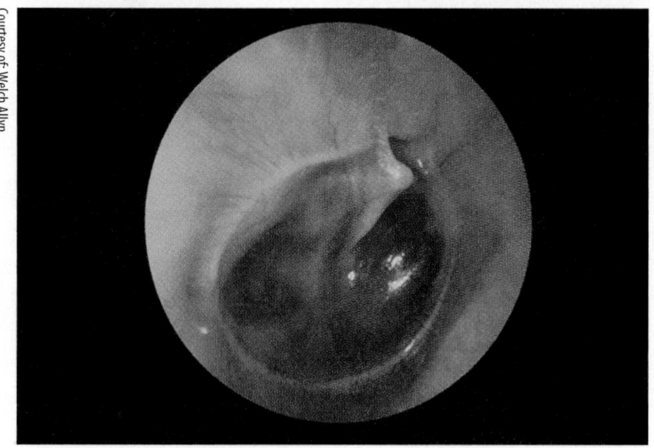
Courtesy of: Welch Allyn.

FIGURE 8-61 Serous otitis media.

Acute Otitis Externa (see FIGURE 8-58)

In **otitis** externa (OE) the auditory canal becomes infected, resulting in inflammation with erythema, edema, pain, and often hearing loss as the canal narrows. Palpation prior to otoscopy should alert the provider to the need for caution with insertion of the speculum.

Otomycosis (see FIGURE 8-59)

Otomycosis is a fungal infection of the auditory canal with cottony-appearing exudate.

Otitis: inflammation of the ear referred to as otitis externa for inflammation of the external ear and otitis media for inflammation of the middle ear

Acute Otitis Media (see FIGURE 8-60)

This is one of the most common infections of the ear, especially in children. The tympanic membrane loses the light reflex and becomes erythematous. With progression, the TM bulges toward the external canal and may result in perforation. Patients relate progressively worsening pain, a sudden pop or release of pressure with decreased intensity of pain, and the appearance of exudate.

Serous Otitis Media (see FIGURE 8-61)

In contrast, serous otitis media is associated with negative inner ear pressure, resulting in retraction and immobility of the TM with accentuation of the ossicles. Effusion or bubbles can often be seen behind the TM.

Tympanostomy Tube (see FIGURE 8-62)

Tympanostomy tubes are often encountered on examination of the ear. These tubes are surgically inserted in cases of chronic otitis media.

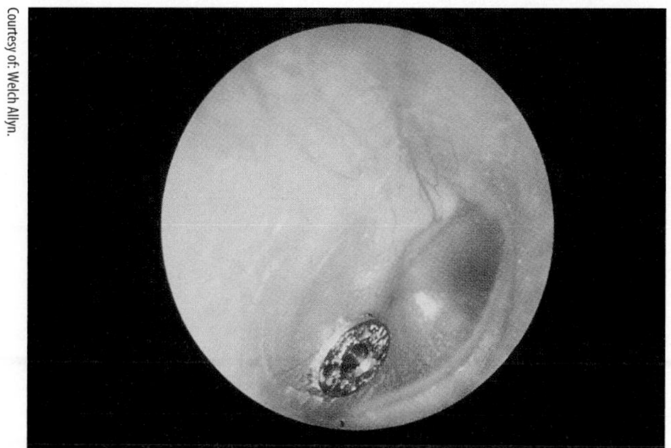
Courtesy of: Welch Allyn.

FIGURE 8-62 Tympanostomy tube.

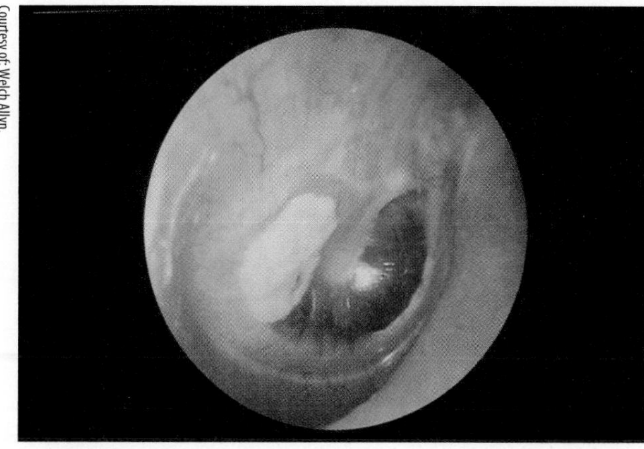
Courtesy of: Welch Allyn.

FIGURE 8-64 Tympanosclerosis.

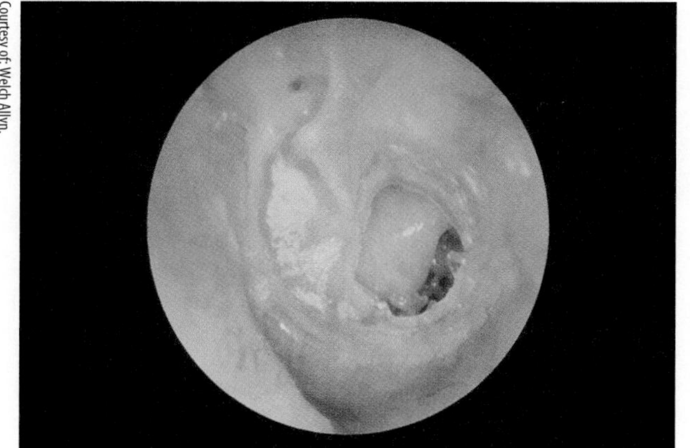
Courtesy of: Welch Allyn.

FIGURE 8-63 Tympanic membrane perforation.

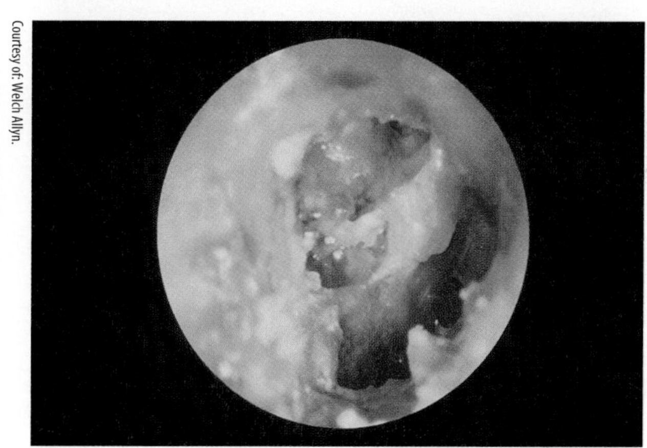
Courtesy of: Welch Allyn.

FIGURE 8-65 Cholesteatoma.

Perforation of the Tympanic Membrane (see FIGURE 8-63)

Perforations may be associated with OM or traumatic injury.

Tympanosclerosis (see FIGURE 8-64)

Tympanosclerosis appears as scar tissue where the normally translucent TM becomes opaque and thickened, and is often associated with ear infections.

Cholesteatoma (see FIGURE 8-65)

Cholesteatomas appear as irregular waxy masses; if left untreated, they can cause permanent destruction, as the benign though space-occupying tumor-like cyst advances. These require referral for surgical intervention.

TABLE 8-3 provides a breakdown of the HEENT flow process.

TABLE 8-3 Head, Eyes, Ears, Nose, and Throat (HEENT) Flow

HEAD
Inspection
Size
Symmetry
Trauma
Palpation: tenderness, lesions, and deformity
FACE
Inspection
Lesions
Symmetry: CNVII
Ask the patient to complete a series of facial expression motions:
Please raise your eyebrows
Puff out your cheeks
Show me your teeth
Frown

(continues)

TABLE 8-3 Head, Eyes, Ears, Nose, and Throat (HEENT) Flow *(Continued)*

- SINUSES
  - Inspection via transillumination
    - Frontal sinuses
    - Maxillary sinuses
  - Palpation
  - Percussion
- EYES
  - Function: CNII—optic nerve
    - Assess visual acuity in each eye separately, holding chart at correct distance
    - Assess peripheral fields: 4 quadrants each eye tested separately, crossing midline
  - Inspection
    - Examiner moves to approximately 4 feet in front of patient
      - Ptosis: memory tool: upper lid is held up by the pillar III—CNIII
      - Position of the eye by light reflection—rule out strabismus
      - Extraocular movements (cranial nerves III, IV, and VI)
      - Assess for nystagmus CNVIII—acoustic (vestibulocochlear)
    - Examiner moves closer to approximately 1 foot in front of patient
      - Cornea: clouding, lesions, injection
      - Corneal reflex: cotton ball with lateral approach—CNV—sensory branch
      - Pupil: size, shape
      - Perpendicular light across iris; rule out shallow anterior chamber/glaucoma
      - Iris: lesions
      - Pupillary reflex: direct & consensual—CNII and CNIII (oculomotor)
      - Sclera: injection, icterus, lesion, hemorrhage
      - Conjunctiva: injection, pallor, exudate
    - Ophthalmoscopic examination: R eye to R eye, L eye to L eye.
- NOSE
  - Inspection
    - External nose: lesions, deformity, symmetry of the nares
    - Internal nose
      - Ask patient to tilt the head backward
      - Lift the tip of the nose with the thumb to open the nares
      - Use a nasal speculum or light source
      - Inspect turbinates and septum
      - Inspect for exudate, polyps, bleeding, septal deviation, and foreign bodies
      - Patency: ask patient to breathe through one naris while occluding the other
  - Function: olfactory nerve, CNI assessment
    - Advise patient you will be testing smell
    - Have patient close the eyes
    - Assess smell with two separate samples
- MOUTH/THROAT
  - Inspection
    - Lips for cyanosis, pallor, lesions, inflammation, and cheilitis
    - Utilize light source and tongue blade
    - Evert the lips with tongue blade, inspecting the inner mucosal surface
      - Gingiva: hypertrophy, bleeding, retraction, or inflammation
      - Buccal mucosa
      - Lesions, masses
      - Opening to the parotid duct lateral to the second upper molar
      - Teeth: accretions, cavitation, state of repair, or loss
      - Floor of the mouth
      - Lesions, torus mandibularis
      - Openings of the ducts of the submandibular gland
      - Tongue
        - Distension in midline: hypoglossal nerve, CNXII assessment
        - Identify lesion with the deviation of the tongue going toward the same side
      - Palate: deformity, lesion
      - Tonsillar pillars and tonsils: hypertrophy, exudate, or lesions
        - Ask the patient to say "Ahhhh"
        - Confirm uvula rising in midline, CNX assessment
        - Identify deviation to one side, which suggests a lesion on the opposite side
        - Note sound of phonation for harshness
      - Pharynx: erythema, exudate, postnasal drainage, lesions
      - Gag reflex: glossopharyngeal and vagal nerve assessment, CNIX and X
        - Advise the patient of intent to check gag reflex
        - Depress the blade on the posterior tongue surface
  - Palpation
    - Don latex-free gloves, washing the gloves to remove any residue

TABLE 8-3 Head, Eyes, Ears, Nose, and Throat (HEENT) Flow *(Continued)*

Lips and buccal mucosa
Parotid gland: enlargement or stones
Gingiva
Floor of mouth
Hard palate
Tongue: use dry gauze to hold tip while palpating for lesions with the other hand
EARS
Function
Whispered word
Finger rub
Specialized testing
Weber
Rinne
Inspection of the external ear
Shape, lesions, deformity, lesions
Meatus of external auditory canal for caliber, exudate, or lesions
Palpation of the external ear
Lesions
Tenderness
Otoscopic exam
Depress the tragus and retract the pinnae for tenderness
Invert otoscope with the fifth finger extended, resting against the side of the head
Straighten the ear canal
Adult: lift the ear up, back, and out
Child: pull ear down, back, and out
Inspection
Auditory canal: lesions, foreign bodies, erythema, edema, or exudate
Tympanic membrane
Landmarks
Pars tensa
Pars flaccida
Malleolus
Cone of light
Bulge, retraction, scars, perforation, or masses
Tympanic cavity: fluid, air bubbles, or masses
Insufflation: mobility of TM

The authors would like to express deep appreciation to Welch Allyn in granting permission to extensively reprint sections and photographs from *A Guide to the Use of Diagnostic Instruments in Eye and Ear Examinations* in this chapter's section on ophthalmoscopy and otoscopy.

A Guide to the Use of Diagnostic Instruments in Eye and Ear Examinations
4341 State Street Road, P.O. Box 220, Skaneateles Falls, NY 13153-0220 USA
(p) 800.535.6663 (f) 315.685.3361
www.welchallyn.com
©2006 Welch Allyn, Inc. Printed in USA SM2815 Rev C

References

1. Bushby KM, Cole T, Matthews JN, Goodship JA. Centiles for adult head circumference. *Arch Dis Child.* 1992;67:1286–1287.

CHAPTER 9

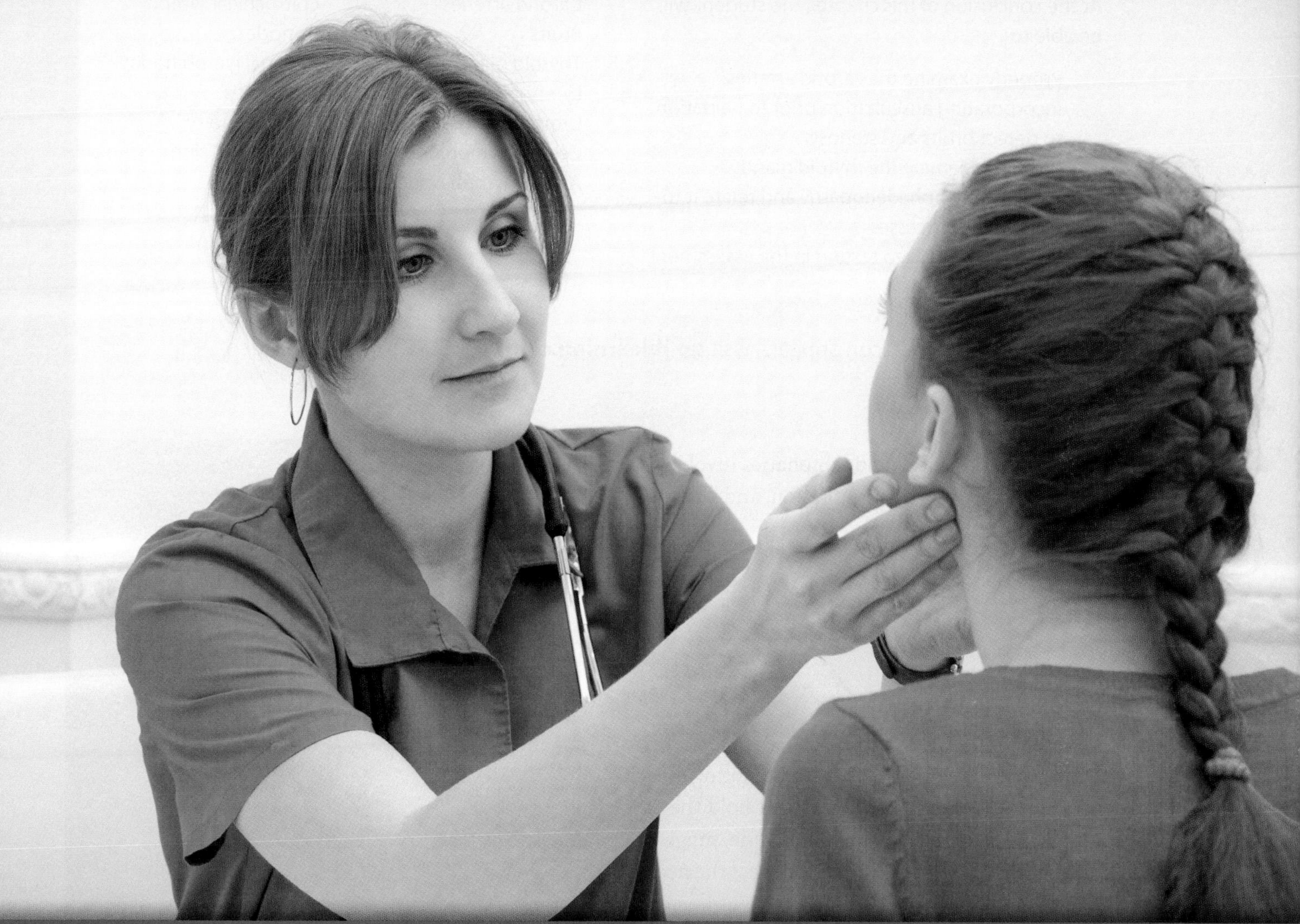

© Capifrutta/ShutterStock, Inc.

Neck and Lymphatic

OBJECTIVES

At the conclusion of this chapter, the student will be able to

1. Properly examine the carotid arteries, incorporating auscultation prior to palpation to detect bruits and stenosis
2. Properly examine the thyroid gland
3. Assess for lymphadenopathy and relate it to pathologic processes
4. Perform specialized testing in the assessment of meningitis

KEY TERMS

Carotid arteries
Bruits
Thyroid gland
Lymphadenopathy
Lymphatics
Cervical lymph nodes
Axillary lymph nodes
Epitrochlear lymph nodes
Inguinal lymph nodes
Meningitis
Nuchal rigidity
Brudzinski's sign
Kernig's sign

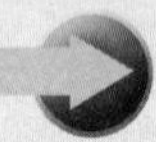

Where this icon appears, visit **go.jblearning.com/HPECWS** to view the video.

Examination of the neck and lymphatics involves the techniques of inspection, auscultation, and palpation.

Neck

INSPECTION

General

Begin inspection with proper exposure of the neck. Inspect the general symmetry of the neck, noting muscle mass (see **FIGURE 9-1**). Does the patient hold the chin in midline or is there deviation to one side, suggestive of torticollis (see **FIGURE 9-2**)? Now inspect the neck in segments: right anterior, left anterior, right posterior, left posterior. Observe for lesions, masses, and the position of the trachea (see **FIGURE 9-3**). Masses may represent lymphadenopathy, thyromegaly, or tumors.

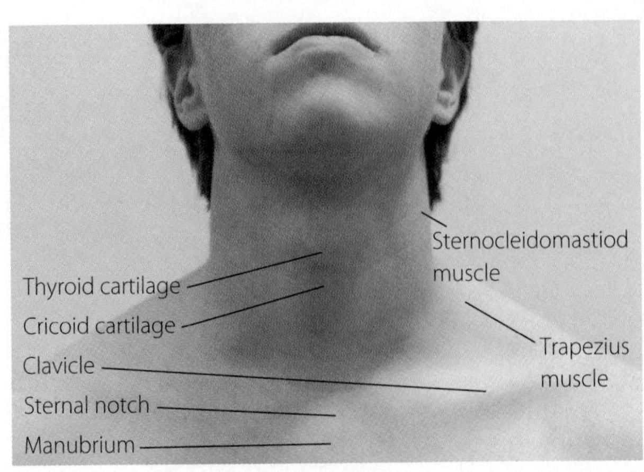

FIGURE 9-1 Anterior neck anatomy.

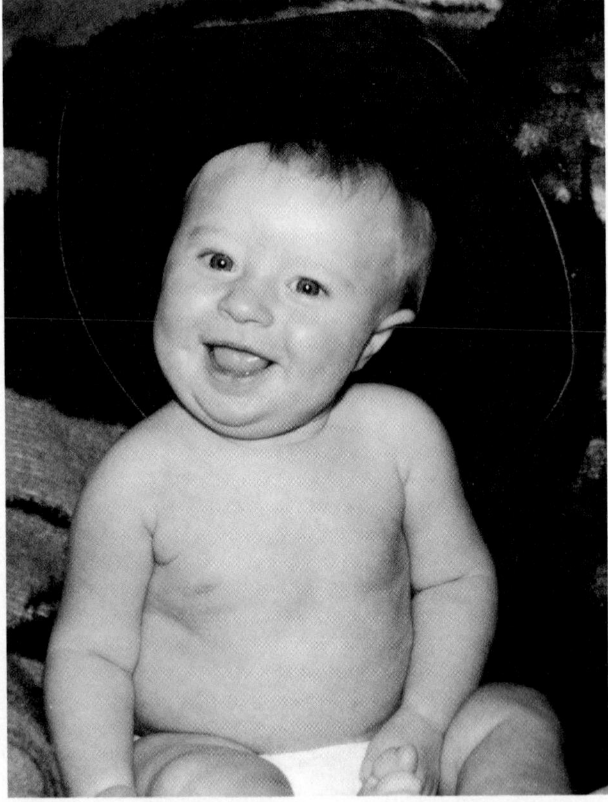

FIGURE 9-2 Left torticollis, a contracture of the sternocleidomastoid muscle from intrauterine positioning, resulting in extension of the neck and rotation away from the involved side.

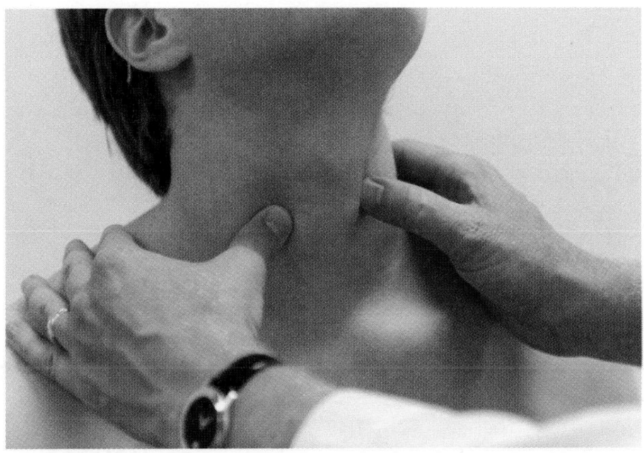

FIGURE 9-3 Palpation of tracheal position.

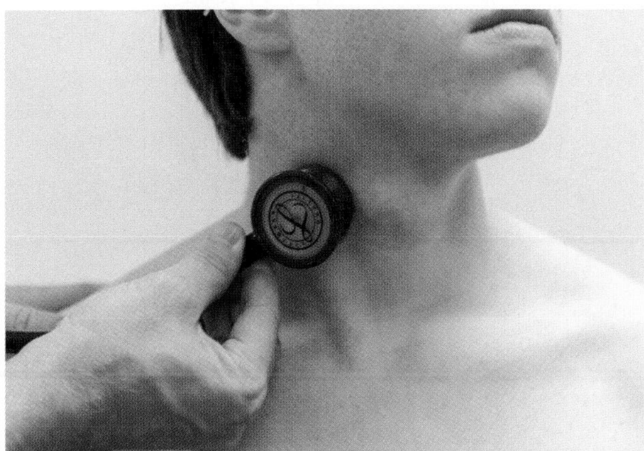

FIGURE 9-4 Carotid auscultation using light pressure and the small head with bell of the stethoscope to detect low-pitched bruits.

Range of Motion

9-1 Standing in front of the patient, assess active range of motion of the neck. Ask the patient to touch his/her chin to the chest (flexion), tilt the head back (extension), rotate the chin to the shoulder (rotation), and bend the ear toward the shoulder (sidebending). Assure that the patient performs sidebending only with the neck, as it is common for the patient to lift the shoulder to meet the ear. If necessary, place your hands on the shoulders, lightly instructing the patient to hold the shoulders still during the maneuver. Demonstrating this when asking the patient to perform the motion aids in understanding.

AUSCULTATION

Always perform auscultation of the neck before palpatory techniques. Auscultate the **carotid arteries** using the bell to detect the low pitch of bruits (see **FIGURE 9-4**). **Bruits** are systolic and represent turbulence of blood flow either due to atherosclerotic narrowing or tortuosity. The carotids lie beneath the sternocleidomastoid (SCM) muscle. Using light pressure, use the chestpiece to slightly displace the SCM posteriorly, allowing improved access to the carotid. Adult-size chestpieces may be difficult to lay flat against the neck over the carotids due to the musculature. This may be avoided by using the smaller pediatric-size chestpiece. After placing the stethoscope, ask the patient to take a breath in, then let it out and hold it. This helps to avoid the sound of air passing through the trachea, which may mask faint bruits. Listen through five or six heartbeats. Allow the patient to breathe regularly for a few breaths, then repeat on the opposite side.

Auscultate the **thyroid gland** for bruits (see **FIGURES 9-5A** and **9-5B**). Thyroid bruits are associated with increased blood flow, found in hyperthyroidism with hyperplasia of the organ. Follow the same technique for breath holding. Listen laterally over the lobes as well as over the isthmus. This assures that the bruit is thyroidal and is not being detected from an underlying carotid.

PALPATION

Provider in Front of Patient

With auscultation complete, the provider may move to palpation. Begin with palpation of the posterior neck anatomy, with the provider standing in front of the seated patient (see **FIGURE 9-6**). Palpate the cervical spinous processes, paravertebral musculature, and transverse processes. At the same time, the provider may assess for occipital and posterior cervical chain **lymphadenopathy**.

Carotid arteries: paired arteries of the neck that supply the greatest amount of blood to the head and neck. Lying beneath the sternocleidomastoid muscles, they are easily auscultated for bruits as an assessment for atherosclerotic disease.

Bruits: low-pitched, systolic turbulence of blood flow either due to atherosclerotic narrowing or tortuosity heard during auscultation

Thyroid gland: a two-lobed endocrine gland located anteriorly along the trachea at the base of the neck, connected by an isthmus crossing over the trachea just below the cricoid cartilage and secreting hormones important in the regulation of metabolism, growth, and development

Lymphadenopathy: pathologic enlargement of the lymphatic system easily palpated when superficial such as when the carotid, axillary, epitrochlear, or femoral areas are involved

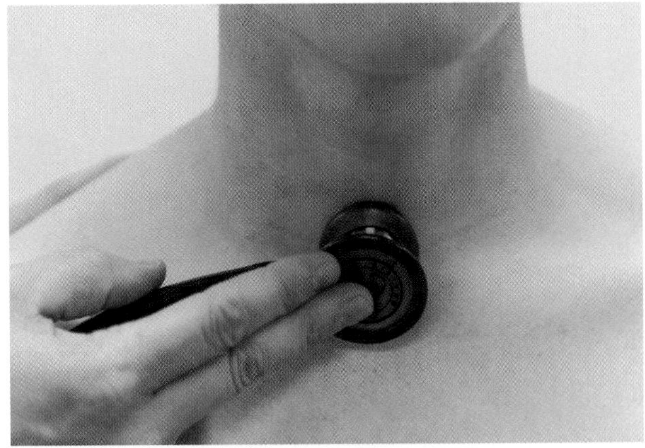

FIGURE 9-5A Auscultation of the isthmus of the thyroid, midline and just below the cricoid cartilage.

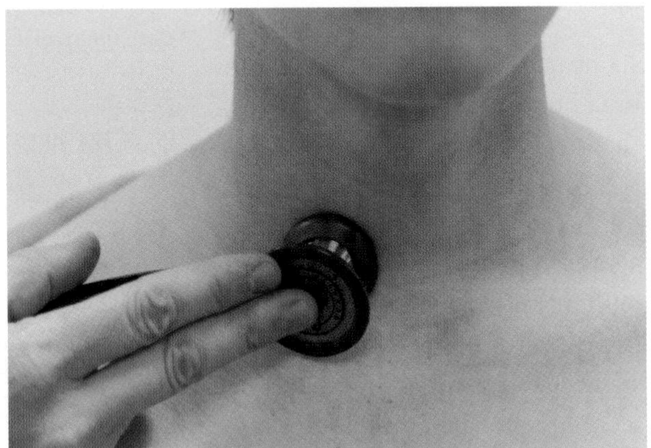

FIGURE 9-5B Auscultation of a lateral lobe of the thyroid.

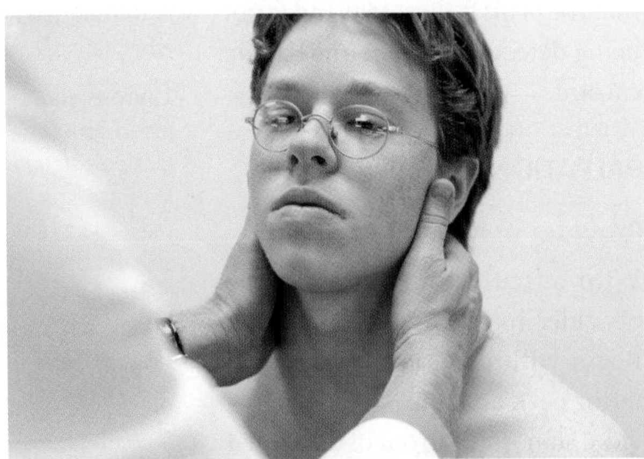

FIGURE 9-6 Palpation of the posterior neck structures with the provider standing in front of the patient.

The tips of the thumbs may be used to gently outline the position of the trachea. Tracheal deviation in nonurgent presentations may reflect mass effect from space-occupying lesions pushing the trachea from midline position. In emergent situations with respiratory distress, the tracheal position should be assessed as the trachea may deviate to the same side with collapse of the lung (pneumothorax) and toward the opposite side when trapped air continues to accumulate without release (tension pneumothorax).

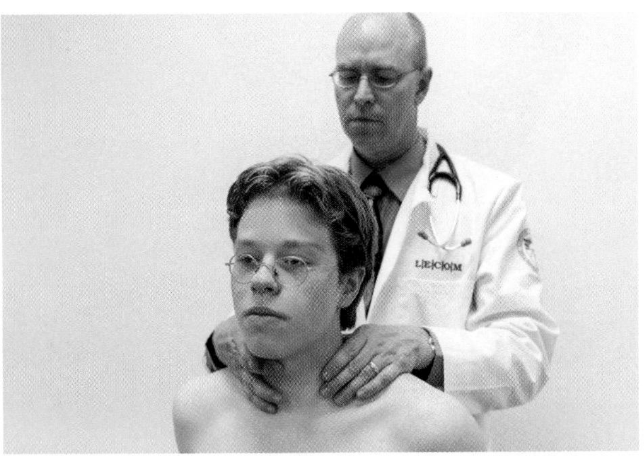

FIGURE 9-7 Palpation of the anterior neck structures with the provider standing behind the patient.

Provider Behind the Patient

If the seated patient is positioned so that you can stand behind him/her, do so to perform the palpation of the anterior neck structures (see **FIGURE 9-7**). If you cannot stand behind the patient, ask the patient to angle to the side and sit beside the patient facing his/her back (see **FIGURE 9-8**). Advise the patient that you will be putting your hands around his/her neck to feel the structures. Though this will not be threatening to most patients,

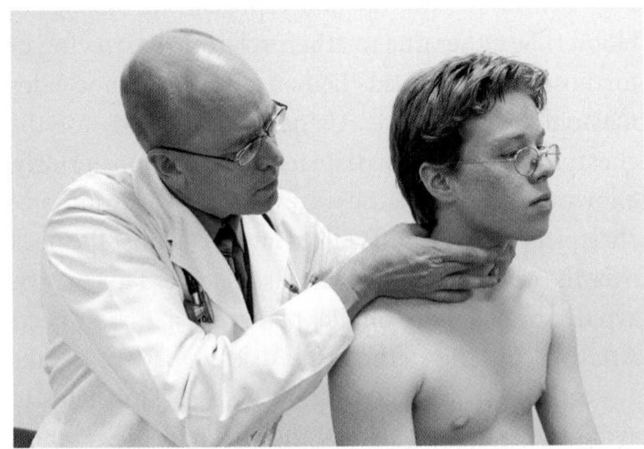

FIGURE 9-8 Palpation of the anterior neck structures with the provider seated beside the patient.

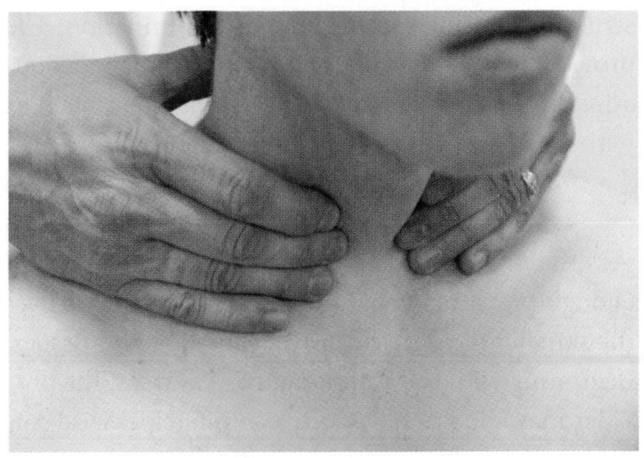

FIGURE 9-9 Palpation of the thyroid gland.

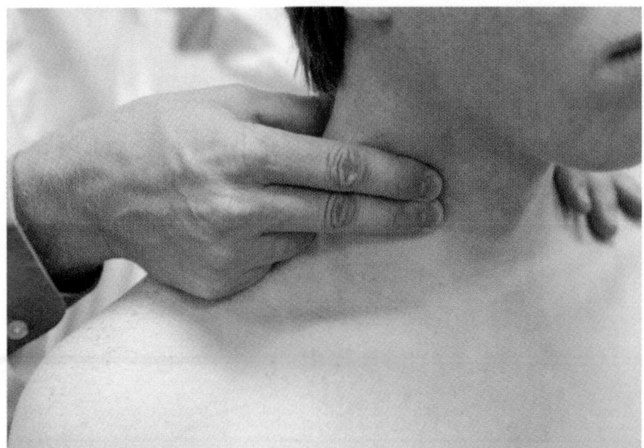

FIGURE 9-10 Unilateral palpation of the carotid by gently retracting the sternocleidomastoid muscle posteriorly.

those with psychiatric disorders or phobias need to be advised of what you plan to do.

Thyroid Gland.

9-2 Palpate the cricoid and thyroid cartilage (see **FIGURE 9-9**). The isthmus of the thyroid gland crosses over the trachea just below the cricoid cartilage. Now slide the pads of your hands laterally from the isthmus to the lobes of the thyroid to test for for enlargement or nodules. To facilitate palpation of the thyroid, ask the patient to swallow. This causes the thyroid to slide up and down beneath your fingers, helping to reveal smaller nodules. If you need to have the patient swallow again, it is best to offer the patient a cup of water with a straw, as most patients will be able to comply with a single swallow but not more without water.

Carotid Arteries.

9-3 Standing to the side of the patient, place two of your fingers flatly on the side of the neck closest to you so that the SCM muscle lies under the distal interphalangeal joints and the fingertips face anteriorly (see **FIGURE 9-10**). Apply light traction to slide the SCM muscle posteriorly, resulting in the pads of the fingers coming into place directly over the carotid artery. Slowly depress the pads to palpate the carotid beneath. The absence of a bruit on auscultation does not guarantee that stenosis of the carotid artery does not exist. If the stenosis is significant enough, the narrowing can be so great that no murmur is heard. For this reason, only gentle pressure should be used to palpate the carotids.

DOCUMENTATION

- Neck: Inspection with symmetry, chin midline. No lesions or masses. Full AROM. Auscultation without carotid or thyroid bruit. Palpation without tenderness, masses, lymphadenopathy, or thyroidmegaly. Trachea midline. Carotid pulses 3/4 b/l.

Lymphatics

The major areas for evaluation of the **lymphatics** include cervical, axillary, and inguinal regions (see **FIGURES 9-11A** and **9-11B**). Inspection of these areas may reveal enlargement of the lymph nodes; however, lymphadenopathy is more commonly found through palpatory techniques.

Lymph nodes may be palpable but not represent pathologic conditions. Normal lymph nodes are typically less than 1 cm, rubbery, and mobile. When lymphadenopathy occurs, it is most commonly associated with infections and malignancy but may also be associated with autoimmune, endocrine, and drug reactions. Assessment and documentation of lymphadenopathy should include location, size, tenderness, consistency, and mobility.

Localized lymphadenopathy is commonly associated with infection processes within the drainage area. Generalized lymphadenopathy is more common with HIV, tuberculosis, and EBV infections.

Lymphatics: deep and superficial conduits that drain lymph from tissues, emptying it into the venous system

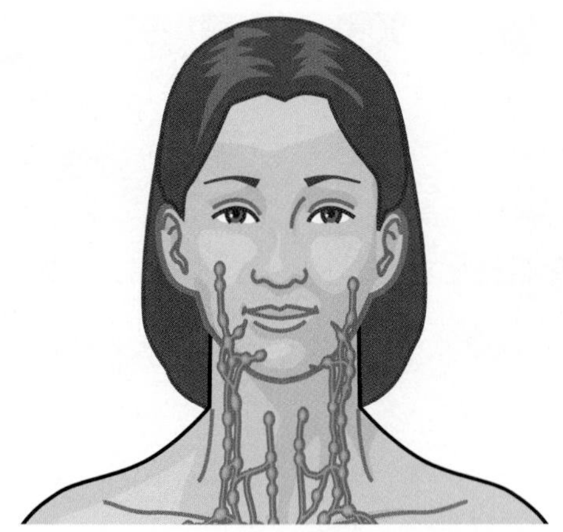

FIGURE 9-11A Lymph nodes of the head and neck.

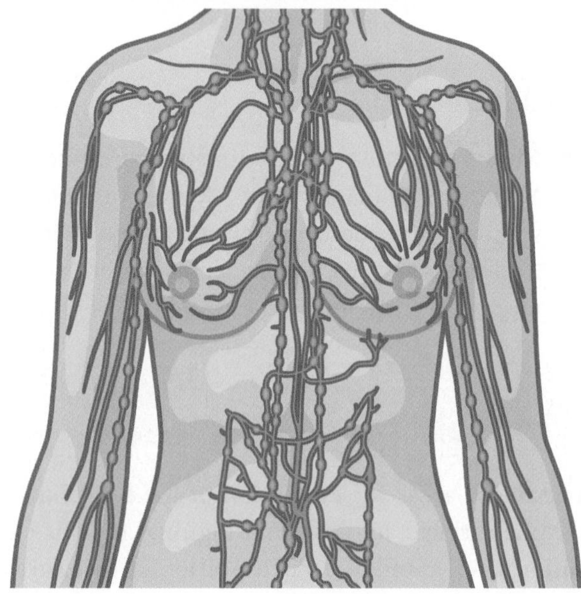

FIGURE 9-11B Thoracic and upper extremity nodes.

Cervical lymph nodes: chain of lymphatics primarily responsible for drainage of the head, neck, and upper thoracic areas

Axillary lymph nodes: lymphatics primarily responsible for drainage of the arms, breasts, and upper areas

Medications such as phenytoin, as well as systemic lupus erythematosus, are also associated with generalized lymph node enlargement.

Enlargement with tenderness is often associated with infectious processes. Enlargement that is nontender, firm, and fixed is more commonly associated with malignancy.

CERVICAL

Palpation of **cervical lymph nodes** should be incorporated simultaneously with palpation of other neck structures during routine physical examination. The provider may also evaluate for cervical lymphadenopathy during problem-specific examinations, such as with a patient with a chief complaint of sore throat.

9-4 Stand in front of the patient and place the fingers flatly against the skin. Keep the fingers flat and massage in a circular motion, applying enough pressure so that the fingers do not slide over the skin but the skin slides over subcutaneous tissues. Beginning with the anterior auricular areas, the provider may choose to work in a counterclockwise pattern to cover all areas of lymphatic drainage. Palpate the following areas:

- Anterior auricular (preauricular)—eye and ear infections
- Parotid—parotid gland malignancy or infection
- Posterior auricular—scalp and ear pathology
- Occipital—scalp infection, particularly tinea capitis
- Posterior cervical chain—head and neck malignancy and infection
- Anterior cervical chain—head and neck infection more common than malignancy
- Submandibular—cheek, salivary gland, lip, tongue, gingiva infections and malignancy
- Submental—floor of mouth, lip, tongue malignancy and infections
- Supraclavicular—suspect malignancy
  - Right side/thorax (mediastinum, lungs, esophagus)
  - Left side/abdomen (stomach, pancreas, kidney, gonads)
- Infraclavicular—breast malignancy and infection

AXILLARY

Axillary lymphadenopathy is most commonly associated with malignancy of the breast, with the majority of the lymphatic drainage from the breast going to the **axillary lymph nodes**. Axillary lymphadenopathy may also be associated with pathology of the arm and thorax.

The provider should wear gloves when palpating axillary lymph nodes. Position patients in a seated position with their arms at their sides. Break the axilla into sections for detailed palpation: anterior fold, chest

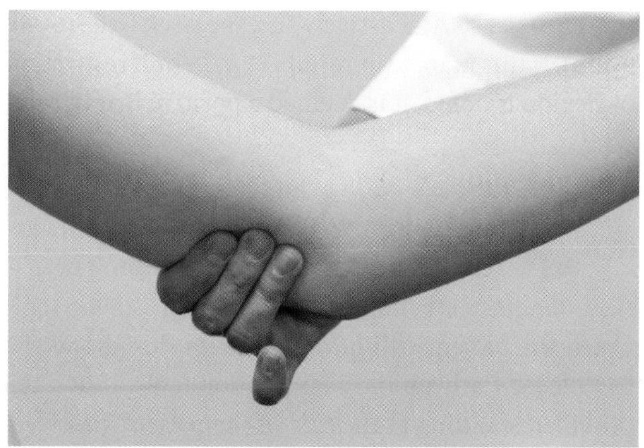

FIGURE 9-12 Palpation of the epitrochlear lymph nodes.

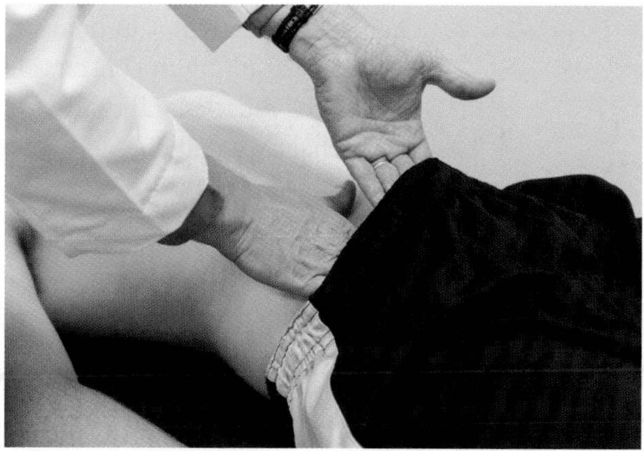

FIGURE 9-13 Palpation of the inguinal lymph node while preserving patient dignity.

wall, posterior fold, and medial arm surface. Use slow rolling motion with the pads of all four fingers.

EPITROCHLEAR

Epitrochlear lymph nodes are normally not palpable but should be sought with any infection of the hand and arm. If axillary lymphadenopathy is found, it is helpful to evaluate for epitrochlear lymph node involvement, which increases the likelihood of localized or systemic infection over that of breast malignancy. Palpate for epitrochlear lymph nodes above the medial epicondyle (see **FIGURE 9-12**).

INGUINAL

Inguinal lymphadenopathy may be present with lower-extremity, genitalia, and abdomen pathology, including malignancy and sexually transmitted infections.

9-5 Assist the patient to the supine position for examination of the **inguinal lymph nodes**. Cover the pelvis with a sheet. During routine examination, the provider may choose not to completely expose the inguinal region for inspection in an attempt to preserve the dignity of the patient. In this case, the provider advises the patient that he/she is about to check for inguinal lymph nodes. Standing at hip level beside the supine patient, the provider can keep the sheet in place, lift the waistband of clothing or undergarments, and slide the hand into position in the inguinal region, palpating for lymphadenopathy and assessing the femoral pulse at the same time without exposure of the genitalia (see **FIGURE 9-13**).

However, with problem-specific complaints such as vaginal or penile discharge, it is more appropriate to expose the inguinal regions for detailed inspection as well as palpation.

Special Testing

SUSPECTED MENINGITIS

- Symptoms associated: neck pain, stiff neck, headache, fever, photophobia, mental status change, nausea and vomiting
- Physical findings: appears acutely ill, often in distress, confused or obtunded, febrile, tachycardia, tachypnea, occasional rash

To assess the likelihood of meningitis, special testing should be performed.

Nuchal Rigidity

With the patient in the supine position, palpate the nuchal cord from occiput to C7 for **nuchal rigidity**. The nuchal cord is firm and bandlike but softens with extension of the neck and is not typically tender. Meningeal irritation can cause

Epitrochlear lymph nodes: lymphatics primarily responsible for drainage of the arms and hands

Inguinal lymph nodes: lymphatics primarily responsible for drainage of the lower-extremity, genitalia, and abdomen

Meningitis: potentially life-threatening inflammation of the membranous covering of the brain and spinal cord, the meninges

Nuchal rigidity: firm, bandlike presentation of nuchal cord found on palpation resulting from contraction of the neck muscles by the patient in an attempt to hold the head still due to meningeal irritation and possible meningitis

Brudzinski's sign: an assessment for meningitis wherein passive flexion of the neck of a patient in the supine position results in flexion of the hip

Kernig's sign: an assessment for meningitis wherein a patient in the supine position with hips and knees flexed experiences pain when the lower extremity is passively extended

the patient to attempt to hold the head still, resulting in contraction of the neck muscles and rigidity of the nuchal cord that does not relax with extension of the neck.

Brudzinski's Sign

To assess for **Brudzinski's sign**, the patient is placed in the supine position with the provider standing at the end of the table at the patient's head. Advise the patient that you will be moving his/her head, asking the patient to relax and avoid assisting in the movement. Cradle the head in your palms with the fingertips placed so that they lightly support the neck (see **FIGURE 9-14A**). Passively flex the neck (see **FIGURE 9-14B**). If this maneuver results in pain or if restriction of flexion is noted, it is deemed a positive Brudzinski.

Kernig's Sign

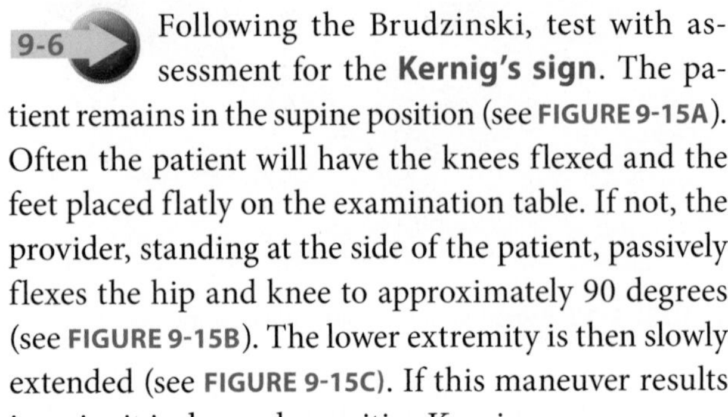

9-6 Following the Brudzinski, test with assessment for the **Kernig's sign**. The patient remains in the supine position (see **FIGURE 9-15A**). Often the patient will have the knees flexed and the feet placed flatly on the examination table. If not, the provider, standing at the side of the patient, passively flexes the hip and knee to approximately 90 degrees (see **FIGURE 9-15B**). The lower extremity is then slowly extended (see **FIGURE 9-15C**). If this maneuver results in pain, it is deemed a positive Kernig.

TABLE 9-1 reviews the neck and lymphatic examination flow.

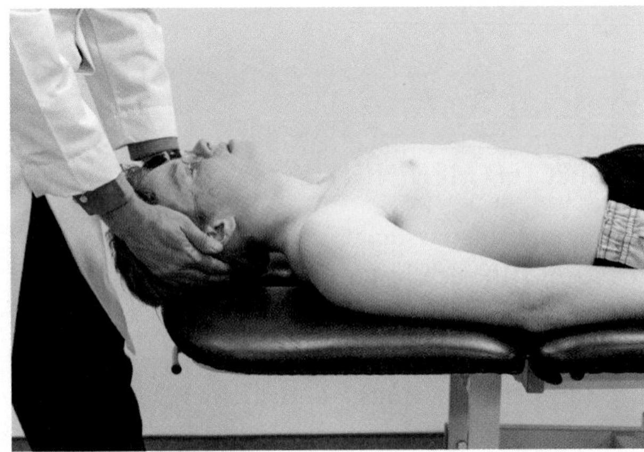

FIGURE 9-14A Cradling the patient's head in preparation of testing for a Brudzinski's sign.

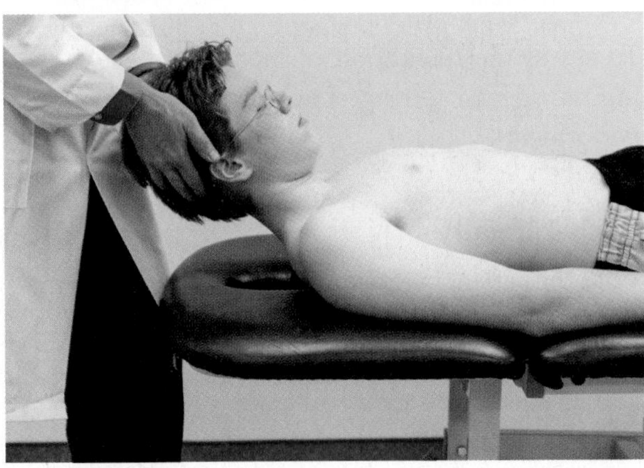

FIGURE 9-14B The provider passively flexes the neck of the patient. If flexion of the hip occurs, a positive Brudzinski's sign is documented.

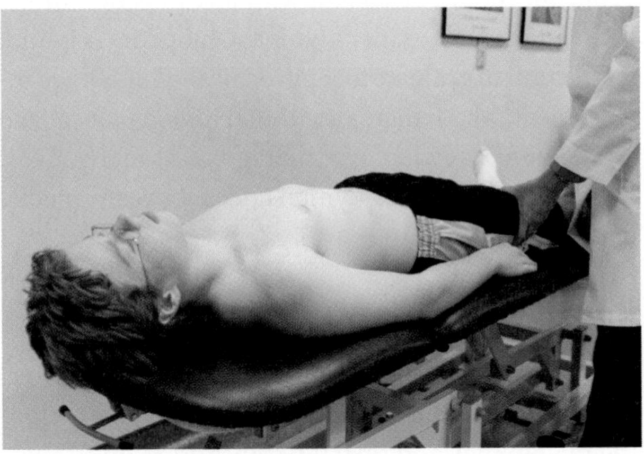

FIGURE 9-15A In testing for a Kernig's sign, the patient is in the supine position.

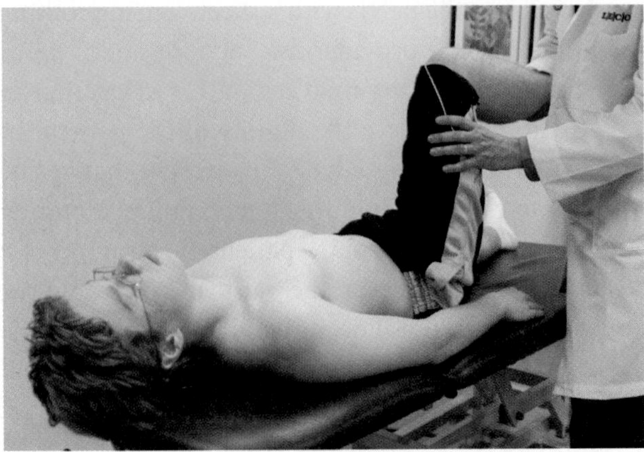

FIGURE 9-15B The hip and knee are passively flexed.

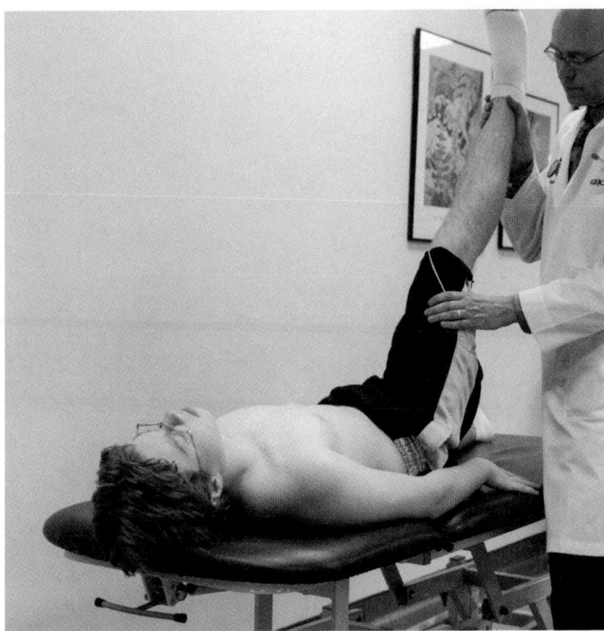

FIGURE 9-15C If pain is experienced as the provider extends the lower extremity, a positive Kernig's sign is documented.

TABLE 9-1 Neck and Lymphatic Flow

Introduces self and explains that physical exam will now be performed
Washes hands for 15 seconds, turning off water with towel
NECK
Inspection
Symmetry
Lesions
Masses
Lymphadenopathy
Tracheal position
Range of motion: flexion, extension, sidebending, and rotation
Auscultation prior to palpation
With stethoscope earpieces facing anteriorly
Carotids—for bruit
Thyroid—bruit
Palpation
Provider in front of seated or at head of supine patient
Cervical spinous processes
Paravertebral musculature/transverse processes
Position of trachea
Provider behind patient
Cricoid and thyroid cartilage
Thyroid—have patient swallow
Carotids
LYMPHATICS
Cervical
Anterior auricular
Posterior auricular
Submandibular
Submental
Posterior cervical chain
Anterior cervical chain
Supraclavicular
Infraclavicular
Axillary: wear gloves
Position patient in seated position with arms at sides
Palpation: chest wall, medial arm, anterior and posterior folds
Epitrochlear
Inguinal
Assists patient to supine position
Covers lower extremities with sheet
SPECIAL TESTING
Suspected meningitis
Nuchal rigidity
Brudzinski—patient supine, provider passively flexes neck
Kernig—patient supine, knees bent, provider extends lower leg
Assists patient back to seated position

CHAPTER 10

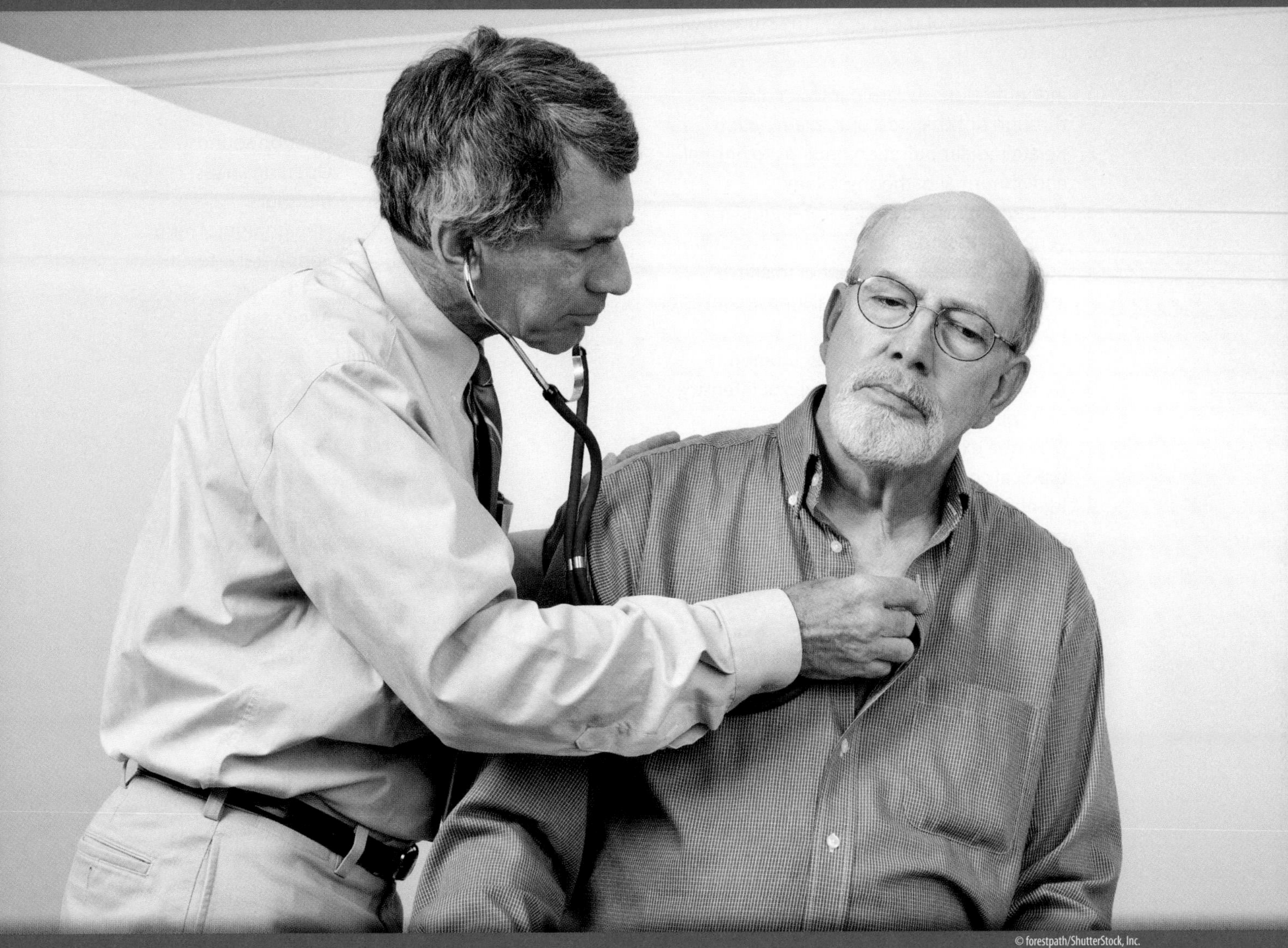

© forestpath/ShutterStock, Inc.

Cardiovascular

OBJECTIVES

At the conclusion of the chapter, the student will be able to

1. Indentify signs of cardiovascular disease through ophthalmoscopic examination
2. Relate jugular pulsation findings to normal and abnormal pathophysiology
3. Properly measure and interpret jugular venous pressures
4. Locate and utilize the point of maximal impulse and pulsations to diagnose causes of displacement
5. Localize valvular areas of auscultation
6. Explain components, variations of intensity, and splitting of S1 and S2
7. Describe extra heart sounds in relation to medical conditions
8. Identify murmurs through their key components
9. Grade murmurs according to intensity
10. Assess for abdominal aortic aneurysm and hepatojugular reflux
11. Grade peripheral edema
12. Assess the extremities for varicosities and peripheral arterial disease
13. Assess and grade peripheral pulses
14. Perform the Allen's test

KEY TERMS

Silver and copper wiring
AV nicking
Jugular pulsations
"a" wave
"v" wave
Jugular venous pressure
Point of maximal impulse
S1
S2
Splitting of S1
Splitting of S2
S3
S4
Ejection sounds
Opening snaps
Murmurs
Hepatojugular reflux
Peripheral arterial disease
Allen's test

Where this icon appears, visit **go.jblearning.com/HPECWS** to view the video.

The cardiovascular system consists of the heart and the arterial and venous systems. When beginning a cardiovascular exam, the provider is tempted to go directly to the heart. It is important to recognize that cardiovascular disease can be detected throughout the body, from the eyes to the feet. Thus, utilizing the head-to-toe sequence, one would encounter the eyes as the first stop for evidence of cardiovascular disease, such as that encountered with hypertension, hyperlipidemia, or diabetes. Begin the cardiovascular exam with the patient in the seated position.

Eyes

Ophthalmoscopic examination of the eyes allows for the only direct visualization of the arteriovenous (AV) system. Any patient diagnosed with hypertension should undergo ophthalmoscopic examination both at onset and on a yearly basis for evidence of pathology related to elevated blood pressure, most commonly hypertensive retinopathy, choroidopathy, and optic neuropathy.[1] Having hypertension also increases the risk of retinal vein and artery occlusion, retinal arteriolar emboli, diabetic retinopathy, glaucoma, and macular degeneration.[1]

A dilated ophthalmoscopic exam is preferred, though it is often not practical in the primary care office. The inability to perform a dilated exam should not negate the examination. Columns of blood in the arterioles are normally seen with a central line of light reflection, the light reflex, of about one-third the total width (see **FIGURE 10-1A**). Inspect for arteriolar narrowing and thickening of the walls, known as **silver or copper wiring**, where the lateral walls of the column narrow and the central light reflex of the arteriole enlarges, appearing as bright wires (see **FIGURE 10-1B**). Arterioles hardened with atherosclerotic plaque cause the appearance of **AV nicking** due to compression of underlying venules by the arteriole, resulting in the venule appearing to be pinched off (see **FIGURE 10-2**). Examine for flame hemorrhages and areas of ischemia, known as cotton-wool spots due to their light appearance. The provider should evaluate the retina for evidence of hypertensive retinopathy (see **FIGURE 10-3**). Then examine the optic nerve for papilledema (see **FIGURE 10-4**).

Silver and copper wiring: narrowing and thickening of the retinal arteriolar walls resulting in the central portion appearing as thin, bright wires on ophthalmoscopic examination

AV nicking: the appearance of retinal venules being pinched off due to compression by overlying arterioles that are hardened with atherosclerotic plaque

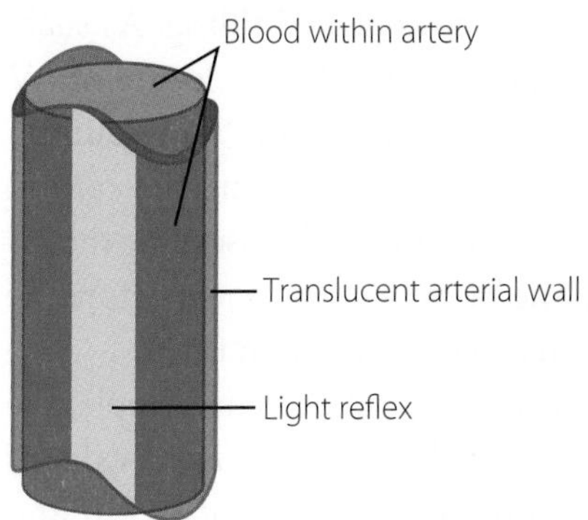

FIGURE 10-1A A normal light reflex is approximately one-third of the width of the blood column of the arteriole.

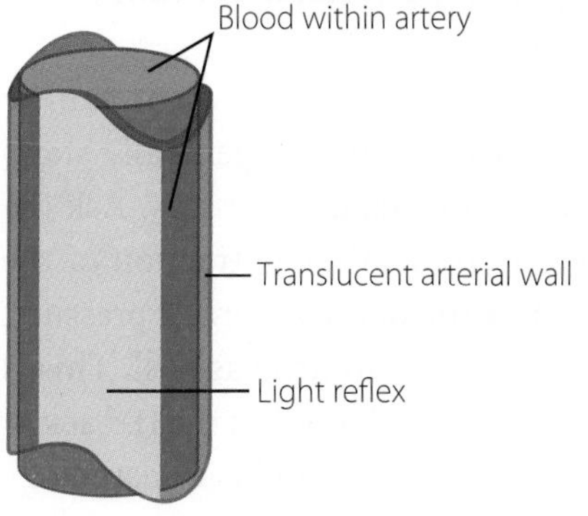

FIGURE 10-1B Copper wiring is seen as an increased width of the central light reflex.

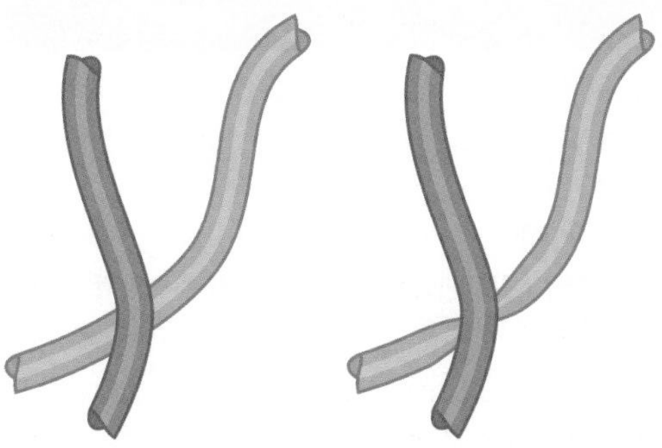

FIGURE 10-2 AV nicking.

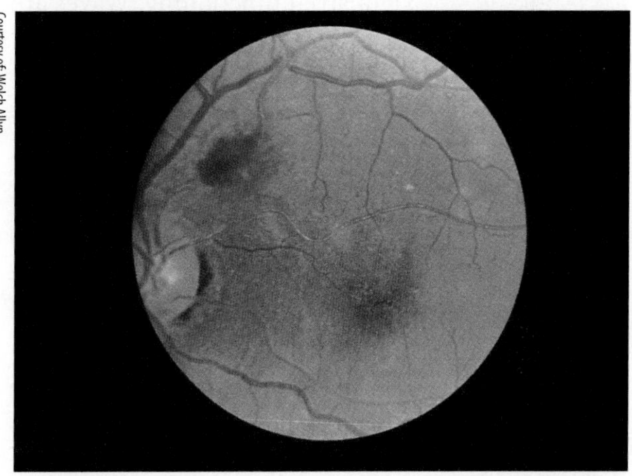

Courtesy of: Welch Allyn.

FIGURE 10-3 Hypertensive retinopathy with exudates and flame hemorrhages.

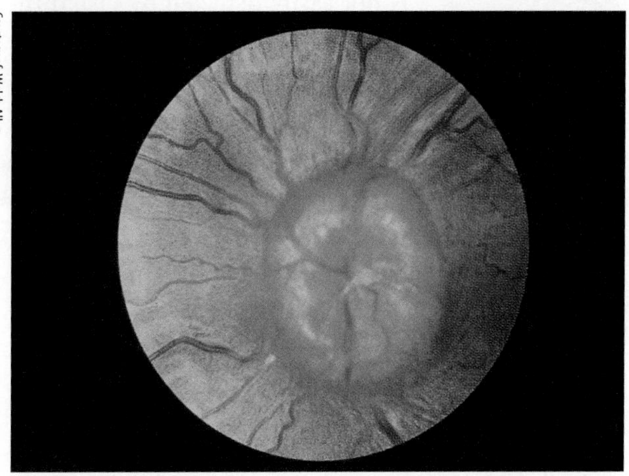

Courtesy of: Welch Allyn.

FIGURE 10-4 Papilledema with an elevated, edematous disc with blurred margins.

DOCUMENTATION

- Ophthalmoscopic exam—No AV nicking, copper or silver wiring, flame hemorrhages, or cotton-wool spots.

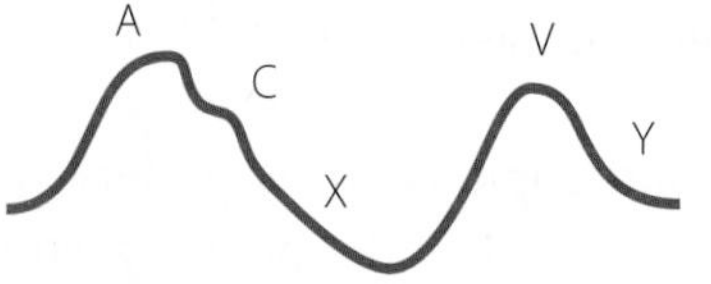

FIGURE 10-5 Jugular pulsation wave.

Neck

As the patient is still seated, inspect the right internal jugular (IJ) vein, which provides the highest correlation to pressure in, and functioning of, the right atrium. Observe for jugular pulsations and distension.

JUGULAR PULSATIONS

10-1 **Jugular pulsations** visible to inspection are the result of pressure waves caused by right atrial functioning. Waves are categorized as positive (a and v) and negative (x and y) (see **TABLE 10-1**). Positive waves are seen as cephalad filling of the vein whereas negative waves are seen as caudad descent of the vein. Each cardiac cycle is accompanied by the double ripple of the a and v waves, though the separation of the two becomes increasingly difficult to observe as the heart rate increases. A "c" wave exists as a slight upstroke occurring on the "x" descent and is a result of right ventricular contraction, but it is not easily detected by visual inspection (see **FIGURE 10-5**).

Jugular pulsations: visible wave-like fluctuations of blood in the jugular veins that reflect right atrial functioning

"a" wave: the first cephalad filling of jugular pulsation, reflecting right atrial contraction

"v" wave: the second cephalad filling of the jugular pulse, reflecting increasing pressure as the right atrium and the vena cava fill behind the closed tricuspid valve

Place the stethoscope on the chest over the tricuspid area. Inspect the IJ to identify the double ripple of the "a" and "v" waves while auscultating. The **"a" wave** is seen during right atrial contraction, which fills the right ventricle but also causes a backflow of pressure up into the jugular, seen as cephalad filling. As such, the "a" wave is seen just before S1, the closure of AV valves, and is heard as the "lump" of "lump/dump." Also confirm identification by palpating the carotid artery on the contralateral side while observing the "a" wave, where again, the "a" wave is seen just before the carotid pulse of ventricular contraction is felt.

Now observe for the second cephalad ripple, the **"v" wave**. This occurs while the tricuspid valve is closed, the right atrium and the vena cava fill and the increasing pressure results in backflow or cephalad filling of the IJ. The "v" wave is seen right before S2, closure of the pulmonic valve, and heard as the "dump" of "lump/dump."

If little upstroke is visible, the patient can be placed in a position of recumbency, generally starting at 45 degrees and lowering as necessary. Ask the patient to take in a deep breath. Contraction of the diaphragm results in a drop of intrathoracic pressure, allowing the venous pressure to drop as well. This is observed as an "inspiratory collapse" of the IJ. Lack of this normal finding can be associated with pathology

TABLE 10-1 Jugular Venous Waves

Wave	Observed	Reflects
A	Inspection: Cephalad IJ filling Auscultation: occurs before the first heart sound (S1) Palpation: occurs before the carotid pulse	Right atrial contraction
X	Inspection: Caudad IJ descent	Right atrial relaxation
V	Inspection: Cephalad IJ filling Auscultation: occurs just before S2 Palpation: occurs on the downslope of the carotid pulse	Right atrial and venous filling during right atrial relaxation and right ventricular contraction
Y	Inspection: Caudad IJ descent Auscultation: just after S2 or at the S3 if present	Opening of tricuspid valve with right atrial emptying

that prevents right-sided filling, such as constrictive pericarditis, pulmonary embolism, and right ventricular infarction.[2]

High-Amplitude "a" Waves

Examine the "a" wave for amplitude. If an exaggerated "a" wave is encountered, consider the anatomy and remember that the "a" wave represents a transmitted wave of increased pressure caused by atrial contraction. What anatomic abnormality could occur that would cause an increase in the pressure exerted by the atrium during contraction? The answer is any process that obstructs the flow of blood from the right atrium to the right ventricle through the tricuspid valve, such as tricuspid stenosis, or myxoma. Therefore it is important to note other evidence of tricuspid disease, such as an opening snap or murmur.

Moving through the cardiac anatomy, increased resistance could next be seen with decreased compliance of the right ventricle. If the right ventricular wall fails to stretch during filling, the pressure rises more quickly, increasing the intensity of the backflow and the "a" wave. Decreased compliance could be found with right ventricular hypertrophy or infarct.

The next structure encountered would be the pulmonary valve. If the pulmonary valve is diseased, it may impede blood flow, resulting in delayed emptying of the right ventricle and backflow, increasing right atrial pressure. Assess for disease of the pulmonic valve by auscultating for an associated systolic murmur, which would be heard greatest over the pulmonic area. In addition, emptying across a diseased valve means that the right ventricle takes longer to contract, delaying the closure of the pulmonary valve (P2), resulting in a split S2.

Moving past the pulmonary artery, resistance could next be encountered in the setting of pulmonary hypertension or with a large pulmonary embolism.

Absent "a" Waves

The finding of absent "a" waves should prompt the provider to consider which disease processes cause a lack or inefficiency of atrial contraction. Most commonly this would reflect atrial fibrillation, but it could also reflect dilated right atrial cardiomyopathy, such as that found with excessive alcohol intake.

High-Amplitude "v" Waves

Now examine the "v" waves for amplitude, which is typically slightly less than the amplitude of "a" waves. Remembering that the "v" wave represents right atrial and venous filling during atrial diastole and ventricular contraction, if an exaggerated "v" wave is encountered, consider which processes would result in increased atrial pressures as it fills. This would most commonly be caused by tricuspid regurgitation, the backflow of blood from the right ventricle into the right atrium. Auscultate the tricuspid area for a systolic murmur. As this murmur occurs during ventricular systole, the "v" wave created can be noted to occur between S1, the closure of the AV valves, and S2, the closure of the semilunar valves, and is simultaneous with the palpated carotid pulse.

JUGULAR VENOUS PRESSURE

Just as the "a" and "v" waves reflect right atrial pressure, so does the height of jugular vein filling, referred to as **jugular venous pressure** of jugular venous distension.

Technique of Measurement

Help the patient to the supine position, then elevate the head of the bed to 45 degrees and stand on the right side of the patient. Ask the patient to look slightly to the left to aid in exposure of the right internal and external jugular veins. Assure appropriate lighting, utilizing a tangential source if necessary. Though measurement is more accurate by utilizing the internal jugular, the external jugular can also be used. However, if the external jugular is used for measurement, the provider must compress the external jugular vein at the edge of the mandible to reveal the top of the column as it drains.[2]

Identify the top of jugular venous filling. If the jugular vein is distended but fills entirely to the angle of the mandible, elevate the patient to 60 degrees. If still fully distended, continue to elevate the head of the bed to 75, and finally 90 degrees, stopping when the top of the column can be observed. Severe elevation of venous pressure should be suspected if the patient is at 90 degrees and the jugular vein

Jugular venous pressure: visible distension of the jugular vein as a reflection of right atrial pressure

continues to fill to the edge of the mandible; however, superior vena cava obstruction such as from a mass could cause similar findings.

If the top of the column cannot be seen at 45 degrees, reverse the process and lower the patient to 30 degrees, 15 degrees, and then fully supine, again stopping when the top of the filling is seen.

10-2 Once the top of the column has been identified, the height is measured in centimeters (cm) from the sternal angle. This is accomplished by placing a cm ruler perpendicularly against the patient's chest at the sternal angle and bisecting it with a straightedge laid parallel to the floor at the top of the column of filling in the jugular (see **FIGURE 10-6**). The number of centimeters of elevation is read at the point of bisection. The sternal angle is used, as it represents the level that is considered to be 5 cm above the right atrium. Therefore 5 cm is added to the measurement taken for the total estimated venous pressure for patients lying at 30 degrees recumbency or less[2,3] Because the sternal angle has been determined to be closer to 10 cm above the atrium when patients are elevated at 45 degrees or more, 10 cm should be added to the measurement to more accurately reflect venous pressure. Normal venous pressure ranges from 1 to 10 cm.[2,3]

DOCUMENTATION

- Neck—Inspection with identifiable "a" > "v" wave internal jugular venous pulsation. 2 cm JVD at 30 degrees recumbency.

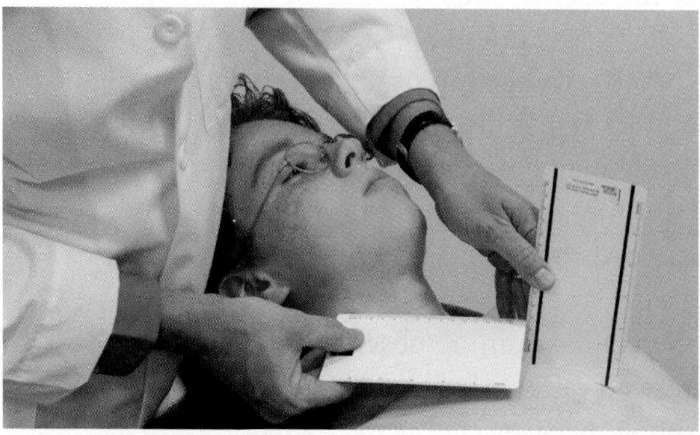

FIGURE 10-6 JVP measurement.

Elevated Jugular Venous Pressure

Barring obstruction of the superior vena cava, elevated jugular venous pressure typically indicates increased pressure in the right atrium. Picture the right atrium anatomically and consider which processes would result in increased pressure; resistance to outflow would be a primary cause. Similar to the exaggerated "a" wave, any obstruction or resistance to right atrial emptying can lead to elevated jugular venous pressure, such as with pulmonary hypertension, pulmonary embolism, pericarditis, pulmonary or tricuspid valvular disease, or noncompliance of the right ventricle from hypertrophy, ischemia, or infarct with diminished contractibility. Left-sided heart failure can cause increased pulmonary vascular pressure ultimately resulting in elevated right atrial and venous pressures. Elevated jugular venous pressure with concurrent edema is often associated with heart or renal failure.

Superior vena cava obstruction should be considered when the column of jugular venous pressure lacks "a" and "v" waves, which cannot exist in this instance as the superior vena cava obstruction prevents the back pressure from the right atrium. This finding should prompt the provider to inspect for associated venous prominence of the upper thorax and arms.

Low Jugular Venous Pressure

If the patient must be lowered to the supine position before the jugular venous column can be identified, the jugular venous pressure is low, which may reflect low-volume status, as can be found with dehydration or anemia.

Chest

Continuing to work caudally, you have now reached the chest. Examination may begin in the seated position, though the supine position allows for a more comprehensive evaluation by providing unobstructed exposure for improved inspection.

INSPECTION

Examination of the chest should be performed with the provider standing on the right-hand side of the patient. This position allows the provider to scan across the precordium tangentially rather than have the more perpendicular view from the left side and provides unobscured inspection of the right jugular veins. Proper exposure is essential. Assure that the patient is in a gown. Men should have their shirts removed. Women may leave bras on to preserve dignity unless removal is essential. Help the patient to the supine position and cover the pelvis with a sheet. Elevating the head of the bed to 45 degrees during the examination allows for concomitant examination of JVP. Then ask the patient permission to drop the gown to expose the chest.

Shape of the Chest

Note the shape of the chest wall in relation to how it might displace the heart. Pectus excavatum may shift the heart to the left, while the depressed diaphragms of COPD may shift the heart to the right.

Point of Maximal Impulse

Inspect the precordial area (see **FIGURE 10-7**), noting any visible **point of maximal impulse** (PMI). The PMI is the location where the apex of the heart, the tip of the left ventricle, taps against the anterior chest wall during systole and is usually located in the 5th intercostal space (ICS) in the midclavicular line (MCL). The PMI is often not visible except in patients who are thin unless the PMI is hyperdynamic.

Displacement inferiorly and to the left is found with hypertrophic cardiomyopathy as seen with chronic hypertension or aortic stenosis, where increased contractility causes thickening of the heart muscle. This can be pictured in the same way as doing repeated biceps curls with weights resulting in enlargement of the biceps. Left displacement may also be seen with mitral regurgitation, pulmonary fibrosis, and right-sided tension pneumothorax.

Displacement to the right and inferiorly is a common finding in COPD, where the flattened diaphragm allows the heart to shift medially. Noting a PMI on the right side of the chest would likely indicate the presence of dextrocardia.

Pulsations

Other pulsations may be visible. Inspect each of the valvular areas as well as the epigastrium, correlating the anatomic position of the heart under the precordium with the likely cause of pulsations. Begin with the aortic area, where a pulsation may suggest aneurysm of the ascending aorta. Observe the suprasternal area, which would relate to an aneurysm of the aortic arch. Pulsation in the pulmonic area may relate to pulmonary artery dilation. Pulsation along the left sternal border may reflect a hyperdynamic right ventricle. Pulsations in the epigastric area can be caused by right ventricular hypertrophy or aortic aneurysm.

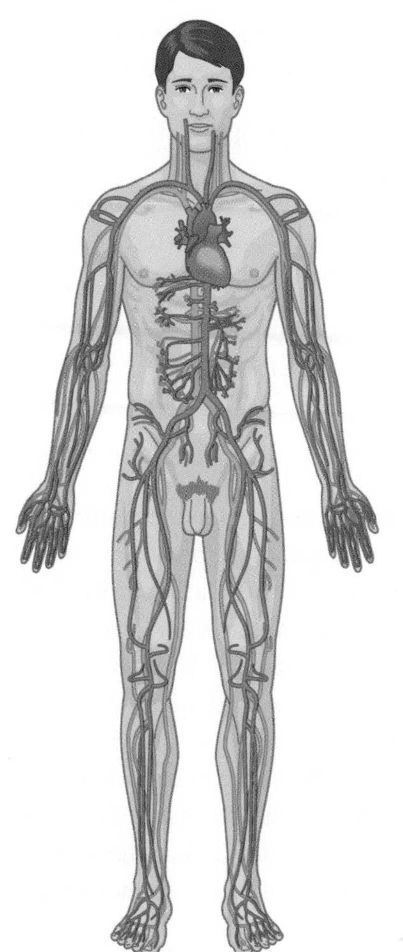

FIGURE 10-7 The cardiovascular system.

Point of maximal impulse: the location where the apex of the heart, the tip of the left ventricle, taps against the anterior chest wall during systole

DOCUMENTATION

- Chest—Inspection. No chest wall deformity. No visible PMI or precordial pulsations.

AUSCULTATION

Place the stethoscope in the ears with the earpieces angled slightly anteriorly in the natural direction of the external auditory canals. Auscultate each of the valvular areas in consistent order (see **FIGURE 10-8**):

- Aortic: 2nd right intercostal space (ICS) along the sternal border
- Pulmonic: 2nd left ICS along sternal border
- Tricuspid: 4th or 5th left ICS along sternal border
- Mitral: 4th or 5th ICS mid-clavicular line

Rate and Rhythm

Assess rate and rhythm.

Valve Closure

The sound of valve closure carries the nomenclature of **S1** and **S2**, corresponding to the commonly used "lump" and "dump" of the heart sounds. Both are high-frequency and best auscultated by using the diaphragm of the stethoscope head. S1 is sound created by the closure of the atrioventricular (AV) valves and marks the onset of ventricular systole, where contraction of the ventricles causes the mitral and tricuspid valves to shut. Simultaneous closure of these two valves results in a single audible heart sound (S1) but is composed of the sounds of mitral closure and tricuspid closure, which can be denoted as M1 and T1, respectively.

S1: closure of the atrioventricular valves marking the onset of ventricular contraction, systole

S2: closure of the semilunar valves marking the onset of ventricular relaxation, diastole

S2 is created by the closure of the semilunar valves, marking the onset of ventricular diastole, and the closure of the aortic and pulmonic valves.

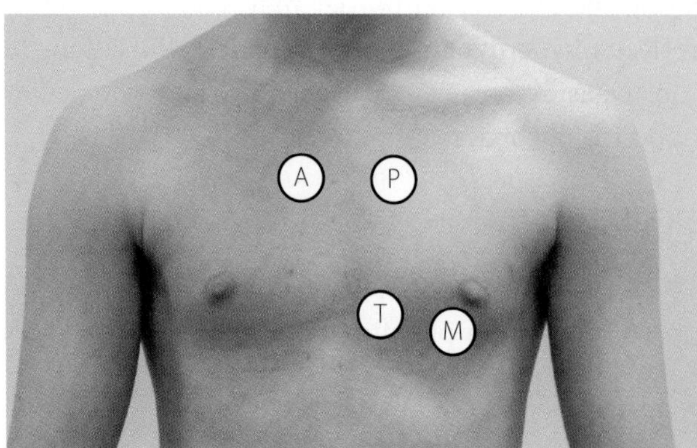

FIGURE 10-8 Aortic, pulmonic, tricuspid, and mitral valve areas of auscultation.

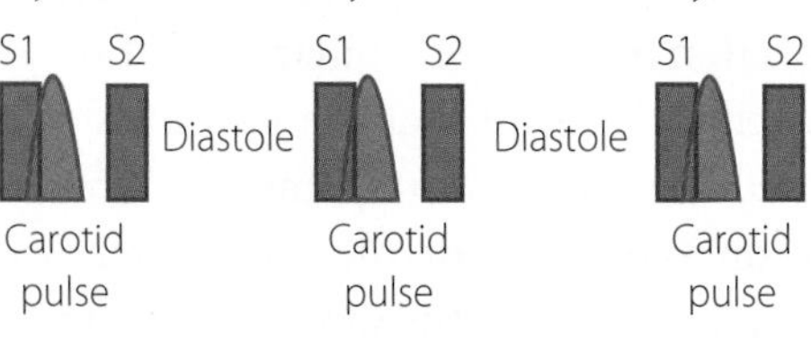

FIGURE 10-9 S1 can be identified by palpating the carotid artery. S1 occurs just before the carotid pulse is felt.

It is easier to distinguish between S1 and S2 with heart rates in the normal range as the length of diastole is twice as long as systole, creating the pattern of:

- Lump (S1), dump (S2), pause, lump (S1), dump (S2), pause, lump (S1), dump (S2), pause

Discerning between S1 and S2 is more difficult with tachycardia, where the pause is less obvious. In these cases, palpate the right carotid artery while auscultating (see **FIGURE 10-9**). The heart sound that occurs directly before or concurrently as the upstroke is palpated correlates to the S1 of ventricular contraction.

S1

Using a logical approach, normally, in which of the four areas of cardiac auscultation is S1 heard loudest? S1 (see **FIGURE 10-10**) represents the closure of the mitral and tricuspid valves, meaning it would be heard loudest over these areas of auscultation. The mitral valve normally closes under more force and is louder than tricuspid closure. Closure of the mitral valve occurs just an instant before tricuspid, but the overlap is so close that the sounds are commonly heard as one.

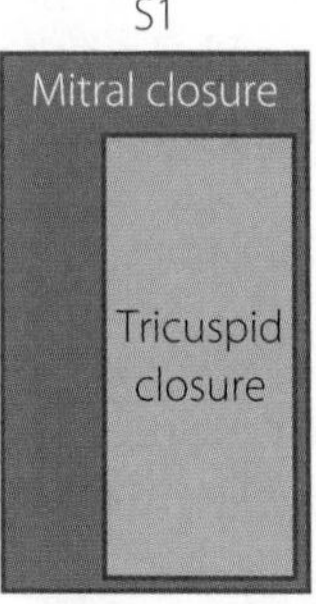

FIGURE 10-10 A normal S1 is comprised of combined sounds of the closure of the louder mitral and softer tricuspid valve.

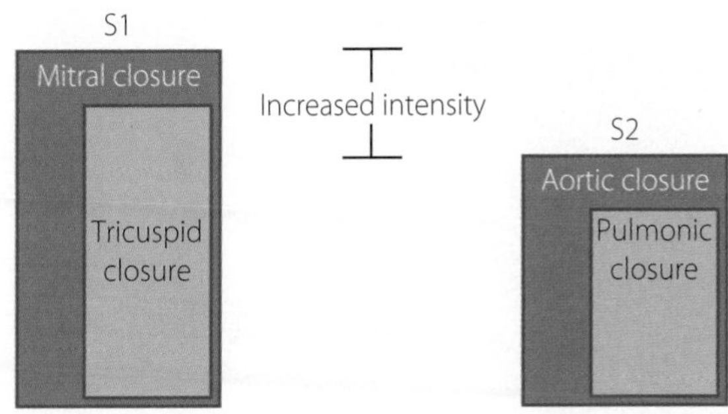

FIGURE 10-11 Increased S1 intensity as compared to S2.

The strength of left ventricular contraction is greater than that of right ventricular contraction, resulting in S1 being heard best over the mitral area as opposed to the tricuspid area.

Increased S1 Intensity.

If S1 is perceived to be louder than normal, confirmation can be gained by listening over the aortic and pulmonic areas, where S2 would be expected to be louder than S1. If S1 is found to be equal to or louder than S2 in these areas, S1 should be deemed to be of increased intensity (see **FIGURE 10-11**). Envision the mitral and tricuspid valves as doors. What processes would cause an increase in S1 intensity, slamming shut of the mitral and/or tricuspid doors?

First, this could be observed if the door was left widely open. Picture being in a hurry and attempting to close a door when it slips from your hand. If it slips just 1 inch from being closed, there wouldn't be much of an increase in intensity of noise. However, if it slips from 2 feet out, the door would slam with a deafening sound. So what process leaves the mitral or tricuspid valves widely open? Valvular obstruction either by stenosis of the valve or atrial myxoma allows the door to be held more ajar by transvalvular flow. This also occurs with a left-to-right shunt, as with ventricular septal defect. The chordae tendineae function to prevent prolapse of the mitral and tricuspid valves. If compromised, the valves slam shut with an increased S1 and possible prolapse of the valve.

For practice purposes in being able to note increases in S1, enlist a health partner and listen to the intensity of S1 compared to S2. Have the partner exercise, such as with 20 to 30 jumping jacks or pushups. Then auscultate again. The intensity of S1 should be increased as exercise increases the force of ventricular contraction and shortens diastole, correlating with a hyperdynamic contraction.

Splitting of S1: separation of closure of the atrioventricular valves so that closure is no longer simultaneous but separates so that closure of the mitral and tricuspid valves can be heard independently

Decreased S1 Intensity.

If the degree of mitral or tricuspid stenosis is significant, the immobility of the valve can result in slowing of the valve closure and a decrease in intensity of S1, even to the point of absence (see **FIGURE 10-12**). Stenosis may also prevent the valves from opening widely, meaning the door is already partially closed and has less distance to travel as it swings shut. Decreased S1 intensity is also found in the presence of reduced ejection fraction.

Variable S1 Intensity.

When the intensity of S1 varies between beats, it typically represents variability in filling pressures, commonly found with premature beats, heart block, or arrhythmia such as atrial fibrillation.

Splitting of S1.

Splitting of S1 occurs when the closure of the mitral and tricuspid valves no longer occur close enough so that only one sound is detected (see **FIGURE 10-13**).

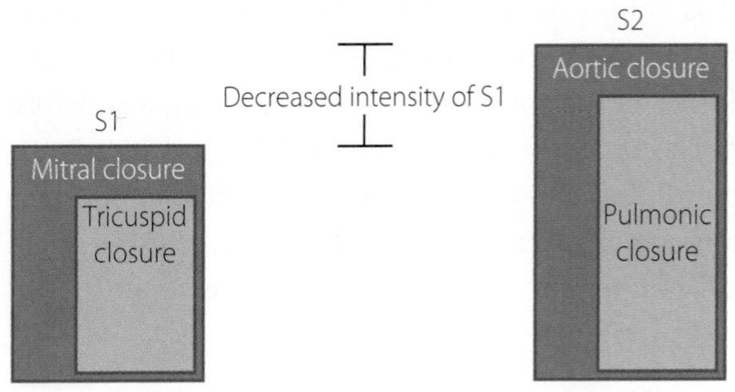

FIGURE 10-12 Decreased S1 intensity as compared to S1.

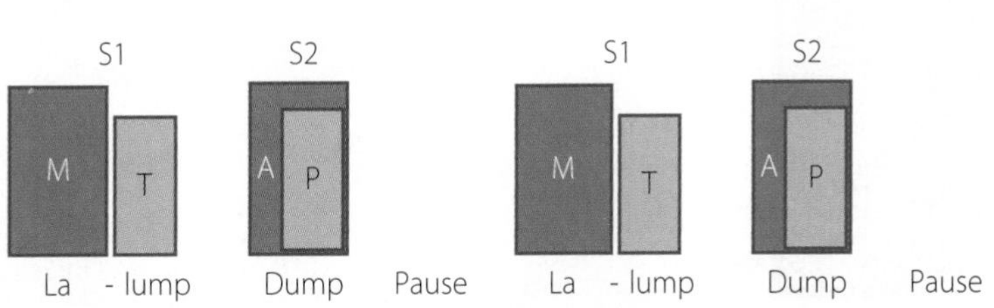

FIGURE 10-13 Splitting of S1 with separate closure of the mitral and tricuspid valves creating two distinct sounds.

- Lump, dump, pause, lump, dump, pause, lump, dump, pause

becomes

- La-lump, dump, pause, la-lump, dump, pause, la-lump, dump, pause

Important to note is that each sound is of high frequency and somewhat sharp character as the valve slaps shut.

When any split occurs, two major causes should be considered: conduction abnormalities and pressure differences between the two sides of the heart. An example of conduction delay is seen in bundle branch blocks. If a right bundle branch block is present, electrical impulse to the left ventricle occurs first, resulting in closure of M1 before T1. The louder M1 will be heard, followed by the softer T1. A left bundle branch block would delay mitral closure, resulting in a split where the softer T1 is heard before the louder M1.

Another common cause of a split S1 is found when there is delay of tricuspid closure due to pressure differences. This may occur with atrial left-to-right shunts, where excessive right atrial filling represents a counterforce to closure of the tricuspid as the ventricular contraction begins. Other causes of delayed closure include tricuspid stenosis or right atrial myxoma.

S2

S2 is sound made by the closure of the semilunar valves. Again, this is typically simultaneous with the closure of the aortic valve (A2), occurring just before the closure of the pulmonic valve (P2), creating a single sound (S2) (see **FIGURE 10-14**). As ventricular contraction comes to an end, the pressure within the aorta and pulmonary artery becomes greater than that of the left and right ventricles. This results in the backflow of blood and forces the semilunar valves to close, thus preventing regurgitation back into the ventricles. By palpation the S2 would be heard on the downslope of the carotid pulse.

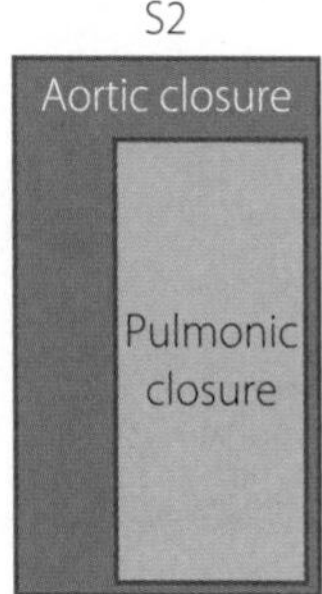

FIGURE 10-14 A normal S2 is comprised of combined sounds of the closure of the louder aortic and softer pulmonic valves.

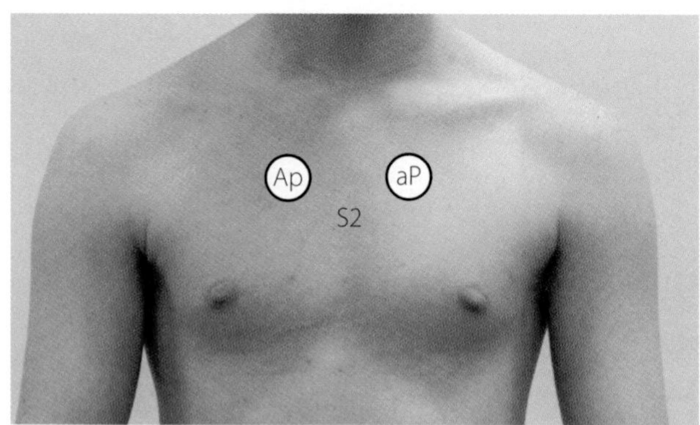

FIGURE 10-15 A2 is heard loudest over the 2nd right ICS. P2 heard best of the 2nd left ICS.

S2 is heard best over the 2nd right and left intercostal spaces along the sternal borders. A2 is loudest over the aortic area, whereas P2 would be better appreciated over the pulmonic area (see **FIGURE 10-15**). Transmission occurs easily to the right carotid due to the anatomic proximity of the aortic valve.

Intensity of S2.

Just as the M1 is characteristically louder than T1, so A2 is louder than P2, with P2 being hard to detect except in the pulmonic areas of auscultation. This is partially due to increased pressure in the aorta as compared to the pulmonary artery. Changes in intensity of S2 can be divided into changes of each component (see **TABLE 10-2**).

TABLE 10-2 Changes in S2 Intensity

Change in S2	Association
Increased A2	Hypertension
	Aortic obstruction (coarctation, aneurysm)
Decreased A2	Aortic regurgitation
	Aortic stenosis
	Hypotension
Increased P2	Pulmonary hypertension
	Atrial septal defect
Decreased P2	Pulmonary valve stenosis

Splitting of S2.

Splitting of the S2 is much more common than splitting of the S1 (see **FIGURE 10-16A**).

- Lump, dump, pause, lump, dump, pause, lump, dump, pause

becomes

- Lump, da-dump, pause, lump, da-dump, pause, lump, da-dump, pause

Induce splitting by having the patient take slow, deep inspirations while auscultating over the pulmonic area. One mechanism by which this physiologic splitting occurs is that with deep inspiration, pulmonary vascular resistance declines, resulting in less pressure to slam shut the pulmonary valve, delaying closure of P2 and resulting in an appreciable split. In addition, as the diaphragm contracts during inspiration, negative intrathoracic pressure is induced, allowing for increased venous return. This increased venous return increases right ventricular stroke volume. Increased volume requires longer time for ejection, thereby delaying closure of the pulmonic valve.

Widely split S2. If a split S2 is detected, ask the patient to take slow, deep breaths. If the split fails to resolve with expiration, a wide S2 split is diagnosed (see **FIGURE 10-16B**). This finding can be caused by conduction delays such as a right bundle branch block, which results in delayed contraction of the right ventricle and hence the delayed closure of the pulmonary valve. P2 can also be delayed in conditions that result in prolonged right ventricular contraction: chronic pulmonary hypertension, acute increases in pulmonary pressure such as with pulmonary embolism, or any outflow obstruction from the right ventricle, such as pulmonary stenosis.

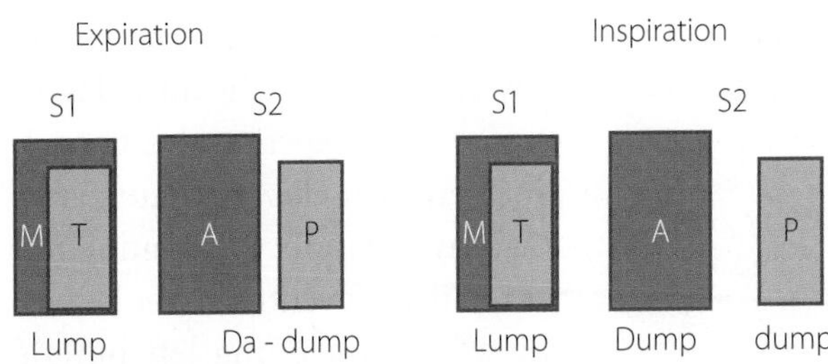

FIGURE 10-16B A widely split S2 is heard in expiration but increases with inspiration.

Other causes of asynchronous contraction of the ventricles should also be considered, such as Wolff-Parkinson-White syndrome, where pre-excitation of the left ventricle causes early contraction of the left ventricle as compared to the right, resulting in an early A2. An early A2 can also be seen with mitral regurgitation and ventricular septal defect, as left ventricular ejection is hastened by alternative outflow tracts, resulting in an early end to left ventricular contraction.

Splitting of the S2: separation of closure of the semilunar valves so that closure is no longer simultaneous but separates so that closure of the aortic and pulmonic valves can be heard independently

With the above examples, splitting is wide but still has some narrowing with inspiration. An S2 split that remains fixed, equidistant in inspiration and expiration, is more commonly associated with right ventricular failure or atrial septal defect.

Paradoxical split S2. As the term suggests, a paradoxical split S2 is one in which P2 occurs prior to A2. Unlike the physiologic splitting, wherein inspiration makes the split more pronounced, in paradoxical splitting the split becomes more pronounced during expiration and may completely disappear with inspiration (see **FIGURE 10-16C**).

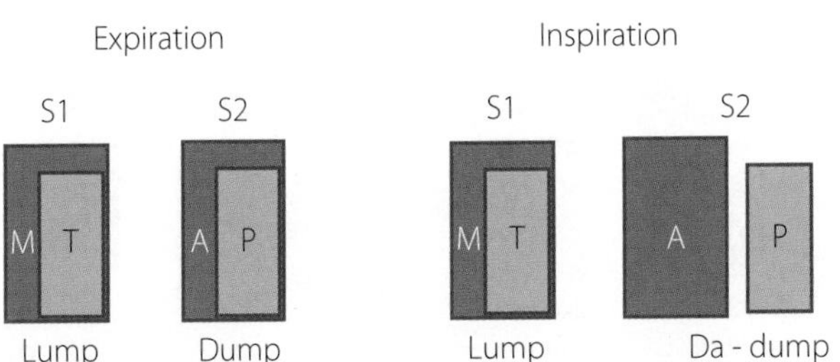

FIGURE 10-16A A physiologic split S2 occurs with deep inspiration.

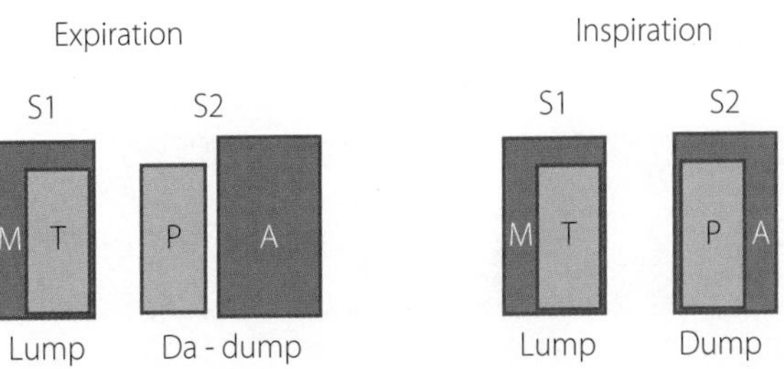

FIGURE 10-16C A paradoxical split S2 is heard in expiration instead of inspiration.

S3: a low-frequency sound occurring early in ventricular diastole as a result of turbulence created by atrial emptying against a noncompliant left ventricular wall

S4: a low-frequency sound occurring late in ventricular diastole as a result of turbulence created by resistance to filling by ventricular noncompliance

Ejection sounds: high-frequency, sharp, clicking sounds occurring during ventricular systole commonly related to stenotic semilunar valves or dilation of the root of the aorta or pulmonary artery

Consider the processes that may result in significant delay in closure of the aortic valve to such an extent that closure occurs after P2. Any delay in the conduction within the left ventricle would have this effect, including left bundle branch block. Conditions prolonging the left ventricular ejection time also delay closure of A2. This can be seen with aortic stenosis or hypertrophic cardiomyopathy as the ventricle fights against the outflow obstruction.

Conversely, early conduction in the right ventricle, such as by an ectopic pacing, would have the same result: earlier contraction followed by earlier closure of the pulmonary valve, P2 before A2.

Extra Sounds

S1 and S2 are normal heart sounds representing closure of the heart valves. In addition to these sounds, extra heart sounds may be heard in association with pathologic processes.

S3.

As opposed to the sharp, high-frequency closure of valves, an **S3** is a low-frequency "shoo" best heard with the bell of the stethoscope. The S3 occurs early in ventricular diastole, immediately following the S2. As the left ventricle relaxes, the semilunar valves close, the mitral valve opens, and left atrial blood rapidly begins to fill the ventricle. If this flow of blood meets a noncompliant left ventricular wall, turbulence, the S3, is created (see **FIGURE 10-17**).

- Lump, da-shoo, pause, lump, da-shoo, pause, lump, da-shoo, pause

The "da-shoo" represents a gallop comprising the sharper, high-frequency component of aortic valve closure combined with the low-frequency swoosh of blood against a noncompliant ventricle. The S3 of left ventricular origin is best detected by auscultation at the mitral area. If an S3 is suspected, place the patient in the left lateral decubitus position, which brings the left ventricle closer to the anterior chest wall, accentuating the S3.

An S3 can be the result of enlargement of the chamber of the ventricles, such as caused by mitral and aortic valve regurgitation, and is associated with heart failure, but it can also be a normal finding in the younger patient. The left-sided S3, heard best over the mitral area, is more common than the right ventricular S3, heard best over the tricuspid area.

S4.

An **S4** is also a low-frequency "shoo," again best heard with the bell. It occurs late in ventricular diastole, directly before S1 during atrial contraction (see **FIGURE 10-18**).

- Shoo-lump, dump, pause, shoo-lump, dump, pause, shoo-lump, dump, pause

The S4 occurs at the end of atrial contraction when the atrial kick provides one final thrust of blood to fill the ventricles. Again, as resistance to filling is met by ventricular noncompliance, turbulence is heard as the S4, which is found more commonly in the left ventricle. This noncompliance is commonly seen as aging occurs, but unlike an S3 it is not common in younger patients and merits evaluation. An S4 may indicate presence of left ventricular hypertrophy, such as is associated with hypertension and aortic valve stenosis.

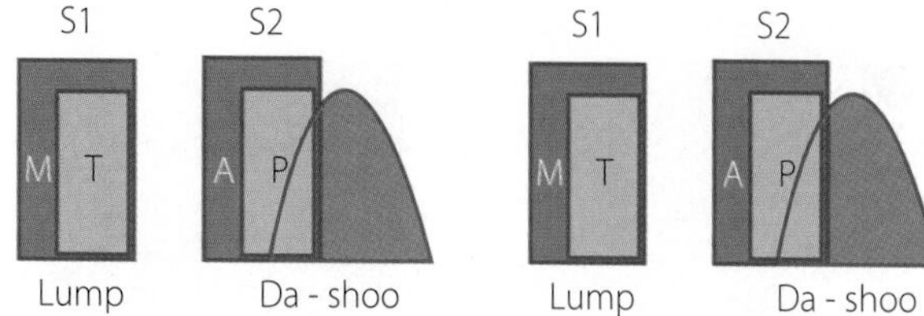

FIGURE 10-17 A low-frequency S3 begins at the end of and immediately follows S2.

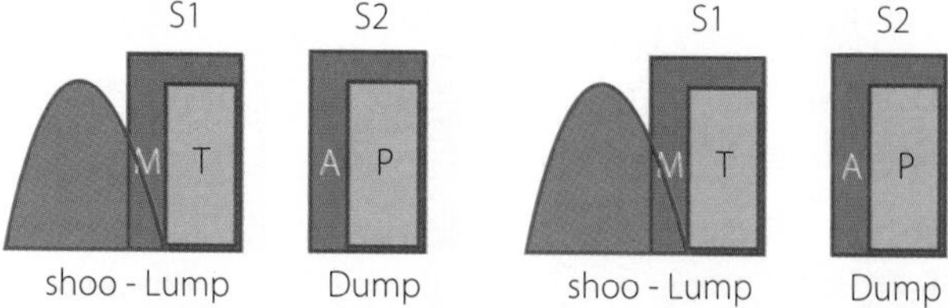

FIGURE 10-18 A low-frequency S4 begins just before and continues into early S1.

EJECTION SOUNDS/CLICKS.

The word "ejection" suggests contraction of the cardiac muscle. **Ejection sounds** can then be remembered to occur during systole (ventricular contraction), when contraction is greatest. "Click" describes the high-frequency, sharp quality of the sound created, helping the provider to remember to use the diaphragm in its evaluation. An aortic ejection sound occurs as a stenotic aortic valve suddenly clicks open under force from left ventricular contraction. This can also occur with bicuspid aortic valves or dilation of the root of the aorta.

Similarly, pulmonary ejection sounds are related to pulmonary valve stenosis or pulmonary artery dilation.

MIDSYSTOLIC CLICK.

As the name implies, a midsystolic click is found midway through ventricular systole (see **FIGURE 10-19A**). The midsystolic click is found with mitral and tricuspid valve prolapse, mitral being more common. Auscultation over the valvular areas will show an increase in intensity over the corresponding valve affected.

OPENING SNAP.

Opening snaps occur during diastole (see **FIGURE 10-19B**). Again, look at the words themselves. The only things that "open" within the heart are the valves. "Snap" itself is a sharply pronounced word, describing the high-frequency sound produced as the valve opens. Occurring in ventricular diastole, one must envision the contraction of the atria and the valves being opened that of the mitral and tricuspid. Normally these valves begin to open spontaneously as ventricular contraction ends and the residing pressure in the atria begins to fill the ventricles passively. In the diseased states of mitral and tricuspid stenosis, opening is delayed but then occurs rapidly as the atria contract, creating the sound of the snap.

Opening snaps: high-frequency sounds occurring during ventricular diastole, commonly related to the snapping open of stenotic mitral and tricuspid valves

Murmurs: the sound of turbulence as blood flows over the valves or structural defects of the heart

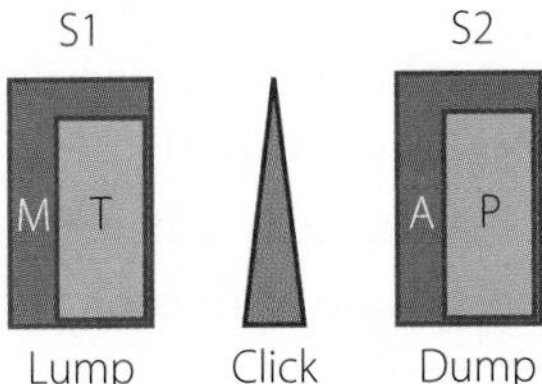

FIGURE 10-19A A midsystolic click occurs between S1 and S2.

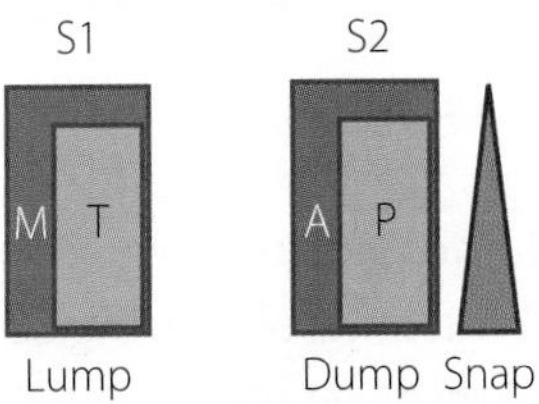

FIGURE 10-19B An opening snap occurs immediately after S2.

Murmurs

Murmurs represent the sound of turbulence as blood flows over the valves or structural defects of the heart. Accurate diagnosis can be made through identifying key components of the identified murmur, including location, radiation, intensity, pitch, quality, timing, and shape.

LOCATION.

One of the easiest components of the murmur to identify is location. Identify in which area of auscultation the murmur is heard with greatest intensity. When documenting the location, do so by identifying intercostal space such as:

- Parasternal 2nd R ICS (Aortic)
- Parasternal 2nd L ICS (Pulmonic)
- Parasternal 4th L ICS (Tricuspid)
- Apical 5th ICS L MCL (Mitral)

RADIATION.

Following identification of location, search for associated radiation of the murmur. Common patterns of radiation include:

- Parasternal 2nd R ICS (Aortic)—Carotid
- Apical 5th ICS L MCL (Mitral)—Axilla

INTENSITY.

Intensity of murmur is defined through a grading system representing both the volume of blood and the velocity at which it flows over the structural disorder.

- Grade 1—Faint, may not be heard with each contraction

- Grade 2—Quiet but heard easily
- Grade 3—Moderately loud
- Grade 4—Loud with palpable thrill
- Grade 5—Loud with thrill, may be heard with stethoscope partially off of the chest
- Grade 6—Loud with thrill, may be heard with stethoscope off of the chest

When identifying a murmur, the provider should auscultate each area of auscultation to identify where the intensity of the murmur is greatest. Listen first to see if the murmur can be heard with each cardiac cycle. If so, it is at least a grade 1. Though this is subjective, if the provider considers the murmur to be faint but easily heard, it is a grade 2, whereas if it is considered moderately loud, it is a grade 3. To distinguish between a grade 3 and 4, palpate the area with the metacarpal phalangeal (MCP) joint or ulnar aspect of the hand (see **FIGURES 10-20A** and **10-20B**). If a palpable vibration, or thrill, is felt, it is at least a grade 4 and should be considered loud. Return the stethoscope head to the chest, but tilt it so that it rests partially off the chest. If the murmur is still present, it is a least a grade 5. Lift the head of the stethoscope so that it hovers over the chest. If still audible, it is a grade 6.

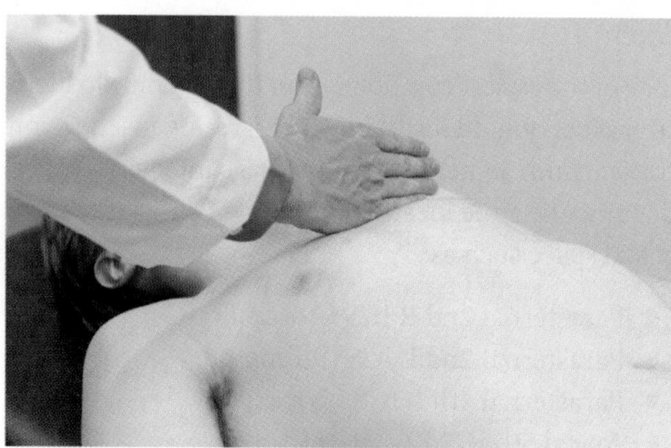

FIGURE 10-20A Palpation of thrill with the lateral aspect of the hand.

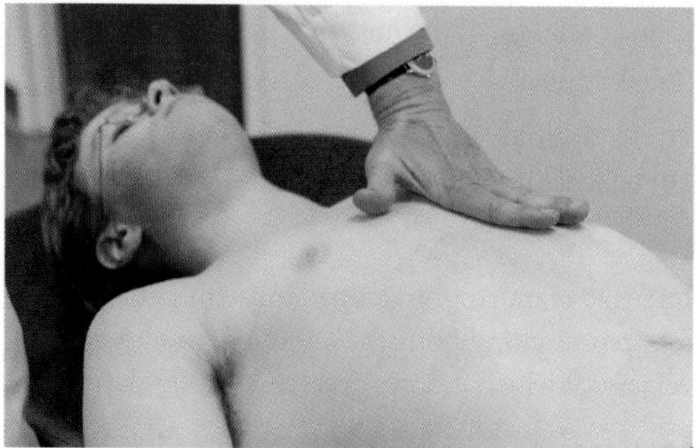

FIGURE 10-20B Palpation of thrill with the MCP joint.

Pitch.

Pitch of murmur refers to whether the murmur is of high or low frequency. This is determined by auscultating with both the bell and the diaphragm, noting which allows the murmur to be better heard; the bell accentuates low-frequency murmurs and the diaphragm high-frequency murmurs. Low-frequency murmurs are more often associated with valvular stenosis, whereas high-frequency murmurs are more common with valvular incompetency resulting in regurgitation.

- Low-frequency murmurs
  - Mitral stenosis
  - Tricuspid stenosis
- High-frequency murmurs
  - Pulmonic regurgitation (PR)
  - Tricuspid regurgitation (TR)
  - Aortic regurgitation (AR)
  - Mitral regurgitation MR)

Quality.

Quality is a descriptive term that characterizes the sound of the murmur. Terms commonly used include mechanical, blowing, musical, harsh, and rumbling.

Timing.

The timing of the murmur refers to which part of the cardiac cycle the murmur occurs in: systolic, diastolic, or both (continuous). Auscultate the murmur while palpating the right carotid pulse to identify the timing in relation to S1 and S2. Then identify when the murmur starts and stops within systole or diastole.

Systolic murmurs. Systolic murmurs occur between S1 and S2 but may obscure either. Depending on the side of the heart causing the murmur, A2 or P2 is obscured in murmurs that end at S2 (see **FIGURE 10-21**).

- Early systolic: early onset obscuring S1 but ending before S2
- Midsystolic: onset after S1 and ends before S2
- Late systolic: onset after S1 but ends obscuring S2
- Holosystolic/Pansystolic: early onset obscuring S1 and ends obscuring S2

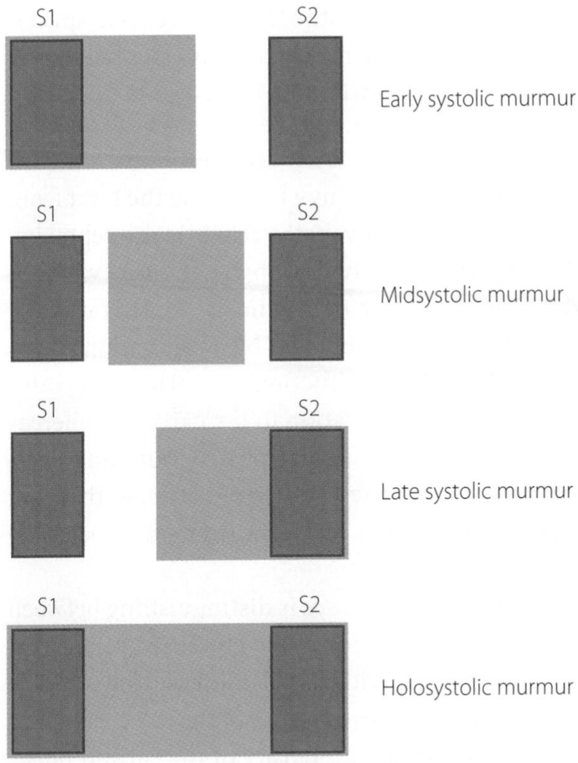

FIGURE 10-21 Timing of systolic murmurs.

Diastolic murmurs. Diastolic murmurs occur between S2 and S1 (see **FIGURE 10-22**).

- Early diastolic: early onset obscuring S2 and ending before S1

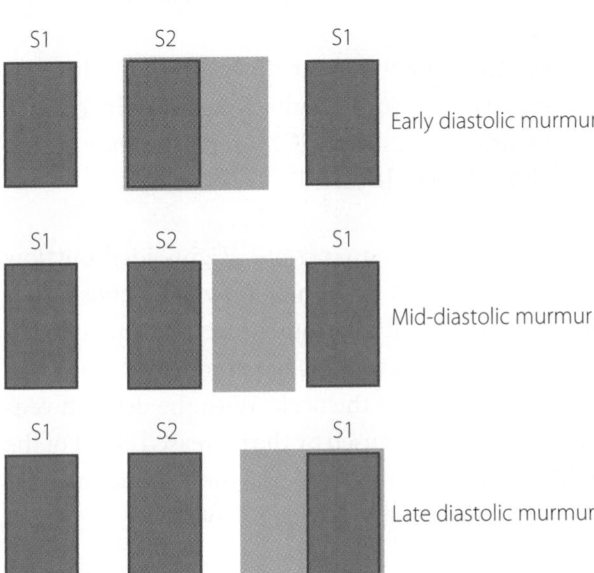

FIGURE 10-22 Timing of diastolic murmurs.

- Mid-diastolic: onset after S2 but ends before S1
- Late diastolic: onset late in diastole close to S1 and ends obscuring it

Continuous murmurs. These murmurs begin in systole but continue through to diastole.

Shape.

Shape of the murmur refers to the configuration made by the intensity of the murmur over time (see **FIGURE 10-23**).

- Crescendo: rising intensity over time
- Decrescendo: falling intensity over time
- Crescendo-decrescendo: rising then falling intensity over time
- Plateau: flat intensity without rise or fall

Types of Murmurs.

Bringing all of these components together allows the provider to identify which abnormality is most likely to be contributing to the finding. Grouping of possible causes is best accomplished by beginning with timing.

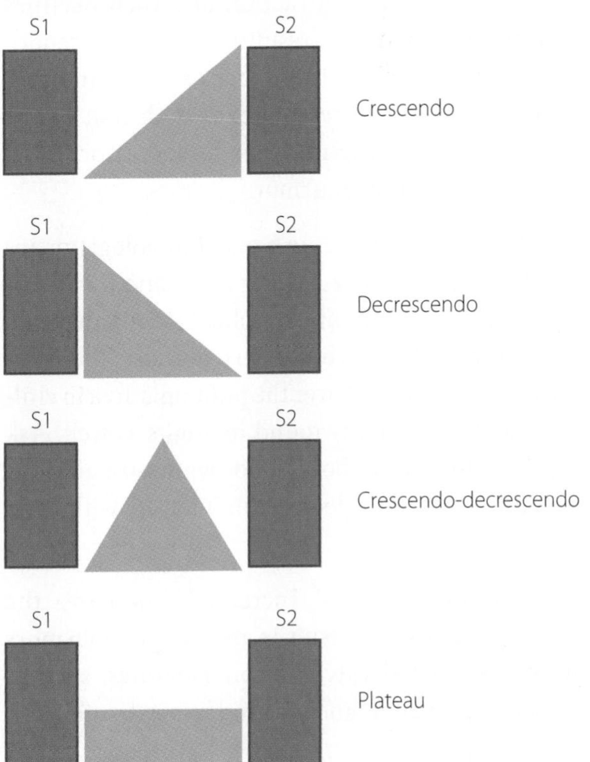

FIGURE 10-23 Shape of murmurs.

Early systolic murmurs. Consider physiologically what is occurring at early systole. The ventricles begin to contract, forcing the tricuspid and mitral valves to close. Therefore a murmur heard from blood passing over these valves must be related to failure of the valves and resultant regurgitation into the atria. These murmurs start at S1, are decrescendo with high velocity, and flow at onset but taper as ventricular and atrial pressures equalize in the case of MR and TR, and end before S2. What other defects would allow early outflow of blood from the ventricles? Ventricular septal defect (VSD) would do so. VSD also follows the decrescendo shape due to decreasing left-to-right shunt toward the end of systole.

Midsystolic ejection murmurs. Reviewing the components of systole, as ventricular contraction begins, S1 occurs with the closure of the AV valves. Pressure begins to rise in the ventricles but does not force open the AV valves until it exceeds that in the aorta and pulmonary artery. For this reason, onset of midsystolic murmur, created by turbulence over the semilunar valves, begins only after ejection of blood from the ventricles occurs, which preserves S1.

Intensity of the murmur at first builds under the force of ventricular contraction and then declines as the contraction eases, resulting in the crescendo-decrescendo shape. Outflow stops as aortic and pulmonary artery pressure equalizes with that of the ventricles, causing the murmur to end prior to S2, hence the midsystolic murmur.

Physiologic or innocent murmurs. Physiologic or innocent murmurs, those lacking association with abnormal pathology, are midsystolic, soft, and have no other associated abnormal heart sounds. These are most commonly found over the pulmonic area in children but are commonly found in adults as well. Ask the patient to squeeze both hands while auscultating. These murmurs often decrease in intensity with hand grip.

Increased flow murmurs. Increased flow across the semilunar valves can result in midsystolic murmurs without associated valvular abnormalities, such as seen with pregnancy, anemia, and hyperthyroidism.

Structural defects. Structural defects of the aortic and pulmonic valves may also result in the midsystolic murmur greatest over the 2nd intercostal spaces. When detecting these murmurs, it is essential to rule out outflow tract obstruction.

Left-sided outflow obstruction. Left-sided outflow obstruction can occur anywhere along the tract from hypertrophic cardiomyopathy (HCM) with septal hypertrophy and subvalvular obstruction to valvular and aortic supravalvular stenosis. Localization of obstruction can be predicted by auscultation of the carotids. Valvular obstruction, as with aortic valve stenosis, may have radiation to the carotids, whereas this is absent in subvalvular obstruction. Supravalvular stenosis may have greater radiation to the right verses the left carotid. These murmurs may be musical or harsh.

Of greatest importance is distinguishing between outflow tract obstruction caused by HCM versus that of valvular disease. With valvular disease, the ventricle must work against the resistance of the valve, resulting in delay and decreased intensity of the carotid pulse. This delay does not occur with HCM.

To further distinguish between the two, special testing should be utilized.

- Have the patient squat while you do the same. Place the stethoscope over the aortic area, noting the intensity of the murmur. Ask and assist the patient to a standing position while continuing to auscultate. An increase in intensity is consistent with HCM, whereas a decrease is found with valvular disease.
- Ask the patient to bear down (the Valsalva maneuver) while you auscultate. Again an increase in intensity occurs with HCM, and a decrease occurs with valvular disease.

Pulmonic outflow obstruction. Right-sided outflow obstruction caused by pulmonary valve stenosis does not have the benefit of carotid pulse assessment to aid in diagnosis. However, this harsh murmur may radiate to the left side of the neck. With the delay in ventricular emptying caused by the increased effort of the right ventricle to force blood past the stenotic valve, P2 is delayed, resulting in a wide S2 split.

Late systolic murmurs. Late systolic murmurs begin well after S1 and extend into S2, obscuring it. These murmurs are related to prolapse of the mitral or tricuspid valves. These are high-pitched murmurs best heard with the diaphragm.

Mitral valve prolapse (MVP). Best heard over the mitral area, MVP is often associated with a click that is heard at the onset of the murmur as the valve snaps back into the atria. MVP can also be accentuated by auscultating the mitral area while the provider assists the patient in a squat.

Pulmonary valve prolapse. This murmur has similar physiology to MVP. Prolapse of the pulmonary valve is best heard over the 2nd left ICS.

Holosystolic murmurs. A holosystolic murmur begins at S1 and ends at S2, partially obscuring both. These are typically regurgitant murmurs of the mitral or tricuspid valve or VSD.

Mitral regurgitation. MR is high-pitched and is heard best with the diaphragm. With the stethoscope over the mitral area, ask the patient to roll from the supine position into the left lateral decubitus, which brings the left ventricle closer to the chest wall. Radiation may occur to the left axilla, to the neck, or to the back below the left scapula.

Tricuspid regurgitation. TR is best heard along the left sternal border and may radiate into the epigastrium.

Ventricular septal defect. The murmur of VSD is secondary to the left-to-right shunt created by left ventricular pressure's being greater than right ventricular pressure. As such it is auscultated over the ventricular septum, which is typically left 2nd to 4th ICS, being higher when the defect is in the superior aspect of the septum and lower when inferior.

Diastolic murmurs. When a diastolic murmur is encountered, consider what is occurring during diastole. The ventricles have relaxed, allowing the pressure in them to drop below the pressure in the aorta and pulmonary artery. Backflow of blood caused the aortic and pulmonic valves to close, resulting in the S2. The atria at first empty passively but then contract toward the end of diastole, filling the ventricles.

Early diastolic murmur. Early diastolic murmurs would then correlate with closure of the aortic and pulmonic valves. Failure to close properly would result in regurgitation (see Figure 10-22).

Aortic regurgitation. The AR murmur would have an onset at A2. This murmur is decrescendo in nature as the pressure in the aorta drops during diastole. It is often described as "blowing" but is of low intensity and is best heard over the aortic area. Just as MR and TR murmurs are high-pitched, so is the AR murmur. Radiation may occur toward the apex of the heart following the direction of regurgitation. AR murmur typically ends prior to S1.

AR can be accentuated by having the seated patient lean forward, breathe out completely, and hold his/her breath.

Pulmonic regurgitation. PR begins at P2 and again ends before S1. It shares the same characteristics of AR but is heard over the pulmonic area.

Mid-diastolic murmurs. The semilunar valves have closed, resulting in S2, and there is a brief period of silence followed by the onset of a diastolic murmur. What is occurring at this time? Filling of the ventricles is occurring; therefore murmurs associated must reflect flow over the mitral and tricuspid valves.

Mitral stenosis. The murmur of MS is described as "rumbling." It is low-frequency, meaning best heard with the bell. Again, to bring the left ventricle closer to the chest wall, the patient may be placed in the left lateral decubitus position. With stenosis, the stiff mitral valve must be forced open, often resulting in an opening snap at onset of the murmur. It ends with S1.

Tricuspid stenosis. Tricuspid stenosis also has a rumbling character but is found at the tricuspid area of auscultation. Ask the patient to take a deep breath, which will increase the intensity. An opening snap may also be found with this murmur.

Late diastolic murmurs. Both mitral and tricuspid stenosis may have late diastolic murmurs in addition to the midsystolic murmur. This occurs with end atrial contraction. Atrial myxomas may also cause late diastolic murmurs when they cause obstruction of the AV valves.

Continuous murmurs. Continuous murmurs begin in systole but extend beyond S2 into diastole and represent flow from a high to a low pressure, such as is seen with patent ductus arteriosus, with flow from the high-pressure aorta into the low pressure of the pulmonary artery. Continuous murmurs are often described as machinery-like. Atrial septal defect and arteriovenous fistulas are also examples of defects that are associated with continuous murmurs.

DOCUMENTATION

- Cardiac Auscultation—S1, S2 without splitting, S3, S4, ejection click or opening snap. III/VI holosystolic murmur, best heard with the diaphragm over the mitral area with radiation to the left axilla.

Summary of Auscultation Technique

10-3 Approach auscultation of the heart in the same deliberate stepwise manner of examination used elsewhere. Following a head-to-toe approach to the valvular areas and examining each area with the chronological approach of the cardiac cycle allows for a comprehensive examination.

1. Place the stethoscope in your ears and tune the head to the diaphragm.
2. Locate the aortic area by palpating the sternal notch and then moving down to the sternal angle. Slide your fingers laterally off the sternum to the 2nd rib, which attaches at the sternal angle. Drop inferiorly to the 2nd ICS.
3. Place the stethoscope directly on the skin at the aortic area in the 2nd ICS along the sternal border.
4. Identify S1 and S2 by concurrent palpation of the carotid pulse. S1 occurs just before the upstroke. Identify which is louder.
5. Using a chronological approach:
   a. Focus on S1, noting any splitting.
   b. Focus on the systole represented by the space between S1 and S2, noting:
      i. Systolic murmurs
      ii. Ejection clicks
   c. Focus on S2.
      i. Note splitting
      ii. Identify which component has greater intensity: A2 or P2
   d. Focus on diastole.
      i. Note murmurs
      ii. Opening snaps
      iii. S3
      iv. S4
   e. Palpate to identify the location, then repeat the process of auscultation in each consecutive area. Repeat with the bell.
      i. 2nd ICS LSB—Pulmonic area
      ii. 3rd ICS LSB
      iii. 4th ICS LSB—Tricuspid area
      iv. 4th or 5th ICS MCL—Mitral area
   f. Return to areas of greatest intensity for each abnormality found.
   g. Perform special testing to identify likely etiologies.

PALPATION

Point of Maximal Impulse

If the PMI cannot be seen on inspection, it may be identifiable through palpation. Placing the fingers along the intercostal spaces with the ribs running between the fingers allows for a palpable scanning of the area (see **FIGURE 10-24**). As a generalized tap is felt under one of the fingers, reposition the pads of the fingers over the area to achieve a more precise location. Document the location by identifying the ICS where it is located and measure the distance from the right sternal border.

- PMI 5th ICS 6 cm from the LSB (left sternal border)

Alternatively, anatomic lines can be used to document the lateral distance.

- PMI 5th ICS MCL (midclavicular line)

Also document if the PMI is felt to be hyperkinetic.

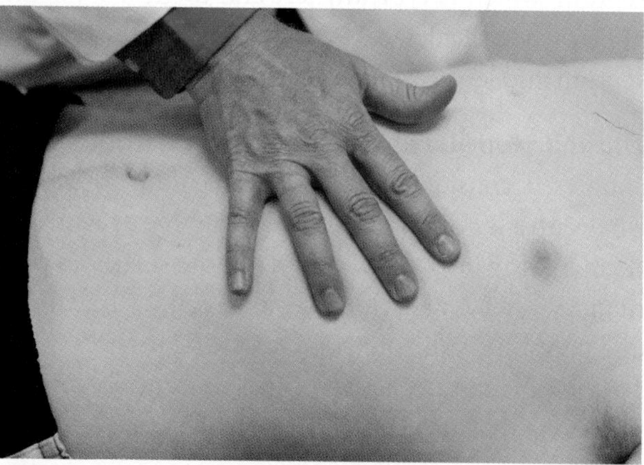

FIGURE 10-24 Palpation of the PMI with the provider's fingers aligned in the intercostal spaces.

Thrills

If a murmur was identified, palpate the area to ascertain if a thrill is present. A thrill is the vibratory sensation found with increased force of turbulent flow across the defect. If a thrill is present, the murmur is at least a grade 3.

Pain

When a patient presents with chest pain, do not forget to include palpation of the chest wall as part of the examination. If palpating the chest wall results in significant reproduction of the pain, musculoskeletal etiology becomes most likely in the differential diagnosis.

Immediately after inspection and palpation of the heart is completed, regown the patient to preserve dignity.

DOCUMENTATION

- Cardiac palpation—PMI at 5th ICS 5 cm from left sternal border. Nontender without heaves or thrills.

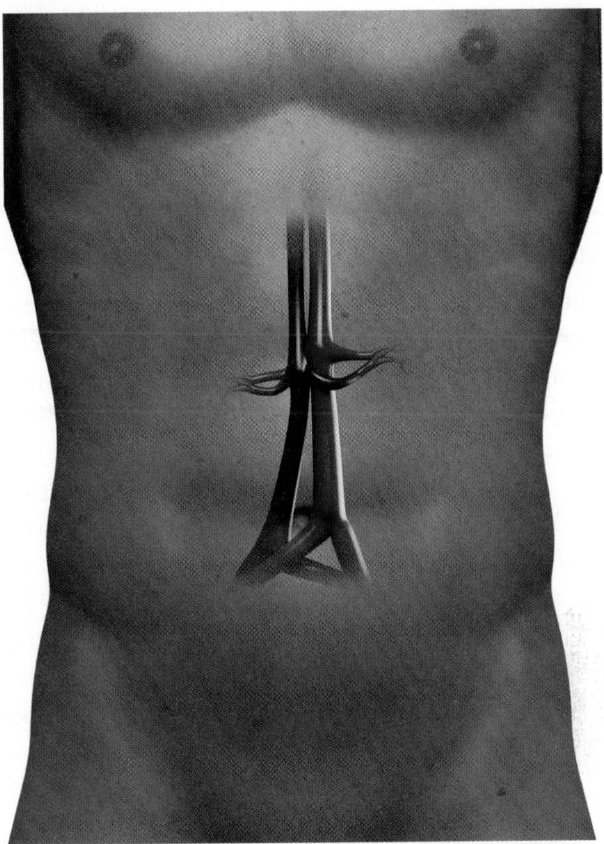

© Sebastian Kaulitzki/ShutterStock, Inc.

FIGURE 10-25 Abdominal vascular anatomy with the renal arteries and bifurcation of the aorta at the level of the umbilicus.

Abdomen

Consider which components of the abdominal exam would be included in the cardiovascular system as you leave the chest and move to the abdomen (see **FIGURE 10-25**).

Continuing our examination, the patient is already in the supine position with a gown covering the thorax and a sheet over the pelvis. Ask permission to expose the abdomen. Lift the gown to just under the breasts and position the sheet to just above the suprapubic area, allowing examination of all four quadrants. A common mistake made by early practitioners of medicine is to expose only to the level of the umbilicus, resulting in examination of only the upper two quadrants.

INSPECTION

Standing on the right side of the patient, inspect the abdomen for visible pulsations that may be associated with an abdominal aortic aneurysm. The presence of venous dilations (caput medusa) is reflective of portal hypertension, mostly associated with end-stage liver disease.

AUSCULTATION

The abdominal aorta lies just left of midline, exiting from under the xiphoid process and bifurcating at the umbilicus, becoming the iliac and then the femoral arteries. Atherosclerotic narrowing and aneurysm can occur at any of these areas.

Using the bell to detect the low frequency of bruits, auscultate:

- Aorta—halfway between the xiphoid and umbilicus
- Iliac arteries—halfway between the umbilicus and inguinal canal
- Femoral arteries—over the inguinal canal

Exposure of the femoral area is not necessary for auscultation of the artery. Simply advise the patient that you will be listening and feeling the femoral artery and slide the head of the stethoscope under the sheet, covering the patient just medial to the midline of the inguinal canal.

PALPATION

Abdominal Vasculature

Immediately after auscultation of the femoral arteries, palpate the pulse. The femoral artery is at its shallowest in the inguinal region; however, it still lies somewhat deeply and may require some depth of palpation to locate it. Compare bilaterally.

10-4 Moving back up, palpate the iliac arteries for strength of beat and aneurysm. To palpate the abdominal aorta, place the hands flatly on the abdomen approximately 5 cm from each side of the aorta about halfway between the xiphoid and the umbilicus. The aorta lies directly over the body of the vertebrae and may be difficult to palpate in nondilated states except in thin individuals.

Advise the patient to tell you if he/she experiences pain. Laying the hands flatly distributes the pressure exerted as you push downward, lessening the discomfort of the exam (see **FIGURE 10-26A**). Palpate for a pulsatile mass pressing downward simultaneously on both sides until reaching about half the thickness of the abdomen (see **FIGURE 10-26B**). If no pulsation is felt, lift the hands, move medially about 1 cm each, and recheck. Continue this process until a tap is felt against the edge of the index finger. This is usually felt first in the right hand of the provider, as the aorta lies just left of midline. Keeping the right hand in place, continue to move the left hand medially 1 cm at a time until the other wall of the aorta is encountered (see **FIGURE 10-26C**). Note the size of the aorta in centimeters. Abdominal aortic aneurysm is diagnosed with measurements above the normal size, approximately 2 cm.

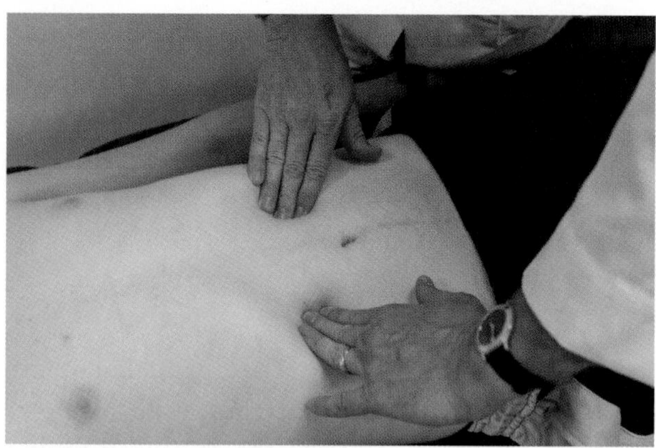

FIGURE 10-26A Assessment for an abdominal aortic aneurysm begins the far lateral palpation.

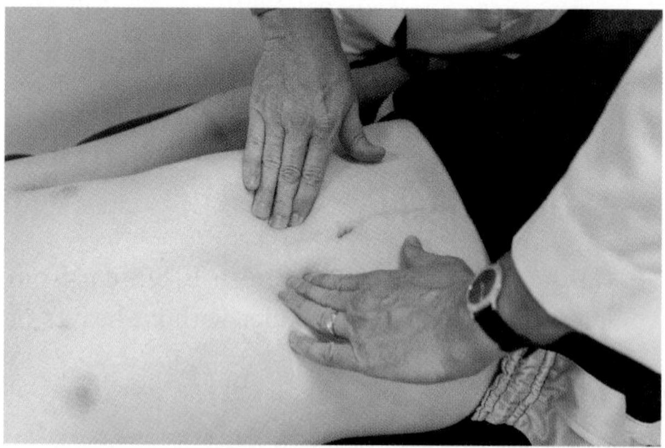

FIGURE 10-26B The provider's hands move medially in 1-cm increments.

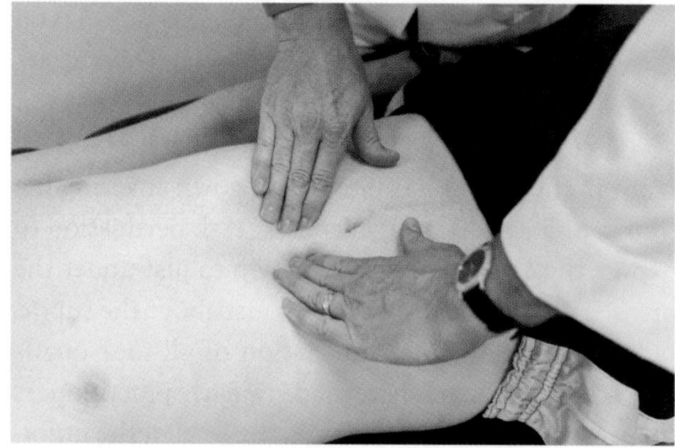

FIGURE 10-26C When the pulsatile sides of the aorta are encountered, the distance between the two sides is measured.

Hepatojugular Reflux

Hepatojugular reflux: increased venous pressure resulting in jugular distension with pressure exerted on the liver during deep palpation

Performing the **hepatojugular reflux** exam accentuates the jugular venous pulse for examination and is useful in assessing increased venous pressure, such as in a state of heart failure or dilated cardiomyopathy.

With the patient in the supine position, the provider places a hand flatly on the right upper quadrant directly below the costal margin. Firm pressure is applied steadily for 10 seconds while observing the right jugular vein.

This technique adds in assessment of the jugular venous pulse by elevating it a centimeter or two so that pulsations can be more clearly observed. This response is greatly exaggerated in patients with heart failure. A positive would be documented as "Positive" or "6 cm hepatojugular reflux."

DOCUMENTATION

- Abdomen—Inspection without visible pulsation or caput medusa. Auscultation without bruits. Palpation without pulsatile masses. Aorta 2 cm diameter. No hepatojugular reflux.

Re-cover the abdomen immediately following completion of the exam.

Extremities

INSPECTION

Edema

Expose the lower extremities by raising the sheet while keeping the pelvis covered.

Inspect for edema of the lower extremities, comparing bilaterally. One prior method for quantifying the amount of edema was for the provider to press a finger or thumb against the extremity, pitting it, and then count how long it took for the pit to disappear. This result is too subjective, since providers count at different speeds. A more accurate method is to quantify the amount of edema according to how far up the extremity the edema extends. This is scaled as:

- 1+ edema = edema at the ankle
- 2+ edema = edema to the mid tibia
- 3+ edema = edema to the mid femur
- 4+ edema = edema to the sacrum

This is most accurate for patients who can ambulate or be in the seated position. For patients who are in the supine position for extended periods, the sacrum may become edematous first, as this is the most dependent body site.

Varicosities

The extremities should also be inspected for varicosities. If varicosities are found, an assessment should be made to determine if the valvular incompetency of the communicating veins is present.

With the patient in the supine position, raise the leg to allow drainage of the venous system. You may assist venous drainage by encircling the leg with your two hands, starting at the ankle and milking to the upper thigh. Place a tourniquet around the upper thigh, tight enough to obstruct venous flow but not arterial flow.

Now assist the patient to a standing position. Filling of the veins should proceed from the ankle upward. If rapid filling occurs with the tourniquet in place, incompetence of the communicating veins is diagnosed.

If slow filling is occurring, release the tourniquet. If rapid filling now occurs, this demonstrates incompetence of the valves of the superficial veins.

Valvular incompetency may lead to stasis dermatitis. This condition results from insufficiency of venous return with increased pressure in the venous system, causing capillary permeability with leak of fluids into the tissues. This skin appears tight, with erythematous to brown pigmentation from hemosiderin deposition, increased warmth, and thickening. Progression may lead to chronic ulceration.

Peripheral arterial disease: narrowing of the distal arterial system resulting in poor perfusion to the extremities commonly caused by atherosclerotic disease

Peripheral Arterial Disease (PAD)

In contrast, **peripheral arterial disease** may be suspected with skin that appears waxy, accompanied by hair loss. If hair loss if found, the patient should be questioned about hair loss and shaving habits. The lower extremities may appear dusky, pale, or cyanotic.

Nails

Moving distally, examine the nails for pallor and cyanosis and splinter hemorrhages. Splinter hemorrhages may be found with endocarditis with embolism. Assess capillary refill by pressing the nail, with the thumb on the nail and the middle phalanx of the index finger underneath for several seconds, which results in blanching of the nail. Now release the nail and observe for pinking of the bed. The nail should perfuse within 2 seconds. Perfusion that takes longer than 2 seconds is suggestive of poor arterial perfusion. For general screening of capillary refill, one digit from each extremity is appropriate; however, for assessment of local perfusion such as after cast placement, each digit should be assessed.

PALPATION

Peripheral Arteries

With the patient still in the supine position, palpate the peripheral arteries, comparing bilaterally. Use the pads of the fingers to simultaneously assess the brachial and radial arteries, dorsalis pedis, and posterior tibialis. Always palpate on bare skin, never through clothing.

The femoral arteries were previously palpated during the abdominal examination. Popliteal arteries are deep-seated within the popliteal fossa, and are best assessed one at a time. Place the thumbs on the patella and encircle the knee, with the pads of the fingers pressing anteriorly from the dorsal surface. Bending the knee to 30 degrees may assist in locating the artery.

Strength of peripheral pulses is scaled from 0 to 4:

- 0 = no palpable pulse
- 1 = faint or weak intensity of pulse
- 2 = easily felt, moderate intensity pulse
- 3 = moderately increased intensity of pulse
- 4 = high intensity, bounding pulse

Re-cover the lower extremities with the sheet and assist the patient to the seated position.

DOCUMENTATION

- Extremities—Inspection without edema, varicosities, or hair loss. Palpation—warm to touch bilaterally. Peripheral pulses 2/4 throughout.

SPECIAL TESTING

Allen's Test

The **Allen's test** assures dual blood supply to the hand through the radial and ulnar arteries. Patency of these arteries must be proven before performing an arterial blood gas (ABG). An ABG requires needle insertion into the radial artery. If perfusion is provided by only the radial artery and a thrombus develops at the site of ABG, the hand will become ischemic. For this reason it is not only imperative to perform the Allen's test prior to performing the ABG; it would be negligent not to do so.

Allen's test: technique for assessment of dual blood supply to the hand through the radial and ulnar arteries

Technique.

1. With the patient's palm up, the provider holds the wrist with both hands, the pads of the fingers over the radial and ulnar arteries. 10-5
2. Palpate the pulse of the radial and ulnar arteries (see **FIGURE 10-27A**).
3. Have the patient clench his/her fist.
4. Compress radial and ulnar arteries simultaneously to obstruct perfusion to the hand (see **FIGURE 10-27B**).
5. Ask the patient to open and relax the hand.

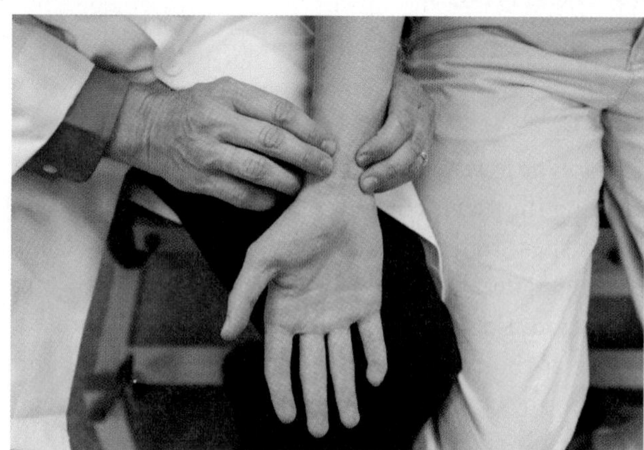

FIGURE 10-27A An Allen's test begins with the provider simultaneously compressing the radial and ulnar arteries.

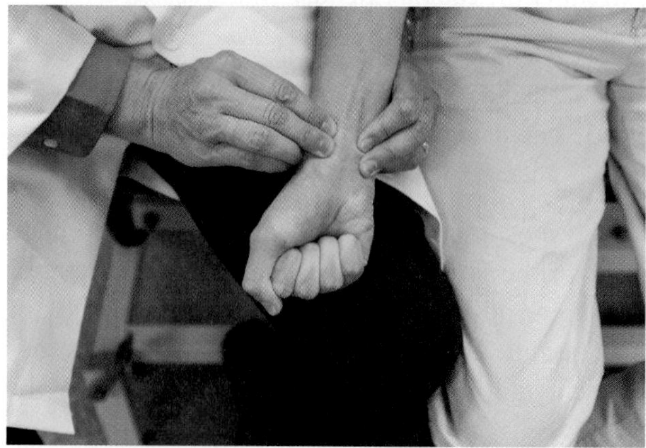

FIGURE 10-27B The patient clenches the hand, evacuating the blood from the palm.

6. Observe the palm, which should be blanched (see **FIGURE 10-27C**). If not blanched, begin the procedure over again, repositioning the fingers over the arteries.

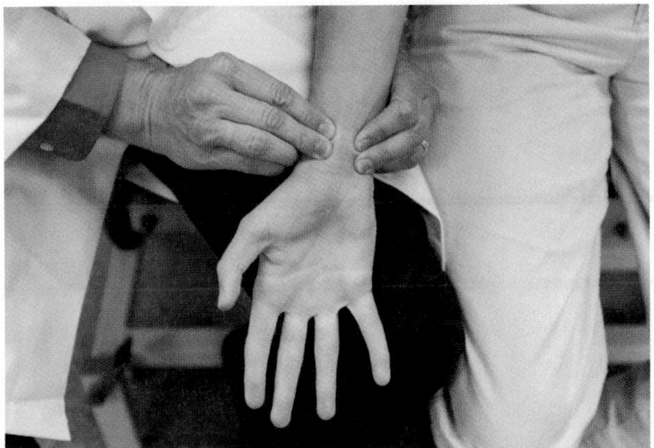

FIGURE 10-27C The provider observes palmar pallor.

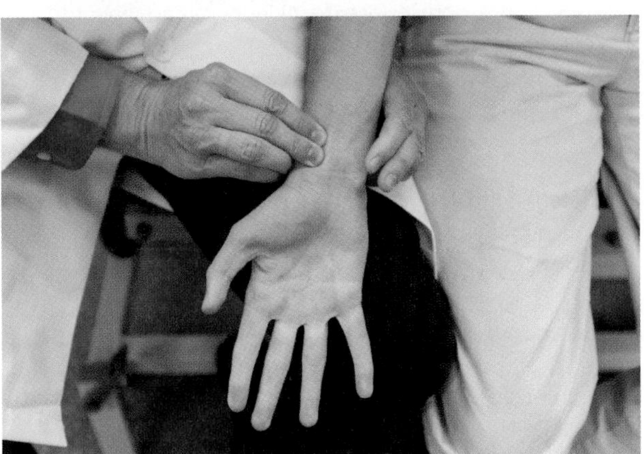

FIGURE 10-27D Release the ulnar artery.

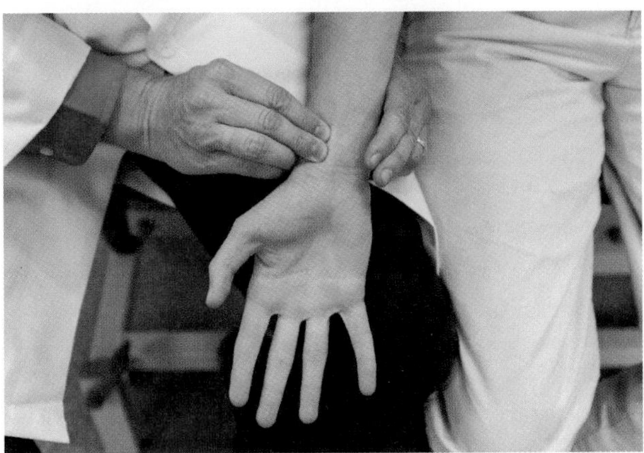

FIGURE 10-27E The provider observes perfusion, which should occur within 3 to 5 seconds.

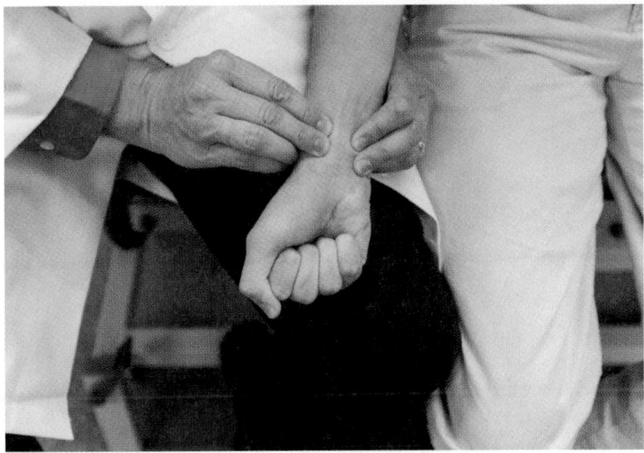

FIGURE 10-27F The provider again compresses both arteries, and the patient clenches the fist to evacuate blood.

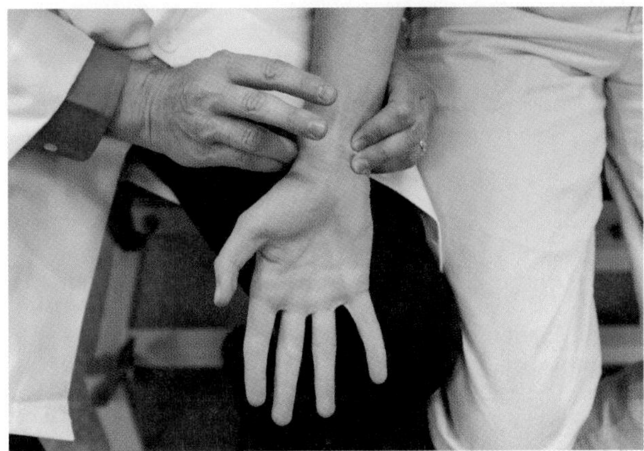

FIGURE 10-27G The provider releases the radial artery and observes for flushing of the palm indicating radial artery patency.

7. Release ulnar artery (see **FIGURE 10-27D**).
8. Observe perfusion, seen by pinking of the palm, which should occur within 3 to 5 seconds (see **FIGURE 10-27E**).
9. Have patient clench again to assess the radial artery (see **FIGURE 10-27G**).

If the palm does not pink, perfusion to the hand does not occur through the ulnar artery and the ABG should not be performed on that extremity. Check the other hand to assess if an ABG can be performed on that extremity.

10-6 If perfusion is intact to both hands but there is a noticeable difference in the rate of perfusion between the two, use the one with the faster perfusion.

See **TABLE 10-3** for the cardiovascular flow.

TABLE 10-3 Cardiovascular Flow

Introduces self and explains that physical exam will now be performed
Washes hands for 15 seconds, turning off water with towel
EYES: Ophthalmoscopic examination for hypertensive retinopathy. R eye to R, L to L
Assists patient to supine position
Drapes lower extremities with a sheet
NECK
Inspect for JVD: State "would elevate as needed to measure JVD if present"
Auscultate for bruits prior to palpation
Palpate the carotids separately
CHEST
Inspection
Stand on right side of patient
Properly expose the chest by dropping gown and keeping sheet in place
Examine for shape of chest wall, PMI, and pulsations
Auscultation: stethoscope placed correctly in the ears
Correct valvular areas
Aortic—2nd right intercostal space (ICS) along sternal border
Pulmonic—2nd left ICS along sternal border
Tricuspid—4th or 5th left ICS along sternal border
Mitral—4th or 5th ICS midclavicular line
Note rate and rhythm
S1—closure of AV valves (marks onset of systole)
S2—closure of the semilunar valves (aortic, pulmonic). Marks onset of diastole
Assess splitting of S2
Extra sounds (may state ejection click, opening snap, S3, S4, murmur)
Murmurs: facilitators, prompt student to describe scale of murmurs
Grade 1—Faint
Grade 2—Quiet but heard easily
Grade 3—Moderately loud
Grade 4—Loud with palpable thrill
Grade 5—Loud with thrill, may be heard stethoscope partially off of chest
Grade 6—Loud with thrill, may be heard with stethoscope off of the chest.
Bell—used for low pitch (S3, S4, mitral stenosis)
Diaphragm—used for high pitch (S1, S2, AR, MR, rubs)
Special Positions: must perform and describe (type of sound accentuated)
Left lateral decubitus (mitral stenosis, S3, S4)
Palpation at valvular areas noted above
Thrills using metacarpal phalangeal joints
Point of maximal impulse (PMI)
Regown chest of patient
ABDOMEN
Expose 4 quads of abdomen by lifting gown to chest and lowering sheet to pelvis
Auscultation
Aorta and renal arteries
Iliac and femoral arteries
Palpation
Size of aorta for aneurysm (in cm)
Hepatojugular reflex (hold for 10 sec)
Re-cover abdomen
EXTREMITIES
Inspection: expose lower extremities by raising sheet to keep pelvis covered
Edema—state scale (1 = ankle, 2 = tibia, 3 = femoral, 4 = sacrum)
Varicosities
Stasis dermatitis pigmentation and ulcerations (valvular incompetency)
Hair loss or waxy skin (peripheral arterial disease)
Nail beds (splinter hemorrhages with endocarditis)
Palpation
Compare pulses bilaterally—brachial to brachial, radial to radial, etc.
Use pads of fingers, not thumbs
Brachial
Radial
Femoral
Dorsalis pedis
Posterior tibialis (may use thumb pad)
Capillary refill—one digit each extremity, normal refill is less than 3 seconds
Re-cover lower extremities with sheet
Assist patient to seated position to finalize murmur evaluation
Auscultate aortic area—have patient sitting, leaning forward, breathe out and hold
Identify that this position would accentuate an aortic regurgitation murmur
Assist patient to standing position
Auscultate mitral area—have patient Valsalva or squat while stabilizing patient

TABLE 10-3 Cardiovascular Flow *(Continued)*

Cardiovascular Flow
Identify that this would accentuate MVP or aortic stenosis murmur
CLINICAL SCENARIOS: Allen Test for hand perfusion prior to ABG performance
Palm up
Have patient clench fist
Compress radial and ulnar artery
Have patient relax hand
Observe pale palms
Release ulnar artery
Explain findings
Normal = pinks in 3–5 seconds
If abnormal—repeat, releasing radial artery

References

1. Wong TY, Mitchell P. The eye in hypertension. *Lancet*. 2007;3610:425–435.
2. Chatterjee K. Examination of the jugular venous pulse. In: Otto CM, ed. *UpToDate*. Waltham, MA: UpToDate; 2012.
3. Devine PJ, Sullenberger LE, Bellin DA, Atwood JE. Jugular venous pulse: window into the right heart. *South Med J*. 2007;100(10):1022–1027.

CHAPTER 11

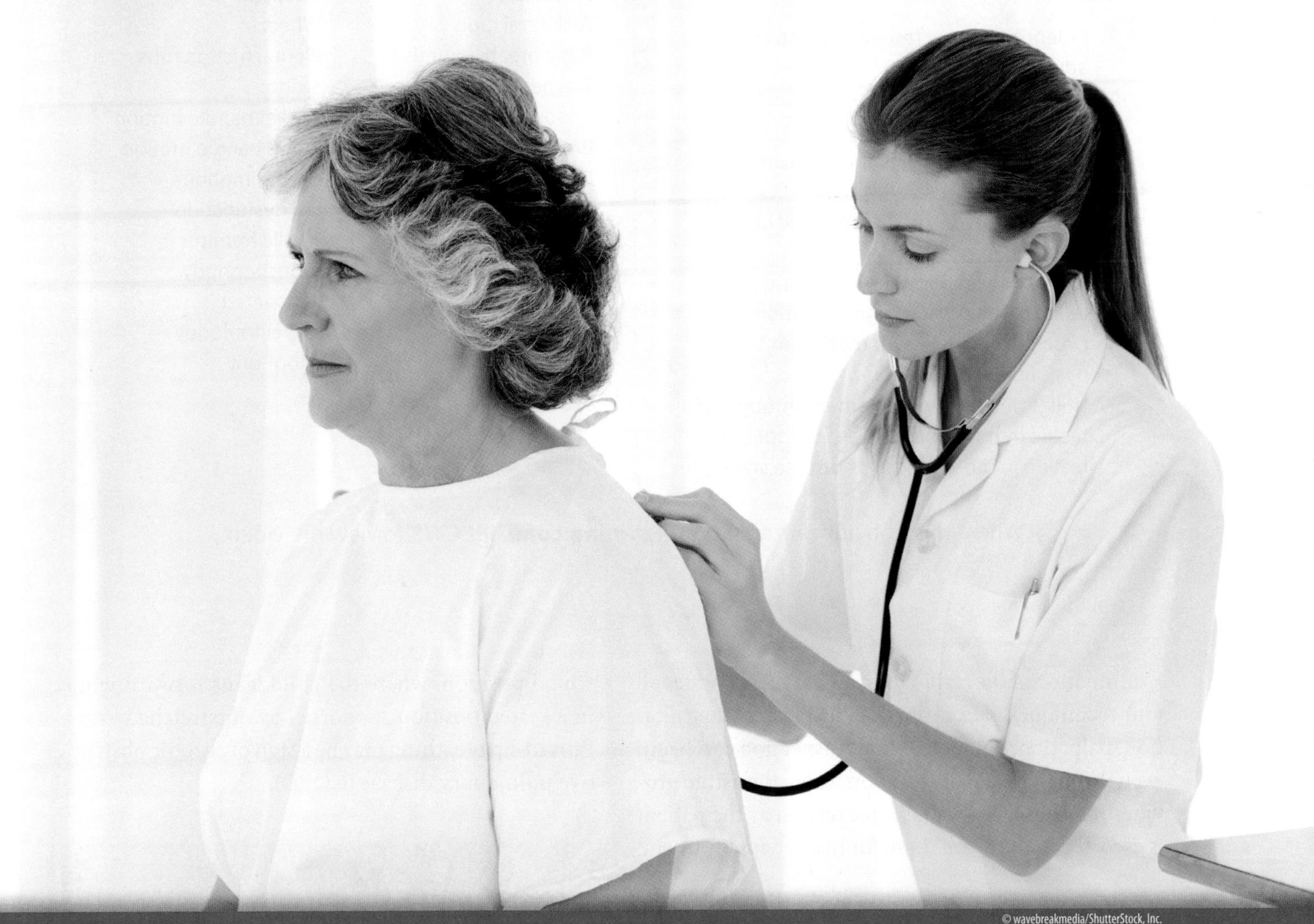

© wavebreakmedia/ShutterStock, Inc.

Respiratory Examination

John Czarnecki, MD, MPA, MPH
Mark Kauffman, DO, MS (Med Ed), PA

OBJECTIVES

At the conclusion of this chapter, the student will be able to

1. Indentify signs of respiratory distress in adults and children
2. Relate direction of tracheal deviation to causative pathology
3. Diagnose chest wall deformities and alterations of AP:lateral ratios
4. Describe the distribution of basic breath sounds
5. Identify adventitious breath sounds and relate them to pathologic conditions
6. Describe and assess rib motion and dysfunction
7. Utilize findings on assessment through tactile fremitus, percussion, and special testing in the diagnosis of disease states

KEY TERMS

Respiratory distress
Flail chest
AP:lateral ratio
Basic breath sounds
Tracheal breath sounds
Bronchial breath sounds
Bronchovesicular breath sounds
Vesicular breath sounds
Adventitious lung sounds
Crackles
Rhonchi
Wheezes
Pleural friction rubs
Stridor
Bucket handle motion
Pump handle motion
Caliber motion
Rib dysfunction
Tactile fremitus
Bronchophony
Whispered pectoriloquy
Egophony

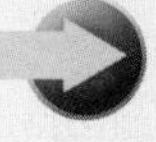 Where this icon appears, visit **go.jblearning.com/HPECWS** to view the video.

Examination of the respiratory system incorporates all four techniques of examination: inspection, auscultation, palpation, and percussion. Inspection can begin even through casual observation where the astute provider may observe dyspnea on exertion as the patient is escorted to the exam room for his/her appointment.

Inspection

GENERAL ASSESSMENT

General assessment of the patient for distress is one of the very first examination techniques with every patient encounter and allows for immediate intervention should obvious signs of acute **respiratory distress** be encountered. In the adult patient these signs include accessory muscle use, intercostal retractions, forward leaning, and deep, exaggerated, or labored breathing (see **FIGURE 11-1**).

Respiratory distress: Inability to obtain adequate oxygenation

Respiratory distress in infants can be manifested by nasal flaring, while in toddlers and older children (see **FIGURE 11-2**) it can be displayed by a tripod position, where the child leans forward while in a seated position supported by outstretched arms. Pursed-lip breathing may be a sign of chronic obstructive pulmonary disease (COPD).

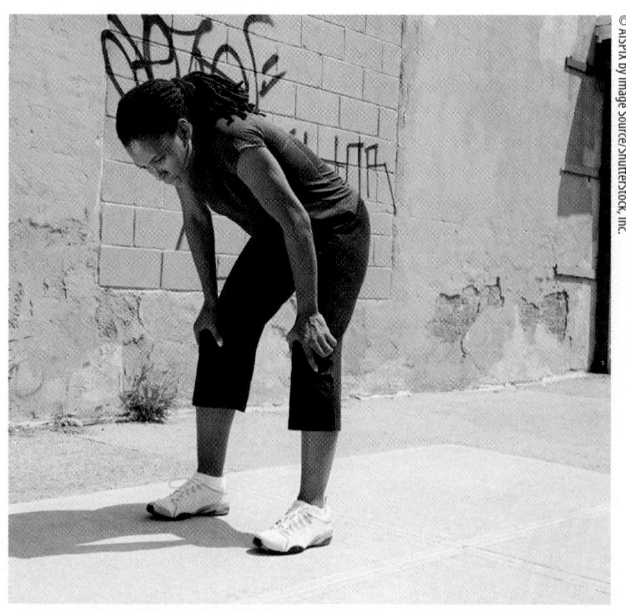

© AISPIX by Image Source/ShutterStock, Inc.

FIGURE 11-1 Respiratory distress in the adult.

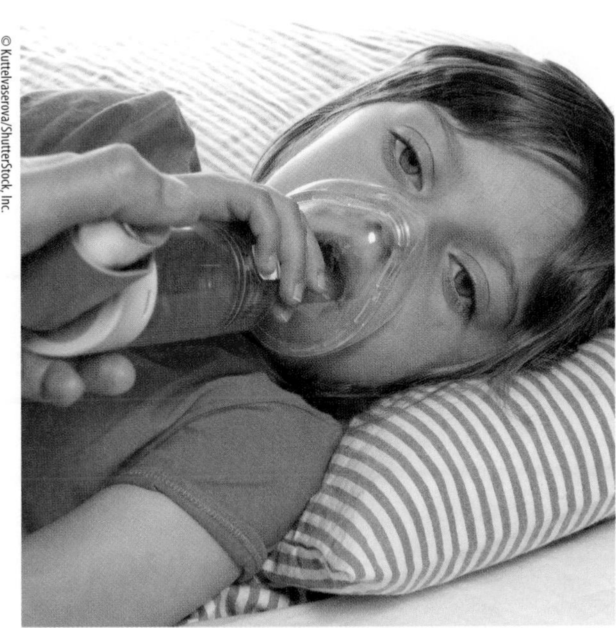
© Kuttelvaserova/ShutterStock, Inc.

FIGURE 11-2 Respiratory distress in the child.

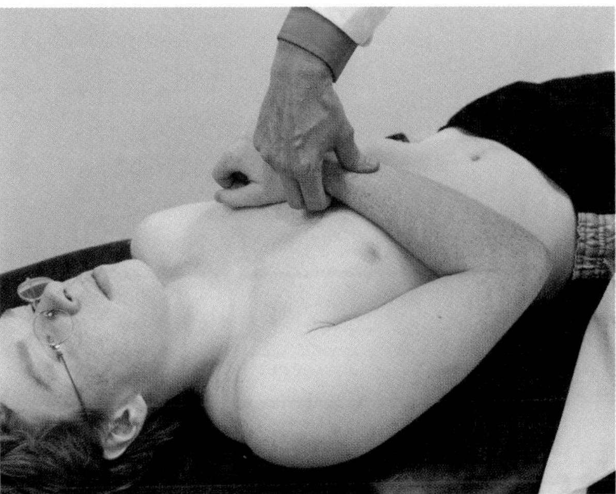

FIGURE 11-3 Respiratory distraction technique with the patient's arm placed over the chest allowing the provider to appreciate rise and fall of the chest.

Note the patient's position of comfort. Is the patient sitting calmly or is he/she working to breathe? Does the patient avoid lying down, sitting up even though the top of the bed is in a flat position, in an effort to keep fluids in the lungs at the bases instead of pooling throughout all lobes as would occur if supine?

DOCUMENTATION

- Patient supine with head of bed elevated to 60 degrees without respiratory distress.

VITAL SIGNS: RESPIRATORY RATE AND RHYTHM

Assess the rate of respiration. Observe the rise and fall of the chest wall, counting the number of breaths per minute. Normal respiratory rate is from 12 to 20 breaths per minute. Patients may inadvertently alter their breathing pattern when they know an observer is watching them breathe. One technique to distract patients is to palpate the radial artery, holding the patient's wrist against the chest while looking at your watch (see **FIGURE 11-3**). While you can assess pulse at the same time, this technique allows you to first count the respiratory rate, feeling and seeing the chest rise with peripheral vision. If you are unable to observe respirations with this technique, you can either auscultate the trachea and count the number of breaths or put your stethoscope on the sternum, feel the rise and fall of the chest wall, and count the respiratory rate.

Determine the respiratory rhythm.

DOCUMENTATION

- Respirations—12 bpm, regular rhythm, inspiration equals expiration.

INTEGUMENTARY

Observe the patient's skin and look for abnormal signs such as cyanosis, pallor, erythema, or cherry redness. Cyanosis is more easily detected around the patient's lips, where the epithelium is thin, and distally in the nail beds of the fingers and toes. Pallor, a sign of possible anemia or hypoperfusion, should be sought by observing the palpebral conjunctiva by everting the lower eyelid and by assessing the skin and the nail beds.

Fingers and toes may also reveal chronic pulmonary or cardiovascular problems manifested through clubbing. Clubbing of the nail is seen by loss of the normal angle of the nail and thickening of the distal portions of the finger (see **FIGURE 11-4**). Diffuse cherry redness is associated with carbon monoxide poisoning.

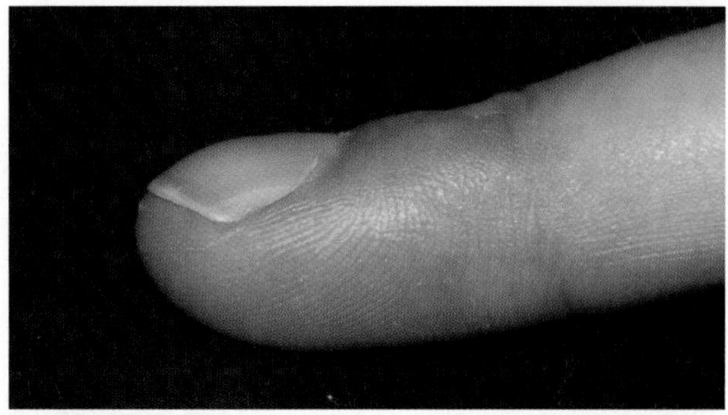

FIGURE 11-4 Clubbing of the nail.

DOCUMENTATION

- Skin pink without cyanosis, pallor, or erythema. Extremities without clubbing.

NECK

Moving caudally, observe for tracheal deviation. Normally the trachea is midline; however, a deviated trachea suggests pathology. A trachea that deviates *toward* the side of pathology can be caused by atelectasis, pneumothorax, agenesis of lung, pneumonectomy, or pleural fibrosis. A deviated trachea that is *away* from the pathologic side can be caused by tension pneumothorax, pleural effusion, large chest wall mass, or a tracheal mass. In emergent situations with respiratory distress, a deviated trachea suggests acute pathology such as pneumothorax. If tracheal deviation is found on general examination with nonurgent presentation, mass effect is more likely.

DOCUMENTATION

- Neck—Trachea midline

CHEST

Inspection of the chest wall requires that the patient be properly exposed. Provide a gown and ask the patient to remove his/her shirt. Female patients may be allowed to keep their brassiere on, because of the importance of preserving the dignity of the patient. When ready to inspect the chest, ask the patient to lower the gown. **FIGURE 11-5A** and **FIGURE 11-5B** show the interior anatomy of the chest. Observe for intercostal retractions and for symmetrical rise and fall

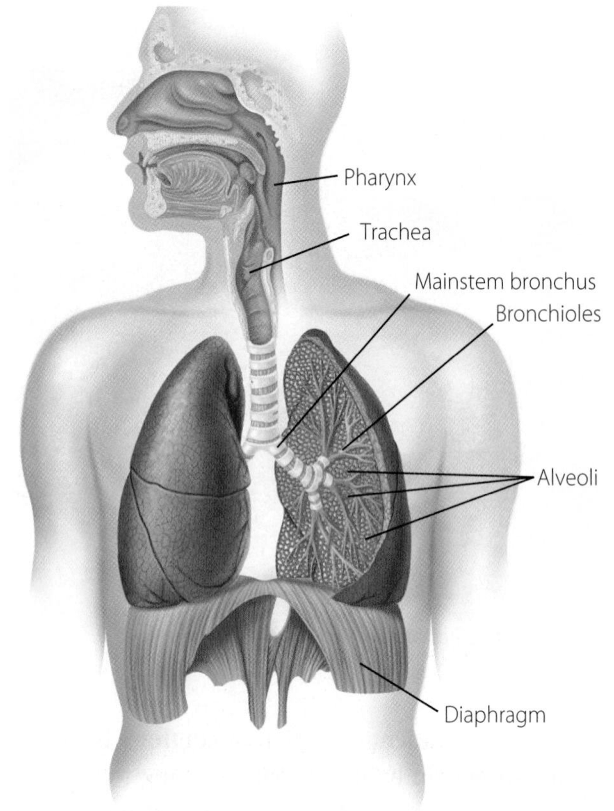

FIGURE 11-5A Diagram of chest anatomy.
© leonello calvetti/Shutterstock, Inc.

© Dim Dimich/ShutterStock, Inc.

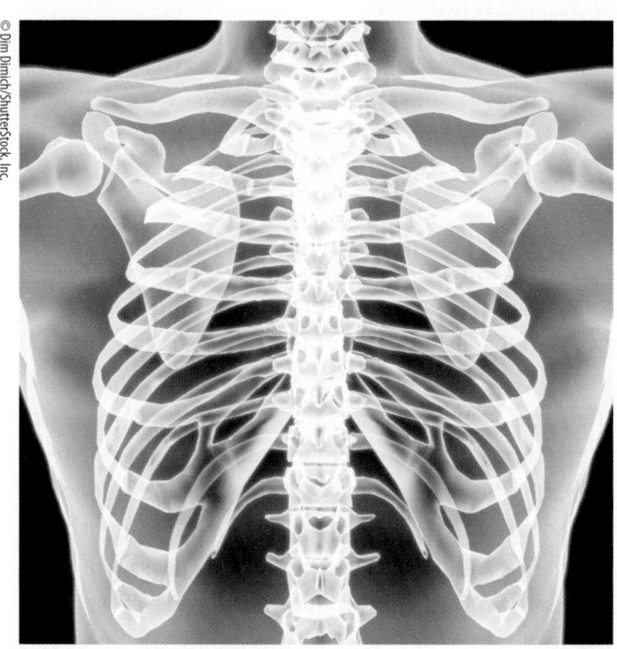

FIGURE 11-5B X-ray of chest anatomy.

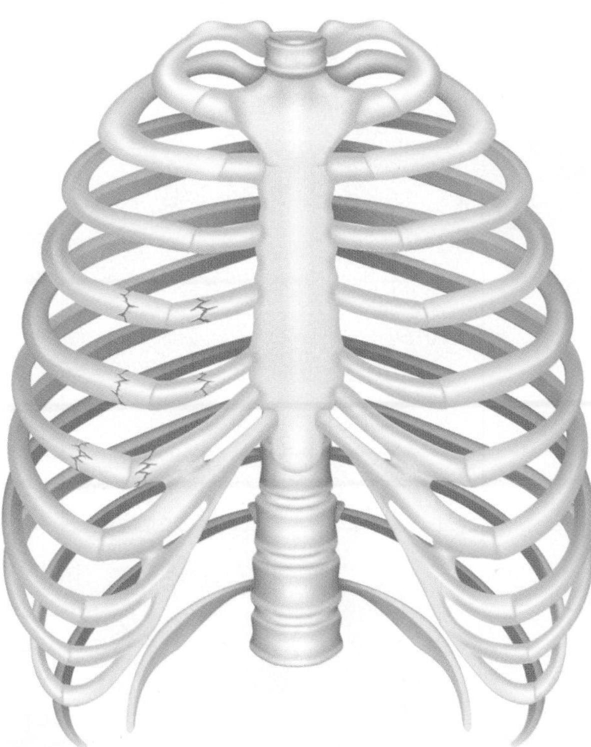

FIGURE 11-6 A flail chest involves three ribs each fractured at two locations, allowing inward retraction with inspiration.
© Oleksii Natykach/ShutterStock, Inc.

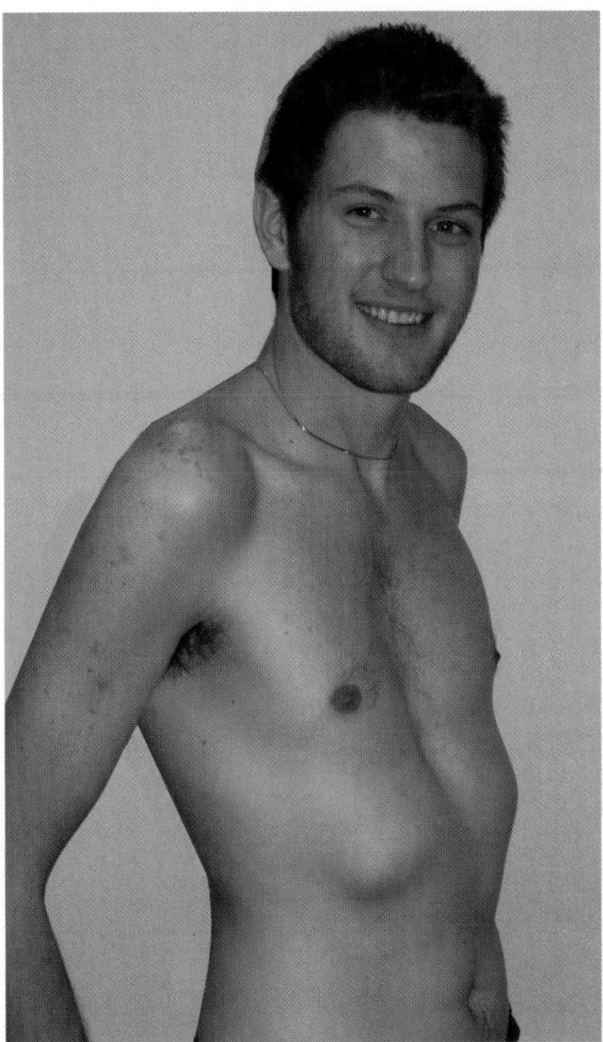

FIGURE 11-7 Pectus excavatum.

of the chest wall. Asymmetrical rise and fall of the chest wall may suggest respiratory pathology, such as a pneumothorax, tumor mass, phrenic nerve damage, or rib dysfunction. Trauma to the chest wall may result in **flail chest**, the paradoxical movement of the chest wall, retracting inward during respiration instead of rising, as a result of three more ribs being fractured at two locations each (see **FIGURE 11-6**).

Chest wall deformities such as pectus excavatum (see **FIGURE 11-7**), pectus carinatum (see **FIGURE 11-8**), and bony deformities such as rotational scoliotic changes (see **FIGURE 11-9**) should be noted. Rachitic rosary are bony knobs at the costochondral joints found in patients with calcium deficiency, such as seen with hypoparathyroidism or rickets. The name is derived from their having the appearance of large beads in the form of a rosary.

Note the width of the chest wall laterally from the chest wall just below the axilla, side to side. Compare this to the anterior-posterior (AP) depth, the distance between the front of the chest wall and the back. Normally the lateral width is greater than AP depth, with 1½ to 2 AP depths equal to 1 lateral width or a 1.5:1 or 2:1 **AP:lateral ratio** (see **FIGURE 11-10**).

11-1 When the AP depth increases, it nears the width of lateral diameter resulting in a decreased, or 1:1 ratio, commonly referred to as a barrel chest (see **FIGURE 11-11**), suggesting chronic respiratory pathology such as COPD.

Flail chest: paradoxical movement of the chest wall, retracting inward during respiration instead of rising, as a result of three or more ribs being fractured at two locations each

AP:lateral ratio: comparison of depth to width of the chest wall

DOCUMENTATION

- Chest symmetrical without deformity. 2:1 AP:lateral ratio.

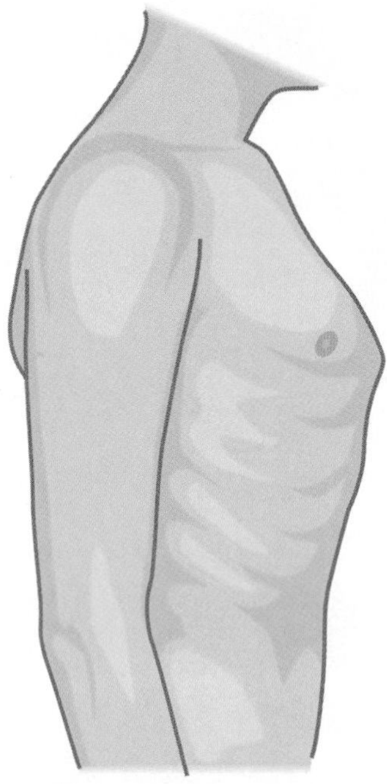

FIGURE 11-8 Pectus carinatum.

Adapted from: American Academy of Orthopaedic Surgeons (AAOS). *First Responder: Your First Response in Emergency Care.* Sudbury, MA: Jones and Bartlett Learning; 2007: 344.

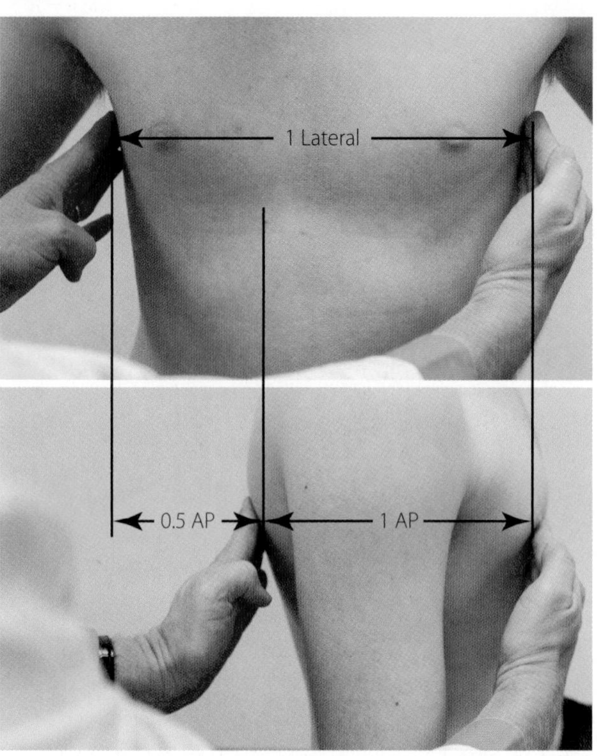

FIGURE 11-10 1.5:1 AP:lateral ratio, where one and one half depths front to back of the chest is required to equal one width from side to side.

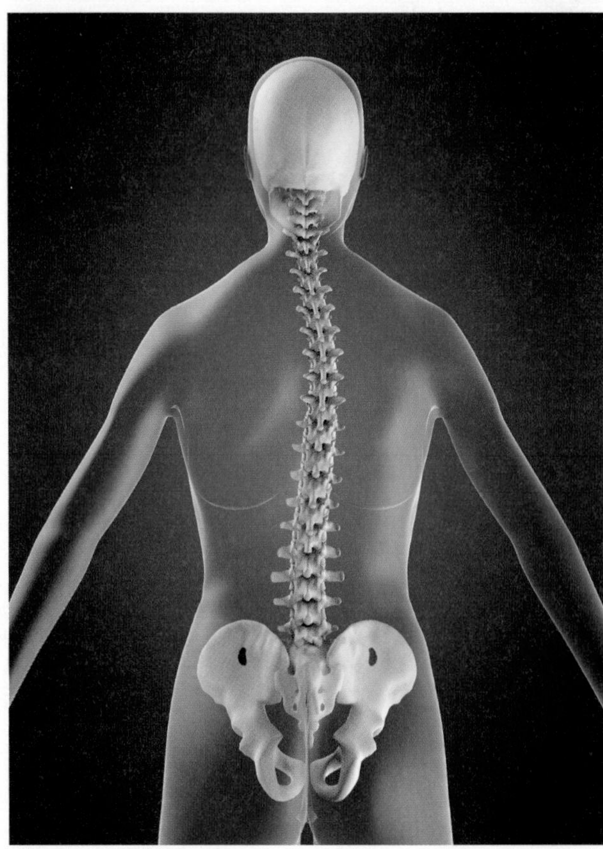

FIGURE 11-9 Scoliosis.

© Sebastian Kaulitzki/ShutterStock, Inc.

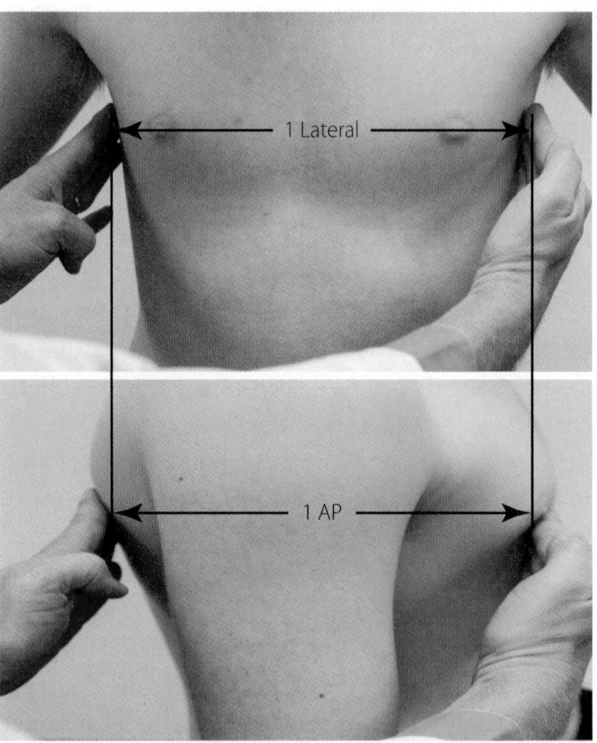

FIGURE 11-11 1:1 AP:lateral ratio, also known as a barrel chest, with the depth of the chest increasing to equal the width of the chest.

Auscultation

TECHNIQUE

Auscultation of the respiratory system is most commonly completed with the patient in the seated position. It should always be completed on bare skin and never through clothing, as fine abnormalities may be missed.

Place the stethoscope in your ears with the earpieces angled forward, since this conforms to the natural anatomy of the ear canal. Use the diaphragm of the stethoscope with the head held by the lateral edges between index and middle fingers. Instruct the patient to take slow, deep breaths through the mouth, as nasal breathing creates distortion of transmitted sounds. At each area of auscultation, be sure to listen throughout the entire respiratory cycle, complete inspiration followed by complete exhalation. Patients will breathe more rapidly than their natural rate if you move your stethoscope from one area to the next too quickly.

11-2 Anteriorly, start at the supraclavicular level to assess the apex of the lung. Then move symmetrically to the opposite side to allow for comparison of upper lobe to upper lobe (see **FIGURE 11-12**). Move inferiorly to approximately the 2nd intercostal space (ICS) in the midclavicular line (MCL) and again compare side to side. Move inferiorly to the 4th or 5th ICS MCL and repeat the side-to-side comparison. Do not move down one side of the chest then back up to the top and down the other side, as this does not allow for detection of small differences between comparable lobes.

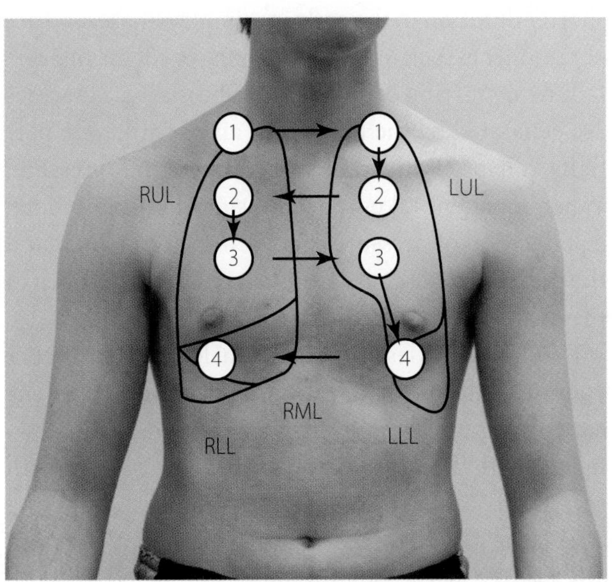

FIGURE 11-12 Anterior areas of respiratory auscultation.

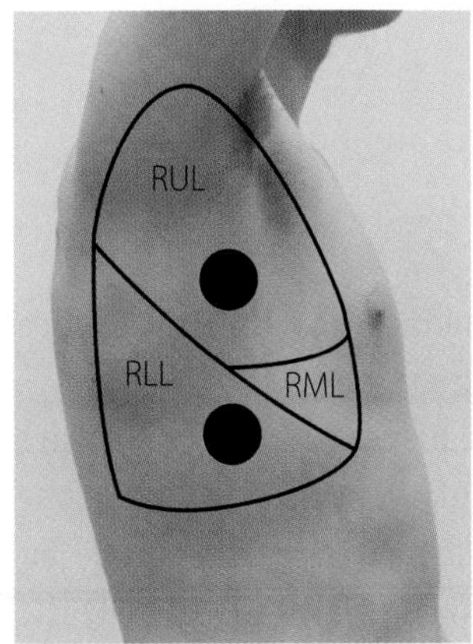

FIGURE 11-13A Right lateral areas of auscultation.

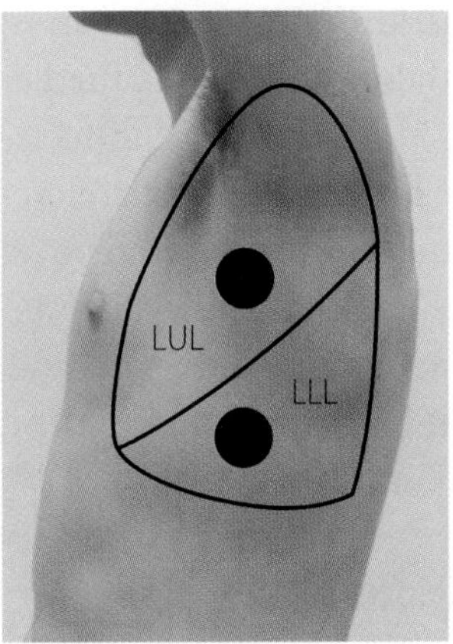

FIGURE 11-13B Left lateral areas of auscultation.

Ask the patient to slightly lift the arms away from the sides, and auscultate in the midaxillary line at the level of the inferior axilla on one side, then move to the opposite side at the same level (see **FIGURES 11-13A** and **11-13B**). Remaining on the same side in the midaxillary line, drop down to the level of the xiphoid, then compare to the opposite side, completing the lateral examination.

Begin posterior auscultation superiorly, with the stethoscope between the scapula and spine. Complete three levels of auscultation, starting superiorly and moving symmetrically side to side at each level before moving inferiorly to the next level (see **FIGURE 11-14**).

A minimum of three levels anteriorly, two levels laterally, and three levels posteriorly should be assessed.

DOCUMENTATION

- Clear to auscultation throughout.

RESPIRATORY SOUNDS

Respiratory sounds are generated by the turbulence of air as it moves through the large and small airways and the vibrations that it causes. The vibrations are transmitted to the lung tissue and thoracic wall to the chest surface, where they can be assessed through auscultation of the chest wall. Respiratory sounds can be categorized as either basic or adventitious (or extra) lung sounds. Each of these categories is further subgrouped, as shown in FIGURE 11-15. **Basic breath sounds** are created by the movement of air over the corresponding area of the respiratory tract and include **tracheal**, **bronchial**, **bronchovesicular**, and **vesicular breath sounds**.

Basic breath sounds: lung sounds created by movement of air through the respiratory tract, including tracheal, bronchial, broncho-vesicular, and vesicular

Tracheal breath sounds: the sound of air movement heard over the trachea

Bronchial breath sounds: the sound of air movement heard over large airways

Bronchovesicular breath sounds: the sound of air movement heard over transitional areas between the larger airways and peripheral areas of alveoli

Vesicular breath sounds: the sound of air movement heard over peripheral lung fields dense with alveoli

Adventitious lung sounds: added sounds superimposed on the basic breath sounds

Crackles: short, nonmusical, high-pitched, discontinuous breath sounds that can be described as explosive or popping in nature; thought to be the sudden opening of small airways and alveoli during inspiration that were previously collapsed due to fluid or exudate

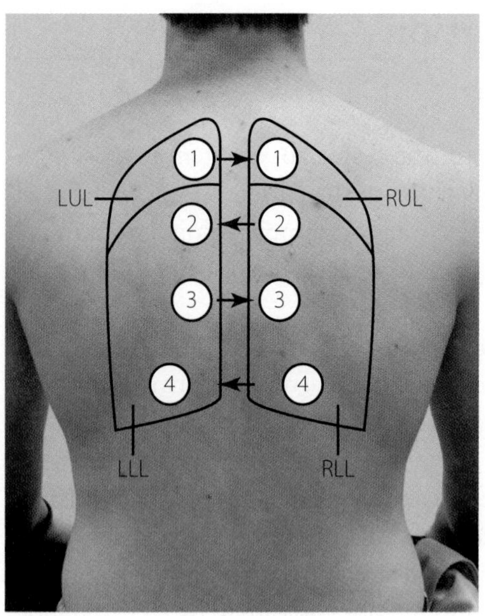

FIGURE 11-14 Posterior areas of auscultation.

Adventitious Lung Sounds

Adventitious lung sounds are *added sounds* superimposed on the normal breath sounds. The most common are crackles, rhonchi, wheezes, and rubs.

Crackles.

Crackles are short, nonmusical, high-pitched, discontinuous breath sounds that can be described as explosive or popping in nature, and are heard mostly in the inspiratory phase. Crackles sound very similar to fresh wood logs on an open fire or the opening of a Velcro strap. The sound can be imitated by holding approximately a quarter-inch of hair and auscultating while rubbing the ends of the hairs against the diaphragm.

The mechanical basis of crackles is thought to be the sudden opening of small airways and alveoli during inspiration that were previously collapsed due to fluid or exudate and can be heard as a "popping sound." Crackles are more commonly heard during inspiration but can be detected less frequently in expiration. They are also more commonly associated with pathology but occasionally can be heard in the bases of normal lungs after either maximal expiration or sustained recumbent position.

Crackles can be categorized as either fine or coarse. Fine crackles are differentiated from coarse crackles by being of higher pitch, softer volume, and shorter duration in the early inspiratory phase, and are commonly associated with pulmonary edema of heart failure or scarring of pulmonary fibrosis. Late crackles are generated by the peripheral airways that are partially collapsed due to increased interstitial pressure. When a patient takes a deep inspiration, the sudden equalization of pressures between the bronchioli and the peripheral airways results in the snapping-open of the distal airways, resulting in crackles.

Coarse crackles are generally of lower pitch, louder volume, and longer duration, and are heard in the early inspiratory phase. They are caused by air flowing through the larger airways, which are covered with secretions, and are comparable to a harsh bubbling sound, or a Velcro-like sound. These can be generally cleared with coughing and are associated with bronchitis.

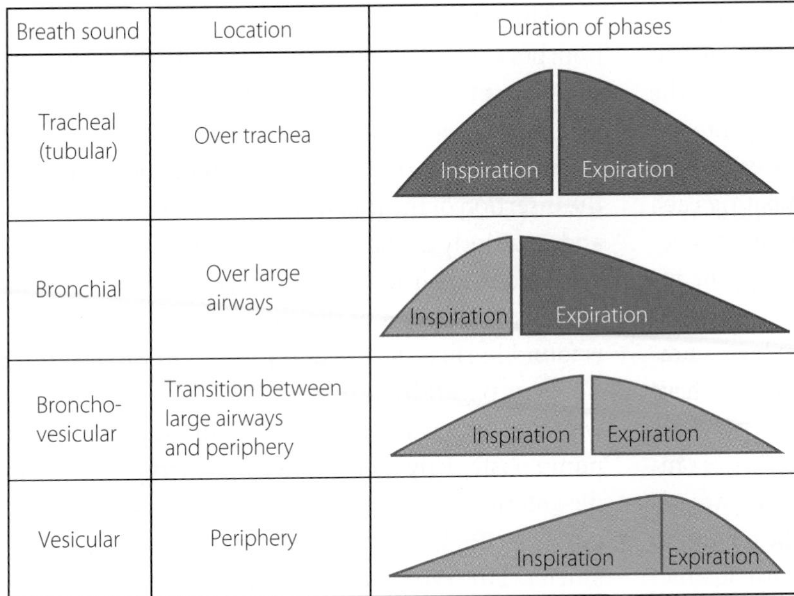

Breath sound	Location	Duration of phases
Tracheal (tubular)	Over trachea	Inspiration / Expiration
Bronchial	Over large airways	Inspiration / Expiration
Broncho-vesicular	Transition between large airways and periphery	Inspiration / Expiration
Vesicular	Periphery	Inspiration / Expiration

FIGURE 11-15 Types of basic breath sounds.

Crackles may also reflect atelectasis, inflammation, and infection, as with bronchitis, bronchiectasis, pneumonia, or acute respiratory distress syndrome.

Rhonchi.

Rhonchi are coarse, low-pitched, continuous sounds with a snoring-like quality, produced on exhalation. The sounds are due to secretions in the bronchial airways and usually clear with coughing. Conditions associated with rhonchi are COPD, bronchitis, bronchospasm, inflammation, or tumor obstructing the larger airways.

Wheezes.

Wheezes are high-pitched, with a somewhat musical quality. They are heard during expiration or both inspiration and expiration when airways are constricted or partially obstructed. Some pathologies that may cause wheezes are bronchospasm, asthma, COPD, and bronchitis.

Pleural Friction Rubs.

Pleural friction rubs occur when inflamed visceral and parietal pleura rub together, producing a harsh scratching or crinkling sound. Pleural friction rubs can result from many etiologies including pleurisy, neoplasm, pulmonary infarction, pneumonia, asbestosis, thoracic surgery, tuberculosis, or systemic lupus erythematosus.

Stridor.

Stridor is a high-pitched sound that is often audible without the aid of a stethoscope. It is generally heard only in inspiration and should alert the provider to the possibility of a medical emergency. Stridor suggests the presence of obstruction or stenosis. Common causes of stridor are epiglottic or tracheal obstruction, often by a foreign body. Other causes include whooping cough, neoplasm, cysts, laryngeal inflammation, diphtheria, and tracheomalacia. Stridor heard in exhalation suggests a lower airway obstruction, most commonly from a foreign body.

DOCUMENTATION

- Auscultation—End expiratory wheezes bilateral lower lobes posteriorly.

Palpation

Palpation of the chest wall focuses on structure and function.

STRUCTURE

Chest pain is a common presenting complaint. Most important is the differentiation between visceral cardiac pain associated with acute coronary syndrome, and musculoskeletal pain, which is often reproducible. Pain from herpetic zoster is also commonly encountered.

Again, exposure of the chest is required. Begin palpation of the chest by using the pads of the four

Rhonchi: coarse, low-pitched, continuous sounds of snoring-like quality, produced on exhalation due to secretions in the bronchial airways; often found in COPD, bronchitis, bronchospasm, inflammation, or tumor obstructing the larger airways

Wheezes: high-pitched, musical sound heard mostly during expiration as a result of constricted or partially obstructed airways; often found in bronchospasm, asthma, COPD, and bronchitis

Pleural friction rubs: sound occurring when inflamed visceral and parietal pleura rub together, producing a harsh scratching or crinkling sound; often found with conditions such as pleurisy, neoplasm, and pulmonary infarction

Stridor: a high-pitched sound, often audible without the aid of a stethoscope that is generally heard only in inspiration; should alert the provider to the possibility of obstruction or stenosis of a large airway and should be considered a medical emergency

Bucket handle motion: lateral, cephalad motion of the ribs that occurs during inspiration and can be visualized as the handle of a bucket being lifted with attachments posteriorly at the insertion of the transverse processes and vertebrae and anteriorly at the sternum

Pump handle motion: motion of the ribs which can be visualized as the spine representing a pump posteriorly with the sternum acting as the handle anteriorly. As inspiration occurs, the handle of the pump is lifted, resulting in an increase in the AP diameter

Caliber motion: the motion of ribs 11 and 12 where inspiration results in an increasing angle like the motion of calibers due to the lack of anterior attachment

fingers of both hands simultaneously, applying enough pressure to contact the bony structure of the chest wall. Divide the chest into anterior, lateral, and posterior sections, methodically palpating each section, starting at the most superior aspect and working to the inferior rib cage.

11-3 If the patient has a complaint of chest pain, have him/her locate the area as precisely as possible and reserve the area indicated for last. Once the area is reached, approach light palpation using only one hand with advancing levels of pressure to assess for reproducibility. Begin with the thought of palpation of the skin level only. As the patient tolerates the exam, advance the amount of pressure. Next palpate the subcutaneous tissue level and then the surface of the rib cage, and then visualize and apply enough pressure to gently move the bony structures inward. Finally, if the patient has tolerated the exam without reproduction of the pain, one hand may be placed over the area of pain with the other hand on the opposite side of the thorax, and slow, gentle pressure applied with both hands. If no pain has occurred, it is considered nonreproducible.

DOCUMENTATION

- Palpation without tenderness.

FUNCTION

The chest wall functions as a protector of thoracic and abdominal organs and as a means of respiration, where muscle contraction expands the chest wall, aiding inspiration. Rib motion during respiration is assessed in three sections:

- Ribs 1 to 3
- Ribs 4 to 10
- Ribs 11 to 12

Three types of rib motion occur during respiration: bucket handle, pump handle, and caliber motion.

Bucket handle motion: The chest wall can be visualized as a bucket, the handles of which are represented by the ribs with attachments posteriorly at the insertion of the transverse processes and vertebrae and anteriorly at the sternum. As inspiration occurs, the handles are lifted, moving outward and increasing the lateral diameter of the chest. This type of motion is found in ribs 1 to 10 but is greatest in ribs 4 to 10.

Pump handle motion: This motion of the chest wall can be visualized as the spine representing a pump posteriorly with the sternum acting as the handle anteriorly. As inspiration occurs, the handle of the pump is lifted, resulting in an increase in the AP diameter. This type of motion is greatest in ribs 1 to 3.

Caliber motion: Ribs 11 and 12 lack anterior attachment and move with caliberlike motion during respiration. With inspiration, the open angle of the calibers increases. The opposite occurs with expiration, with the caliber narrowing the open angle.

Group Motion Assessment

Advise the patient that you will be assessing the motion of his/her ribs, and assist the patient to the supine position. Chest wall motion is assessed for symmetrical expansion in each of the three rib groups.

For anterior assessment, the provider stands to the right side of the patient, facing the patient's head. For group motion in ribs 1 to 3, place the fingers of both hands on the upper chest with the fingertips touching the clavicles and the edges of the index fingers aligned along the edges of the sternum (see **FIGURES 11-16A** and **11-16B**). Ask the patient to take slow, deep breaths. Assess pump handle motion with symmetry of anterior rise as the primary motion in this area, as well as symmetry of slight lateral displacement of bucket handle motion.

Group motion in ribs 4 to 10 is assessed at two levels. The provider abducts the thumbs and places the radial aspect of the index fingers against the chest wall in the third intercostal spaces laterally as the thumbs touch centered at the midsternal line. The palms may lie flat against the chest for male patients (see **FIGURE 11-17**) but should be lifted off the chest for female patients (see **FIGURE 11-18**). Ask the patient to take deep breaths, and watch for symmetrical separation of the

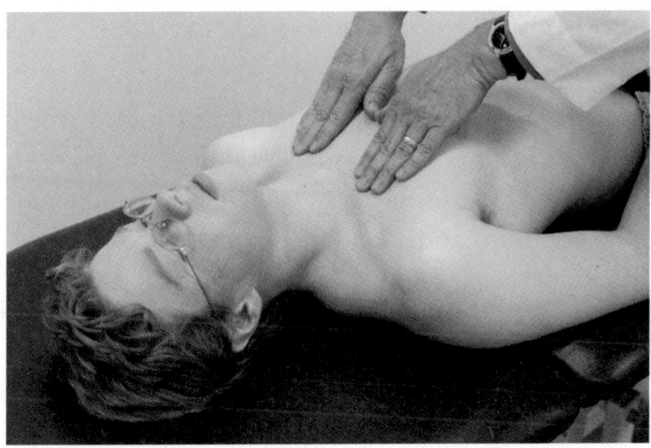

FIGURE 11-16A Hand placement for pump handle motion assessment of the anterior ribs 1 to 3.

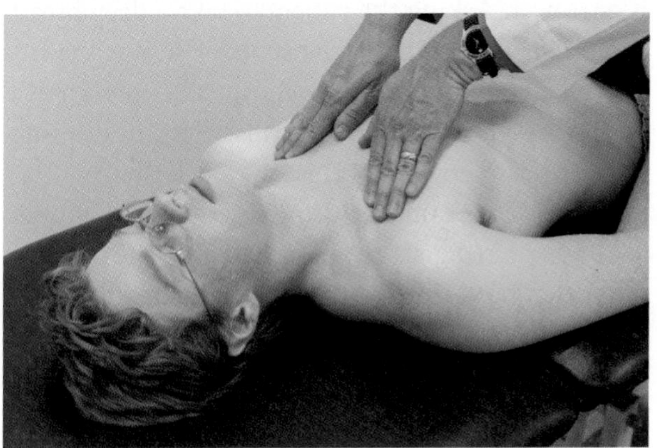

FIGURE 11-16B Hand placement for bucket handle motion assessment of the anterior ribs 1 to 3.

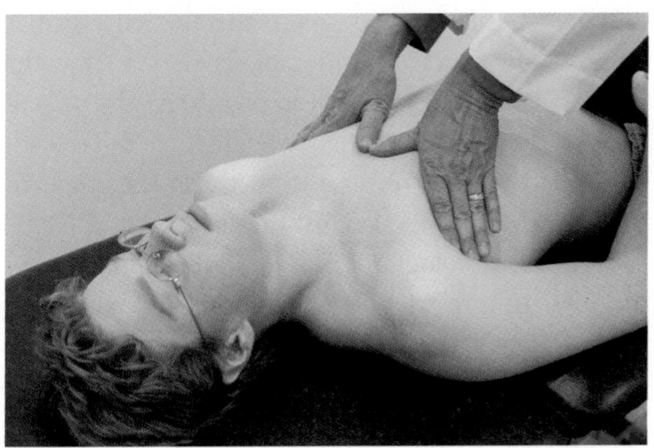

FIGURE 11-17 Superior hand placement for motion assessment of the anterior ribs 4 to 10 in the male patient.

thumbs midline for the primary bucket handle motion of this section and the anterior lift of pump handle motion.

Using the same hand formation, the provider moves the hands so that the thumbs now align just

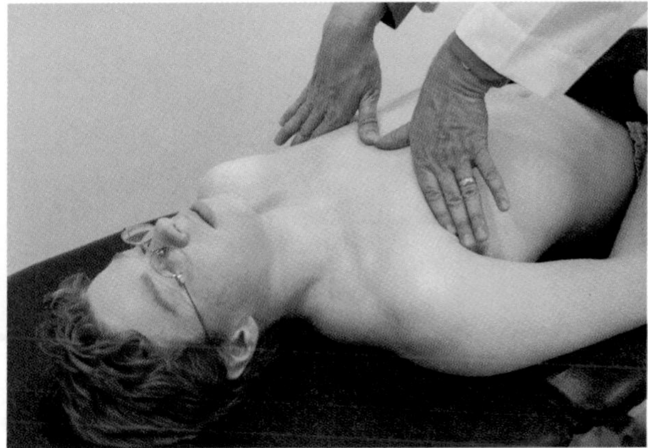

FIGURE 11-18 Superior hand placement for motion assessment of the anterior ribs 4 to 10 in the female patient with palms lifted off the chest.

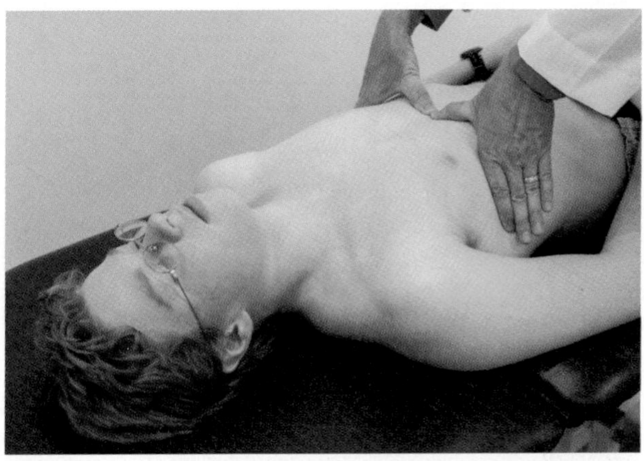

FIGURE 11-19 Inferior hand placement for motion assessment of the anterior ribs 4 to 10.

above the xiphoid process (see **FIGURE 11-19**). In the female patient, hand placement should be just under the breasts. If needed, ask the patient with large breasts to lift them to allow proper hand placement.

An alternative hand placement for female patients is to place the ulnar aspect of the hands vertically approximately 2 cm from each side of the sternum with the fingertips aligned with the clavicle (see **FIGURE 11-20**).

If group motion shows asymmetry, additional levels should be assessed to more finitely define the level of motion dysfunction.

Posteriorly, the process should be repeated with the same hand positioning, thumbs touching over the spinous processes (see **FIGURE 11-21**). Group screening should be completed minimally at three levels, such as

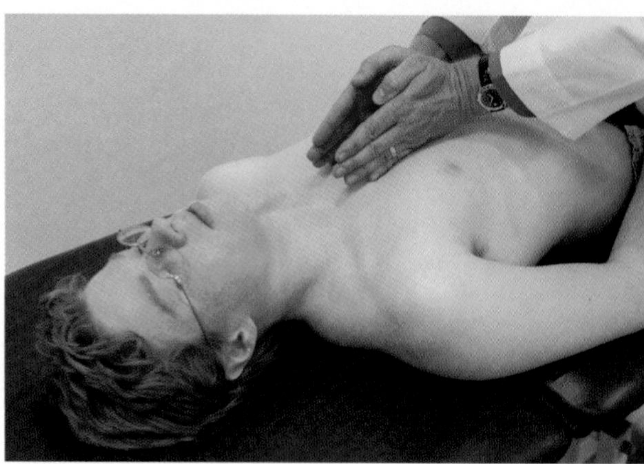

FIGURE 11-20 Alternative hand placement for motion assessment of the anterior ribs 4 to 10 in the female patient.

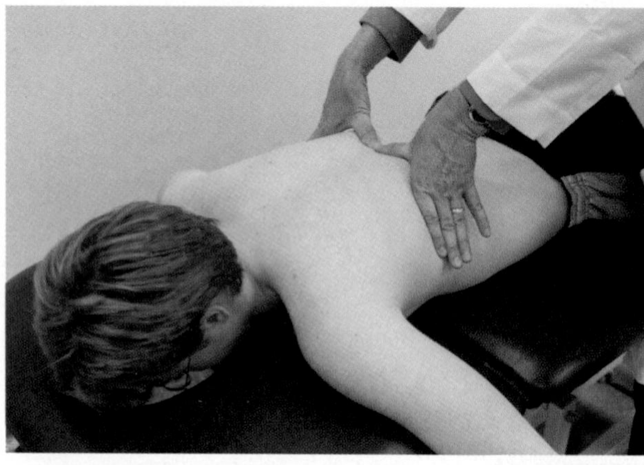

FIGURE 11-21 Hand placement for motion assessment of the posterior ribs.

T2, T7, and T10. Finally, assess the caliber motion of ribs 11 and 12.

11-4 When restriction to group motion is found, assessment of area for rib dysfunction requires a more detailed approach.

Rib Dysfunction

Rib dysfunction occurs when the ribs become restricted in either inhalation or exhalation. Rib restrictions most commonly occur in association with rotation of the vertebrae. Patients may complain of pain, tightness, or the feeling of an inability to breathe in or out completely. To diagnose dysfunction, each rib must be palpated separately, comparing size of the intercostal spaces.

Rib dysfunction: restriction of rib motion in inspiration or expiration

Inhalation Restriction/Exhalation Dysfunction.

An inhalation restriction should be suspected when, on group testing, the provider encounters an area with diminished rise of the chest wall, bucket handle motion, or pump handle motion. Finding the section dysfunction, the ribs and ICSs are palpated individually with bilateral comparison. With an inhalation restriction, the uppermost rib is stuck in a downward, exhalation position. The ICS immediately above the dysfunctional rib is wider than the ICSs above it on the ipsilateral side and the corresponding contralateral ICS. The ICS immediately below the rib dysfunction is narrower. Asking the patient to take a deep breath accentuates widening of the superior ICS as the ribs above expand and move cephalad. The inferior ICS becomes even narrower as the ribs below the dysfunctional rib jam upward against the stuck rib.

11-5 For example, during anterior group motion testing at the midchest level, the provider notes that both sides of the chest fall equally during exhalation but the left side fails to rise as far in both bucket and pump handle motion with inspiration. Upon asking the patient to hold his/her breath briefly at the end of expiration, the 3rd ICS on the left is wider than the 1st and 2nd ICSs above it as well as the 3rd R ICS. The 4th L ICS is narrower than the ICSs above and the 4th R ICS. This suggests that the 3rd left rib is stuck in a downward position of exhalation. Now the patient is asked to take a deep breath. As the patient does so, the 3rd L ICS widens even further and the 4th L ICS becomes narrower as the 4th rib rises upward but is unable to do so against the 3rd rib.

The terminology may be somewhat confusing as an inhalation restriction is also called an exhalation dysfunction. The provider should think:

- The rib is **restricted** from **inhalation** = inhalation restriction
- The rib is **dysfunctional** being **stuck in a position of exhalation** = exhalation dysfunction

Therefore for the case described, we have a L 3rd rib inhalation restriction/exhalation dysfunction.

Exhalation Restriction.

The opposite is true for exhalation restrictions. When the provider detects an area on group motion testing that fails to fall on exhalation, the lowermost rib is stuck in an upward, inhalation position. The ICS immediately below the dysfunctional rib is wider than the ICSs below it on the ipsilateral side and the corresponding contralateral ICS. The ICS immediately above the rib dysfunction is narrower. Asking the patient to exhale completely accentuates widening of the ICS immediately inferior to the dysfunctional rib as the ribs below are drawn downward and together by the intercostal muscle contractions. The ICSs above become even narrower as the ribs above the dysfunctional rib jam downward against the rib, stuck in an upward position.

11-6 For example, during anterior group motion testing at the midchest level, the provider notes that both sides of the chest rise equally during inhalation but the right side fails to fall as far in both bucket and pump handle motion with expiration. Upon asking the patient to hold his/her breath briefly at the end of expiration, the 4th ICS on the right is wider than the 5th and 6th ICSs below it as well as the 4th L ICS. The 3rd R ICS is narrower than the ICSs below and the 3rd L ICS. This suggests that the 3rd right rib is stuck in an upward position of inhalation. Now the patient is asked to take a deep breath, attempting to exhale or empty the lungs completely. As the patient does so, the 4th R ICS widens even further and the 3rd R ICS becomes narrower as the 2nd rib falls downward but is unable to do so against the stuck 3rd rib. The diagnosis is 3rd R rib exhalation restriction/inhalation dysfunction.

The provider should think:

- The rib is **restricted** from **exhalation** = exhalation restriction
- The rib is **dysfunctional** being **stuck in a position of inhalation** = inhalation dysfunction

DOCUMENTATION

- Palpation—Group inspiration restriction right mid thorax with R 3rd rib exhalation restriction/inhalation dysfunction.

TACTILE FREMITUS

Tactile fremitus is the transmission of sound from the bronchial tree to the chest wall as the patient speaks and is assessed by the provider through the palpation of the vibratory sensation transmitted through the chest wall. To visualize the process, imagine a road that runs from the large airway through the alveoli to the chest wall (see **FIGURE 11-22**).

Tactile fremitus: the transmission of sound from the bronchial tree to the chest wall as the patient speaks, which can be assessed by the provider through palpation of the vibratory sensation

11-7 To assess tactile fremitus, the patient is asked to say the word "ninety-nine" while the provider palpates the chest wall with the ulnar aspect of the hand, which has higher sensitivity in detecting vibratory sensations (see **FIGURE 11-23**). Simultaneous side-to-side approach over the same areas for auscultation is used anteriorly, laterally, and posteriorly, with the patient repeating "ninety-nine" at each level. The provider is attempting to detect areas of increased or decreased vibration between the two sides being tested.

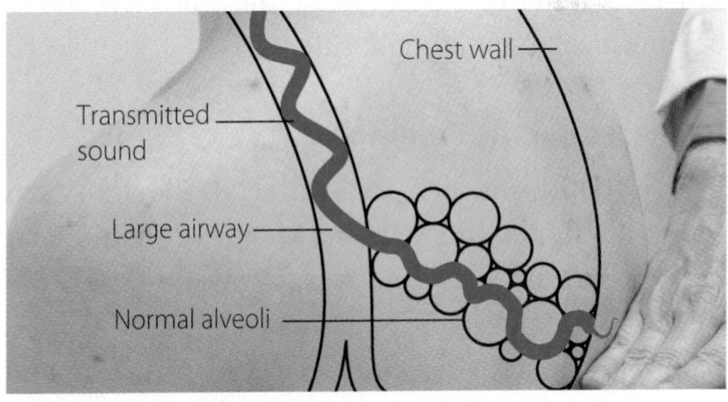

FIGURE 11-22 Tactile fremitus: palpation of vibratory sensation created as the patient speaks as the sound is transmitted through the airways to the provider's hand placed against the chest wall.

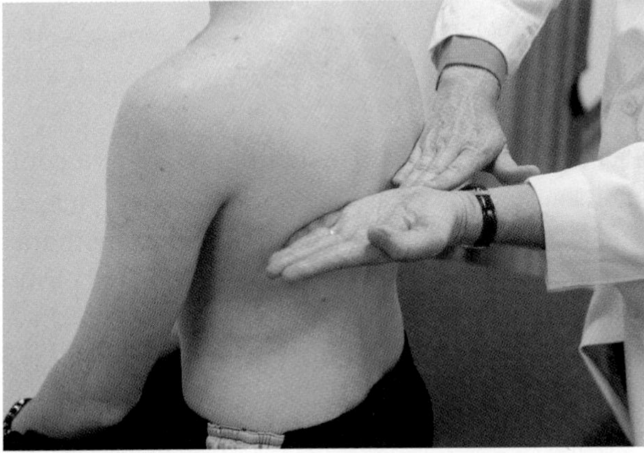

FIGURE 11-23 Bilateral comparison of tactile fremitus assessing one level at a time.

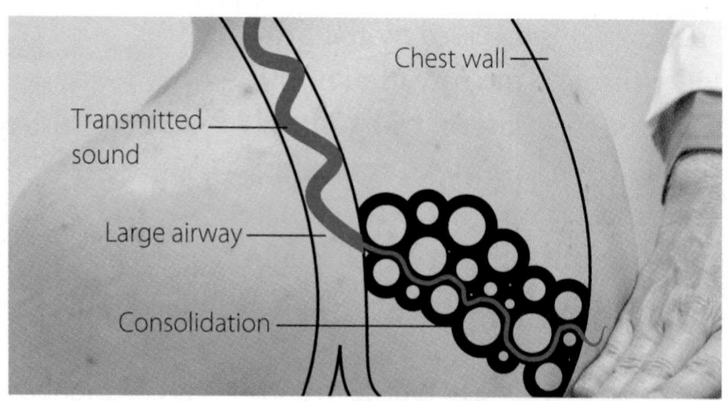

FIGURE 11-24 Increased tactile fremitus as thickened alveoli increase transmission of the vibration.

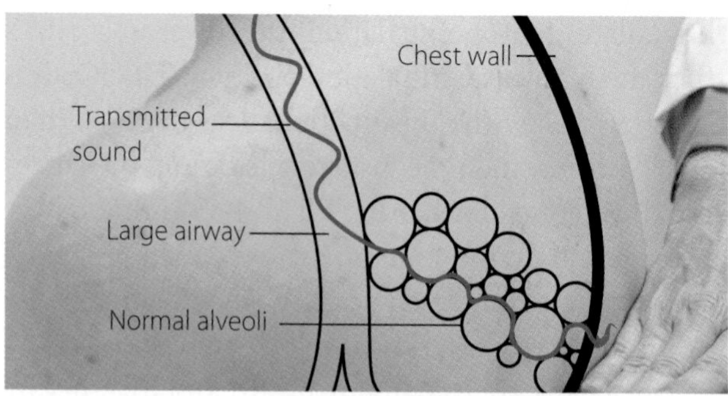

FIGURE 11-25 Decreased tactile fremitus as a wall of fluid or air impedes transmission of the vibration to the provider's hand.

To appreciate this, place the ulnar aspects of your hands along the anterior 4th ICS with your fingertips touching. Say "ninety-nine" several times. In which hand could you detect the greater vibration? You should have detected less vibration in the left hand. Why? Tactile fremitus is decreased in the left side due to decreased transmission of vibration through the heart. If you have dextrocardia, the vibration would be diminished on the right side.

Increased Tactile Fremitus

Tactile fremitus is increased with consolidation such as found in pneumonia. Increase in transmission occurs as a result of sound waves traveling more efficiently through solids than through air. We can picture the road being widened as inflammation and fluids accumulate within the alveoli, providing easier passage of the vibrations. In the case of right middle lobe pneumonia, the provider would detect increased tactile fremitus (vibration) over the right middle lobe (see **FIGURE 11-24**).

Decreased Tactile Fremitus

Pleural effusion and pneumothorax are two common causes of decrease in tactile fremitus. This occurs over areas of pleural effusion or pneumothorax as the space between the parietal and visceral pleura is filled with fluid or air, creating a wall that slows the transmission of vibration. In these cases, as the sound travels along the road, a wall is encountered, slowing transmission, as the vibration no longer has a road to travel on but must work its way through the wall (see **FIGURE 11-25**).

DOCUMENTATION

- Increased tactile fremitus R middle lobe anterior and laterally.

Percussion

Percussion is a technique to assess resonance, dullness, and hyperresonance of the chest wall cavity, as in the beating of a drum. Normal lungs should have a resonance when percussing with air throughout the lung tissues. Solid organs, tumors, and areas of consolidation or fluids will have dullness to percussion. COPD with air trapping and pneumothorax would percuss with hyperresonance.

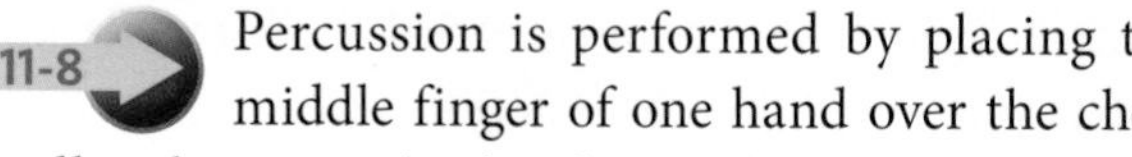

Percussion is performed by placing the middle finger of one hand over the chest wall and tapping the distal interphalangeal joint with the middle finger of the opposite hand. It is important to tap with the action at the wrist and not with the elbow. Tap quickly about three or four times in a row, lifting the tapping finger after each strike to avoid dampening of the sound. The order of percussion should be performed at the same levels and in the same manner as auscultation, starting at the top and comparing one side to the other at the same level before moving downward to the next level. Posteriorly it is important to stay medial, superiorly moving laterally as you work inferiorly to avoid percussion over the scapulae.

Pneumonias and pleural effusions can be thought of as solids and liquids that take up space where air was once found. Percussion over these areas will be less drumlike, with diminished resonance or dullness to percussion. With pneumothorax or air trapping with COPD, there is excess air in the chest. Anytime there is increased air in a container, on percussion it will sound more drumlike or hyperresonant on percussion.

DOCUMENTATION

- Dullness to percussion R middle lobe anteriorly and laterally.

Special Testing

CONSOLIDATION

Consolidation of the respiratory tissues refers to the process of solidification where the lung tissue becomes less airlike through engorgement of the lung tissues with fluids and cells of inflammation. Bronchophony, egophony, and whispered pectoriloquy are three special techniques employed to detect areas of consolidation commonly found with pneumonia.

Bronchophony is abnormal sound transmission where vocal resonance is heard louder and clearer over areas of consolidation. To test for bronchophony, place the diaphragm of the stethoscope over the same areas and order as in auscultation, but instead of asking the patient to breathe a full respiratory cycle, ask the patient to say a word, such as "pencil," at a normal speaking volume of phonation. Hearing the word with a louder, clearer quality—"pencil, pencil, pencil, PENCIL, pencil"—over an area of the lung field suggests consolidation, such as with pneumonia.

Whispered pectoriloquy is similar to bronchophony except that instead of having the patient phonate at a normal level of volume, he/she is asked to whisper the word instead. An increase in volume or clarity represents a positive test: "pencil, pencil, pencil, PENCIL, pencil."

11-9 **Egophony** is a third test for consolidation. With this test, the patient is asked to say "EEEE." When an area of consolidation is encountered, lower-frequency sounds are filtered out so that the "EEEE" becomes "AAAA": "EEEE, EEEE, EEEE, AAAA, EEEE."

DOCUMENTATION

- Auscultation—Positive bronchophony, egophony, and whispered pectoriloquy R middle lobe.

CLINICAL APPLICATIONS

When an area of abnormality, diminished or adventitious breath sounds, is encountered on auscultation, the techniques of tactile fremitus and percussion can be used in combination to differentiate among pneumonia, pneumothorax, and pleural effusion (see **TABLE 11-1**).

Pneumonia exhibits increased tactile fremitus as the alveolar walls become thickened, widening the road of transmission, but with dullness on percussion as air is replaced with fluids and tissue edema.

Pneumothorax shows a decrease in tactile fremitus as a wall of air blocks the road over which vibration travels. This same air results in hyperresonance on percussion.

11-10 Pleural effusion is also associated with a decrease in tactile fremitus, except that the wall is now made of fluids; however, there will be decreased resonance on percussion as air is replaced by fluid.

See **TABLE 11-2** for the respiratory flow.

Bronchophony: technique of assessment for consolidation where vocal resonance is heard louder and clearer over areas of consolidation

Whispered pectoriloquy: technique of assessment where the patient whispers a word that is perceived to have an increase in volume or clarity as the provider auscultates

Egophony: a test for consolidation where the patient is asked to say "E" while the provider auscultates the lungs. An area of consolidation is encountered when the "E" is perceived as an "A"

TABLE 11-1 Clinical Applications

Condition	Tactile Fremitus	Percussion
Pneumonia	↑	Dull
Pneumothorax	↓	Hyperresonant
Pleural effusion	↓	Dull

TABLE 11-2 Respiratory Flow

Introduces self and explains that physical exam will now be performed.
Washes hands for 15 seconds, turning off water with towel
INSPECTION
General Assessment—assess for signs of respiratory distress

(continues)

TABLE 11-2 Respiratory Flow (*Continued*)

Respiratory Flow
Cyanosis
Accessory muscle use
Nasal flaring
Note position of comfort—tripod, leaning forward, head of bed elevated
Assess respiratory rate and rhythm
Skin
Color—pallor, erythema, cherry red
Nails—clubbing, pallor
Conjunctival pallor
Neck—position of trachea
Chest
Drape lower extremities with a sheet
Ask patient to lower the gown, exposing the chest
Intercostal retractions
Wall symmetry with rise and fall
Deformity—pectus excavatum, pectus carinatum, bony deformity, flail chest
Anterior/Posterior–lateral ratio (AP:lat ratio) barrel chest
AUSCULTATION
Instruct patient to take deep breaths, slowly, through the mouth
Place stethoscope in ears with earpieces angled forward
Auscultate through complete inspiration and expiration
Symmetrically, R upper lobe to R upper lobe, etc.
Anteriorly—minimum three levels including supraclavicular
Laterally—minimum two levels
Posteriorly—minimum three levels
Identify adventitious sounds—crackles, rhonchi, wheezes, rubs
PALPATION
Tenderness, tissue texture changes, bony deformity, reproducible pain
Symmetrical expansion/rib dysfunction—anterior and posterior
Tactile fremitus—uses medial hand margin, symmetrical approach
PERCUSSION
Symmetrical approach for each level, anterior, posterior, and lateral
Diaphragmatic excursion—posterior approach with patient seated
Have patient take full inspiration and hold. Percuss caudally until dullness met.
Have patient force full expiration and hold. Percuss caudally until dullness met.
Measure distance of excursion
CLINICAL SCENARIOS:
Consolidation findings—facilitators, prompt student to demonstrate
Bronchophony—sound transmitted louder at area of consolidation
Whispered pectoriloquy—whispered word louder at area of consolidation
Egophony: patient says "e," sounds like "a" at areas of consolidation
Regown patient
Expected findings—facilitators, prompt student to explain findings for:
Pneumonia—increased tactile fremitus, diminished resonance on percussion
Pneumothorax—decreased tactile fremitus, increased resonance on percussion
Pleural effusion—decreased tactile fremitus, decreased resonance on percussion

CHAPTER 12

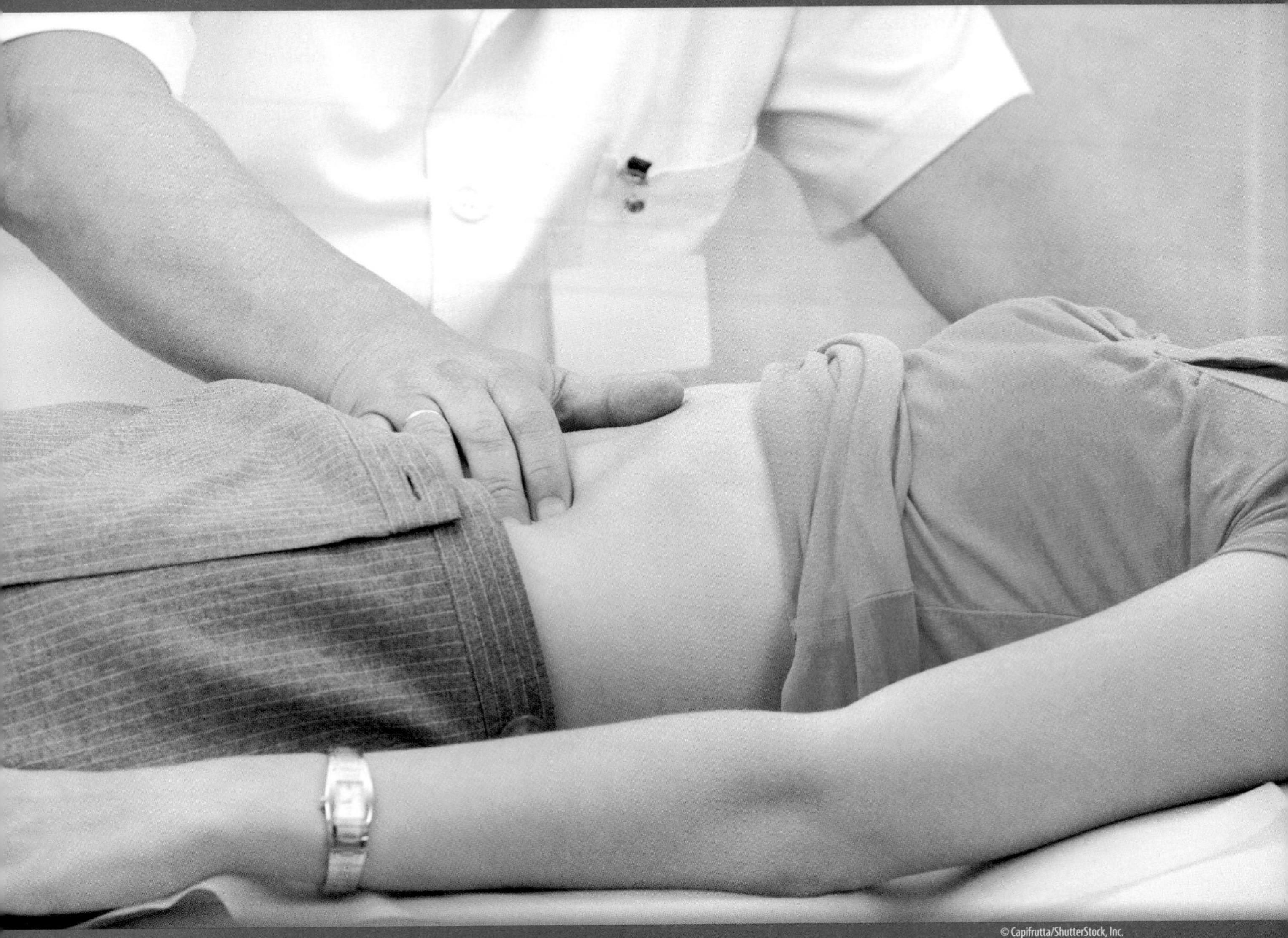

© Capifrutta/ShutterStock, Inc.

Abdominal Examination

Mark Kauffman, DO, MS (Med Ed), PA
Theodore Makoske, MD

OBJECTIVES

At the conclusion of the chapter, the student will be able to

1. Characterize bowel sounds and relate to a differential diagnosis
2. Identify aneurysms and renal artery stenosis through auscultatory and palpatory techniques
3. Correctly demonstrate light and deep palpation of the abdomen
4. Assess for enlargement of the liver, spleen, kidneys, and bladder
5. Assess abdominal and flank pain
6. Assess for ascites

KEY TERMS

Bowel sounds
Light palpation
Deep palpation
Hepatomegaly
Splenomegaly
Kidney catch
Abdominal aortic aneurysm
Rigidity
Rebound tenderness
Appendicitis
Rovsing's sign
Psoas sign
Obturator sign
Cholecystitis
Murphy's sign
Ascites
Fluid wave
Shifting dullness
Lloyd's punch

 Where this icon appears, visit **go.jblearning.com/HPECWS** to view the video.

Examination of the abdomen primarily provides assessment of the gastrointestinal system; however, the genitourinary, renal, and vascular systems are also encountered.

Inspection

PATIENT POSITIONING

The examination begins with inspection of the abdomen (see **FIGURE 12-1**). The provider stands on the right side of the patient, who is in the supine position. Even if the patient is young, fit, and easily able to lie down without any help, it is important to assist him/her with each position change.

Consistently examining from the right side of the patient may not seem important to the beginner, but once embroiled in a busy day, it is much easier not to have to ask, "Which way was Mr. Smith facing when I examined him?" or "Which side was that lesion on?" In addition, examination of the precordium during the cardiovascular examination allows detection of minute chest wall movement if performed on the

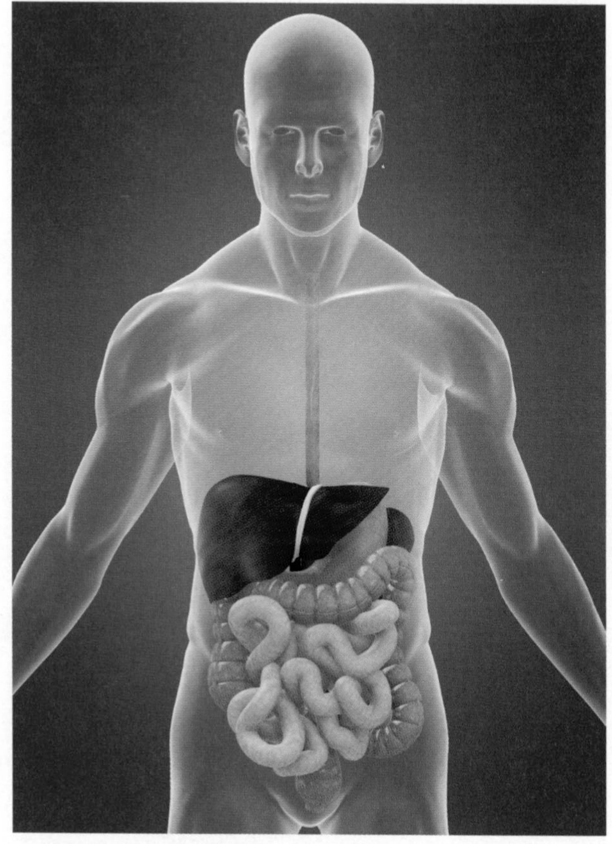

FIGURE 12-1 Abdominal anatomy.
© Sebastian Kaulitzki/ShutterStock, Inc.

patient's right side. The abdominal examination then commonly follows.

12-1 The abdomen must be properly exposed for the examination. Exposure should allow for inspection of all four quadrants from the xiphoid process to the suprapubic area (see **FIGURE 12-2**). To accomplish this while preserving dignity, a sheet should be draped over the pelvis prior to exposing the abdomen. A sheet should always be used whether the patient is in a gown, shorts, or pants. The patient should then be advised of the intent to expose the abdomen and permission should be sought to do so. Position the sheet at the level of the iliac crests, then lift the shirt or gown cephalad to the level of the xiphoid. Mistakes are sometimes encountered at this point as, with the sheet at the level of the iliac crests and umbilicus, only the upper quadrants are exposed. Push the sheet caudad so that it rests several centimeters above the pubic symphysis.

If the patient is wearing a belt or fastener that needs to be undone, ask the patient to unfasten it and expose the lower abdomen for you.

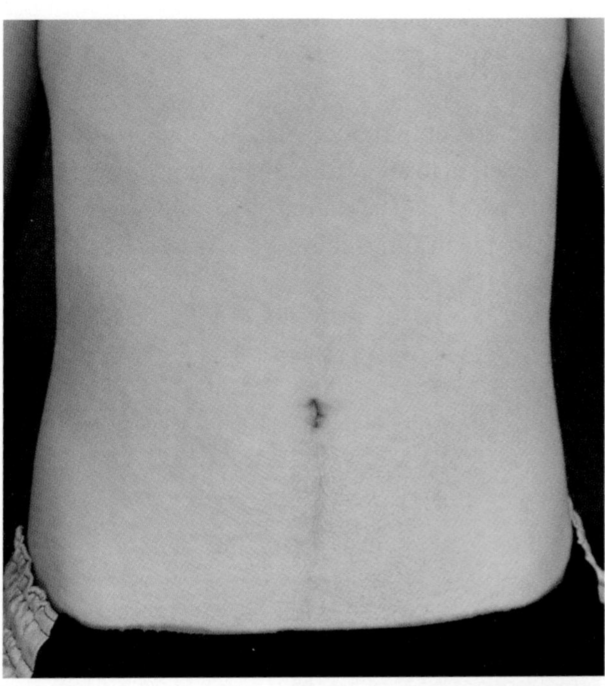

FIGURE 12-2 Abdominal exam exposure from the xiphoid to the symphysis pubis.

ELEMENTS

First inspect the general contour of the abdomen as a whole, often described as either scaphoid (hollowed), flat, or rounded (see **FIGURES 12-3**, **12-4**, and **12-5**). Other descriptive terms include "distended," which is used when an abnormal state of inflation is detected. "Protuberant" may also be used to describe the condition where the abdomen is thrusting forward in a more solid fashion.

Note the general symmetry of the abdomen, inspecting each quadrant for visible masses. Examine

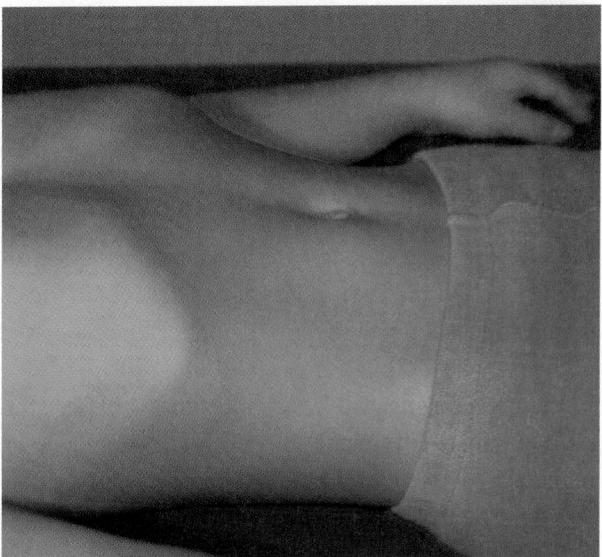

FIGURE 12-3 Scaphoid abdomen.

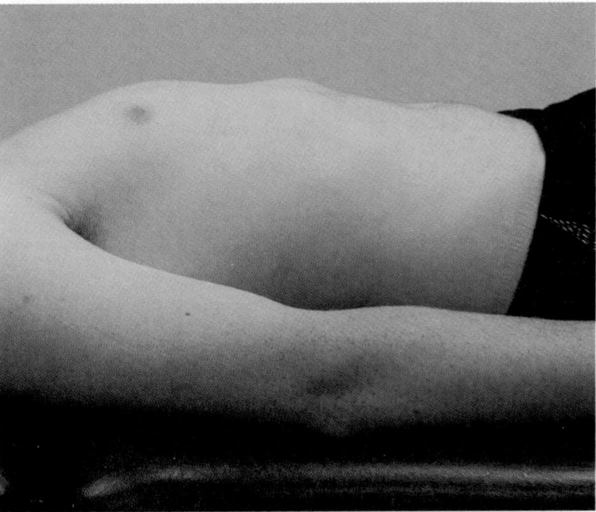

FIGURE 12-4 Flat abdomen.

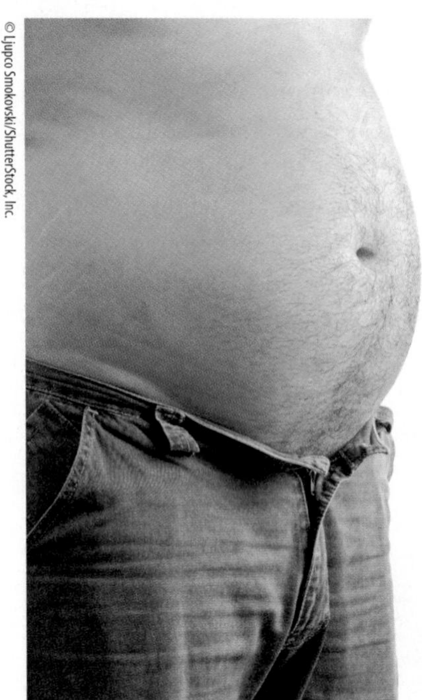
© Ljupco Smokovski/ShutterStock, Inc.

FIGURE 12-5 Rounded abdomen.

the skin for lesions, scars, and striae. Observe for dilated veins around the umbilicus, called caput medusa, which suggests portal hypertension, often associated with cirrhosis of the liver (see FIGURE 12-6).

Inspect for the visible wavelike motion of peristalsis. Peristalsis is typically not visible and when seen may be associated with bowel obstruction.

Ask the patient to bend forward as if doing a sit-up, providing a little support behind the uppermost back as he/she does so. This maneuver increases intra-abdominal pressure and may reveal hernias or rectus diathesis, the separation of rectus abdominis muscles with central linear bulging (see FIGURE 12-7).

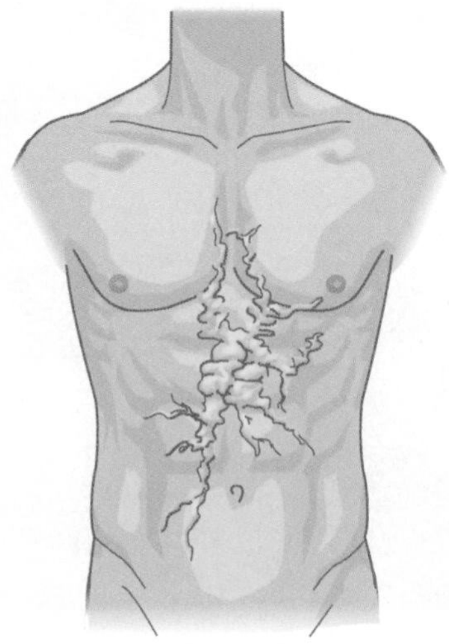

FIGURE 12-6 Caput medusa.

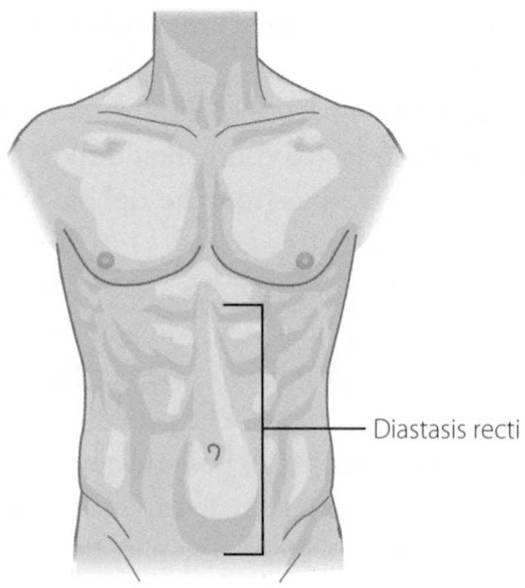

FIGURE 12-7 Rectus diathesis.

DOCUMENTATION

- Abdomen rounded without visible peristalsis, masses, suspicious lesions, scars, or striae. No caput medusa, hernia, or diathesis recti with flexion.

Auscultation

Auscultation of the abdomen is always performed before palpation to allow for proper assessment of bowel sounds, which can be altered by palpatory techniques. All four quadrants should be assessed (see FIGURE 12-8).

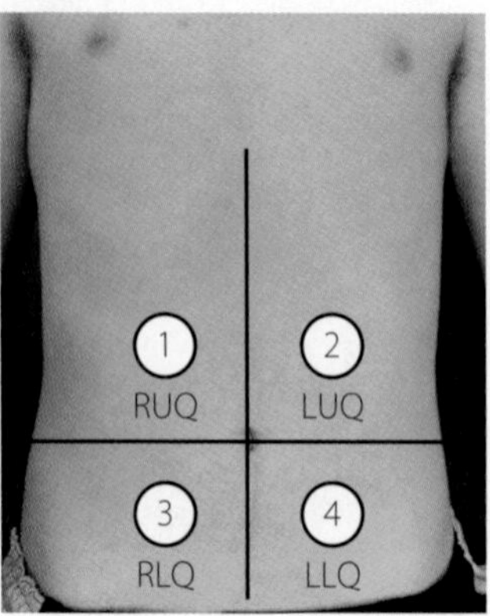

FIGURE 12-8 Location for auscultation of the four quadrants of the abdomen.

BOWEL SOUNDS

Bowel sounds are the result of peristalsis, where the contents of the bowel are being moved through the alimentary tract, producing intermittent clicks and gurgles. The range for normal frequency of bowel sounds is wide: 5 to 34 sounds per minute. At this frequency they are considered to be normoactive. The familiar audible rumbling, gurgling sound of air passage through the fluids of the large bowel is called borborygmus, and it is also part of the everyday sounds of healthy bowel function.

Hypoactive Bowel Sounds

If bowel sounds are not quickly appreciated, auscultation for up to two minutes may be required to confirm that they are diminished to less than five sounds per minute or completely absent. Hypoactive sounds are found with ileus, paralysis of the bowel, and peritonitis. Complete absence of bowel sounds could indicate ischemic or infarcted bowel, where the bowel has essentially died.

Hyperactive Bowel Sounds

Hyperactive bowel sounds, greater than 34 sounds per minute, may be present in a patient with irritation, infection, or inflammation of the bowel, and may result in diarrhea. Hyperactive, high-pitched, or tinkling sounds, reminiscent of a fountain, are found with bowel obstruction and are a result of intestinal air and fluid being under pressure as the bowel works to push contents past the area of obstruction. Rushes of high-pitched sounds are often accompanied by cramping abdominal pain.

Borborygmus may be absent in patients with ileus or obstruction from bowel torsion, volvulus, or strangulation.

DOCUMENTATION

- Normoactive BS × 4 quads

BRUITS

Auscultate for bruits in the large arteries of the abdomen working superiorly to inferiorly (see **FIGURE 12-9**). In a patient who does not have any narrowing of these vessels, the flow of blood should be silent. If turbulent flow is heard, a bruit, atherosclerosis, and narrowing should be considered. The aorta lies just left of midline and directly above the vertebral column. Bifurcation of the aorta occurs at L4, the level of the iliac crests and umbilicus. Therefore auscultation for aortic bruits should be performed approximately halfway between the xiphoid process and the umbilicus, which is approximately the L2 level. This is the level at which the renal arteries branch off from the aorta. Place the stethoscope 1 cm left of midline and slowly depress approximately one-half the depth of the abdomen to assess for bruits, which would indicate atherosclerosis of the aorta. Faint heart sounds are sometimes perceivable but should not be confused with the "whoosh" of the bruit, which occurs after S1.

Bowel sounds: sounds created as a result of peristalsis, where the contents of the bowel are being moved through the alimentary tract, producing intermittent clicks and gurgles

At the same L2 level, move the stethoscope laterally approximately 2 cm and repeat, listening over the renal arteries for a bruit, suggestive of renal artery stenosis. Repeat on the opposite side. As the kidneys lie retroperitoneally, posterior auscultation at the costovertebral angles improves the ability to auscultate renal bruits.

The common iliacs begin at the bifurcation of the aorta and course slightly medial to the midline of the inguinal canal to become the femoral arteries.

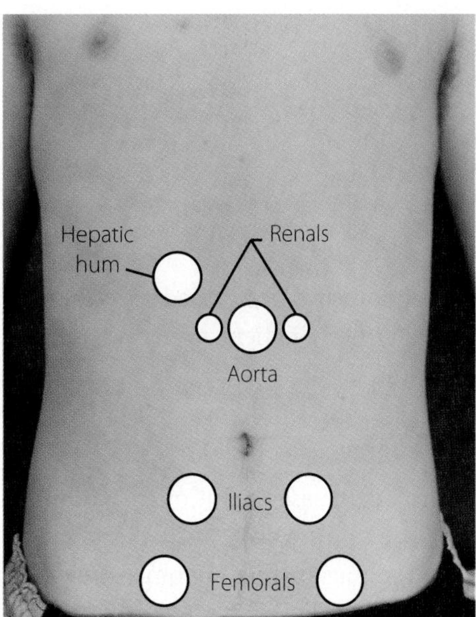

FIGURE 12-9 Location for auscultation of the abdominal vasculature.

Light palpation: technique of examining the abdomen where the provider places one hand flatly against the abdomen and uses a circular motion to assess the skin and subcutaneous tissue for tenderness or masses

Deep palpation: palpatory technique of abdominal examination where the provider places one hand on top of the other, applying slow, deliberate pressure from the top hand into the lower one in a rolling, kneading motion to assess for tenderness and the deep structures of the abdomen

Auscultate at a point midway between the umbilicus and the inguinal canal and again slightly medial to midline directly over the inguinal canal, assessing for bruits of the iliacs and femoral arteries, respectively.

12-2 Auscultate over the liver to assess for a venous hum, a continuous low-grade humming associated with increased circulation between the portal and venous vessels in patients with cirrhosis of the liver. In the patient with possible peritonitis, a friction rub, grating or rasping sounds audible in the upper abdomen due to the motion of the diaphragm with respiration, indicates inflammation of the peritoneum and may be associated with tumor, infection, abscess, or splenic infarct.

In summary:

- First auscultate the four quadrants of the abdomen for bowel sounds.
- Assess the aorta, renal arteries, iliacs, and femoral arteries for bruits.
- Auscultate the right upper quadrant (RUQ) for venous hums.

DOCUMENTATION

- Auscultation without aortic, renal, iliac, or femoral bruits.

Palpation

Palpation of the abdomen is performed with the provider on the right side of the patient, under two degrees of pressure: light and deep.

LIGHT PALPATION

12-3 Always begin assessment of the abdomen with **light palpation**, with the provider placing one hand flatly against the abdomen and using the pads of the fingers, moving in circular motion to feel the skin and subcutaneous tissue for tenderness or masses (see **FIGURE 12-10**). The provider should

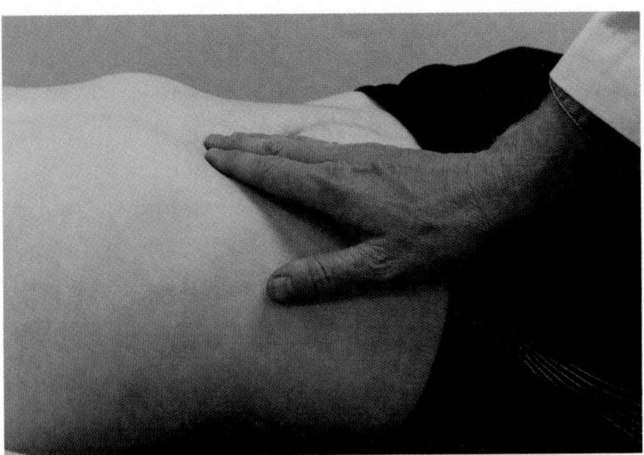

FIGURE 12-10 Light abdominal palpation is preformed with one hand, palpating only to the depth of the subcutaneous tissues and muscle fascia.

consistently watch the patient's face for grimacing or flinching, signs of pain or discomfort, during the examination and adjust the technique appropriately. Assess all four quadrants.

It is not uncommon to encounter a patient who is ticklish to the point that he/she cannot relax the abdominal muscles for palpation. Attempts at distraction of the patient through conversation or questioning unrelated to the physical examination can be made. It may also be helpful to ask the patient to place her hands on her own abdomen, the provider's hands then being placed on top of hers. After several palpatory maneuvers, ask the patient to slide her hands out from under yours, at which point the process can often continue without undue sensitivity interfering.

DEEP PALPATION

12-4 If light palpation is tolerated, progress to **deep palpation**. Deep palpation should be performed with slow, deliberate, cautious technique, keeping the hand flat to disperse the applied pressure and avoid jabbing or poking the patient with just the fingertips. Deep palpation is completed by the provider placing one hand on top of the other. The top hand applies pressure into the lower one in a rolling motion, kneading the hand deeply into the abdomen with deliberate screening of each quadrant (see **FIGURE 12-11**). The provider should envision palpating with the intent of locating intra-abdominal organs and masses. As you approach each quadrant, think of which abdominal organs are in the area. If the

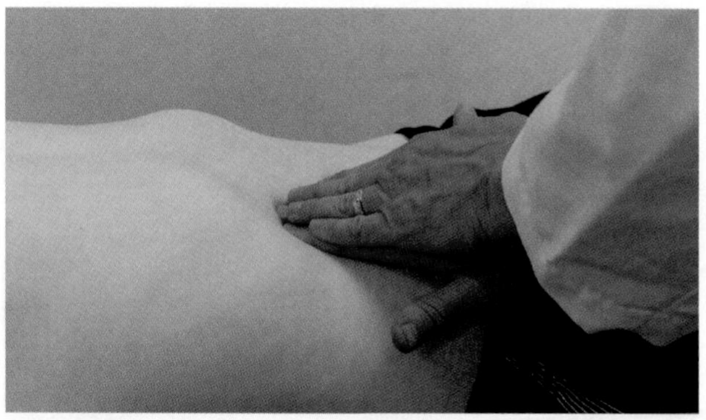

FIGURE 12-11 Deep abdominal palpation with one hand placed on top of the other to assess deep abdominal structures.

abdominal wall is too tense to allow easy palpation, it may be helpful to have the patient bend the knees to 90 degrees, flexing the hips and placing the feet flat on the examination table, to take tension off of the rectus muscles (see **FIGURE 12-12**). Palpation may be limited by body habitus with central adipose.

DOCUMENTATION

- Nontender to light and deep palpation × 4 quads. No masses.

LIVER

12-5 The liver border may be just palpable below the costal margin in the right midclavicular line (MCL) in a normal state. Enlargement greater than this is considered to be **hepatomegaly**. In an attempt to palpate the liver border, use one hand and begin palpation in the right lower quadrant (RLQ) at about the line of the umbilicus, with the hand placed perpendicular to the MCL (see **FIGURE 12-13A**). Roll the hand from the ulnar to the radial aspect, depressing the abdomen approximately 5 to 10 cm, less with thinner abdominal girth, more with thicker (see **FIGURE 12-13B**). After each roll, slide the hand 1 cm cephalad, staying in the MCL, repeating the series until you encounter the liver border or the inferior costal margin.

Hepatomegaly: enlargement of the liver

To experience what a liver border feels like, open a large book and place one hand near the spine. Cover the hand with approximately 30 pages. Palpate on top

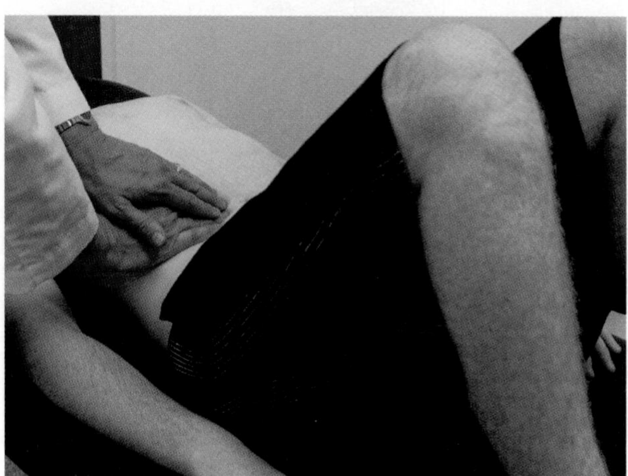

FIGURE 12-12 Patient position for palpating the tense abdomen.

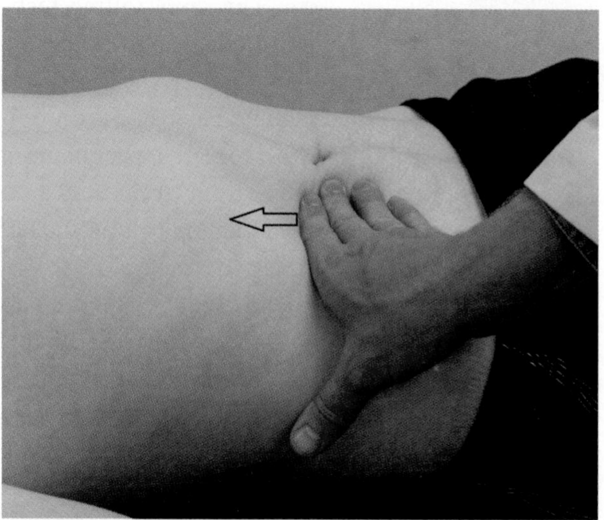

FIGURE 12-13A Palpation of the liver beginning near the level of the umbilicus and moving cephalad in the mid-clavicular line.

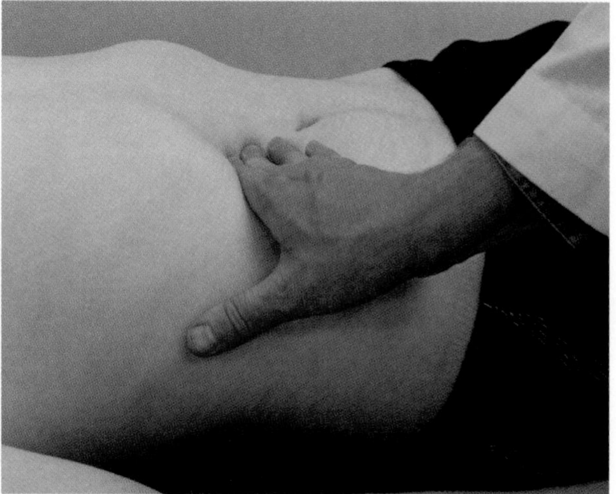

FIGURE 12-13B Palpation of the liver ending at the costal margin.

Splenomegaly: enlargement of the spleen

Kidney catch: technique for assessment of the size of the kidney where the provider places one hand behind the costovertebral angle with the other hand just below the anterior costal margin as the patient is asked to take a deep breath, with the intent of the diaphragm displacing the kidney caudad. At the end of deep inspiration, the provider applies pressure between the hands in an attempt to catch the kidney between the hands.

of the pages with the other hand, using the same rolling method as described, and working from the outer edge of the book toward the buried hand. The palpable characteristic is very similar to the rubbery feel of a liver border.

Hepatomegaly has a host of etiologic causes, of which infections (EBV, viral hepatitis), cancers, early cirrhosis, fatty infiltration, and alcohol abuse are but a few.

SPLEEN

12-6 The same rolling technique is used to palpate the spleen; however, the line of approach should begin at the umbilicus and move diagonally across the left upper quadrant (LUQ) to the inferior costal margin (see **FIGURES 12-14A** and **12-14B**). Placing the left hand behind the left lower ribs and lifting may help to displace the spleen toward the palpating right hand. The spleen is not palpable unless splenomegaly is present. Any palpable enlargement of the spleen is abnormal and should be investigated.

Splenomegaly is caused by conditions that result in increased functioning of the spleen, such as EBV infection (mononucleosis); anemias where red blood cells are trapped within the spleen; increased blood flow, as with portal hypertension from cirrhosis; and infiltration, as with leukemias or lymphomas.

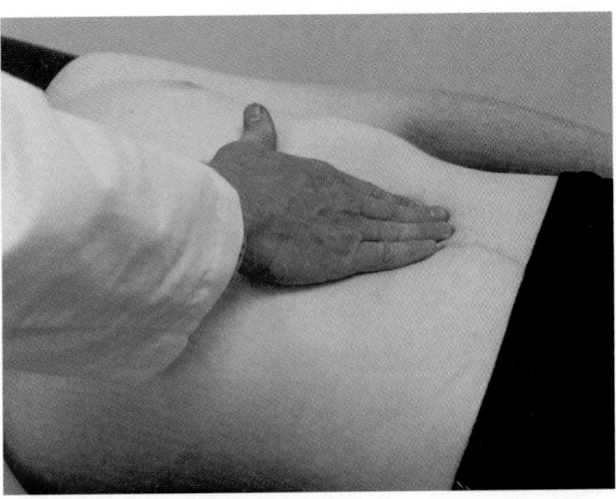

FIGURE 12-14B Palpation of the spleen ending at the costal margin in the anterior axillary line.

DOCUMENTATION

- No hepatosplenomegaly.

KIDNEY

12-7 Both sides of the abdomen can then be palpated for enlargement of the kidneys. A "**kidney catch**" is performed by placing one hand behind the costovertebral angle with the other hand just below the anterior costal margin (see **FIGURE 12-15**).

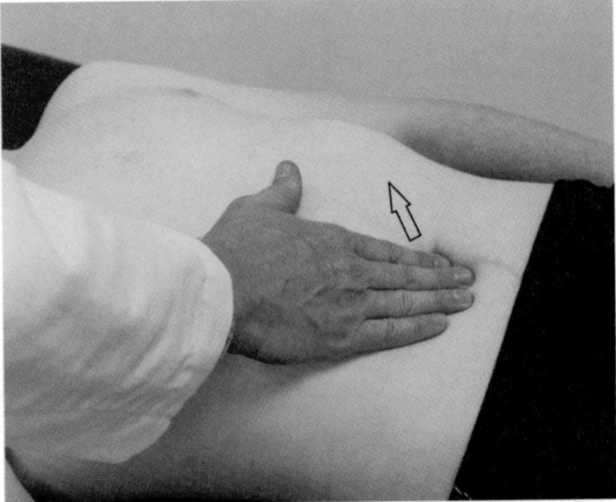

FIGURE 12-14A Palpation of the spleen beginning at the umbilicus and moving diagonally toward the costal margin in the anterior axillary line.

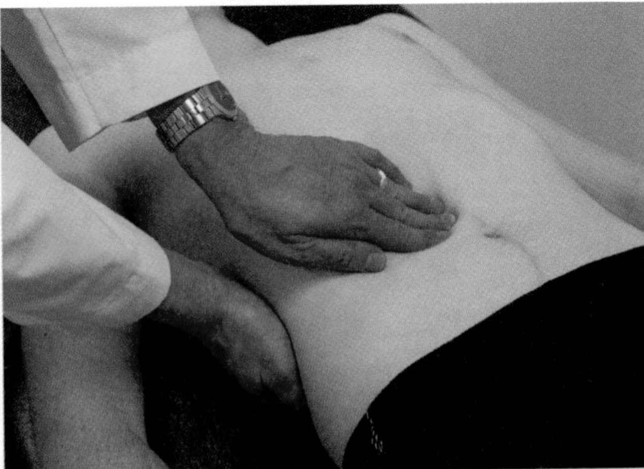

FIGURE 12-15 The "kidney catch" with palpation of the kidney, where the provider attempts to "catch" the kidney between the dorsal and ventral hands.

The patient is asked to take a deep breath, with the intent of the diaphragm displacing the kidney caudad. At the end of deep inspiration, the provider applies pressure between the hands in an attempt to catch the kidney between his/her hands, allowing an estimation of its size.

DOCUMENTATION

- Kidneys nonpalpable

BLADDER

12-8 Palpate for bladder distension or enlargement with a gentle rolling motion, starting just above the umbilicus and moving in midline toward the symphysis pubis.

DOCUMENTATION

- Bladder nonpalpable.

AORTA

Abdominal aortic aneurysm (AAA) is a common condition, with incidence rising with age in the sixties and a history of smoking. It is commonly asymptomatic and is first detected on general physical examination, which highlights the importance of including assessment for AAA in every adult examination on at least a yearly basis.

12-9 The most common location for AAA is below the renal arteries (see **FIGURE 12-16**). As the aorta bifurcates approximately at the level of the umbilicus and iliac crests, place both sides in the lower half of the area between the umbilicus and xiphoid, with the hands approximately 5 cm from midline on each side and the fingers pointing toward the patient's head. Slow, deep pressure is applied, remembering that the aorta lies deeply against the spine. The provider is attempting to palpate the wall of the aorta, detecting the pulse as it courses through. If no beat is felt, lift the hands slightly and move each medially 1 cm, then depress again. Continuing this pattern, the pulse is typically felt first in the provider's right hand as the aorta lies just left of midline. When encountered, keep that hand in place and move the left hand medially 1 cm at a time until the right wall is encountered. Now measure the width of the aorta.

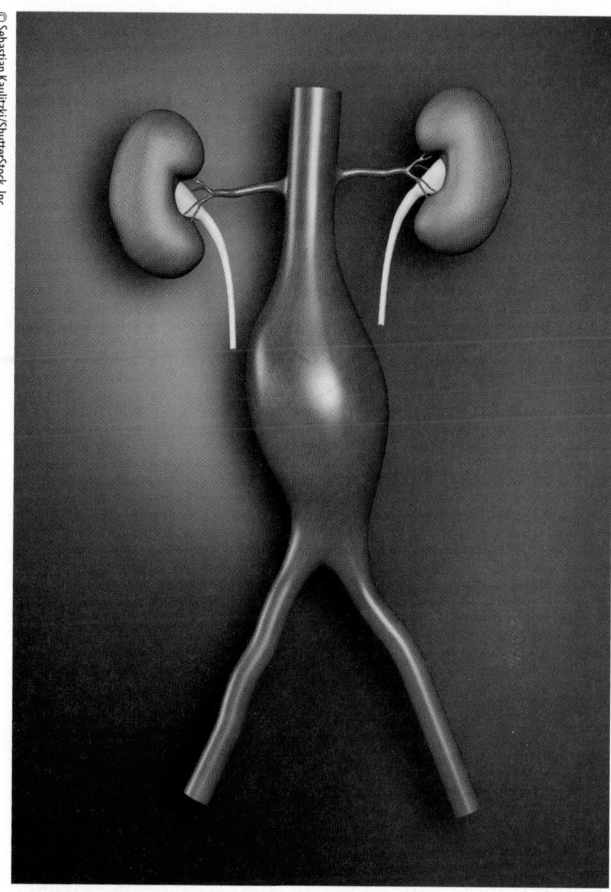

© Sebastian Kaulitzki/ShutterStock, Inc.

FIGURE 12-16 Abdominal aortic aneurysm.

A normal aorta is approximately 2 cm, with enlargement considered to be a width greater than 3 cm. With increasing abdominal girth, the aorta may not be palpable, in which case the provider can document "abdominal aorta is not palpable" or "no pulsitile masses."

DOCUMENTATION

- Aorta 3 cm by palpation.

PAIN

When a patient presents with the complaint of abdominal pain, the examination must be tailored to allow completion of as much of the exam as possible while causing the least amount of pain possible.

Before beginning palpation, ask the patient to locate where the

Abdominal aortic aneurysm: dilation and enlargement of the abdominal aorta, beyond approximately 2 cm, most commonly as a result of atherosclerotic disease

pain is most intense. Begin palpation with the quadrant diagonally from the area identified, saving that quadrant for last. Perform light palpation first, then deep palpation. Apprehension, the fear that the provider's palpation of the abdomen will cause pain, may be encountered. If the abdomen is profoundly tender, such as with peritonitis, the patient may exhibit guarding or involuntary movements to stop the examiner from pressing on the tender area.

In some cases of fictitious pain, the patent may exaggerate intolerance, not allowing the provider to palpate the abdomen. In these cases, the provider should advise the patient that he/she will not palpate but must still listen to the abdomen. Place the head of the stethoscope lightly on the abdominal wall, release it, and raise the hand so that the patient can see it is lifted. Listen for a few seconds then move to a second quadrant, repeating the hand lift. Move the stethoscope to the next quadrant but leave the hand on the head of the stethoscope. Ask the patient to be very quiet and intently listen, even closing your eyes as if trying to hear very faint sounds, and add a little pressure. Now move to the next quadrant and repeat again, adding a bit more pressure. This method will allow at least a measure of palpation in a patient with true pain. The provider may find that he/she can palpate nearly to the posterior abdominal wall in patients whose pain is fictitious.

Percussion

12-10 Percussion of the abdomen is accomplished with the nondominant hand being placed against the patient, fingers spread, with the third digit over the area of investigation (see **FIGURE 12-17**). The dominant hand is held in a curved position and a wrist action is then used to strike the proximal phalanx to generate a sound of resonance. Air creates drumlike resonance, whereas liquids and solids are dull on percussion. Resonance is increased in areas where intestinal gas has collected, commonly the gastric air bubble and over the transverse and descending colon. Solid organs, masses, stool-filled bowel, and intra-abdominal fluid collections percuss with dullness. Percuss over each of the four quadrants.

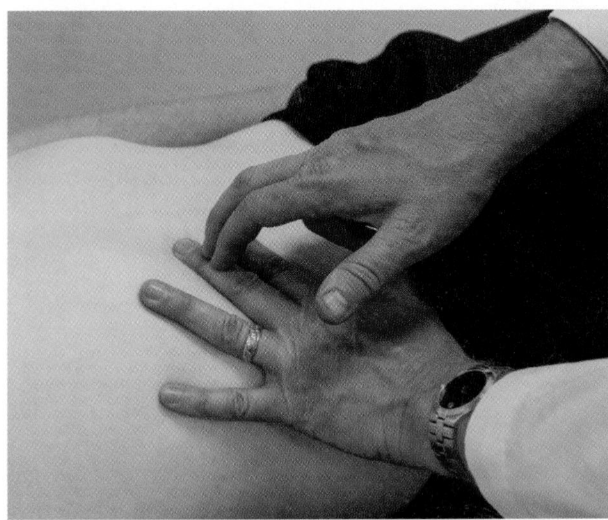

FIGURE 12-17 Hand positioning flatly against the abdomen during percussion.

LIVER SPAN

12-11 Percussion allows the provider to measure the span of the liver. Begin superiorly by percussing at approximately the 5th R ICS in the MCL (see **FIGURE 12-18A**). Move caudad 1 cm at a time until the hyperresonance of the air-filled lung becomes dull at the top margin of the liver (see **FIGURE 12-18B**). Note the level either by a natural landmark, by indenting the skin with a pen cap, or by making a light pen mark (see **FIGURE 12-18C**). Then move inferiorly to the level of the umbilicus and begin percussing cephalad, staying in the MCL (see **FIGURE 12-18D**). Again the resonance of

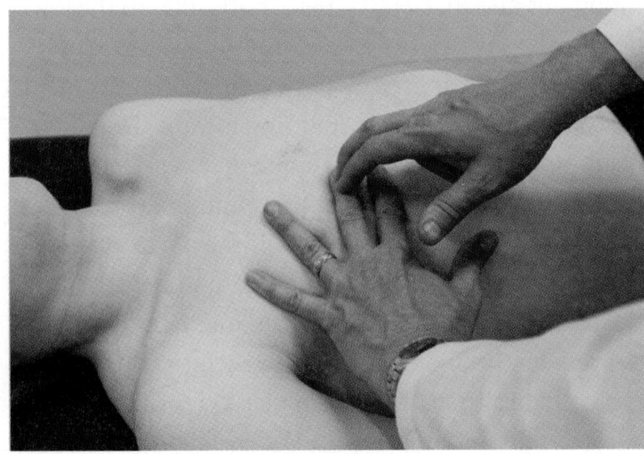

FIGURE 12-18A Percussion of liver span beginning around the 5th ICS to locate the superior border.

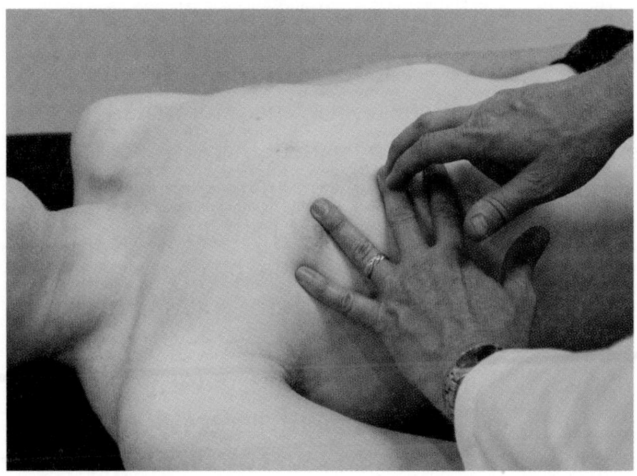

FIGURE 12-18B Percussion of liver span moving caudally.

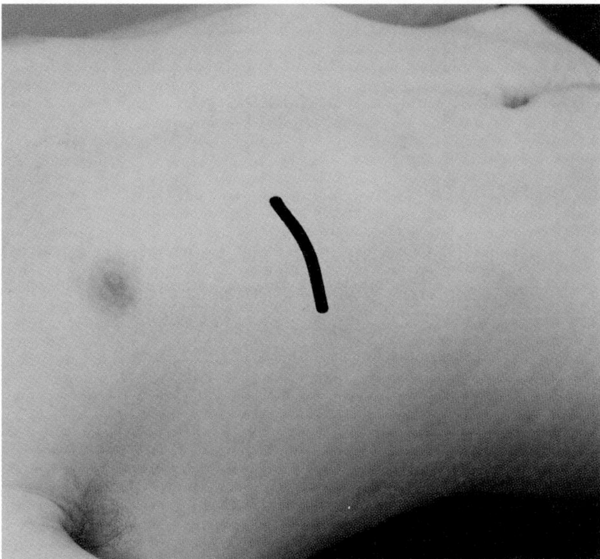

FIGURE 12-18C The level of transition from tympany to dullness is marked.

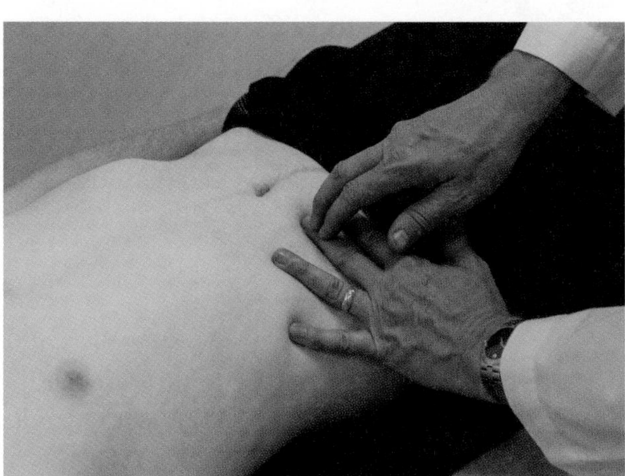

FIGURE 12-18D The hands are repositioned beginning at the level of the umbilicus to locate the inferior border of the liver.

air-filled bowel becomes dull when reaching the inferior margin of the liver (see FIGURE 12-18E).

Remember that one function of the rib cage is to protect the liver from trauma. In the adult, the liver border is typically not palpable, being tucked under the rib cage. Therefore, expect the liver border to be percussed above the costal margin. When locating the inferior edge of the liver, mark the level. Then measure the distance between the two marks (see FIGURE 12-18F). Normal liver span is approximately 6 to 12 cm in the MCL. A liver span that is smaller than 6 cm may indicate cirrhosis, and one larger than 12 cm may indicate hepatomegaly, as can be seen with acute hepatitis.

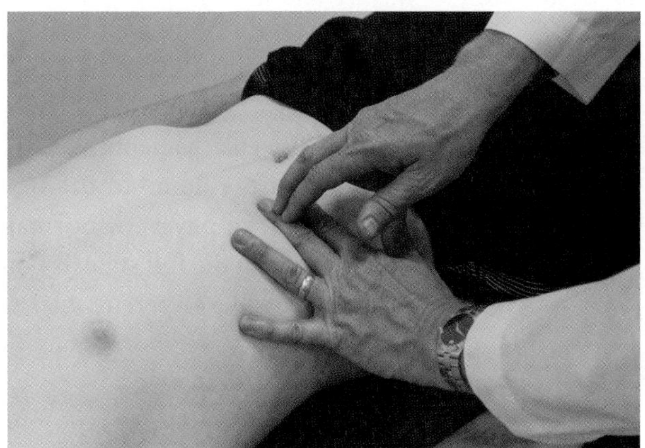

FIGURE 12-18E Percussion then progresses cephalad until dullness of the lower border is identified.

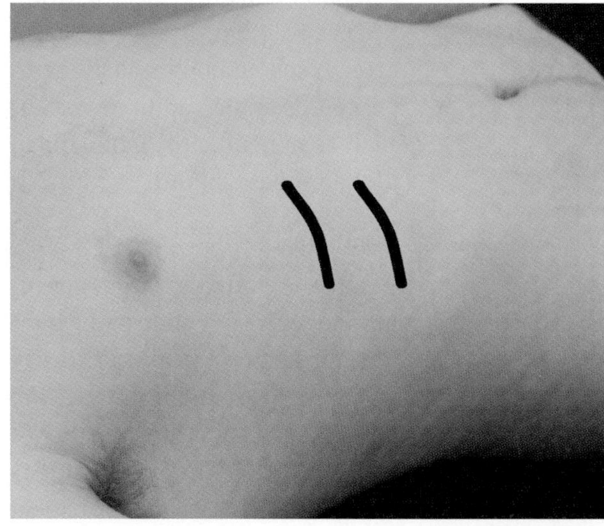

FIGURE 12-18F The distance between the two marks is measured.

DOCUMENTATION

- Tympanic to percussion RLQ and LUQ. Dullness to percussion RUQ and LLQ. Liver 10 cm by percussion R MCL.

Rigidity: sign of acute peritonitis on physical examination where the abdominal muscles are boardlike due to severe irritation of the peritoneum

Rebound tenderness: sign of acute peritonitis on physical examination where the provider compares pain experienced by the patient with deep palpation of the abdomen versus pain experienced with the sudden lifting of the hand off the abdomen from a depressed position. Increased pain with lifting suggests acute peritonitis.

Appendicitis: inflammation of the appendix

Rovsing's sign: sign on physical examination assessed for when a patient presents with RLQ abdominal pain. The provider presses slowly but firmly down on the LLQ. If the RLQ pain worsens, acute appendicitis is suspected.

Psoas sign: sign on physical examination assessed for when a patient presents with RLQ abdominal pain where the provider resists attempted flexion at the hip by the patient. This causes the iliopsoas muscle group to contract, moving the inflamed sheath and causing pain if the appendix is in a retrocecal position.

BLADDER HEIGHT

12-12 Percussion can also be used to find the height of the bladder in a patient who is having problems voiding. Bladder distension secondary to lower urinary tract obstruction may be very painful. Percussion should be performed as gently as possible, starting below the xiphoid process and moving down the midline toward the pubic symphysis. Dullness to percussion is encountered at the dome of the bladder. Measure enlargement in centimeters from the dome to the top of the pubic symphysis. A normal bladder, even in the full state, is not typically palpable or percussible.

Clinical Scenarios

THE ACUTE ABDOMEN

An acute abdomen refers to a sudden onset of pain, typically within the prior 24 hours, and is a term often used synonymously with peritonitis and a ruptured viscous such as appendicitis, gallbladder, ulcer, or diverticulum.

Rigidity

The patient often exhibits guarding and severe irritation of the peritoneum that can result in **rigidity** where the abdominal muscles are boardlike in spite of the patient's efforts to relax. The abdomen may feel hot to the touch, and the patient may flex into the fetal position to decrease stretching of the abdominal wall.

Rebound Tenderness

12-13 Assessment for **rebound tenderness** is a technique used to check for irritation of the peritoneum. Advise the patient that you must palpate the abdomen and that when you do, you want him/her to tell you what causes more pain, pushing down or letting go quickly. Lay your hand on the abdomen and slowly push down as the patient tolerates. Then ask the patient, "What hurts more, me pushing now, or when I let go?" Then quickly lift your hand. The hand must be lifted quickly and completely off the abdomen to jar the peritoneum. Pain greater with lifting is positive rebound tenderness and suggests peritonitis.

A digital rectal examination for tenderness and occult blood should be performed with every acute abdomen evaluation. In a female patient, a pelvic examination should also be completed.

DOCUMENTATION

- Pain in LLQ with light and deep palpation. + rigidity, guarding, and rebound tenderness.

APPENDICITIS

Several common conditions have specialized tests to check for specific tenderness to palpation in the assessment of **appendicitis**.

Rovsing's Sign

12-14 If the patient has RLQ pain and appendicitis is in the differential, the examiner should look for **Rovsing's sign**. The provider presses slowly but firmly down on the LLQ, asking the patient if it causes or worsens the RLQ pain. If so, this is a positive Rovsing's sign and increases the probability of appendicitis.

Psoas Sign

The **psoas sign** may help locate the appendix if it is in a retrocecal anatomic location. In this case the appendix lies on top of the sheath of the psoas muscle, causing increasing irritation as perforation progresses.

With the patient in the supine position, the provider places a hand just above the patient's right knee and asks him/her to lift the leg off the table (see

FIGURE 12-19). This causes the iliopsoas muscle group to contract, moving the inflamed sheath and causing pain if the appendix is in a retrocecal position—a positive psoas sign.

12-15 An alternative would be to have the patient in the supine position, lying close to the edge of the examination table, then lowering the leg slowly off the table, stretching the psoas muscle with passive hip extension, which would again cause pain.

Obturator Sign

12-16 Likewise, if an inflamed appendix lies against the obturator muscle, the location can be detected with the **obturator sign**. With the patient in the supine position, the provider holds the right leg by the ankle and flexes the hip with the other hand along the lateral margin of the knee (see FIGURE 12-20). At 90 degrees of hip flexion the provider internally rotates the hip. This motion moves the obturator muscle, causing pain if the appendix is located at the muscle—a positive obturator sign.

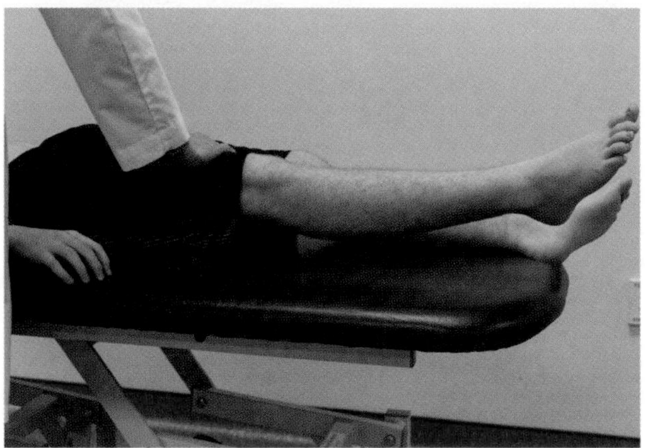

FIGURE 12-19 Assessment for psoas sign as the provider resists hip flexion.

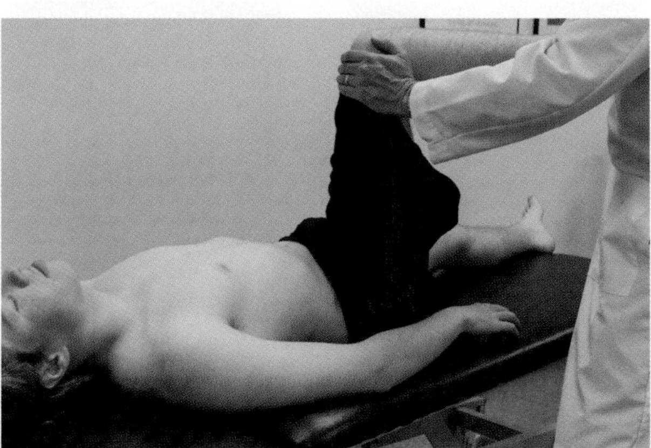

FIGURE 12-20 Assessment for obturator sign with the sheath of the obturator muscle being stretched by internal rotation at the hip.

DOCUMENTATION

- Positive Rovsing's and obturators signs. Negative psoas sign.

CHOLECYSTITIS

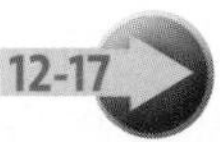

12-17 If **cholecystitis** is suspected due to RUQ pain, **Murphy's sign** should be sought. The provider places the right hand on the abdomen with the fingers parallel to and just below the patient's right costal margin in the MCL (see FIGURE 12-21). The patient is asked to let out a breath and the provider slowly depresses his/her hand several inches. The palpating hand is then held still while the patient is asked to take in a deep breath. As the patient does so, the diaphragm displaces the gallbladder inferiorly against the stationary hand, causing the patient to suddenly halt the breath

Obturator sign: sign on physical examination assessed to help locate the anatomic position of the appendix when acute appendicitis is suspected where the provider places the patient's lower extremity in 90 degrees of flexion at the hip and knee and then introduces internal rotation of the hip. This motion moves the obturator muscle, causing pain if the appendix is located at the muscle.

Cholecystitis: inflammation of the gallbladder

Murphy's sign: sign on physical examination assessed for when a patient presents with RUQ abdominal pain where the provider depresses the abdomen just below the right costal margin and then asks the patient to take a deep breath displacing the gallbladder inferiorly into the provider's stationary hand. Sudden cessation of the breath or increased pain suggests cholecystitis.

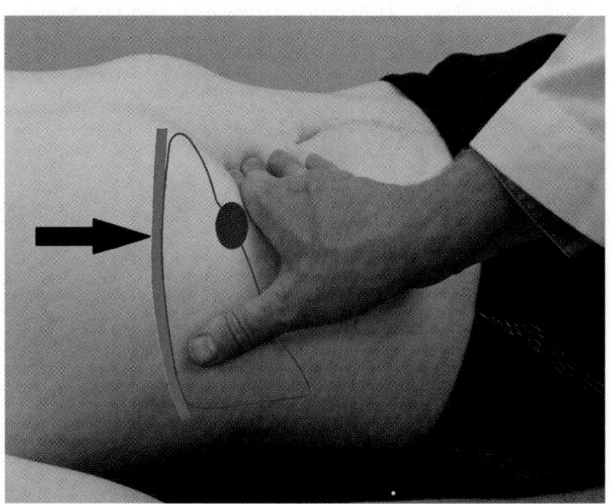

FIGURE 12-21 Murphy's test hand placement just below the right costal margin.

Ascites: accumulation of fluid in the abdominal cavity

Fluid wave: sign on physical examination when assessing for ascites where the patient or an assistant places the ulnar aspect of a hand on the midline of the abdomen as the provider taps sharply on one side of the abdomen, assessing for transmission of the impulse with the opposite hand. Feeling the impulse suggests the presence of ascites.

Shifting dullness: sign on physical examination when assessing for ascites. With the patient in the supine position, the provider begins percussion at the umbilicus working laterally toward the flanks until a level of dullness is encountered. The patient is then placed in lateral decubitus position with the level of dullness reassessed. If ascites is present, the dullness will have shifted to the side against the table while the air will move to the opposite superior side.

or grimace with pain. This is a positive Murphy's sign, showing probable cholecystitis.

DOCUMENTATION

- + Murphy's sign.

ASCITES

In a patient with cirrhosis or heart failure, the abdomen should be assessed for **ascites**, accumulation of fluid in the abdominal cavity. It may be evident with flank bulging but may be more difficult to differentiate from adipose in patients with large abdomens. There are two methods to attempt to determine this.

Fluid Wave

12-18 To assess for a **fluid wave**, either the patient or an assistant places the ulnar aspect of a hand on the midline of the abdomen and depresses 2 to 3 cm. The provider places one hand laterally on each side of the abdomen, then taps sharply on one side while holding the other hand firmly on the opposite side (see FIGURE 12-22). If ascites is present, the fluid wave moves under the hand in midline and the impulse is felt in the provider's opposite hand. With abdominal adipose, the impulse created from the tap stops at the hand placed in midline.

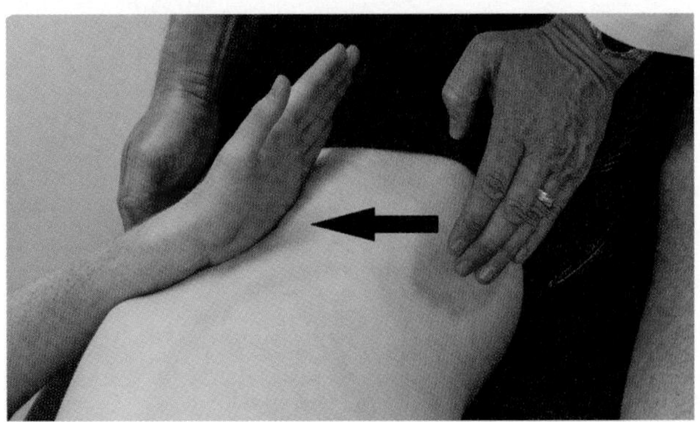

FIGURE 12-22 The provider taps one side of the abdomen while assessing for transmission of the fluid wave impulse passing under a hand placed in midline.

Shifting Dullness

A second test to discern abdominal ascites is the **shifting dullness** test. If the abdomen contains the free fluid of ascites, the principle of gravity dictates that it will pull inferiorly while air rises to the top. With the patient in the supine position, ascites will pool toward the patient's back. Begin percussion at the umbilicus (see FIGURE 12-23A). Note the amount of tympany. Working from the umbilicus, percuss laterally toward the flanks, moving 2 to 3 cm with each step (see FIGURES 12-23B and 12-23C). The umbilical area will be

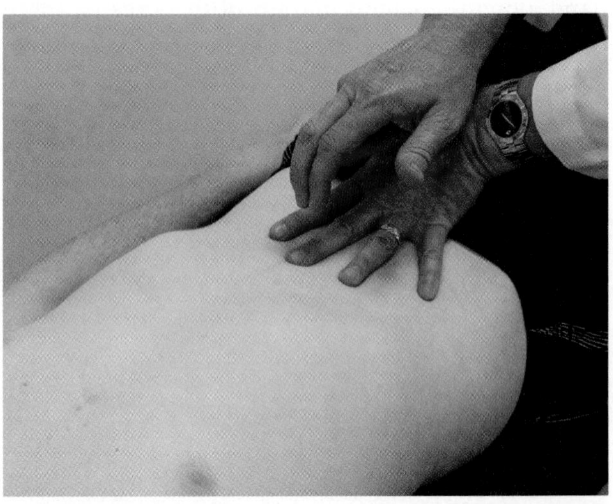

FIGURE 12-23A Assessment for shifting dullness begins with percussion at the umbilicus.

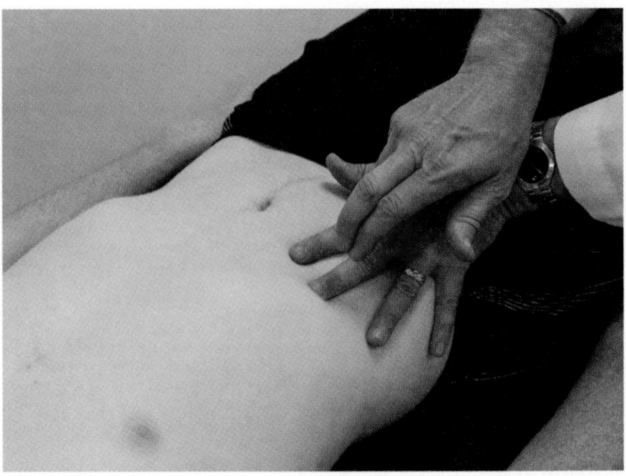

FIGURE 12-23B Percussion continues laterally until a level of dullness is detected.

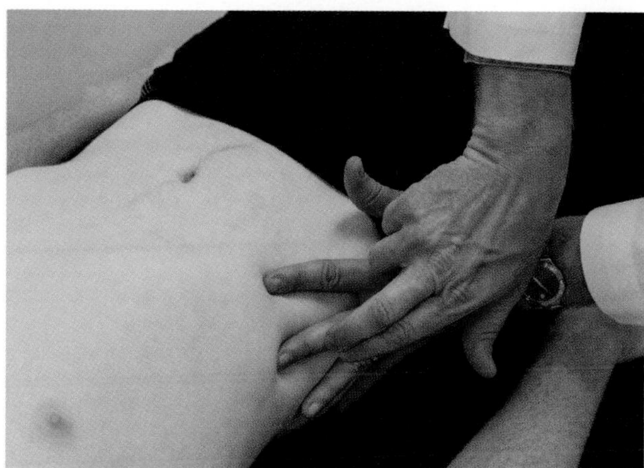

FIGURE 12-23C Percussion ceases when dullness is detected.

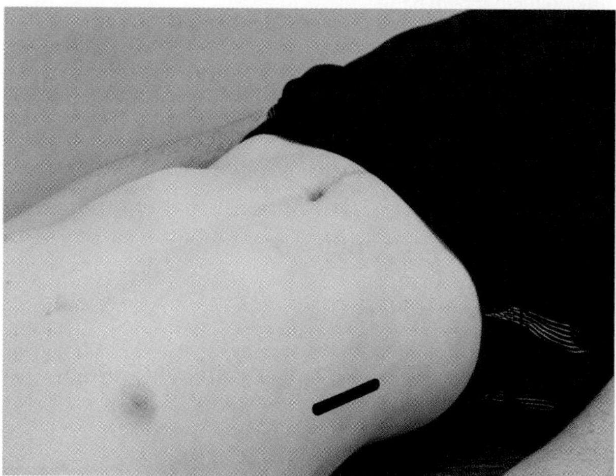

FIGURE 12-23D The level of dullness is marked.

resonant with air accumulation superiorly while dullness will be encountered when the upper level of pooled fluid is reached. Mark the level (see **FIGURE 12-23D**). Now ask the patient to roll into a lateral decubitus position. If free fluid is present, it will now shift to the side against the table while the air will move to the opposite superior side.

12-19 Repeat percussion, this time starting at the patient's superior side (see **FIGURE 12-24A**) and working toward the table (see **FIGURES 12-24B** and **12-24C**). Again mark the level where dullness is encountered (see **FIGURE 12-24D**). If free fluid is encountered, the dullness will shift from the first mark to the second—shifting dullness (see **FIGURE 12-24E**).

DOCUMENTATION

- + shifting dullness and fluid wave.

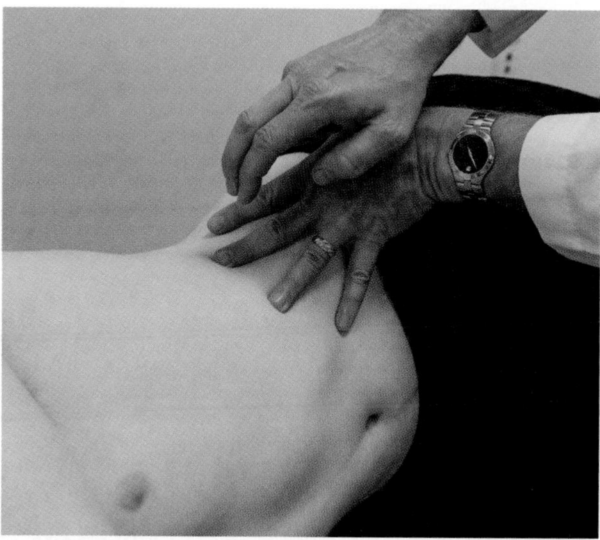

FIGURE 12-24A The patient is placed in lateral decubitus position with percussion beginning again at the top.

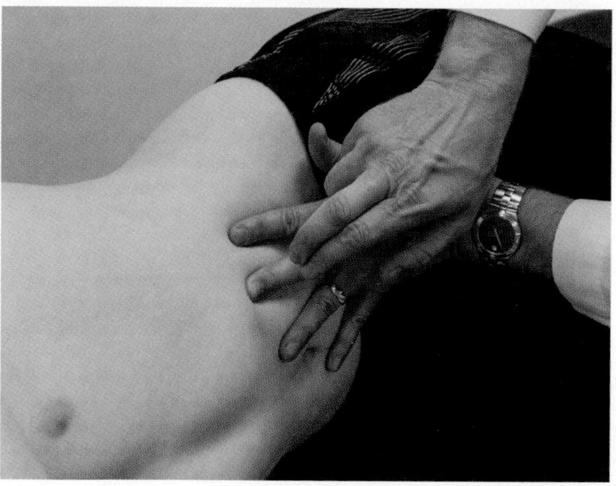

FIGURE 12-24B Percussion continues toward the opposite side.

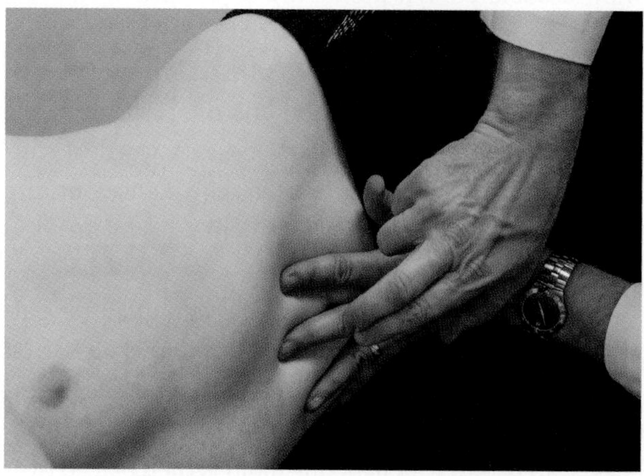

FIGURE 12-24C Percussion ceases when dullness is detected.

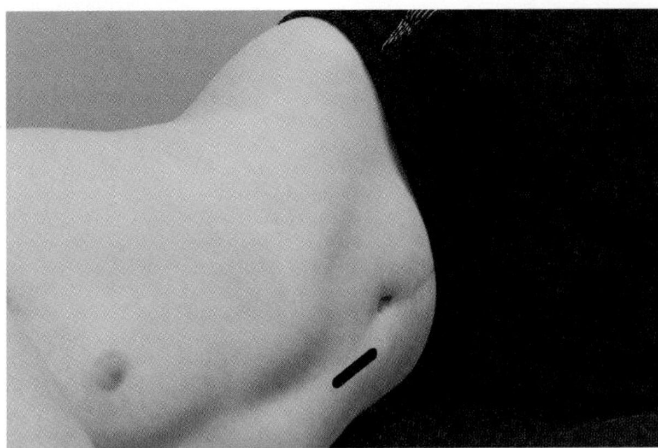

FIGURE 12-24D The level of dullness is marked.

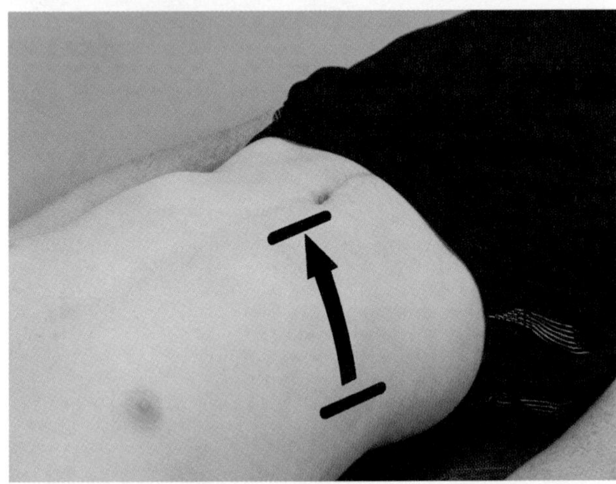

FIGURE 12-24E Ascites is detected when the level of dullness shifts locations.

HYDRONEPHROSIS/PYELONEPHRITIS

Flank pain is the most common symptom associated with hydronephrosis and pyelonephritis. Other common associated symptoms are fever, chills, nausea, vomiting, dysuria, and hematuria.

Lloyd's punch: sign on physical examination when assessing for hydronephrosis and pyelonephritis in a patient with flank pain where the provider places one hand on the costovertebral angle and then strikes the hand sharply, resulting in pain in the presence of distention of the kidney capsule or inflammation

Lloyd's punch is performed to assess for costovertebral angle (CVA) tenderness. A word of caution: This test can cause intense pain in the patient if performed too aggressively.

The provider should first palpate each CVA for tenderness, first with light and then with deep pressure (see **FIGURE 12-25**). If this is tolerated, one hand is then placed over the CVA and gently thumped with the other fist, using the hypothenar eminence. If this is tolerated, another thump can be given with more intensity. Distention of the kidney capsule or the presence of inflammation will cause the patient to experience pain and often jump when struck.

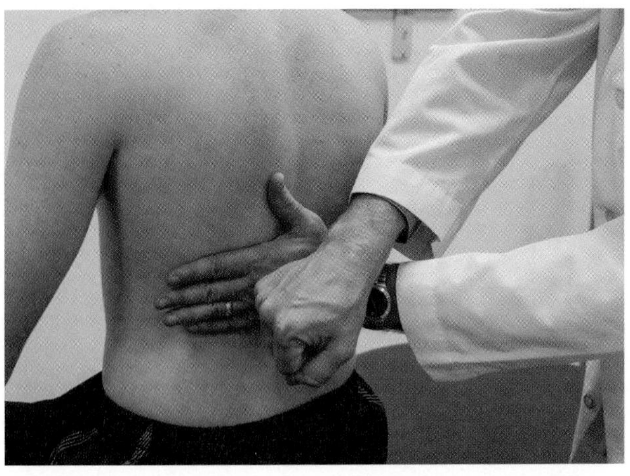

FIGURE 12-25 Lloyd's punch hand position with the provider striking his/her own hand.

DOCUMENTATION

- No CVA tenderness. Negative Lloyd's punch.

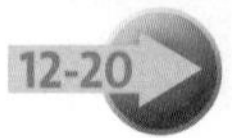

See **TABLE 12-1** for the abdominal flow.

TABLE 12-1 Abdominal Flow

Abdominal Flow
Introduces self and explains that physical exam will now be performed.
Washes hands for 15 seconds, turning off water with towel
INSPECTION
Drape lower extremities with a sheet
Help patient to supine position
Properly expose the abdomen by lifting gown, keeping legs covered with sheet
Provider stands on right side of supine patient
Inspect for
General contour of abdomen—flat, scaphoid, distended
Asymmetry, masses
Lesions, scars
Umbilicus, venous pattern (caput medusa)
Have patient flex forward—assess for hernias, rectus diathesis

TABLE 12-1 Abdominal Flow *(Continued)*

AUSCULTATION
Prior to percussion and palpation
Four quadrants
Identify bowel sound frequency—normoactive, hypoactive, and hyperactive
Bowel sound character—tinkling, borborygmi
Arterial bruits
Aorta—midline—above the umbilicus
Renal arteries—1 to 2 cm lateral to midline anteriorly, flank posteriorly
Iliacs—below umbilicus
Femoral—at inguinal canal
PALPATION
Watch facial expression for grimace during palpation
Demonstrate technique if abdomen tense. Pt bends knees, placing feet flat on the table
Light palpation assessing skin and subcutaneous tissues using finger pads of one hand
Deep palpation assessing visceral structures using one hand on top of the other
Tenderness
Masses
Hepatomegaly—begin in RLQ and roll fingers upward to the right costal margin
Splenomegaly—begin at umbilicus, rolling fingers diagonally to the L costal margin
Uterine height
Bladder distension
Size of aorta—above the umbilicus approaching from lateral to medial
PERCUSSION
Assess pattern of resonance in 4 quadrants
Liver span
CLINICAL SENERIOS
Acute abdomen
Assess for guarding
Rigidity
Rebound—ask patient which hurts more, pushing in (push in slowly but deeply) or letting go (suddenly lift hand from the depressed position)
Rectal exam—state you would perform this exam if your patient was female
Pelvic exam—state you would perform this exam if your patient was female
Appendicitis
Rovsing's sign—pain in RLQ with LLQ pressure
Psoas sign—flexion and extension of hip
Obturator sign—flex hip and internally rotate
Ascites
Fluid wave
Place second provider's or patient's hand vertically on abdomen's umbilical line
Tap side with finger pads while feeling for transmitted pulse on other side
Shifting dullness
Place patient in supine position, percuss from umbilicus laterally to dullness
Roll patient to decubitus position, percuss from highest elevation until dullness
Note shifting of dullness = ascites
Cholecystitis—Murphy's sign
Press deeply into the RUQ
Ask the patient to take a deep breath
Inspiratory arrest (patient stops inspiration due to pain) = positive test
Re-cover the abdomen
Help patient to seated position
Nephrolithiasis, hydronephrosis, pyelonephritis

CHAPTER 13

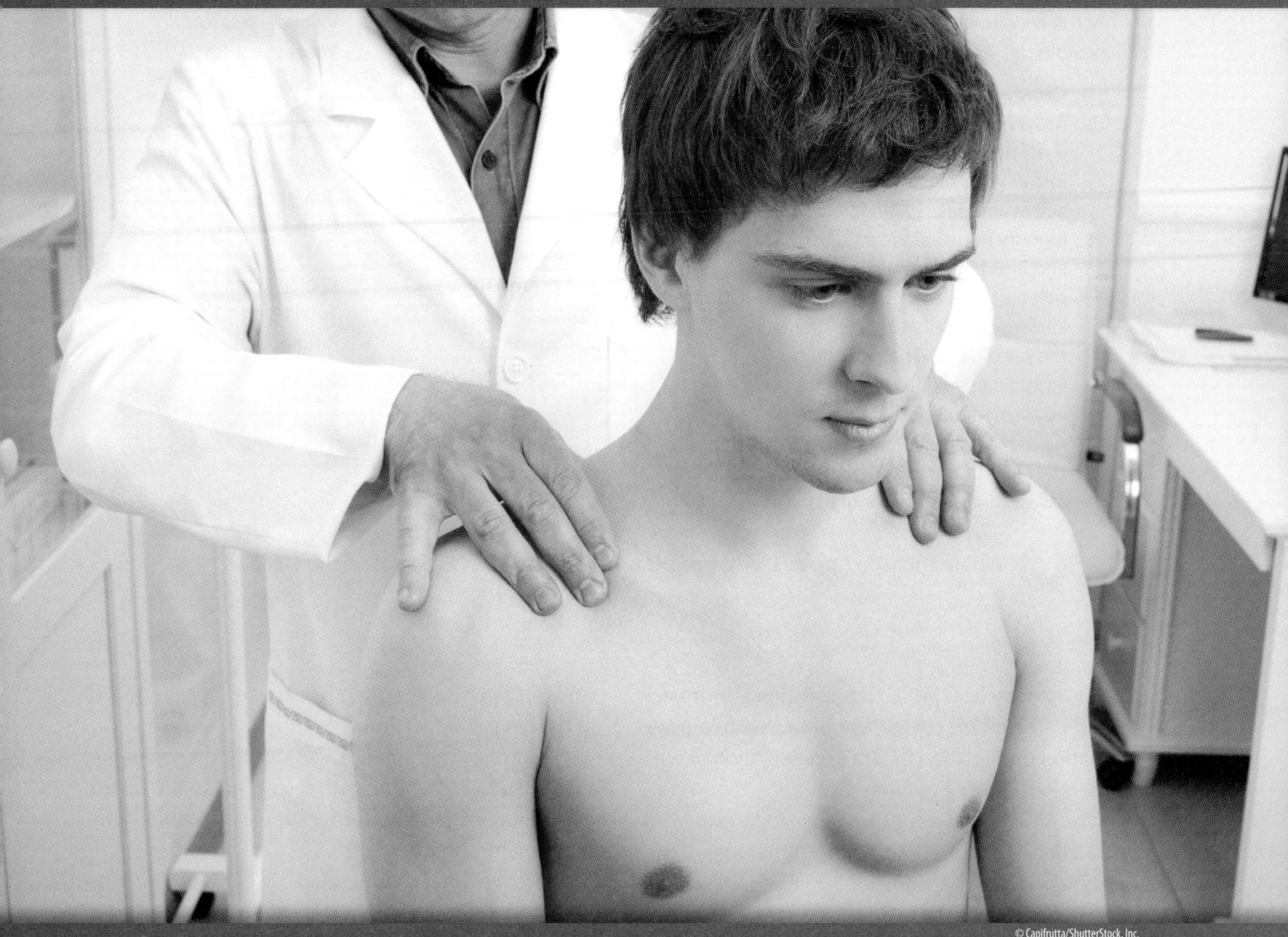

© Capifrutta/ShutterStock, Inc.

Musculoskeletal Examination

OBJECTIVES

At the conclusion of this chapter, the student will be able to

1. Categorize head size
2. Assess the temporomandibular joint for dysfunction
3. Inspect and palpate each joint including active and passive range of motion
4. Identify nodes of the metacarpal phalangeal and interphalangeal joints in relation to osteoarthritis and rheumatoid arthritis
5. Perform a detailed knee examination under the conditions of pain or injury
6. Employ techniques of examination in the assessment of low back pain
7. Assess for carpal tunnel syndrome
8. Describe the structure of the rotator cuff and assess for the presence of tears

KEY TERMS

Active range of motion (AROM)
Passive range of motion (PROM)
Normocephalic
Microcephalic
Macrocephalic
TMJ dysfunction
Heberden's nodes
Bouchard's nodes
Rotoscoliosis
Ballottement
Valgus stress test
Varus stress test
Anterior drawer test
Posterior drawer test
Meniscal tear
McMurray's sign
Straight leg raise
Carpal tunnel syndrome
Phalen's sign
Tinel's sign
Rotator cuff

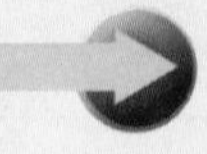
Where this icon appears, visit **go.jblearning.com/HPECWS** to view the video.

The musculoskeletal (MSK) examination is intimately related to the motor component of the neurologic examination through nervous innervation, though separate sections are dedicated to each.

The musculoskeletal examination focuses on muscle and bone structure, particularly joint range of motion. Inspection and palpation are the predominant examination techniques. An important principle is bilateral comparison throughout the examination. When inspecting for range of motion, ask the patient to move the joint being examined actively, in order to determine what is called **active range of motion** (AROM). If AROM is limited, the provider should ask the patient to relax the muscles as the provider moves the joint through **passive range of motion** (PROM).

Active range of motion: action of the patient moving a joint to the greatest degree possible in all planes of motion

Passive range of motion: action of the provider moving a joint of the patient to the greatest degree possible in all planes of motion without the patient assisting with the movement

Compare the size of muscle mass bilaterally, noting any asymmetry, atrophy, hypertrophy, or contracture. Muscle strength testing will be discussed in the neurology section.

Minimize position changes during the screening examination by starting with the patient in the seated position, then moving to the supine and finally the standing position.

Each provider will develop his/her own order of examination for the musculoskeletal system. Some will start at the head and work centrally along the spine and then return to the extremities. Some will choose to work through the extremities first, then return to the spine. The order is an individual preference, but following the same order through each examination helps to assure completeness.

The Seated Position

GENERAL INSPECTION

With the patient in a seated position, inspect the head for size. Assess general body symmetry, comparing bilateral upper and lower extremity length and muscle mass, noting atrophy. Identify limb or bony deformity. Exposure of symmetrical joints is essential. You cannot accurately assess joint dysfunction or injury without comparing to the opposite side, which always requires appropriate exposure. For example, a patient presents with what is likely a sprain of the right ankle. Both socks and shoes must be removed for appropriate comparison of inspection, range of motion, palpation, and examination for joint laxity. An early common mistake in examination is leaving the left sock on, not comparing the normal anatomy of the left side to that of the injured right.

DOCUMENTATION

- Well developed.

THE HEAD

Inspect the head for size (see **FIGURE 13-1A**). **Normocephalic** refers to the size of the head being within one standard deviation of average for the age and sex of the patient. **Microcephalic**, small head, refers to a head circumference that is smaller than two standard deviations below the average. This condition can occur during development and be evident at birth or it can develop over the first several years of life. It commonly occurs with chromosomal abnormalities but may also be related to alcohol use during pregnancy, diabetes, and in utero infections such as varicella, rubella, and cytomegalovirus. Significant developmental delay is commonly associated.

Macrocephalic, large head, refers to a head circumference larger than two standard deviations from the average for the age and sex of the patient (see

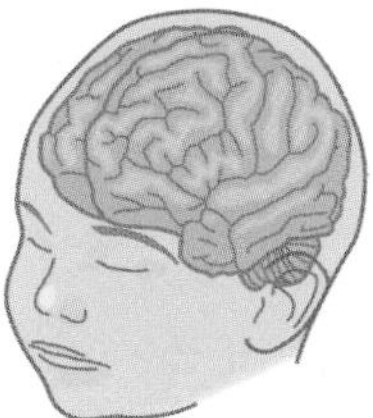
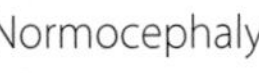
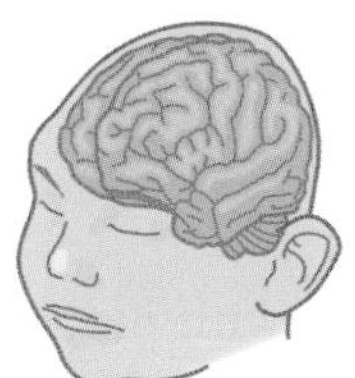

FIGURE 13-1A Normocephalic and microcephalic head size comparison.

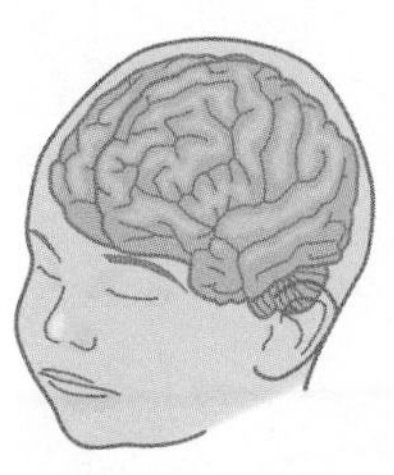
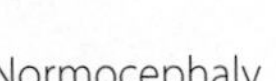
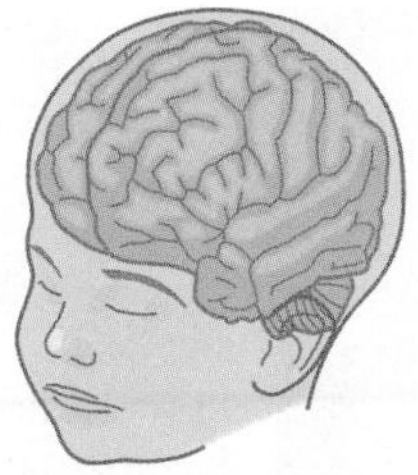

FIGURE 13-1B Macrocephalic head size.

FIGURE 13-1B). This is a common finding with hydrocephalus as well as many genetic conditions such as neurofibromatosis. Developmental delay, autism, and schizophrenia may accompany the condition.

DOCUMENTATION

- Normocephalic.

Though abnormality in the size of the head is commonly apparent at birth and infancy, enlargement can develop in adulthood. Osteitis deformans, or Paget's disease of the bone, can result in enlargement of the skull through thickening of the bone. Other neoplasms such as osteoma may be apparent by inspection.

Palpate the skull for masses. Also note the firmness of the skull above the pinnae. Craniotabes refers to softening of the skull, which can be found with rickets, syphilis, and hydrocephalus.

Normocephalic: size of the head being within one standard deviation of average for others of the same age and sex

Microcephalic: meaning "small head," refers to a head circumference that is smaller than two standard deviations below the average

Macrocephalic: meaning " large head," refers to a head circumference larger than two standard deviations from the average for the age and sex of the patient

TEMPOROMANDIBULAR JOINT

Working head to toe, the temporomandibular joint (TMJ) is the first joint encountered (see **FIGURE 13-2A**).

Inspection

While standing in front of the seated patient, ask the patient to slowly open and close the mouth. Watch for midline tracking of the mandible and listen for audible popping.

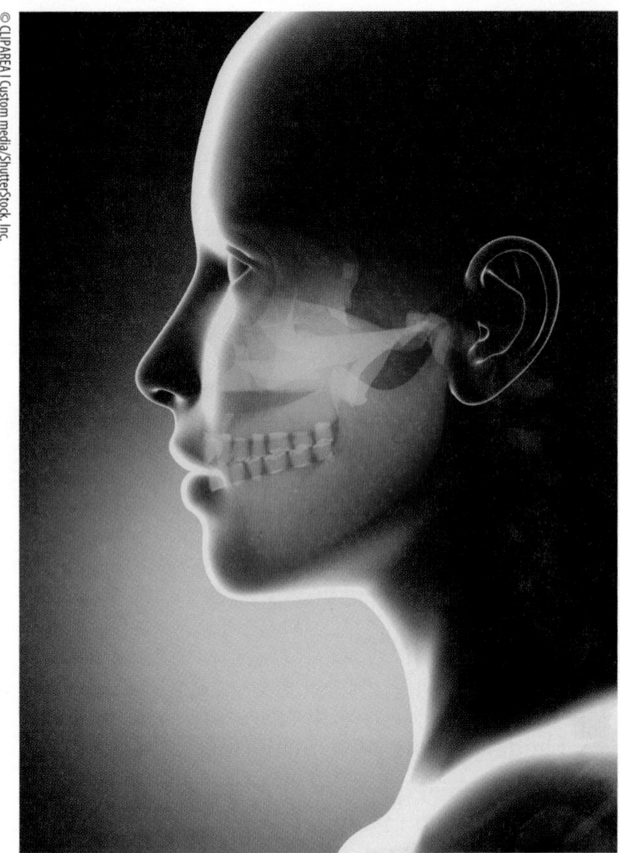
© CLIPAREA l Custom media/ShutterStock, Inc.

FIGURE 13-2A Anatomy of the temporomandibular joint.

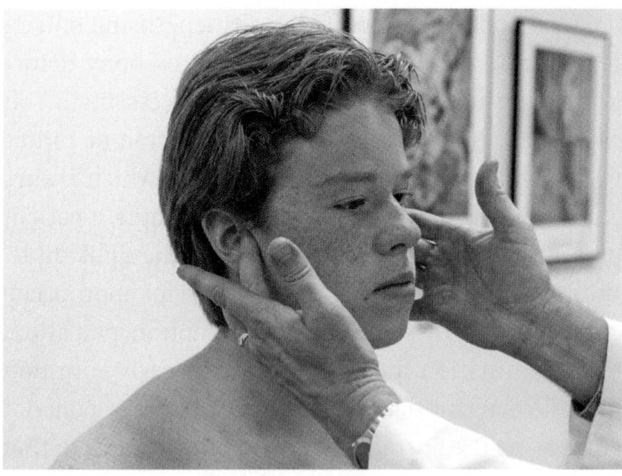

FIGURE 13-2B To palpate for TMJ dysfunction, the provider places the finger pads in the conchal bowls.

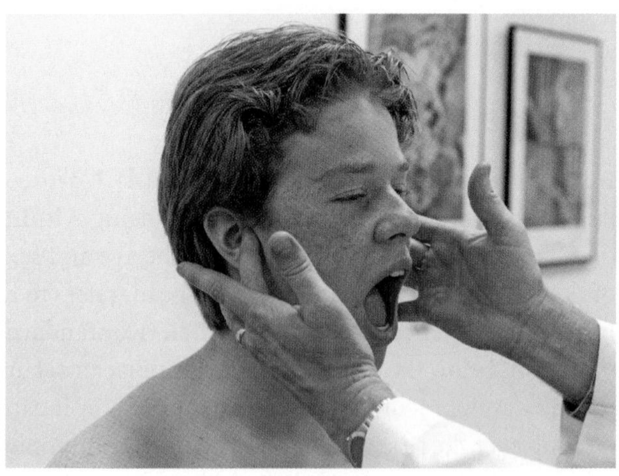

FIGURE 13-2C The patient opens and closes the mouth as the provider observes for deviation and palpates for clicks.

TMJ dysfunction: deviation, popping, or clicking of the temporomandibular joint with range of motion

Inability to open the jaw—trismus or lockjaw—secondary to spasm of the muscles of mastication has greatly decreased in frequency, with widespread immunization efforts contributing to significant decreases in the incidence of tetanus.

Inability to close the jaw may be indicative of TMJ dislocation. The mouth is fixed in an open position with evidence of overbite. This may occur with trauma or excessive opening of the mouth, as with a wide yawn.

Palpation

13-1 Place the pad of each index finger in the conchal bowl behind the tragus (see FIGURE 13-2B). Have the patient open and close the mouth, again palpating for clicking during the range of motion (see FIGURE 13-2C). Deviation, popping, or clicking may reflect **TMJ dysfunction**.

Pain on palpation may indicate rheumatoid arthritis or osteoarthrosis.

DOCUMENTATION

- Mandible moves in midline. TMJ palpation without clicks or tenderness.

NECK

Inspection

Begin inspection with proper exposure of the neck (see FIGURES 13-3A–B, and 13-4). Inspect laterally to identify the degree of cervical lordosis. Note the general symmetry, muscle mass, and alignment of the head.

© CLIPAREA l Custom media/ShutterStock, Inc.

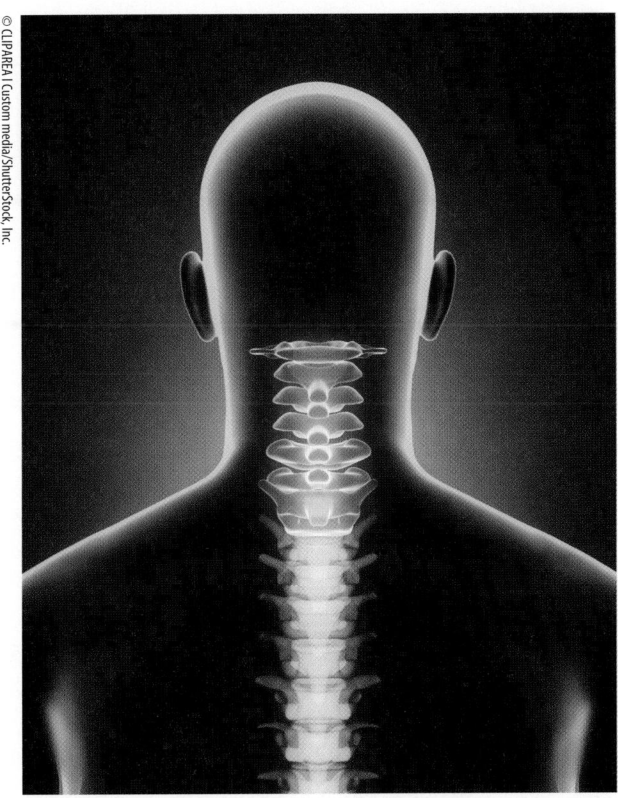

FIGURE 13-3A Posterior view of the cervical spine.

© CLIPAREA l Custom media/ShutterStock, Inc.

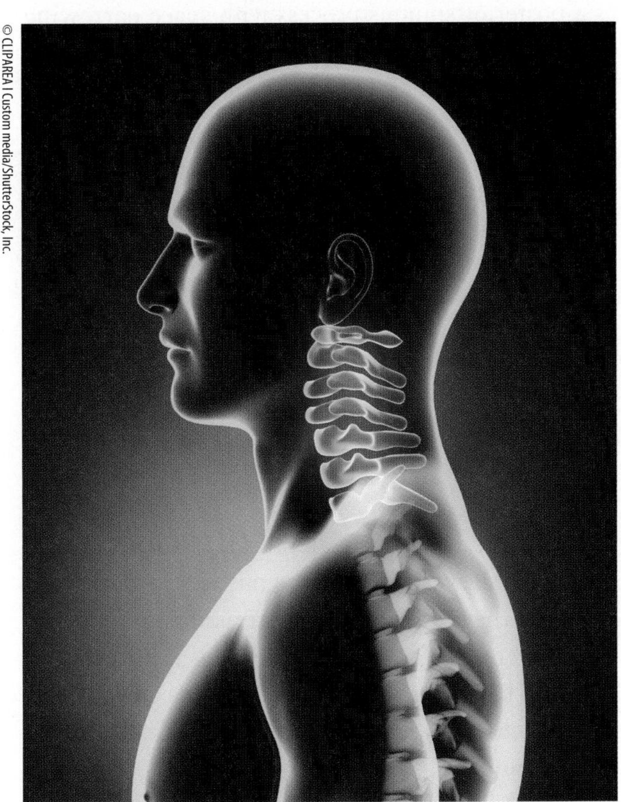

FIGURE 13-3B Lateral view of the cervical spine.

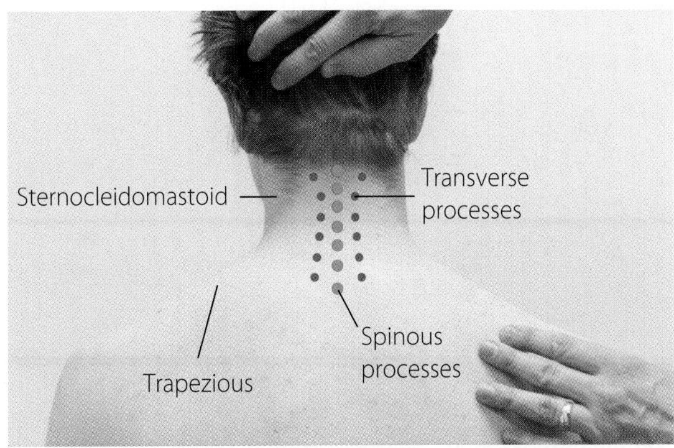

FIGURE 13-4 Posterior neck inspection requires lifting the hair to view posterior landmarks.

Range of Motion.

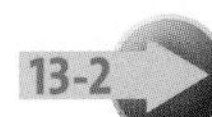

Standing in front of the patient, assess AROM of the neck:

- Flexion (see FIGURE 13-5): The head is bent forward, "Touch your chin to your chest."
- Extension (see FIGURE 13-6): Tilt the head back, "Nose in the air."

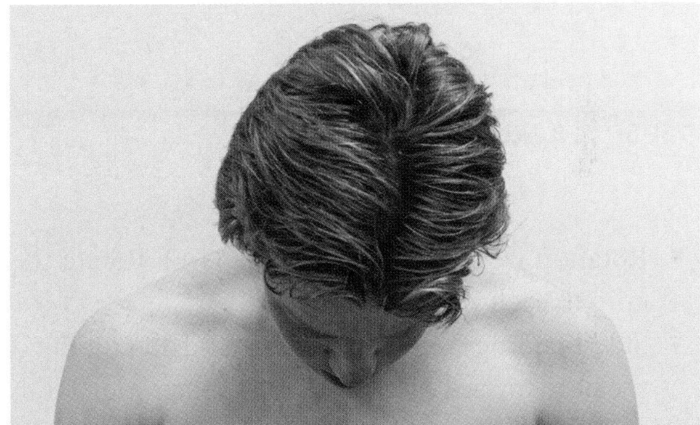

FIGURE 13-5 Neck flexion.

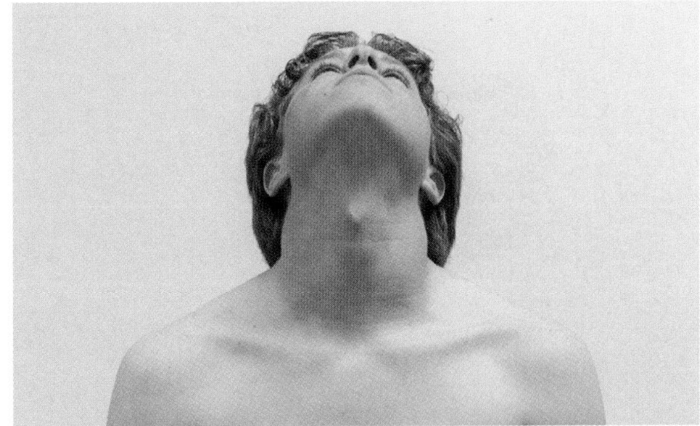

FIGURE 13-6 Neck extension.

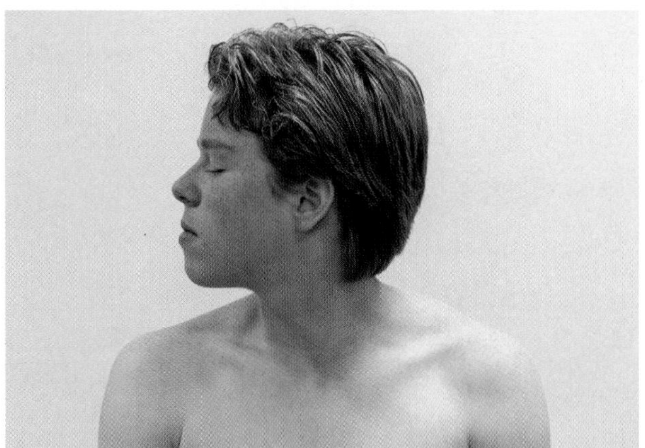

FIGURE 13-7 Neck rotation, right.

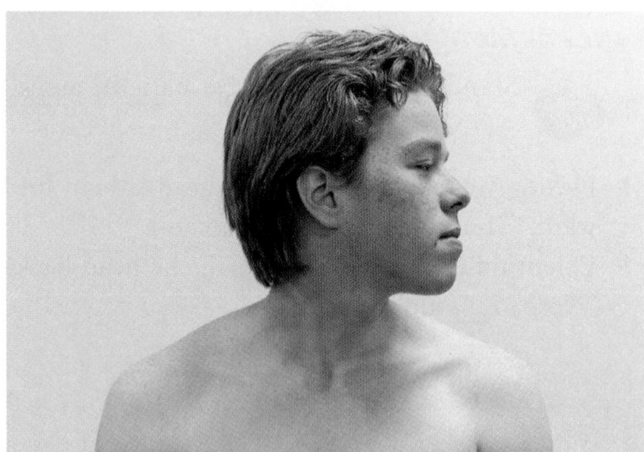

FIGURE 13-8 Neck rotation, left.

- Rotation (see **FIGURES 13-7** and **13-8**): Rotate the chin to each shoulder.
- Side Bending (see **FIGURES 13-9** and **13-10**): Bend the head toward each shoulder, "Touch your ear to your shoulder without lifting the shoulder."

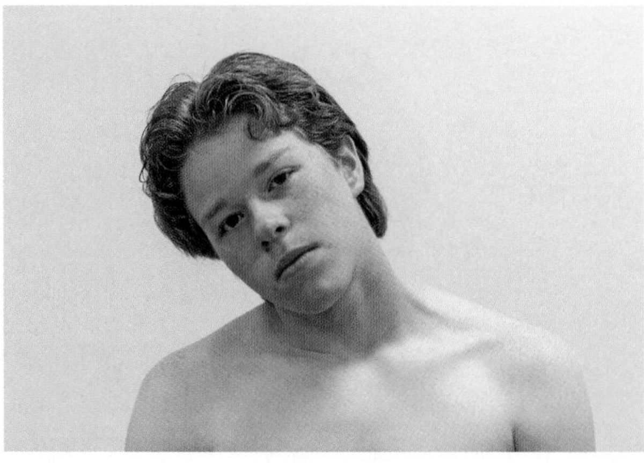

FIGURE 13-9 Neck side bending, right.

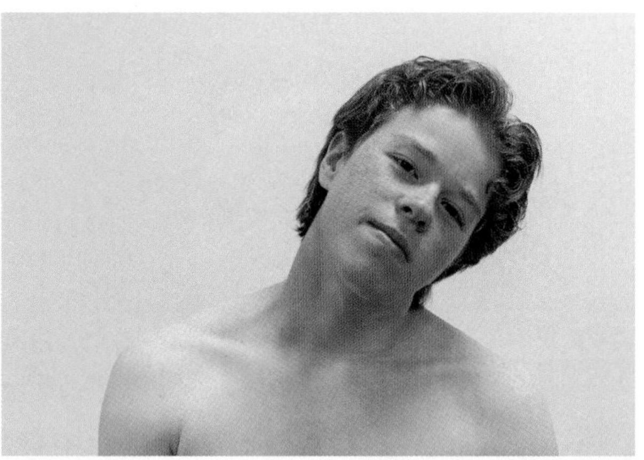

FIGURE 13-10 Neck side bending, left.

Range of motion is commonly limited with arthritis.

Palpation

13-3 Begin at the occiput and palpate the spinous processes for alignment and spacing. Then palpate the transverse processes for spacing and rotation. Rotation of a vertebra will be appreciated as a posterior spinous process with space narrowing or gapping with the adjacent spinous processes. Palpate the paravertebral musculature for tissue texture changes, asymmetry, and tenderness.

DOCUMENTATION

- Neck symmetrical with anticipated lordosis. Head held in midline. No bony deformity. Full AROM. Palpation without tenderness or somatic dysfunction.

SHOULDERS

Inspection

Expose both shoulders bilaterally. If the patient is in a gown, the sleeves can often be pushed upward sufficiently. If they cannot be, ask permission for the gown to be lowered. If the patient is wearing a shirt, ask the patient if he/she can remove it and offer a gown. Carefully watch the patient as the shirt is removed. Can you identify any range of motion restrictions or favoring of one side versus the other while the patient disrobes?

Although inspection can begin with a general comparison, attention to detail is required. Inspection of the shoulder should be broken down into sections: anterior, lateral, and posterior (see **FIGURES 13-11A** through **13-11D**). Compare symmetry of muscle masses—trapezius, rhomboids, supraspinatus, infraspinatus, deltoid triceps, and biceps—noting atrophy, hypertrophy, and asymmetry. Bulging of the biceps over the lower half of the humerus can be associated with rupture of the biceps tendon. Note bony projections, deformity, and the position of the scapula. A posterior "winged scapula" may be caused by muscular or long thoracic nerve dysfunction.

Range of Motion.

13-4 For range of motion assessment, the provider can stand in front of the seated or standing patient and perform the motion that the patient is being asked to do. Run the patient through shoulder ranges of motion testing:

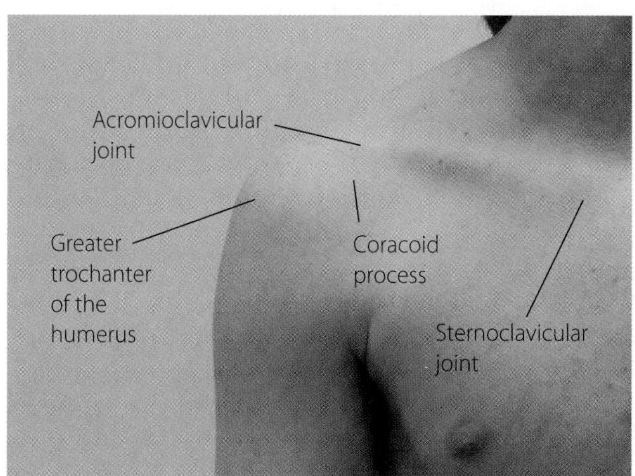

FIGURE 13-11A Shoulder anatomy, anterior.

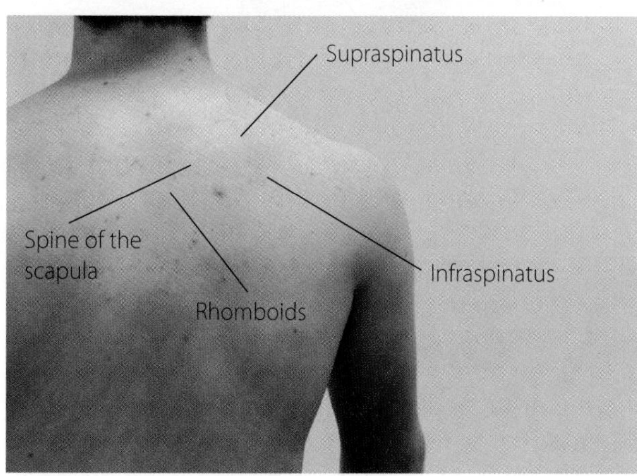

FIGURE 13-11B Shoulder anatomy, posterior.

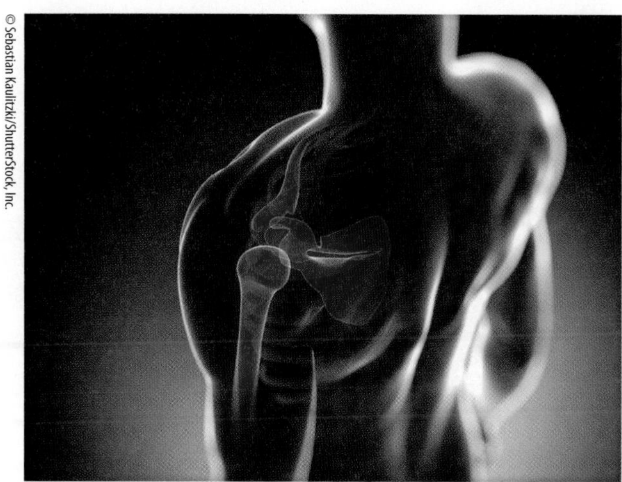

© Sebastian Kaulitzki/ShutterStock, Inc.

FIGURE 13-11C Shoulder anatomy, lateral.

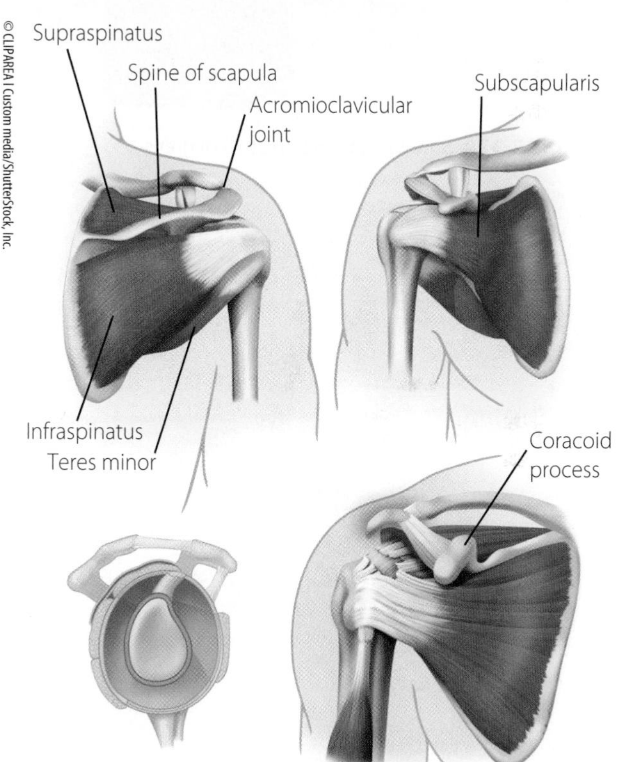

© CLIPAREA l Custom media/ShutterStock, Inc.

FIGURE 13-11D Shoulder anatomy.

- Abduction (see **FIGURES 13-12A** and **13-12B**): The arms move from the sides laterally to touch over the head without bending the elbows.
- Adduction (see **FIGURE 13-13**): The arms move from over the head back to the side and across the thorax.
- Flexion (see **FIGURES 13-14A** through **13-14D**): The arms move from the sides ventrally to over the patient's head without bending the elbows.

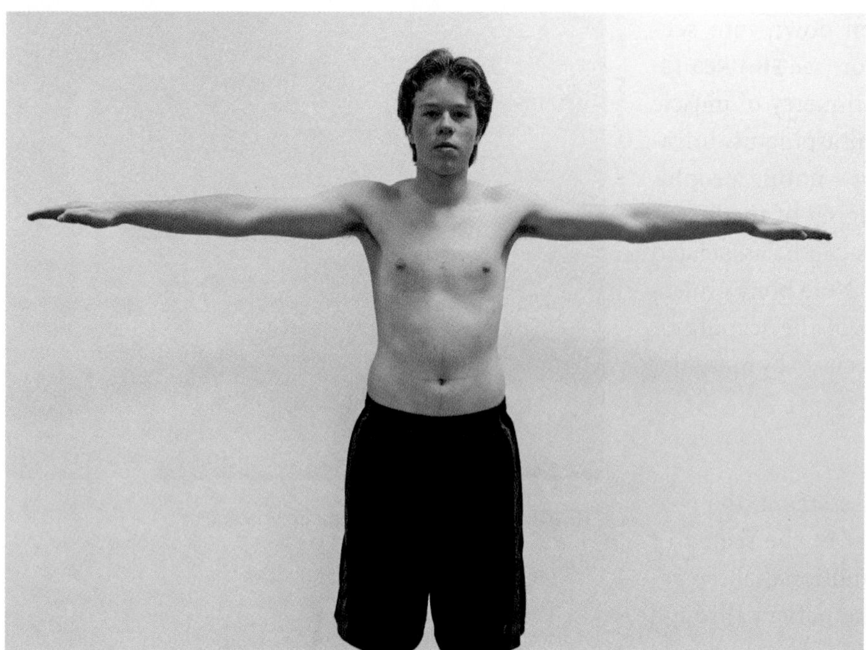

FIGURE 13-12A Shoulder abduction at 90 degrees.

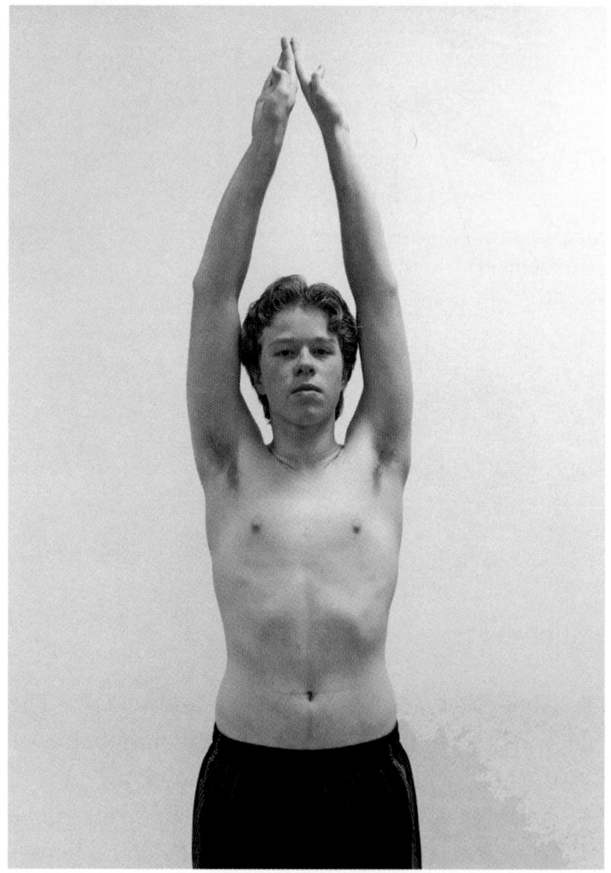

FIGURE 13-12B Shoulder abduction to 180 degrees.

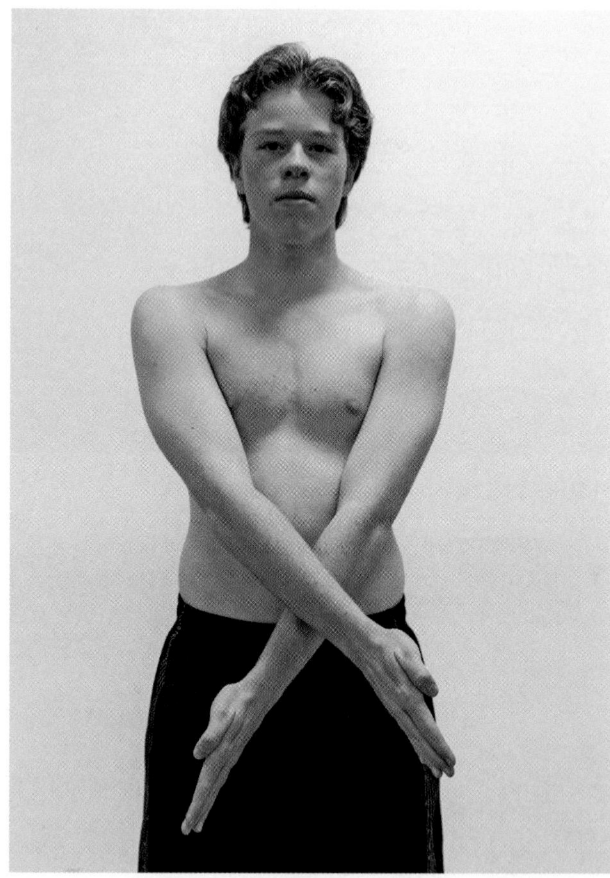

FIGURE 13-13 Shoulder adduction.

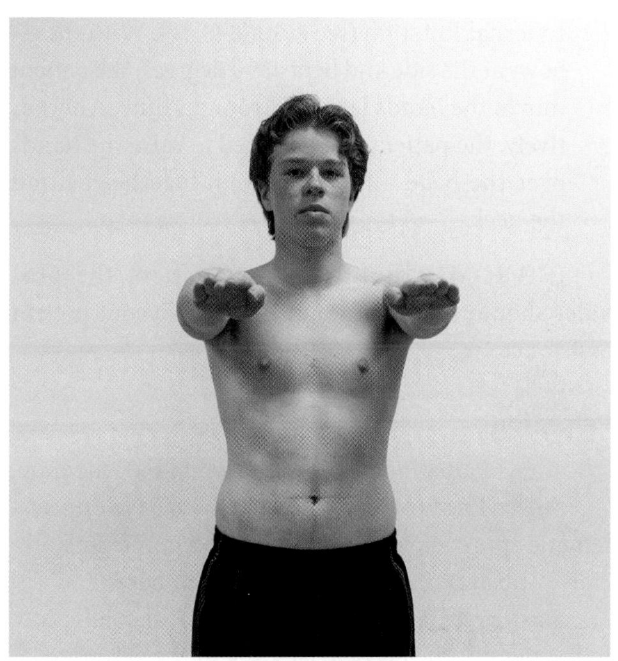

FIGURE 13-14A Shoulder flexion at 90 degrees, anterior view.

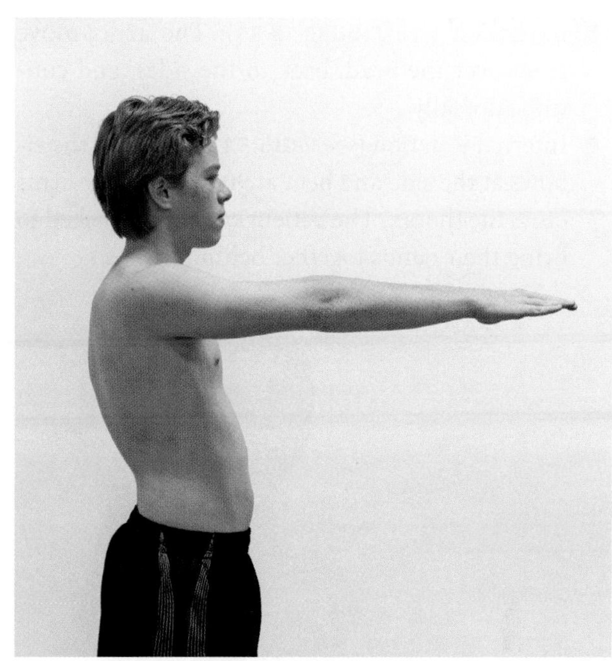

FIGURE 13-14B Shoulder flexion at 90 degrees, lateral view.

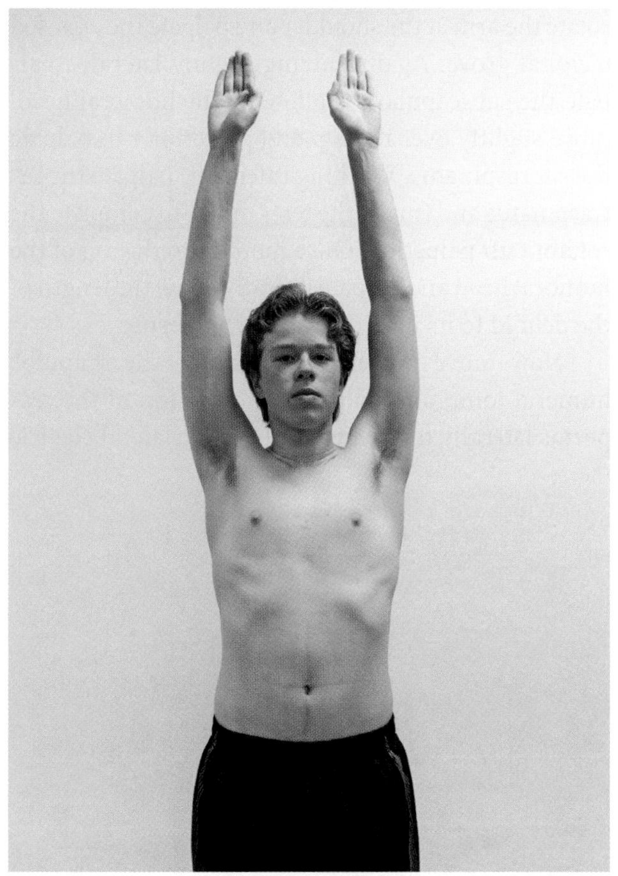

FIGURE 13-14C Shoulder flexion to 180 degrees, anterior view.

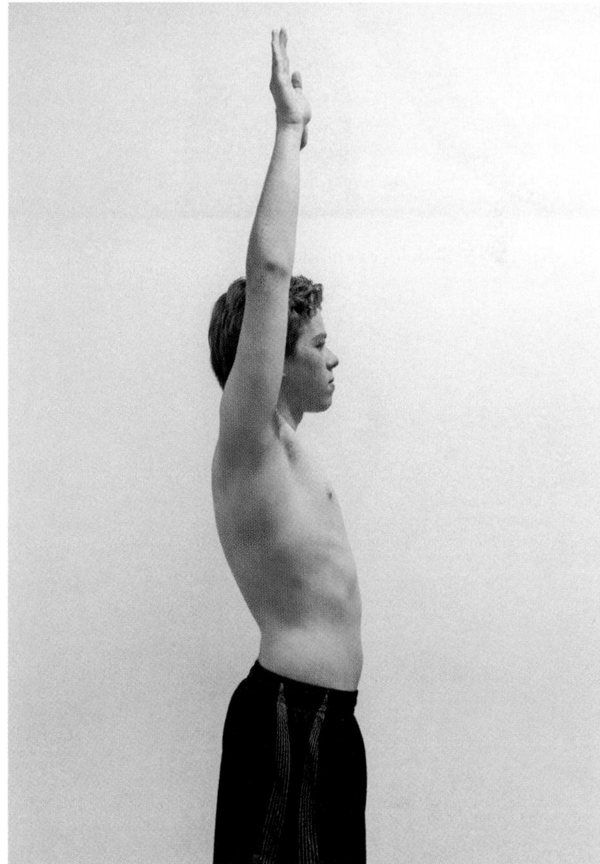

FIGURE 13-14D Shoulder flexion to 180 degrees, lateral view.

- Extension (see FIGURE 13-15): The arms move from over the head, back to the sides, and continue dorsally.
- Internal Rotation (see FIGURE 13-16): With the elbows at the side and bent at 90 degrees, the arms cross the thorax. The patient can then be asked to bring their hands together behind the back.

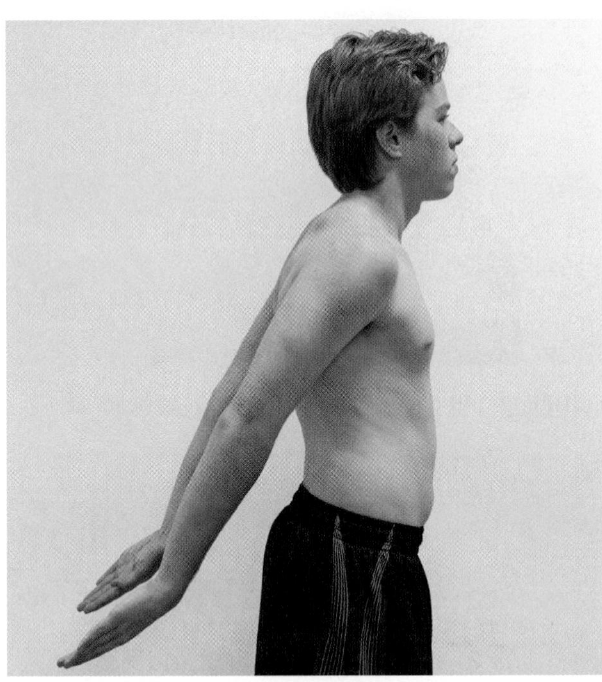

FIGURE 13-15 Shoulder extension.

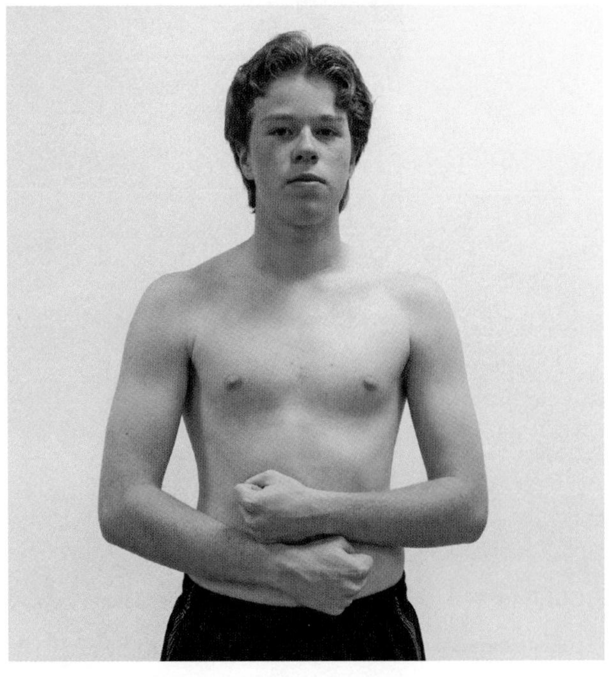

FIGURE 13-16 Shoulder internal rotation.

- External Rotation (see FIGURE 13-17): With the elbows at the side and bent at 90 degrees, the patient moves the hands laterally from midline. Alternatively, the patient can be asked to raise the hands over the head and touch them together behind the neck.

If AROM is limited in any action, the provider should repeat through PROM, without patient assistance.

Palpation

13-5 Palpation of the joint should be deliberate. The provider should strive to develop a systematic approach with a start and end point. An anterior-to-posterior approach is presented here.

Start by palpating the sternoclavicular junction, following out the clavicle laterally to the acromioclavicular (AC) junction. Drop inferiorly to identify the choroid process anteriorly. Have the patient externally rotate the arm at the shoulder and palpate the exposed bicipital grove. Again moving slightly laterally, palpate the subscapularis. Following the humeral head, move slightly over the top and posteriorly to palpate the supraspinatus. Working inferiorly, palpate the infraspinatus and finally the teres minor to complete the rotator cuff palpation. Once more go to the top of the humoral head and palpate laterally down the length of the deltoid to its insertion on the humerus.

Now move posteriorly to assess the scapulohumeral joint, and palpate from the top of the trapezius laterally to the insertion on the lateral clavicle

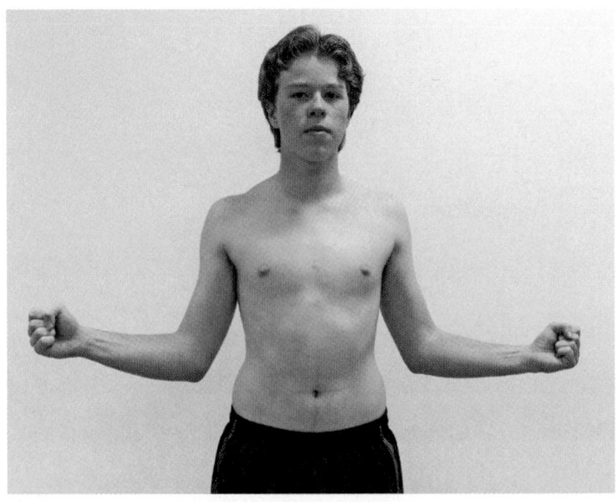

FIGURE 13-17 Shoulder external rotation.

and spine of the scapula. Palpate the body of the supraspinatus and infraspinatus muscles. Repeat in the opposite shoulder.

DOCUMENTATION

- Shoulder inspection symmetrical without deformity. Full AROM bilaterally. Nontender to palpation.

ELBOWS

Inspection

Inspect the elbows bilaterally for erythema, edema, bony deformity, ecchymosis, and bursal swelling (see **FIGURES 13-18A** through **13-18C**). Also look for scaly plaques on the extensor surfaces of the elbows, associated with psoriasis, and on the flexor surfaces, associated with atopic dermatitis (eczema).

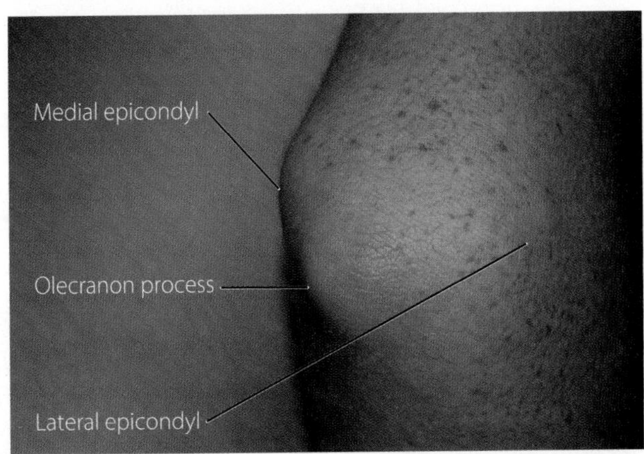

FIGURE 13-18A Surface elbow anatomy.

© Sebastian Kaulitzki/ShutterStock, Inc.

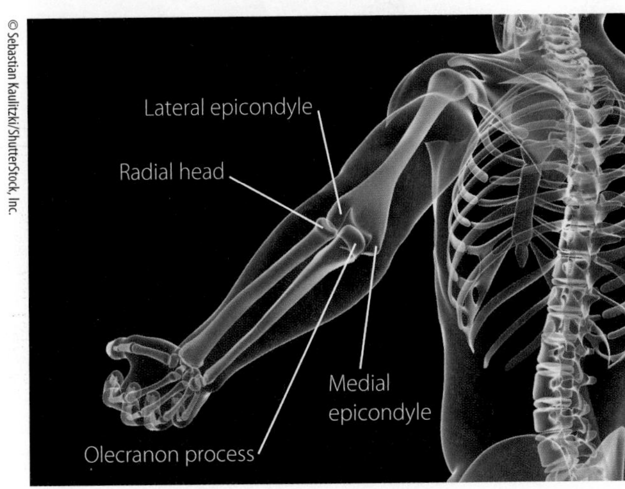

FIGURE 13-18B Skeletal elbow anatomy.

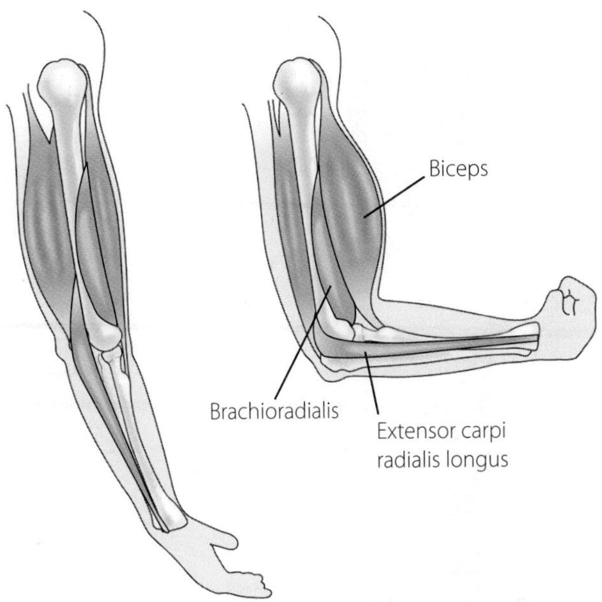

FIGURE 13-18C Muscles involved in elbow movement.

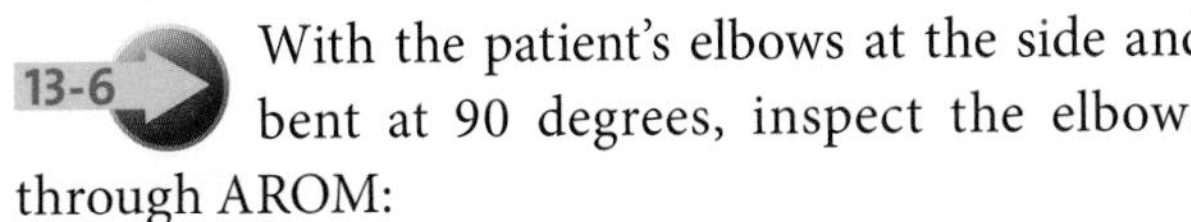

Range of Motion.

13-6 With the patient's elbows at the side and bent at 90 degrees, inspect the elbows through AROM:

- Flexion (see **FIGURE 13-19**): The arms bend at the elbows, bringing the hands to the shoulders.

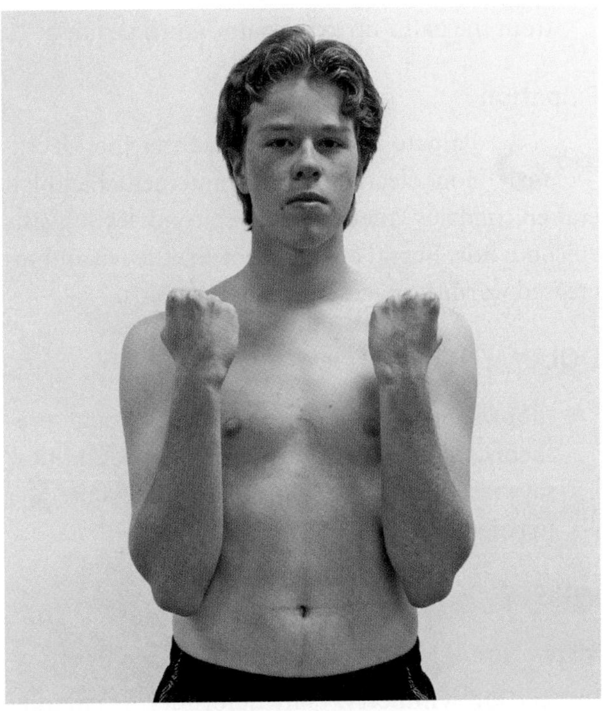

FIGURE 13-19 Elbow flexion.

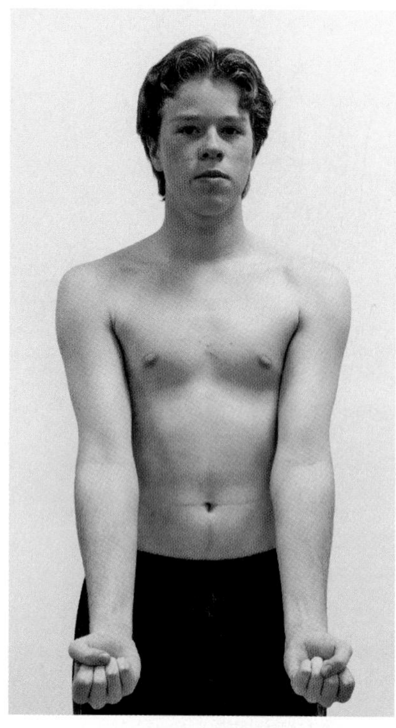

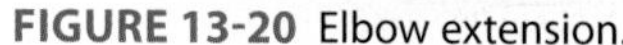

FIGURE 13-20 Elbow extension.

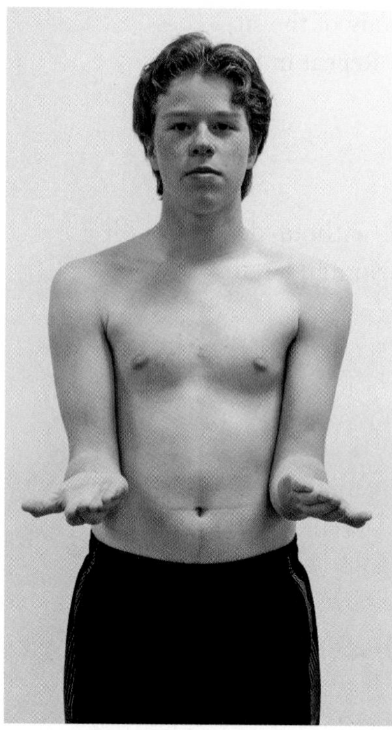

FIGURE 13-21 Elbow supination.

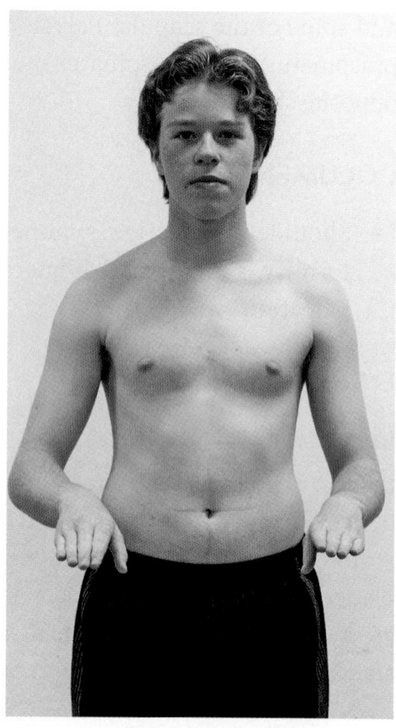

FIGURE 13-22 Elbow pronation.

- Extension (see **FIGURE 13-20**): The arms straighten at the elbows.
- Supination (see **FIGURE 13-21**): The forearms rotate from the palm-down to the palm-up position.
- Pronation (see **FIGURE 13-22**): The forearms rotate from the palm-up to the palm-down position.

Palpation

13-7 Palpate the elbow structure: the olecranon, olecranon bursa, and medial and lateral epicondyles. Tenderness at epicondyles suggests epicondylitis. Bursal enlargement, erythema, and increased warmth suggest olecranon bursitis.

DOCUMENTATION

- Elbows inspection symmetrical without erythema, edema, deformity, ecchymosis, and bursal swelling. Full AROM bilaterally. Nontender to palpation.

WRISTS

Inspection

Inspect for symmetry, bony deformity or enlargement, ecchymosis, edema, and erythema (see **FIGURES 13-23A** through **13-23C**). Small, sessile, round masses over the dorsum of the wrist may represent a ganglione cyst.

© Aaron Amat/ShutterStock, Inc.

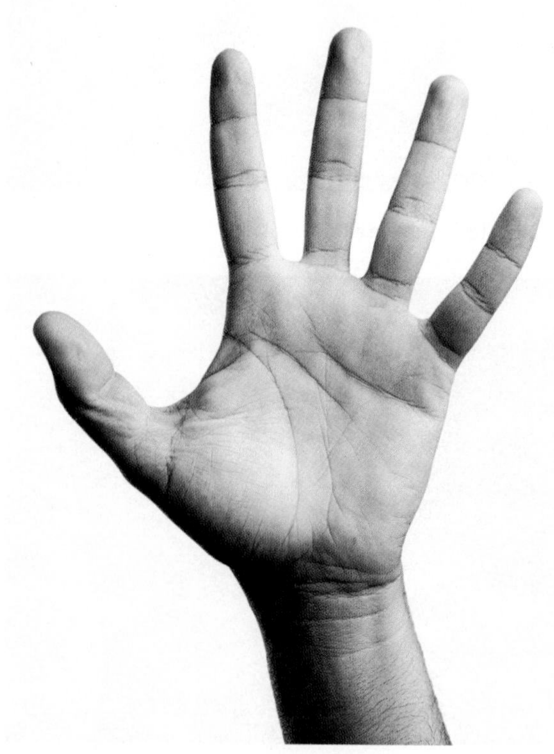

FIGURE 13-23A Anterior wrist.

© ags1973/ShutterStock, Inc.

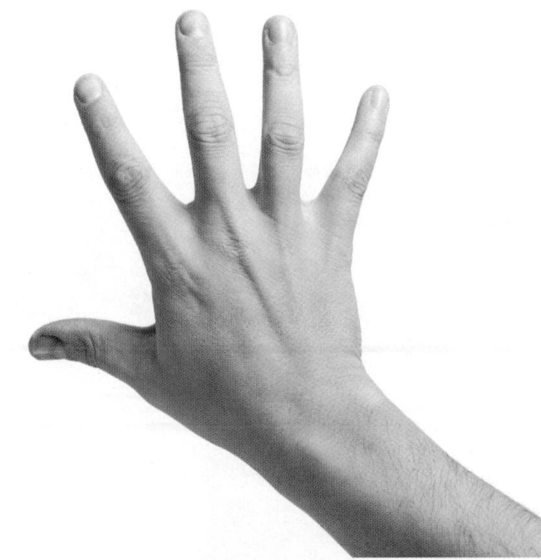

FIGURE 13-23B Posterior wrist.

© Sebastian Kaulitzki/ShutterStock, Inc.

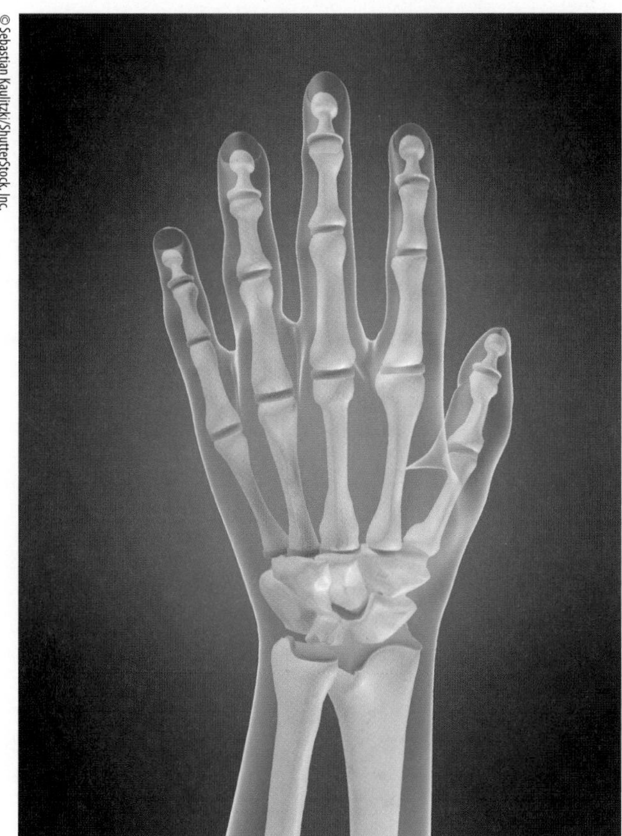

FIGURE 13-23C Wrist anatomy.

Range of Motion.

13-8 With the patient's elbows bent at 90 degrees, start with the wrists straight, the fingers together, and the palms down in pronation, and check the wrists through all ranges of motion:

- Radial Flexion (see **FIGURE 13-24**): Keeping the fingers straight, angle the hand toward the radius.
- Ulnar Flexion (see **FIGURE 13-25**): Keeping the fingers straight, angle the hand toward the ulna.

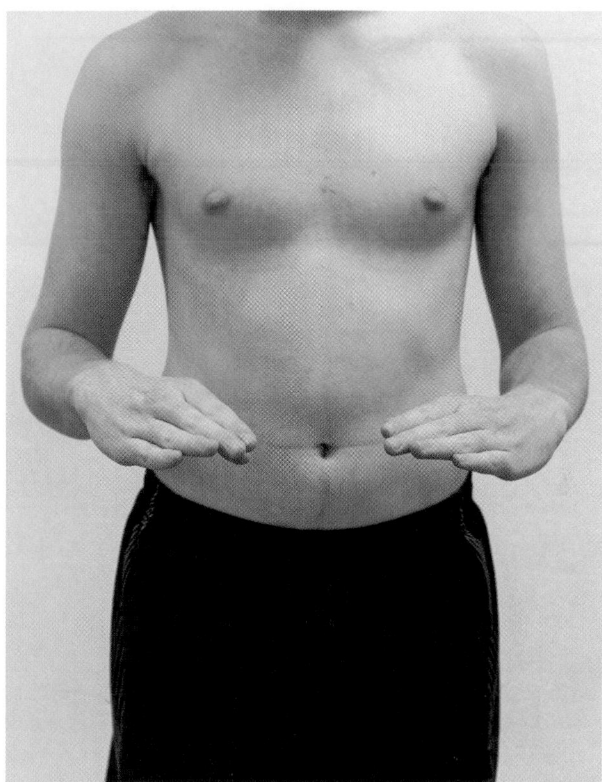

FIGURE 13-24 Radial flexion.

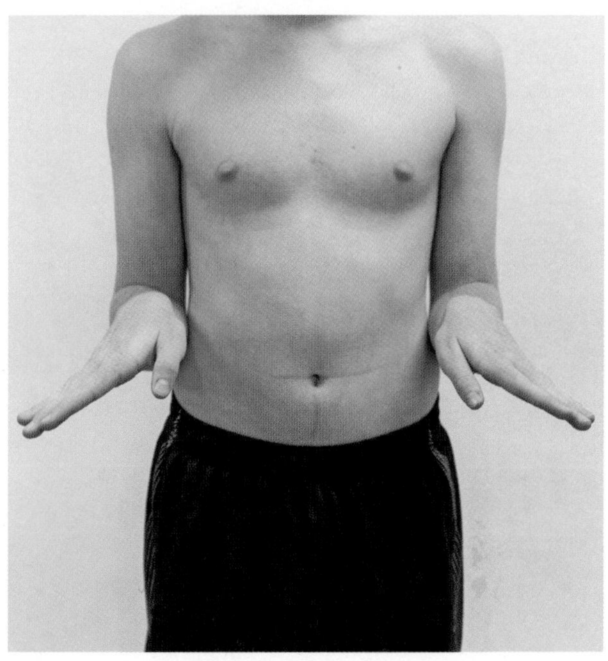

FIGURE 13-25 Ulnar flexion.

- Flexion (Palmar Flexion) (see **FIGURE 13-26**): Bend the hands at the wrist toward the feet.
- Extension (Dorsiflexion) (see **FIGURES 13-27A** and **13-27B**): Bend the hands at the wrist toward the head.

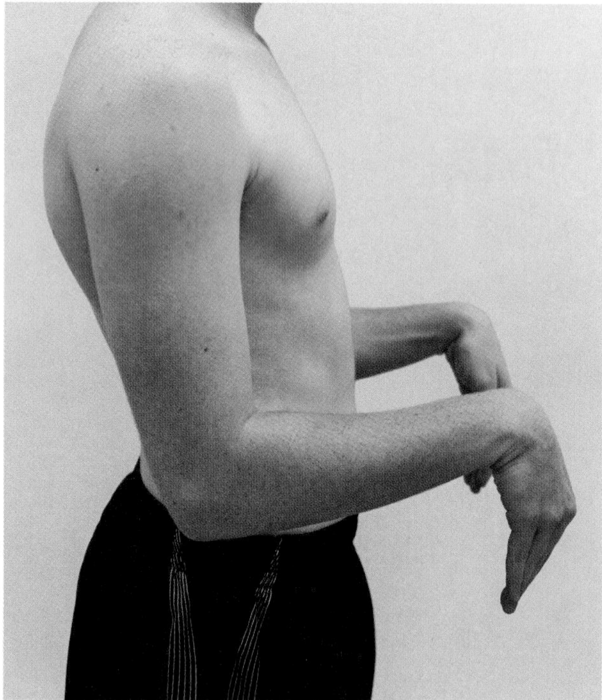

FIGURE 13-26 Wrist flexion.

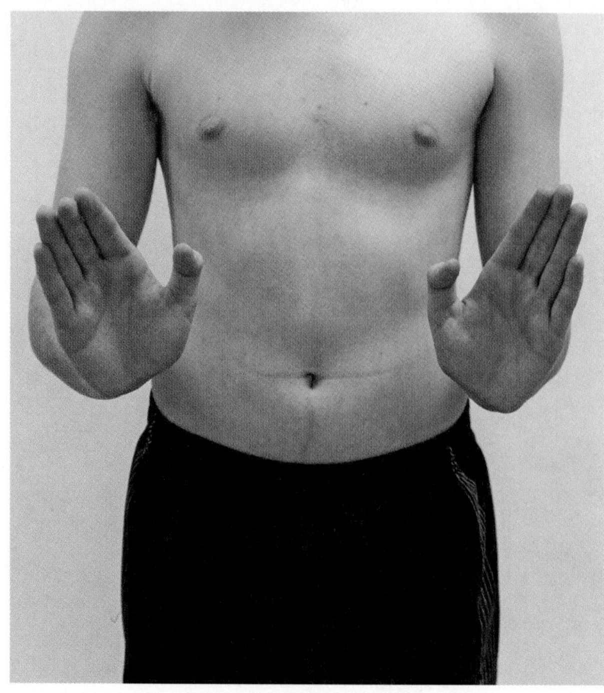

FIGURE 13-27A Wrist extension, anterior view.

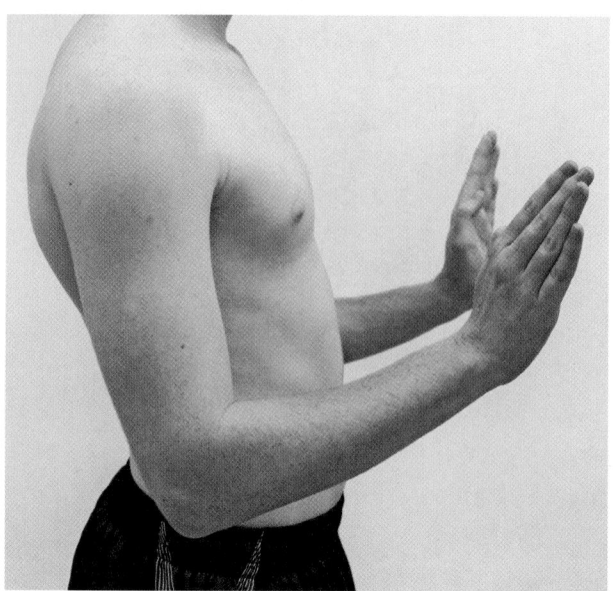

FIGURE 13-27B Wrist extension, lateral view.

Palpation

13-9 Palpate the distal radius and ulna at the articulation with the carpal bones. If a patient complains of pain in the wrist, it is imperative to palpate the anatomic snuff box (see **FIGURE 13-28**). Pain at this location must alert the provider to a possible scaphoid bone fracture. The scaphoid bone has a single distal arterial supply. If a fracture occurs, the proximal scaphoid can become necrotic, hence the need for heightened vigilance.

Chronic pain over the snuff box may represent chronic stenosing tenosynovitis (DeQuervain disease). The patient is asked to flex the thumb to the palm and clench the fingers over it. If ulnar deviation of the hand results in pain, tenosynovitis is likely.

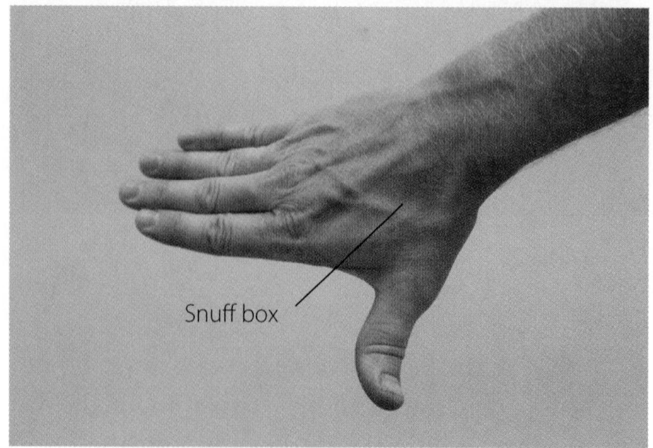

FIGURE 13-28 Anatomic snuff box.

DOCUMENTATION

- Wrists symmetrical without erythema, edema, deformity, ecchymosis. Full AROM bilaterally. Nontender to palpation.

FINGERS

Inspection

Inspect the general size of the hands. Overly large hands may suggest acromegaly. Elongated, slender fingers may be associated with Marfan syndrome. Abnormal elongation must be differentiated from long fingers in proportionally tall individuals. This can be done by asking the patient to fold the fingers over the palmed thumb. The thumb should not typically stick out from under the fifth digit. The patient may also be asked to encircle the wrist with the thumb and finger of the other hand. An overlap of more than 1 cm is considered abnormal. If these tests are positive, the possibility of Marfan should be entertained.

Inspect the fingers, working through each joint from the metacarpal phalangeal (MCP) to the proximal interphalangeal (PIP) and finally the distal interphalangeal (DIP). Note the alignment of the fingers. Ulnar deviation of the fingers is a common finding with rheumatoid arthritis (RA).

Bony enlargement of the PIP and DIP joints are also associated with arthritis. **Heberden's nodes** are found with osteoarthritis (OA) at the distal interphalangeal joints). **Bouchard's nodes** of the proximal interphalangeal joints are associated with both RA and OA (see **FIGURE 13-29**).

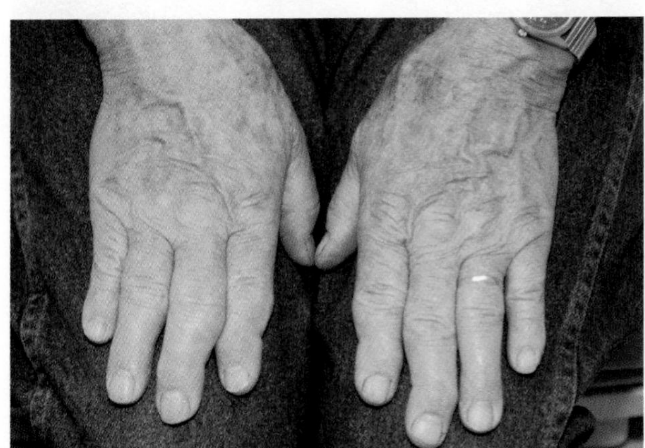

FIGURE 13-29 Heberden's and Bouchard's nodes of osteoarthritis.

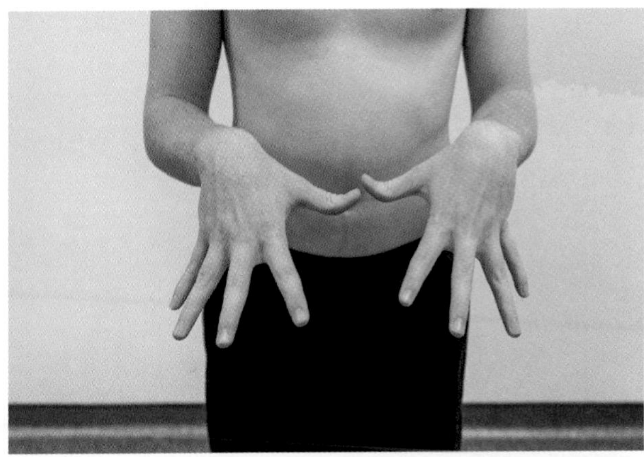

FIGURE 13-30 Finger abduction.

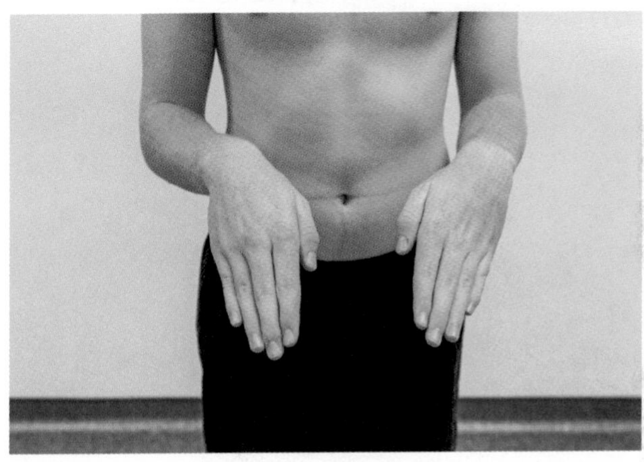

FIGURE 13-31 Finger adduction.

RANGE OF MOTION.

Examine the fingers as a group first, then individually should dysfunction be identified. With the hands out, palm parallel to the floor:

- Abduction (see **FIGURE 13-30**): The fingers are spread open.
- Adduction (see **FIGURE 13-31**): The fingers are brought together.
- Flexion (see **FIGURE 13-32**): The fingers are closed in a grip.
- Extension (see **FIGURE 13-33**): The fingers are lifted back.

Palpation

Palpate each joint for tenderness. Also palpate the palmar surfaces for nodules. A painless nodule or plaque of the palmar fascia can progress to cause retraction and

Heberden's nodes: bony enlargement of distal interphalangeal joints found in osteoarthritis

Bouchard's nodes: bony enlargement of the proximal interphalangeal joints associated with both osteo and rheumatoid arthritis

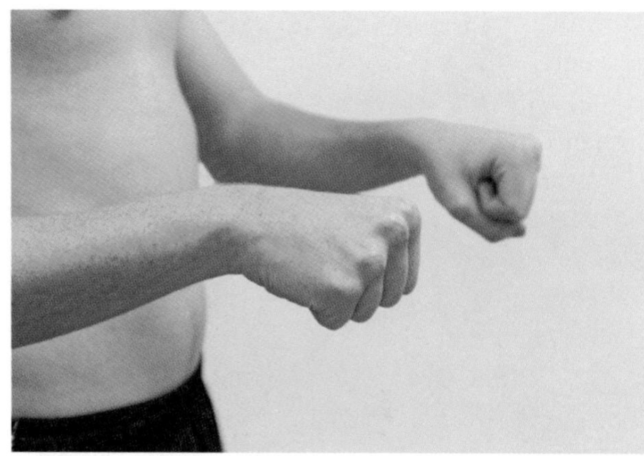

FIGURE 13-32 Finger flexion.

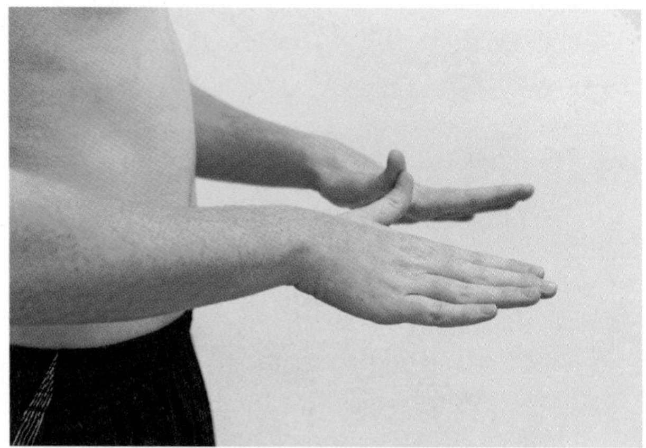

FIGURE 13-33 Finger extension.

flexion of the associated finger, termed Dupuytren contracture.

DOCUMENTATION

- Fingers symmetrical without nodes, erythema, edema, deformity, ecchymosis. Full AROM bilaterally. Nontender to palpation.

KNEES

Before beginning the knee exam, drape the lower extremities with a sheet, lifting it to properly expose the knees.

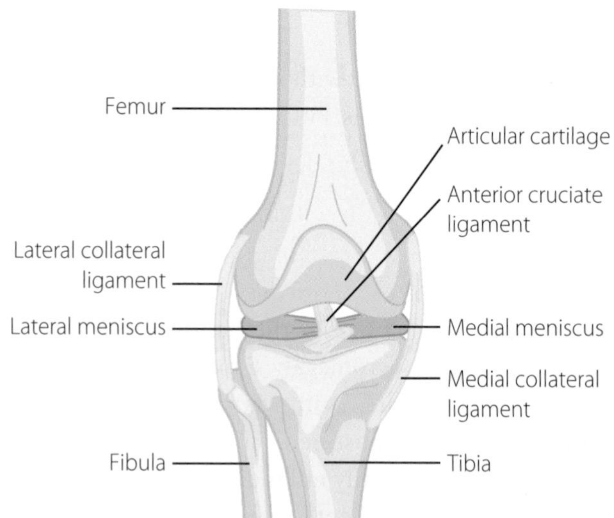

FIGURE 13-34A Knee anatomy.

© Sebastian Kaulitzki/ShutterStock, Inc.

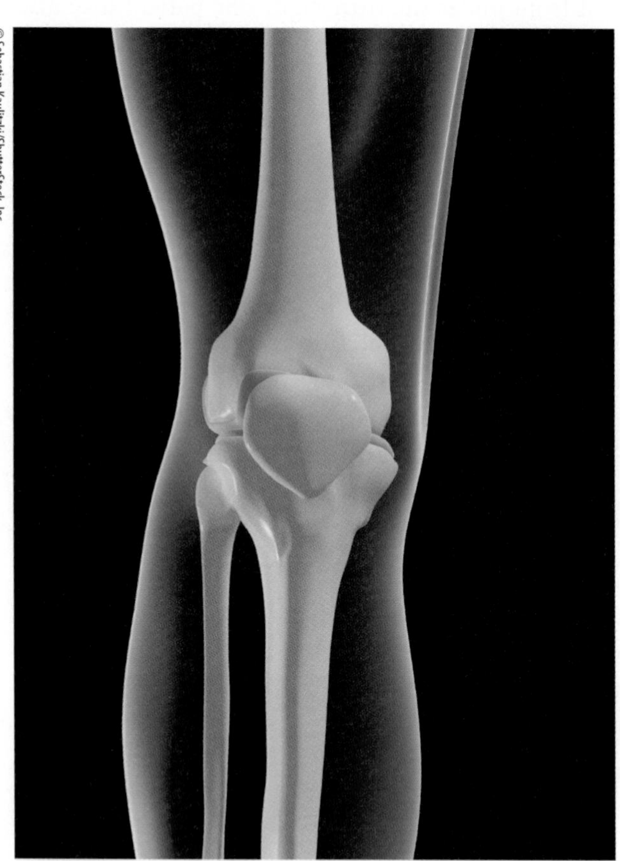

FIGURE 13-34B Skeletal anatomy of the knee.

Inspection

Inspect for symmetry, bony deformity, edema, and evidence of past injury such as surgical scarring (see FIGURES 13-34A and 13-34B). Edema is a common finding with trauma, bursitis, and inflammatory and septic arthritis, and can be seen as increased size in bilateral comparison with loss of peripatellar dimpling.

Range of Motion.

13-10 Ask the patient to slide forward on the table so that about one-half of the upper leg is off the table to allow room for adequate flexion. Inability to fully flex and extend the knee should alert the provider to possible effusion. If flexion is not demonstrated to the full degree, the patient can repeat the range of motion in the standing or supine position.

- Extension (see **FIGURE 13-35**): The lower legs are brought forward, straightening the knee
- Flexion (see **FIGURE 13-36**): From the extended position, the legs are brought back and under the upper leg.

Palpation

13-11 Have the patient slide back to sit fully on the exam table. Palpate bilaterally with the back of the hands as a general screen for increased warmth, indicative of inflammatory processes. Then examine each knee with deliberate palpation. Consider the knee as having three compartments: the central patellofemoral, medial, and lateral compartments.

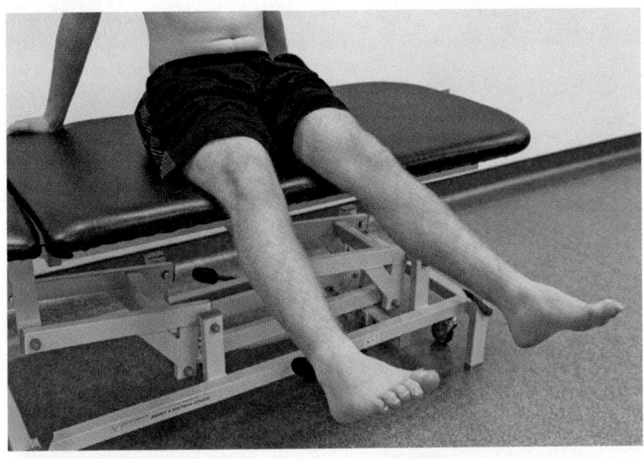

FIGURE 13-35 Knee extension.

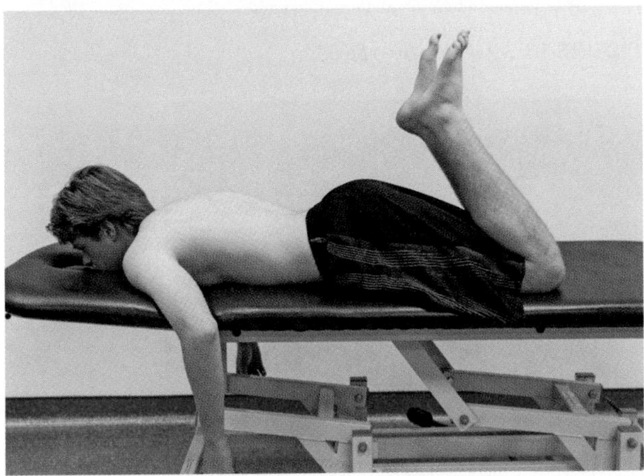

FIGURE 13-36 Knee flexion.

Approach the central patellofemoral compartment first. Starting superiorly, palpate the quadriceps tendon insertion into the patella, the patella, and the peripatellar spaces. Palpate the prepatellar bursa. Inflammation of the bursa is commonly associated with occupations requiring the worker to be on the knees, such as carpet laying, and is caused by repetitive pressure. The bursa may show swelling, warmth, erythema, and tenderness. Follow the patellar tendon inferiorly to the insertion on the tibial tubercle.

With the knees in the bent position, the medial and lateral joint spaces will align at approximately the midpatellar tendon. Palpate each. The medial joint space is a frequent location for pain, being commonly associated with osteoarthritis and medial collateral ligament and medial meniscus injury. The Anserine bursa is located inferiorly to the medial joint line at the insertion of the vastus medialis muscle.

Pain in the lateral joint space may represent iliotibial band syndrome, osteoarthritis, or injury to the lateral collateral ligament or lateral meniscus. These injuries are less common than medial injuries.

Now place a hand lightly on the patella and ask the patient to slowly extend the lower leg. Note the tracking of the patella, which should remain in midline, and the presence of crepitus. Admission of anterior knee pain may represent patellofemoral syndrome, chondromalacia patella (found with osteoarthritis), or prepatellar bursitis. Inferior patellar pain may be indicative of patellar tendonitis. Focal tenderness in children and adolescents at the tibial tubercle where the patellar tendon inserts is associated with Osgood-Schlatter disease.

DOCUMENTATION

- Knees symmetrical without erythema, edema, deformity, ecchymosis. Full AROM bilaterally. Nontender to palpation without masses.

If the patient presents with knee pain or injury, a detailed structural examination should be completed (see Clinical Scenarios later in this chapter for more details).

ANKLES/FEET

Inspection

Finish the lower extremity joint examination with bilateral inspection of the ankles and toes (see FIGURES 13-37A through 13-37C). Ankle sprain injuries are common. Inspect for ecchymosis and edema.

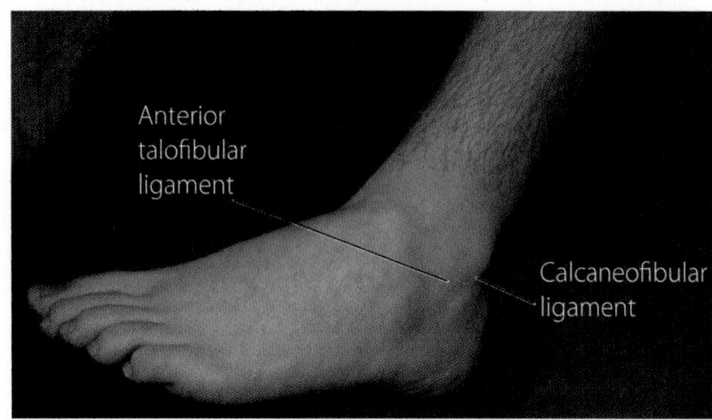

FIGURE 13-37A Surface ankle anatomy.

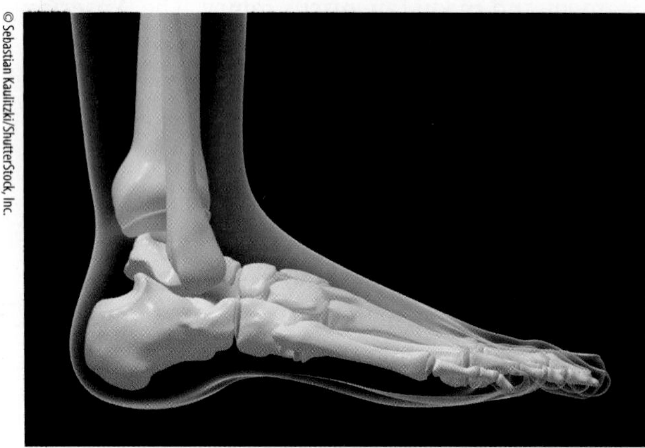

© Sebastian Kaulitzki/ShutterStock, Inc.

FIGURE 13-37B Skeletal ankle anatomy.

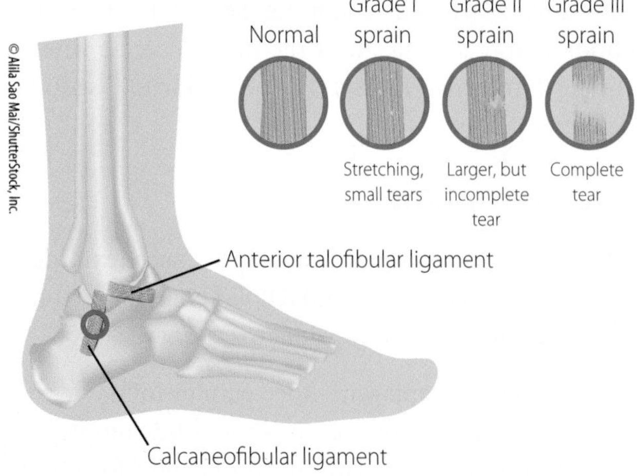

© Alila Sao Mai/ShutterStock, Inc.

FIGURE 13-37C Ligamental ankle anatomy with sprain grades.

Range of Motion.

With the patient still seated on the exam table:

- Plantarflexion (see FIGURE 13-38): The feet are pushed down, "planted," as if stepping on a gas pedal.
- Dorsiflexion (see FIGURE 13-39): The feet are pulled back, putting the "toes in the air."
- Inversion (see FIGURE 13-40): The feet are angled inward as if walking on the outer sides of the feet.

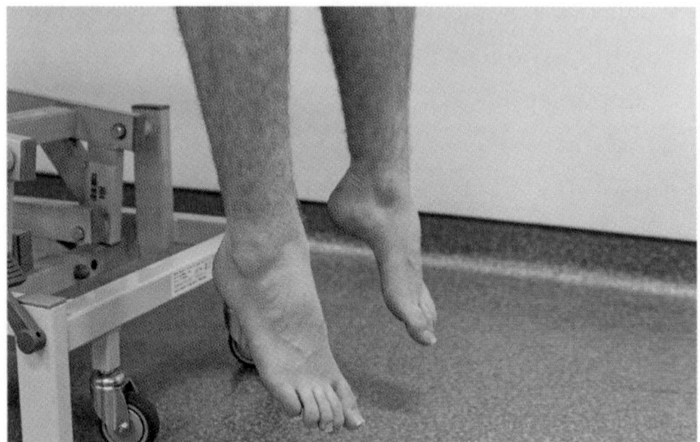

FIGURE 13-38 Ankle plantarflexion.

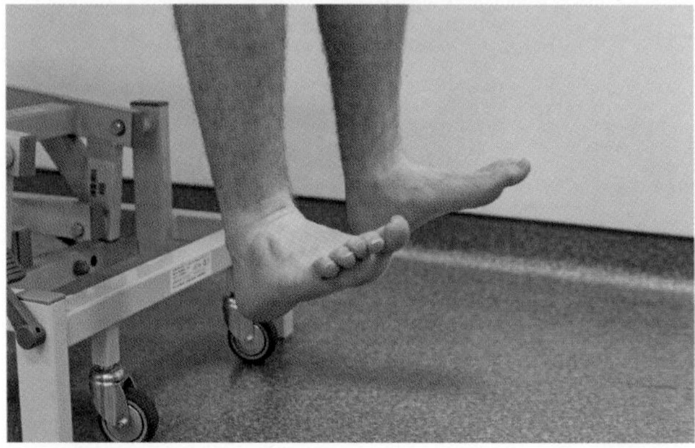

FIGURE 13-39 Ankle dorsiflexion.

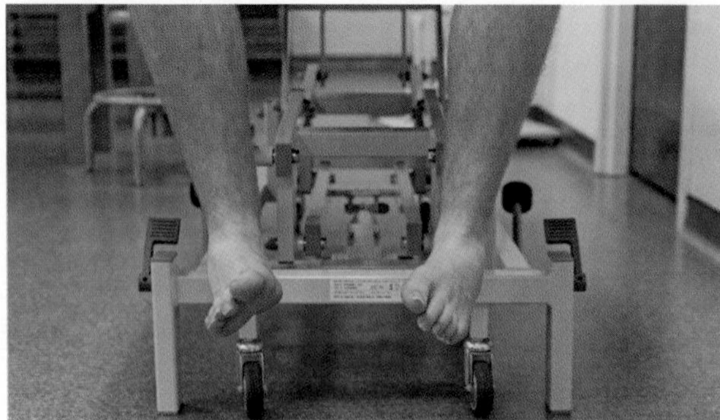

FIGURE 13-40 Ankle inversion.

- Eversion (see FIGURE 13-41): The feet are angled outward as if walking on the inner edges of the feet.
- Internal rotation (see FIGURE 13-42): The feet are rotated inward, bringing the great toes together.
- External rotation (see FIGURE 13-43): The feet are rotated outward, bringing the heals together.

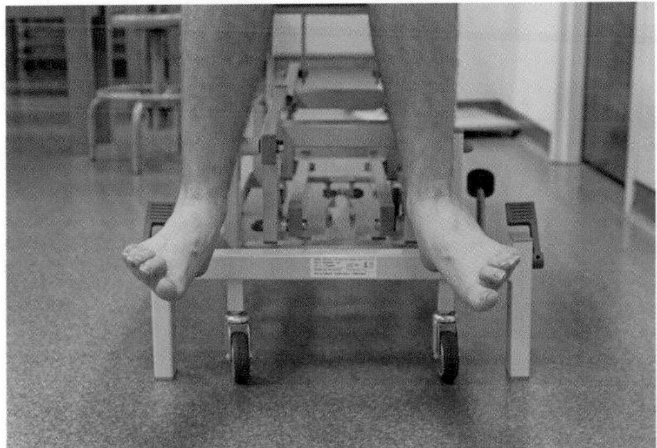

FIGURE 13-41 Ankle eversion.

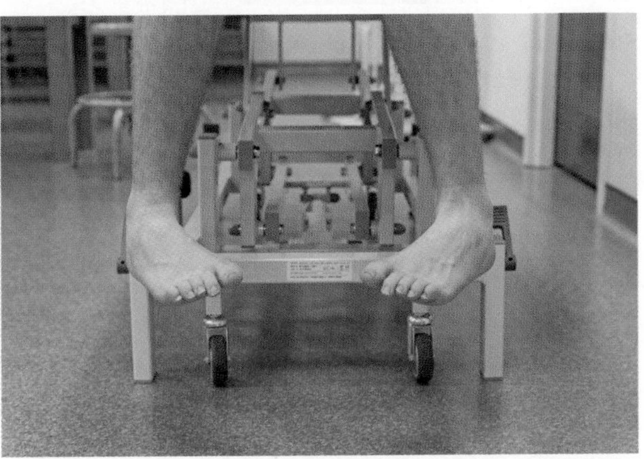

FIGURE 13-42 Ankle internal rotation.

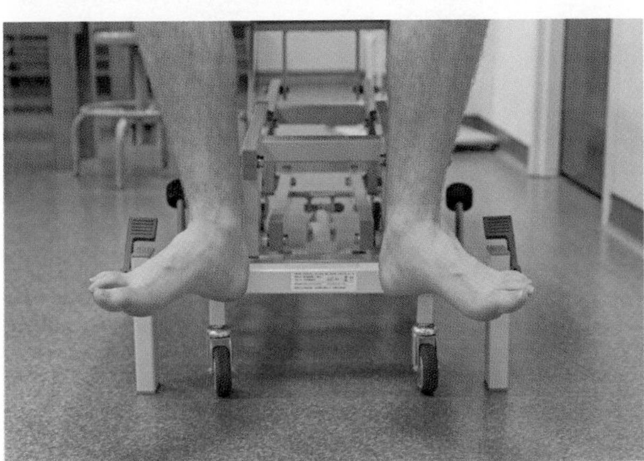

FIGURE 13-43 Ankle external rotation.

Palpation

Palpate the medial malleoli and the deltoid ligament, the site of injury with eversion sprains. Palpate the lateral malleoli and the supporting ligaments, anterior and posterior talofibular, and calcaneofibular ligament. Inversion injuries are the most common sprain mechanism, with the anterior talofibular ligament being the most commonly injured.

Posteriorly palpate the Achilles tendon to its insertion on the calcaneus.

DOCUMENTATION

- Ankles and feet symmetrical without erythema, edema, deformity, ecchymosis. Full AROM bilaterally. Nontender to palpation.

Standing Position

SPINE

With as much examination as possible completed in the seated position, assist the patient to the standing position (see FIGURES 13-44A and 13-44B).

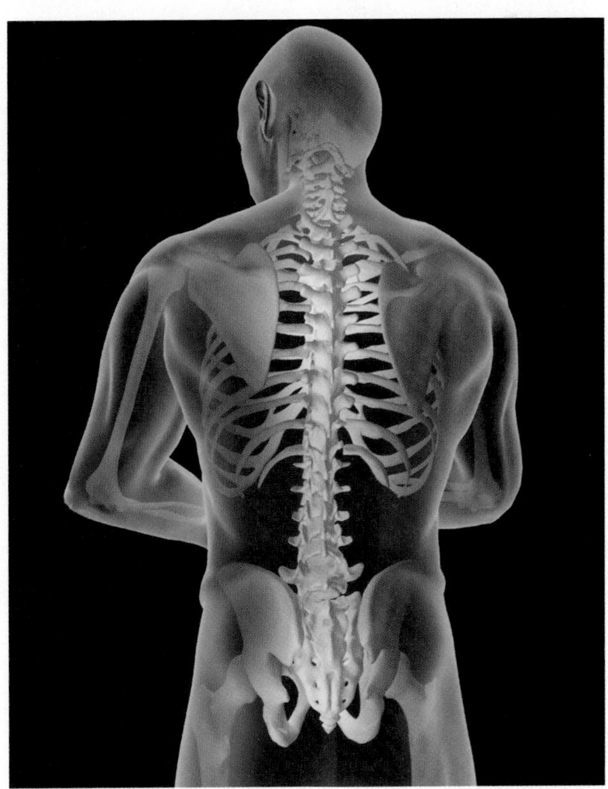

© Sebastian Kaulitzki/ShutterStock, Inc.

FIGURE 13-44A Skeletal anatomy of the spine.

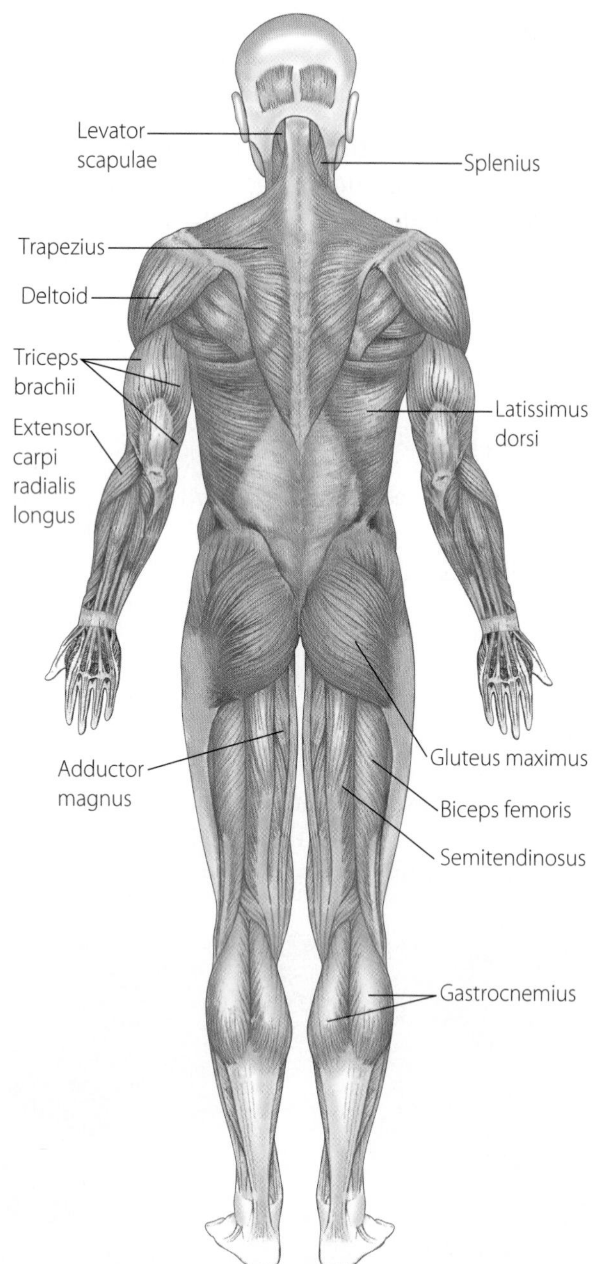

FIGURE 13-44B Posterior musculoskeletal anatomy.

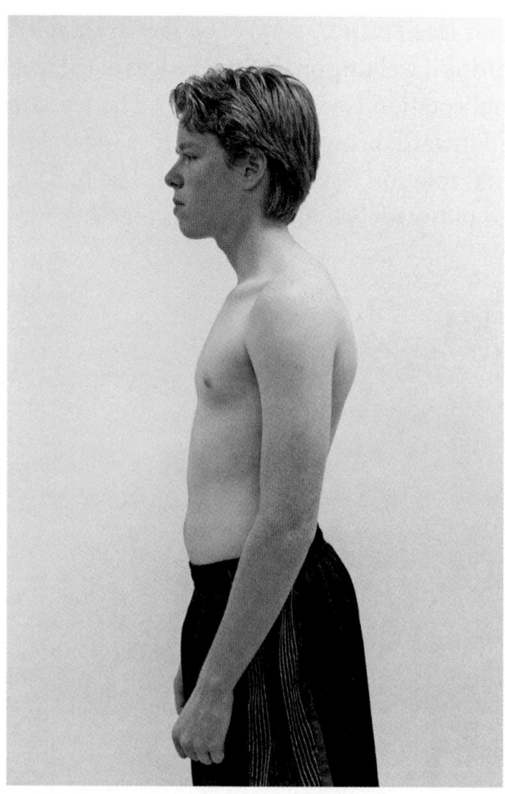

FIGURE 13-45 Lateral spine inspection.

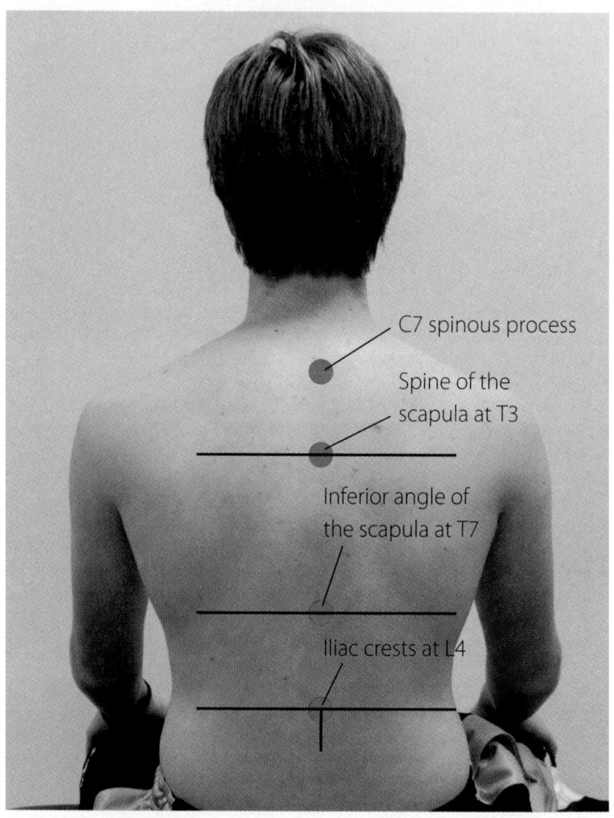

FIGURE 13-46 Posterior inspection of the back with surface anatomy landmarks.

Inspection

Stand several feet from the patient and examine from the side, noting the changes in the suspected cervical lordosis, thoracic kyphosis, and lumbar lordosis (see **FIGURE 13-45**). Note exaggerations or flattening.

Then stand behind and note any lateral curvature suggestive of **rotoscoliosis** (see **FIGURE 13-46**). Identification of slight rotoscoliosis may be aided by noting the space between the patient's side and the

Rotoscoliosis: lateral curvature of the spine

arm hanging loosely at the side, where the space on one side is greater than the other.

Range of Motion.

13-12 Range of motion of the neck was already completed in the seated position. Stand behind the patient to assess general AROM of the thoracic and lumbar spine. If imbalance is detected, stabilize the patient by placing a hand at each hip.

- Flexion (see **FIGURE 13-47**): Bending forward at the waist, "Try to touch your toes."
- Extension (see **FIGURE 13-48**): Bending backward at the waist, "Bend back toward me."
- Side Bending (see **FIGURES 13-49A** and **13-49B**): Lateral bending, "Bend to the side," repeat in the opposite direction.
- Rotation (see **FIGURES 13-50A** and **13-50B**): Rotation at the waist, "Without moving your feet, turn toward me," repeat in the opposite direction.

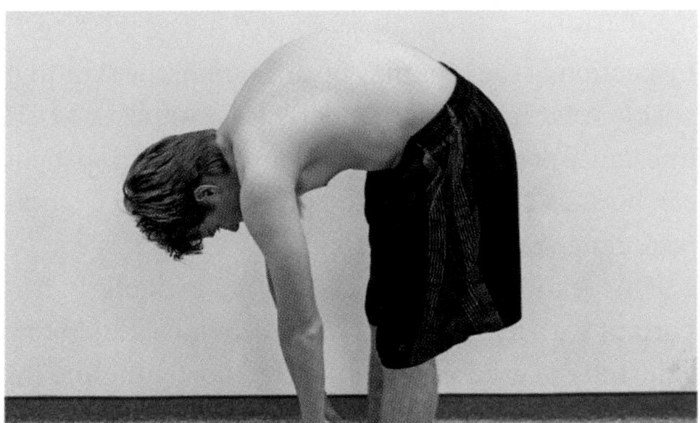

FIGURE 13-47 Waist flexion.

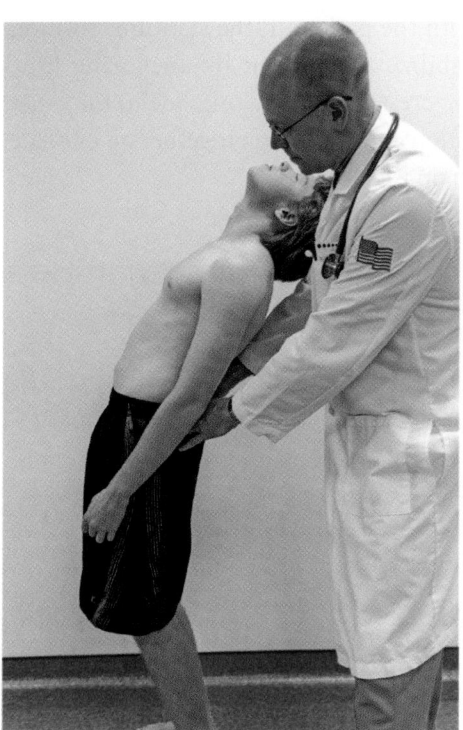

FIGURE 13-48 Waist extension.

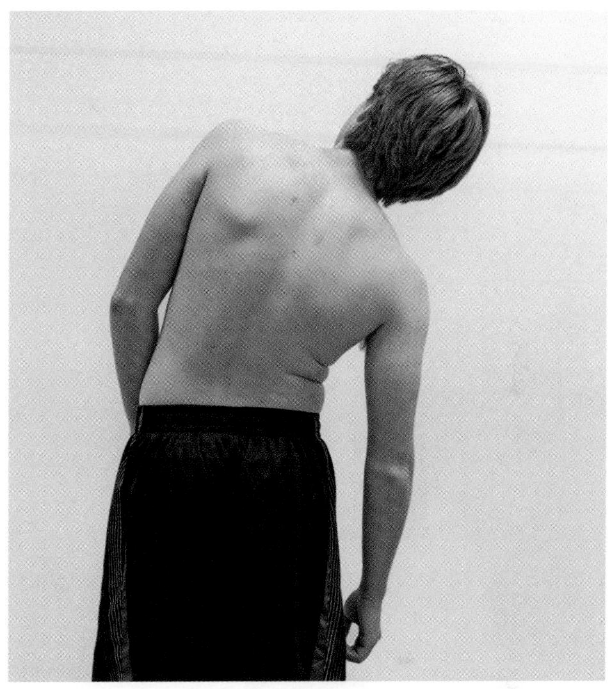

FIGURE 13-49A Side bending right.

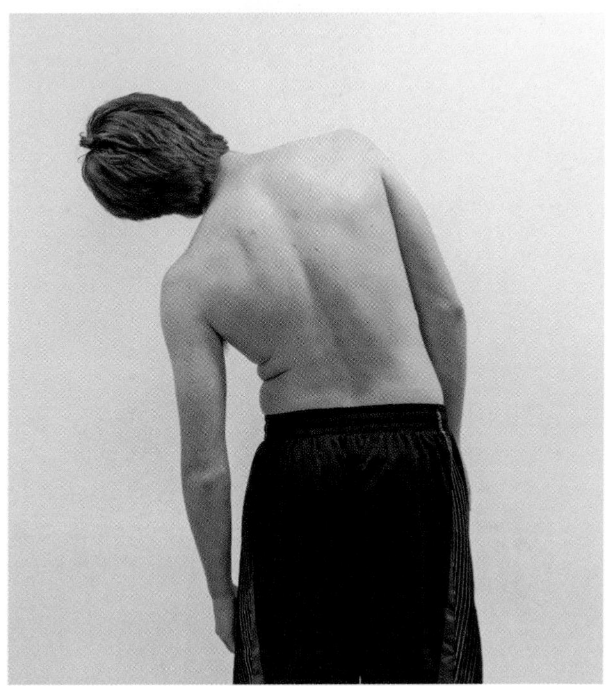

FIGURE 13-49B Side bending left.

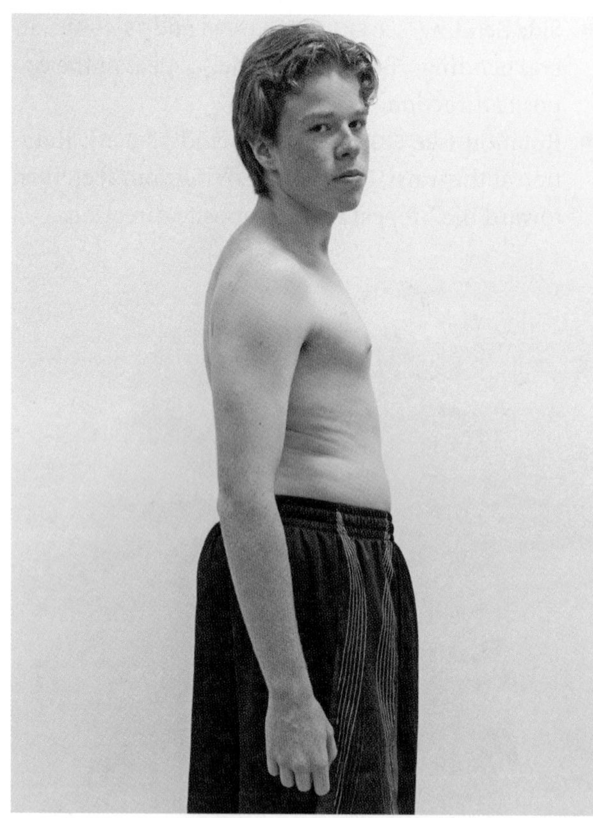

FIGURE 13-50A Rotation right.

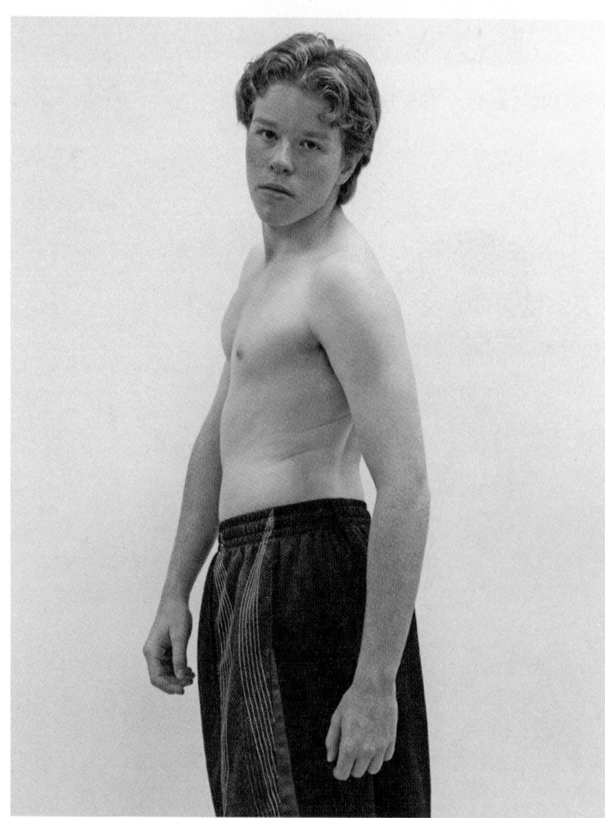

FIGURE 13-50B Rotation left.

Palpation

13-13 Palpate the spinous processes, noting the spaces between each. Palpate the transverse processes bilaterally at each level, noting any posterior positions and narrowing between levels, indicating rotation.

DOCUMENTATION

- Spine with anticipated thoracic kyphosis, lumbar lordosis. No rotoscoliosis. Full AROM. Palpation without tenderness.

HIPS

Inspection

Inspection of the hips may be difficult in the standing position, especially in the elderly (see FIGURE 13-51). If imbalance prohibits adequate examination, the patient can be assisted to supine and prone positions to complete range-of-motion testing.

Inspection of the hip joints is particularly important with a history of a fall. Ecchymosis and bony deformity may be accompanied by shortening and internal rotation of the leg, suggesting fracture.

Range of Motion.

13-14 With the patient in the standing position, stabilize the patient by anchoring him/her at the iliac crests. Compare one side to the other. Group abduction and adduction together on one side, then perform on the other.

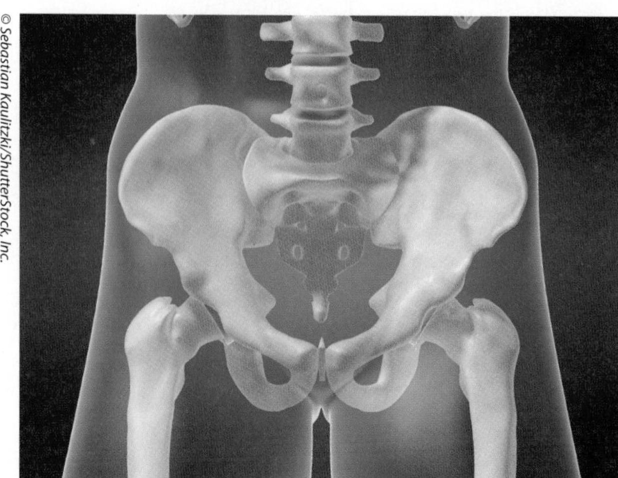

© Sebastian Kaulitzki/ShutterStock, Inc.

FIGURE 13-51 Hip skeletal anatomy.

- Abduction (see FIGURE 13-52): The leg is lifted laterally from the side, "Keeping your knee straight, lift your leg out to the side."
- Adduction (see FIGURE 13-53): The leg is moved back to and across midline in front of the other leg, "Bring your leg back down and cross it in front of the other."
- Flexion (see FIGURE 13-54): The leg is moved ventrally, "Lift your leg in front of you, keeping your knee locked."
- Extension (see FIGURE 13-55): The leg is moved dorsally, "Move your leg behind you, keeping your knee straight."

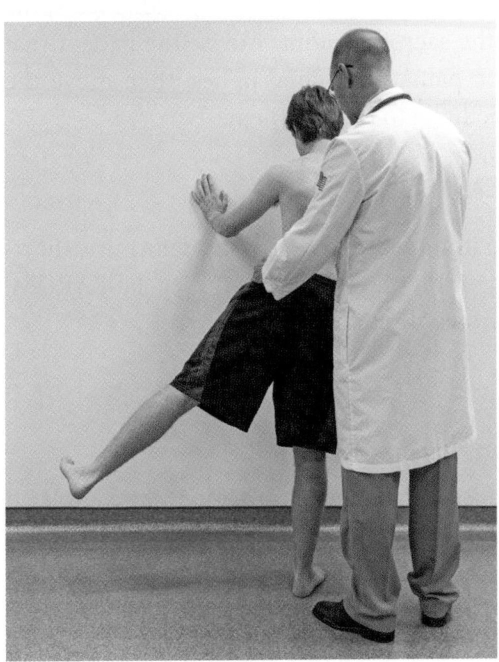

FIGURE 13-52 Hip abduction.

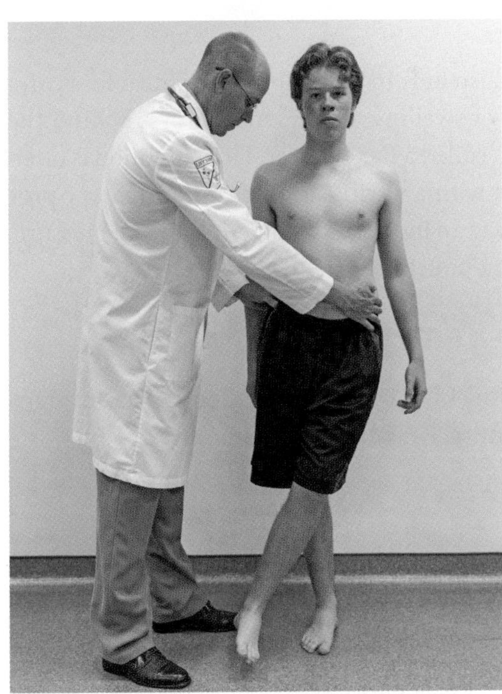

FIGURE 13-53 Hip adduction.

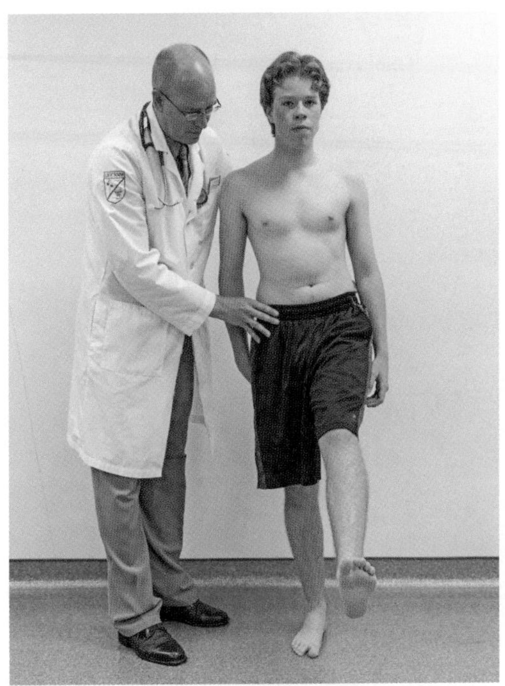

FIGURE 13-54 Hip flexion.

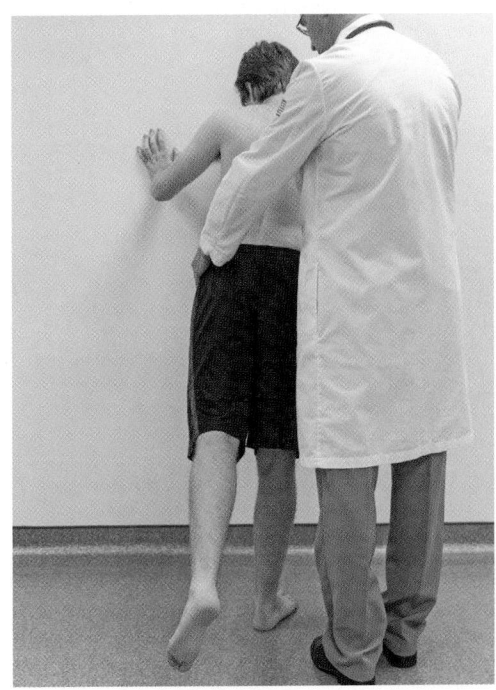

FIGURE 13-55 Hip extension.

- Internal rotation (see **FIGURE 13-56**): The leg is rotated inward, "Turn your knee inward."
- External rotation (see **FIGURE 13-57**): The leg is rotated outward, "Turn your knee outward."

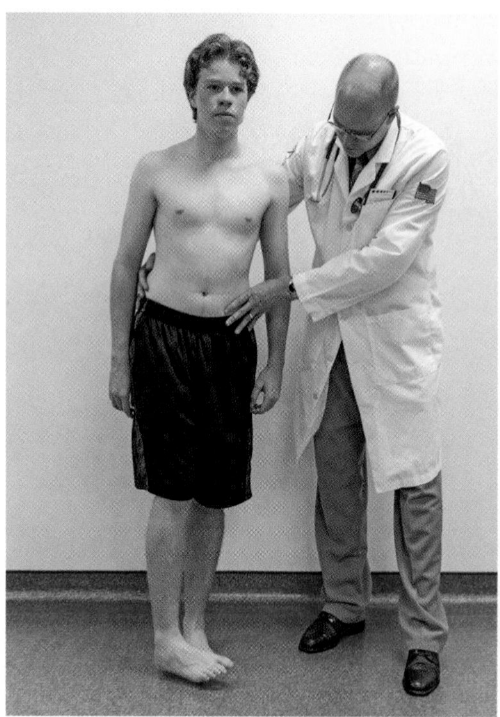

FIGURE 13-56 Internal rotation.

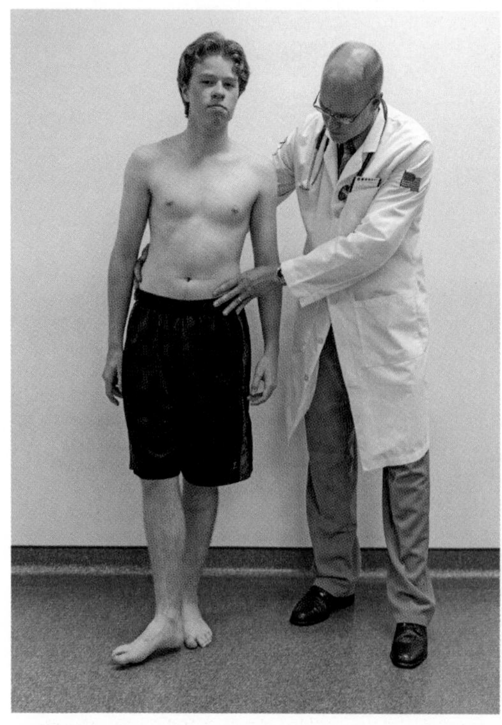

FIGURE 13-57 External rotation.

Palpation

13-15 Begin palpation superiorly at the iliac crest, moving anteriorly to the anterior superior iliac spine. Palpate the muscle mass to the greater trochanter of the femur, then move inferiorly to assess the greater trochanteric bursa.

Beginning again at the top of the iliac crest, palpate posteriorly to the posterior superior iliac spine and then the sacroiliac joint. Advise the patient that you will be palpating ischial bones, then move the thumbs medially to palpate them.

DOCUMENTATION

- Hips without ecchymosis, bony deformity, shortening, or internal rotation of the leg. Full AROM. Palpation without tenderness.

KNEES

Inspection

Though most of the knee examination was completed in the seated position, standing with weight-bearing is necessary for proper evaluation of varus ("bowlegged") or valgus ("knock-kneed") angulation, associated with osteoarthritis. With the provider behind the patient, note angulation at the knees.

Palpation

Standing also aids in palpation of popliteal fossa and detection of swelling of the synovial cyst behind the knee joint, called a Baker's cyst. This condition is often associated with arthritis or other inflammatory process, causing an increase in joint effusion and pressure, resulting in pouching.

DOCUMENTATION

- Standing knee inspection without varus or valgus deformity. Palpation without masses.

FEET

Inspect for flat feet—the loss of the arch, or pes planus (see **FIGURE 13-58**).

DOCUMENTATION

- Feet without pes planus.

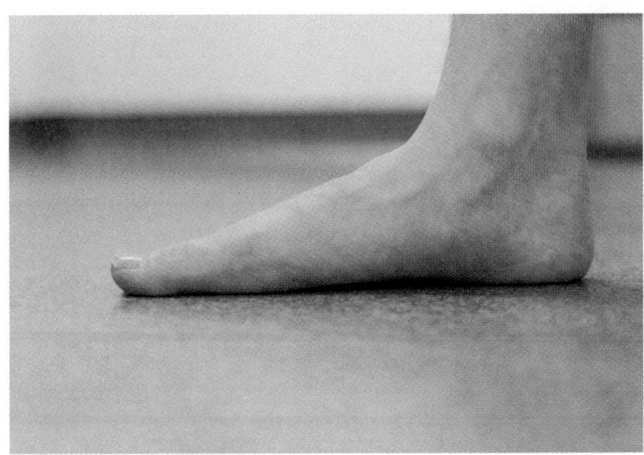

FIGURE 13-58 Pes planus.

Clinical Scenarios

KNEE PAIN OR INJURY

Knee pain with or without known trauma is a common complaint prompting patient visits. Patients complain of pain often associated with swelling, noises, and instability. "Popping" and "clicking" may be normal or associated with meniscal injury or osteoarthritis and chondromalacia patella.

TABLE 13-1 Localization of Pain Helps to Limit the Differential Diagnosis

Location of Knee Pain	Differential Diagnosis
Anterior Knee Pain	Prepatellar bursitis
	Patellofemoral pain syndrome/ chondomalacia patella
	Patellar tendonitis
	Osgood-Schlatter disease
	Osteoarthritis
	Rheumatoid arthritis
	Gout/pseudogout
	Septic arthritis
Medial Knee Pain	Medial collateral ligament injury
	Medial meniscal injury
	Osteoarthritis
	Anserine bursitis
Lateral Knee Pain	Lateral collateral ligament injury
	Lateral meniscal injury
	Osteoarthritis
	Iliotibial band syndrome

Instability most commonly reflects ligamentous injury, where the patient may describe the knee "giving out" suddenly, especially with cutting movements. As a major weight-bearing joint, the knee's structural complexities are susceptible to injury and inflammation. Detailed examination can help the provider to obtain an accurate diagnosis through symptom location, presence of edema, recognition of range-of-motion limitation, and instability (see **TABLE 14-1**).

Ballottement: technique used to identify fluid within the joint space where the provider rapidly taps the patella posteriorly and assesses for its bobbing up if excessive fluid is present

Structural testing should be performed.

Ballottement

13-16 **Ballottement** is a technique used in assessment of fluid within the joint space. This can be caused by an effusion such as that associated with inflammatory or infectious arthritis or with blood after trauma. With the patient in the lying position or seated with the legs extended at the knees, and beginning at the mid-thigh, the provider attempts to milk fluids from the tissues distally several times and stopping just above the patella (see **FIGURE 13-59**). With the last milking, the provider rapidly taps the patella posteriorly (see **FIGURE 13-60**). The patella will depress downward and then bob back up if excessive fluid is present; this is positive ballottement.

Varus and Valgus Stress Tests

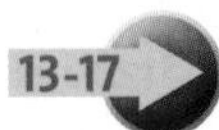

The varus and valgus stress tests assess collateral ligament stability in a patient

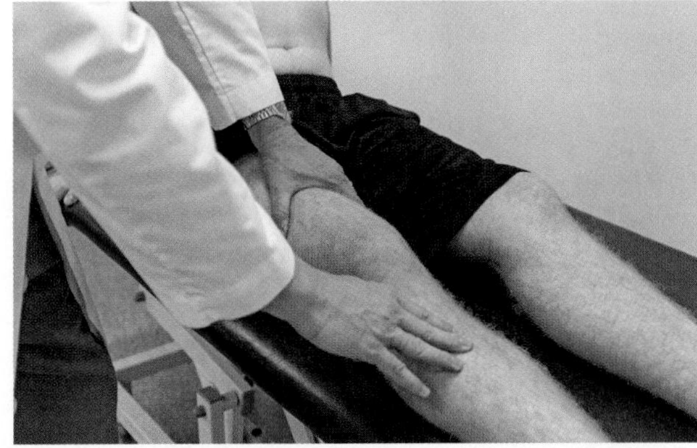

FIGURE 13-59 Ballottement begins at mid-thigh and progressively works caudally, milking toward and stopping just above the patella.

Valgus stress test: assessment technique for medial collateral ligament integrity where the provider holds the supine patient's straightened leg at the ankle and places the other hand along the lateral aspect of the knee. The ankle is pushed laterally as medial pressure is exerted at the knee causing the medial joint space to gap, assessing the medial collateral ligament for laxity.

Varus stress test: assessment technique for lateral collateral ligament integrity where the provider holds the supine patient's straightened leg at the ankle and places the other hand along the medial aspect of the knee. The ankle is pushed medially as lateral pressure is exerted at the knee causing the lateral joint space to gap, assessing the lateral collateral ligament for laxity.

Anterior drawer test: technique for assessment of the stability of anterior cruciate ligament where the patient is placed in the supine position with the knee bent to approximately 60 degrees and the foot anchored. The provider grasps the lower leg behind the knee and applies anterior displacement, noting the amount of shift of the tibia from under the femur.

with a knee injury. For the **valgus stress test**, the provider holds the supine patient's straightened leg at the ankle and places the other hand along the lateral aspect of the knee. The ankle is pushed laterally as medial pressure is exerted at the knee; this is valgus stress (see **FIGURE 13-61**). This causes the medial joint space to gap and is limited by the medial collateral. Compare to the other knee. A larger gap on one side indicates medial collateral laxity.

The lateral collateral is then tested for stability through the **varus stress test**, with the provider changing hands to place one against the medial aspect of the knee. The ankle is then pushed medially as lateral pressure is exerted at the knee; this is varus stress (see **FIGURE 13-62**). This causes the lateral joint space to gap and is limited by the lateral collateral. Compare to the other knee. A larger gap on one side indicates lateral collateral laxity.

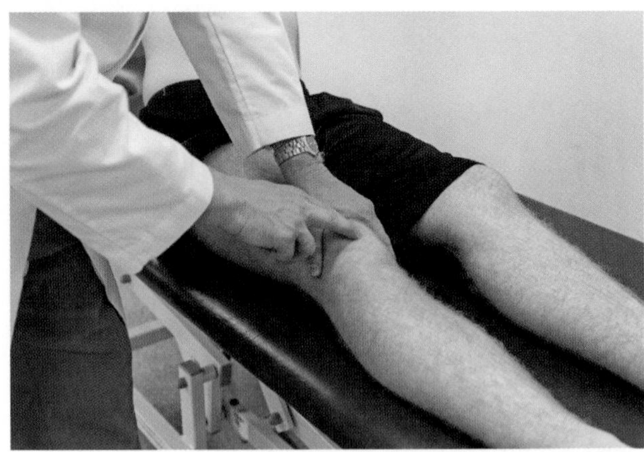

FIGURE 13-60 The patella is rapidly depressed as the provider assesses for it to bob upward against the fingers.

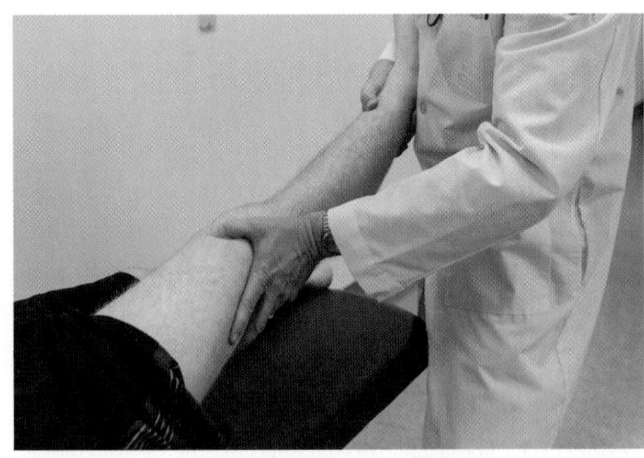

FIGURE 13-61 Valgus stress for medial collateral ligament integrity.

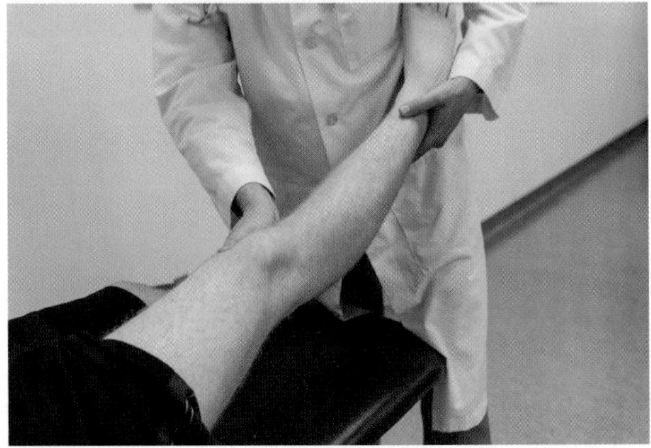

FIGURE 13-62 Varus stress for lateral collateral ligament integrity.

Anterior and Posterior Drawer Tests

13-18 The **anterior drawer test** assesses the stability of the anterior cruciate ligament. A history of trauma is most commonly associated and patients often relate a history of the knee suddenly buckling. With the patient in the supine position and knee bent to approximately 60 degrees, the provider sits on the end of the examination table while anchoring the patient's foot under the provider's upper thigh. The lower leg is grasped with the hands behind the knee so that the thumbs rest anteriorly on the tibial plateau (see **FIGURE 13-63**). The lower leg is then drawn anteriorly toward the provider, who notes the amount of shift, as in a drawer being pulled out. This is compared to the opposite side. An increase in anterior drawer suggests anterior cruciate ligament laxity or tear: a positive anterior drawer.

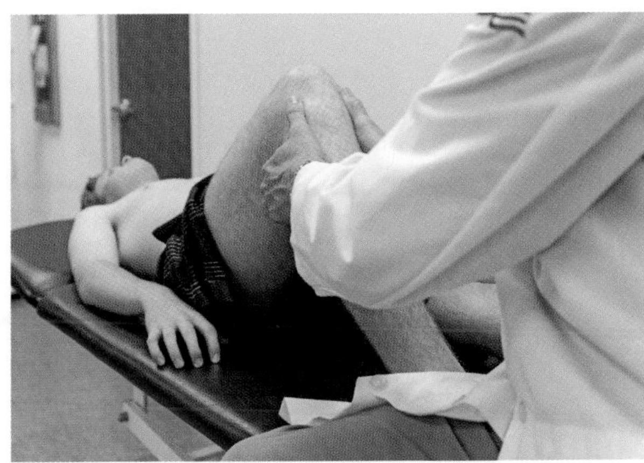

FIGURE 13-63 Anterior drawer for anterior cruciate ligament integrity.

With the hands in the same position, the provider now pushes posteriorly, the **posterior drawer test**, noting the amount of shift, as in a drawer being pushed back in (see FIGURE 13-64). An increase in posterior drawer suggests posterior cruciate ligament laxity or tear: a positive posterior drawer.

Lachman Test

13-19 The Lachman test also assesses the stability of the anterior cruciate ligament. In contrast to the anterior drawer, the knee is placed at 30 degrees of flexion in an attempt to remove the muscular support from the quadriceps. The provider then stabilizes the distal femur with one hand while placing the other hand just below the knee behind the lower leg and pulling forward (see FIGURE 13-65). A positive Lachman would show greater anterior translation as compared to the other side.

Meniscal Tear

McMurray's Sign.

13-20 Assessment of the menisci for tears is indicated with traumatic injury. Patients may indicate popping sounds (crepitus) with knee flexion and extension, as well as the knee locking into place.

To assess for **McMurray's sign**, the provider grasps the supine patient's straightened leg with the palm across the bottom of the foot and places a hand on the lateral aspect of the knee. To test for a medial meniscus tear, the provider then externally rotates the foot and flexes the knee to approximately 90 degrees (see FIGURES 13-66A, 13-66B, and 13-66C). Valgus pressure is then placed on the knee as the leg is extended, palpating the joint for pops (see FIGURE 13-66D). If a pop occurs or the patient experiences pain, a medial meniscal tear should be suspected.

Posterior drawer test: technique for assessment of the stability of posterior cruciate ligament where the patient is placed in the supine position with the knee bent to approximately 60 degrees and the foot anchored. The provider grasps the lower leg behind the knee and applies posterior displacement, noting the amount of shift of the tibia backward under the femur.

Meniscal tear: tear of the medial or lateral menisci of the knee

McMurray's sign: clicking or pain in the knee suggesting a meniscal tear elicited as the provider places the supine patient's lower leg in first internal rotation with varus pressure on the knee while taking the knee and hip through flexion and extension to assess the lateral meniscus and then reversing the forces to externally rotate the lower leg with valgus pressure on the knee to assess the media meniscus

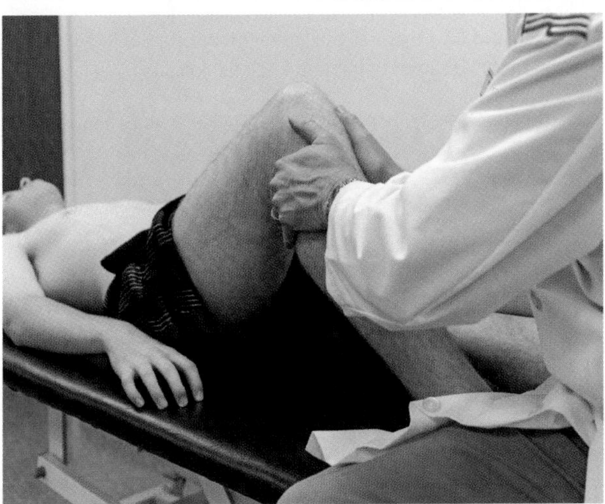

FIGURE 13-64 Posterior drawer for posterior cruciate ligament integrity.

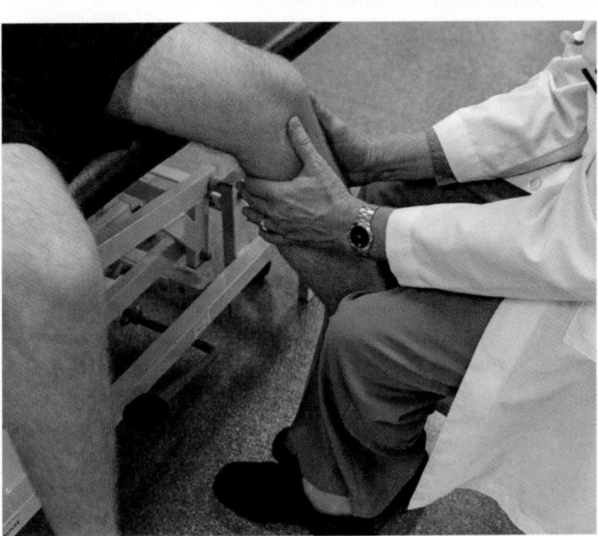

FIGURE 13-65 Lachman test.

The provider then places a hand on the medial aspect of the knee. To check the lateral meniscus, the foot is internally rotated, the knee is flexed, and varus pressure is applied as the leg is once again straightened (see **FIGURES 13-67A, 13-67B, 13-67C,** and **13-67D**). Pain or popping indicates a possible lateral meniscal tear.

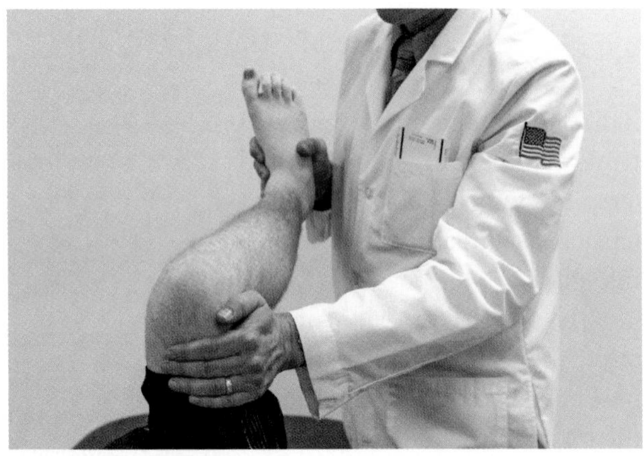

FIGURE 13-66A The McMurray test begins with the hip and knee flexed at 90 degrees.

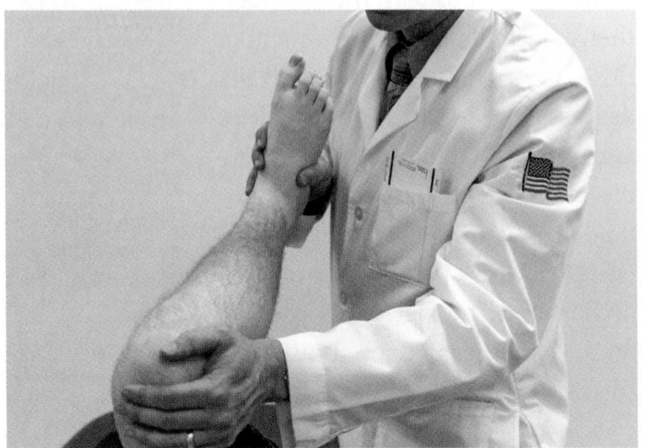

FIGURE 13-66B The provider externally rotates the lower leg.

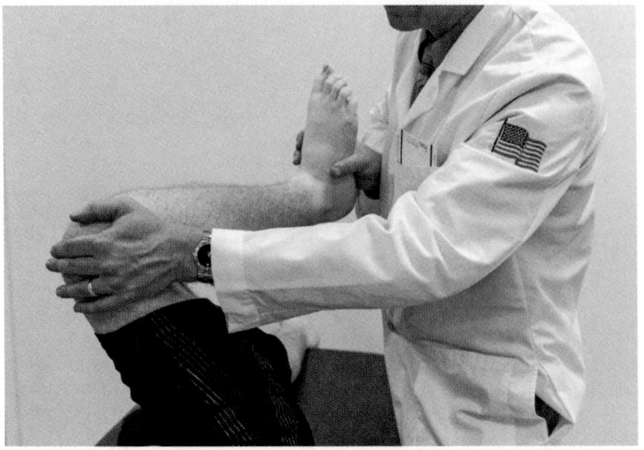

FIGURE 13-66C Valgus pressure is placed on the lateral aspect of the knee, stretching the medial meniscus.

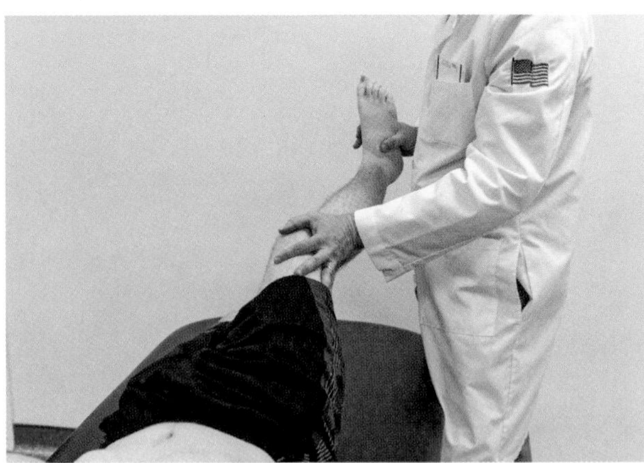

FIGURE 13-66D Pain or clicking with extension suggests a medial meniscus tear.

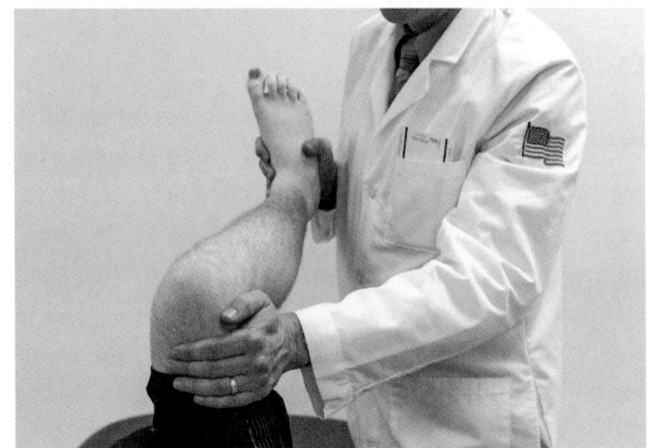

FIGURE 13-67A To assess the lateral meniscus, the leg is returned to 90 degrees of hip and knee flexion.

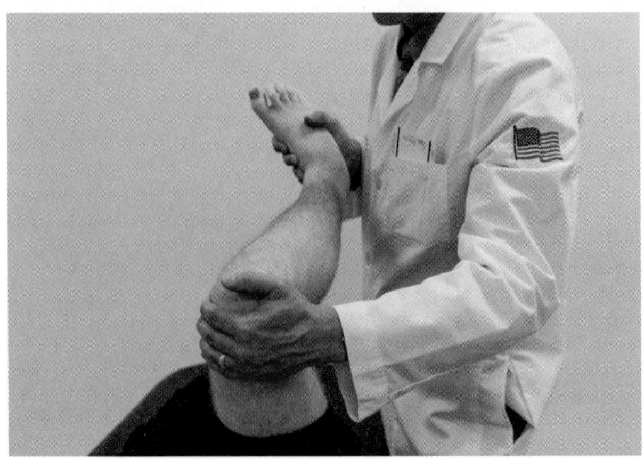

FIGURE 13-67B The lower leg is internally rotated.

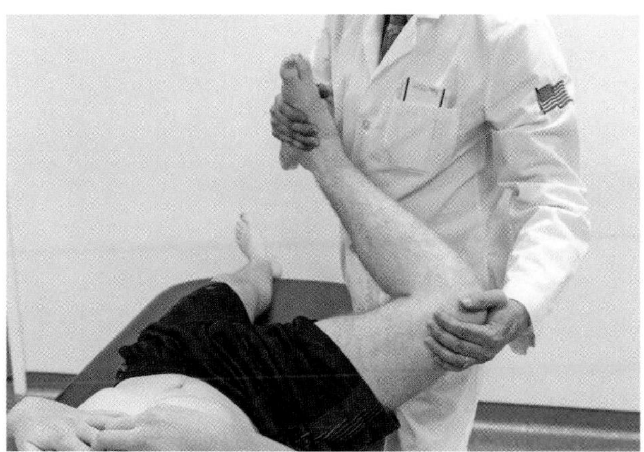

FIGURE 13-67C Varus pressure is placed against the medial aspect of the knee, stretching the lateral meniscus.

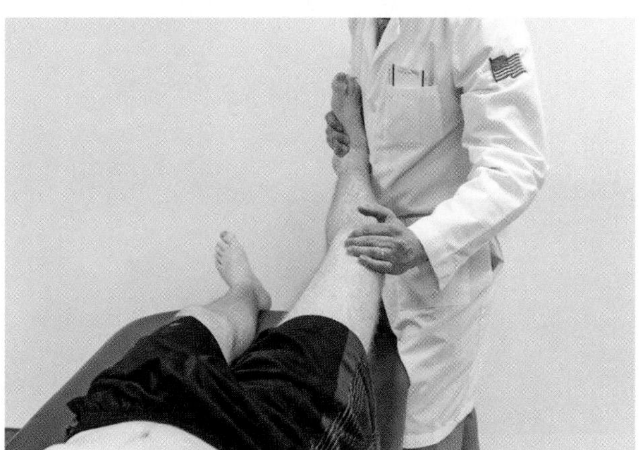

FIGURE 13-67D Pain or clicking with extension of the leg suggests a lateral meniscus tear.

Apley Grind.

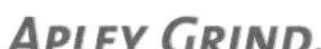

13-21 Another exam technique used to detect a meniscal tear is the Apley grind test. The patient is assisted to the prone position with the knee flexed to 90 degrees, perpendicular to the floor. The provider places one hand between the table and the knee. The other hand holds the mid-foot. Pressure is then exerted through the foot toward the knee while the provider internally and externally rotates the foot, feeling for grinding or popping indicating a possible meniscal tear (see FIGURE 13-68).

DOCUMENTATION

- Bilateral knees with negative ballottement, varus/valgus stress, anterior/posterior drawer, McMurray, and Apley grind.

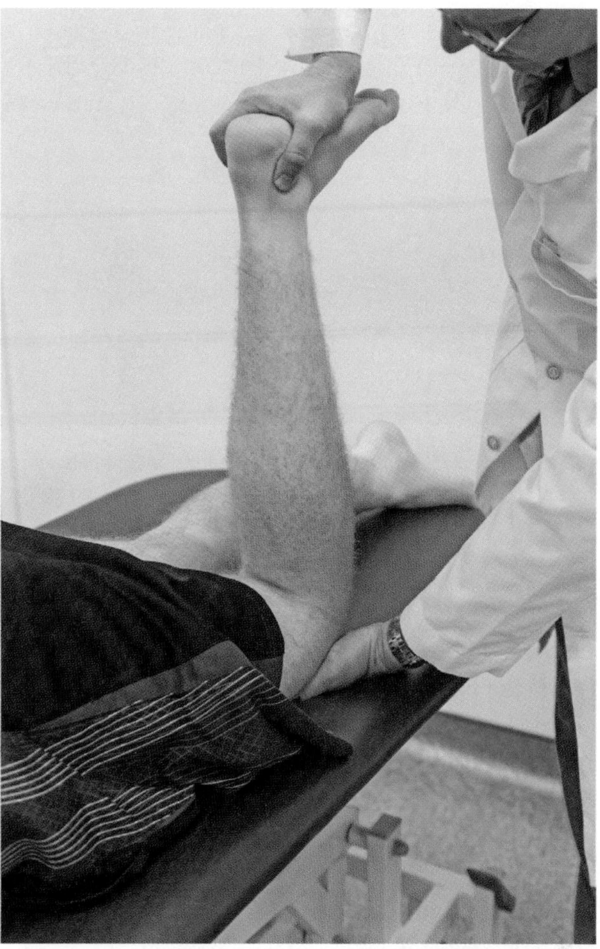

FIGURE 13-68 Apley grind test.

LOW BACK PAIN

Low back pain can be a serious, acute, or chronic condition requiring conscientiousness in care. Unfortunately, back pain is also a common fictitious complaint. Several examination techniques can help the provider differentiate between the two and provide expert care to the patient.

Straight Leg Raise

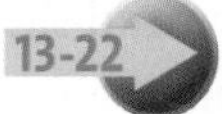

13-22 The **straight leg raise** (SLR) is used to assess the patient for a herniated lumbar disc. With the patient supine, the provider stands at the end of the exam table and places both hands under the patient's heels. The patient is then asked to raise one leg at a time without bending the knee (see FIGURE 13-69). If the patient relates increased pain as the leg is raised, it is

Straight leg raise: technique of examination used to assess for a herniated lumbar disc

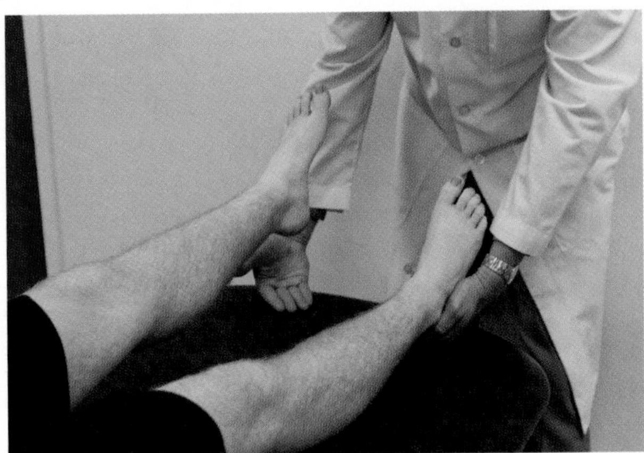

FIGURE 13-69 SLR with the provider's hands under heels. Pressure should increase in the hand under the resting leg as the other is raised, indicating true effort is being exerted.

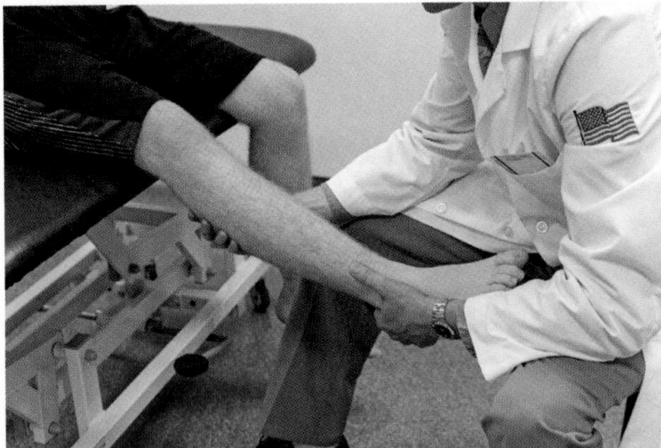

FIGURE 13-70 Seated SLR, lower leg palpation.

considered a positive SLR and a bulging or herniated disc should be considered.

If the patient is lifting the right leg, the provider should be able to appreciate the left heel pressing down into the provider's hand, indicating a true effort in lifting the leg. If no pressure is appreciated, the effort should be considered fictitious.

Seated Straight Leg Raise

13-23 In such cases or if the patient has a positive supine SLR, the provider can also perform a seated SLR. Help the patient to the seated position, with the legs over the side of the exam table. Advise the patient that you will now be checking the lower leg. Palpate the ankle with the leg hanging loosely and ask the patient to tell you if any pain is experienced (see **FIGURE 13-70**). Then ask the patient, "Any pain in the calf?" and palpate it, but extend the lower leg 10 to 20 degrees. Move up to the knee and palpate while extending the knee to 45 degrees. Ask, "How about in the knee?" Finally, slowly extend the lower leg and slide your hand under the lower thigh of the patient, lifting the leg enough that the hip begins to flex and the knee is straight (see **FIGURE 13-71**). At this point, if the patient were supine, the leg would be at 90 degrees of hip flexion or a full SLR. If the patient tolerates this examination without pain but complains of pain with the supine SLR, malingering should be suspected.

Carpal tunnel syndrome: compression of the median nerve as it passes through the carpal tunnel often resulting in numbness, paresthesia, and weakness of the hand

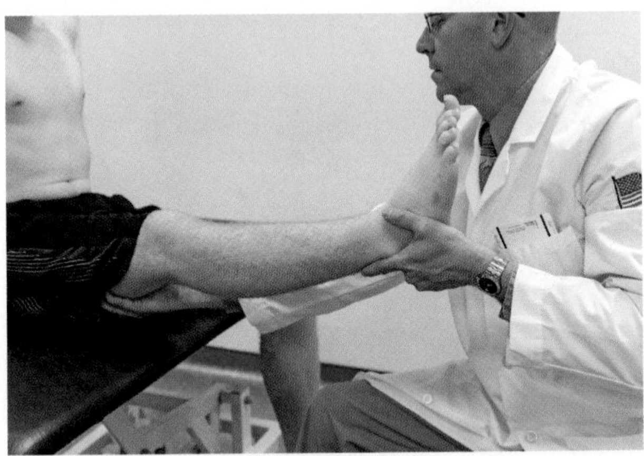

FIGURE 13-71 Seated SLR, upper leg palpation resulting in a straight leg.

SLR testing can also be performed passively, with the provider lifting the patient's leg.

DOCUMENTATION

- Negative SLR and seated SLR bilaterally.

CARPAL TUNNEL SYNDROME

When a patient presents with numbness or tingling in the hand in the first three digits and the lateral aspect of the fourth digit, **carpal tunnel syndrome** should be suspected. Two signs should be sought in an attempt to reproduce the symptoms.

Phalen's Sign

13-24 With the patient seated, have him/her raise the elbows and bring the dorsal aspects of the hand together in midline so that the forearms are

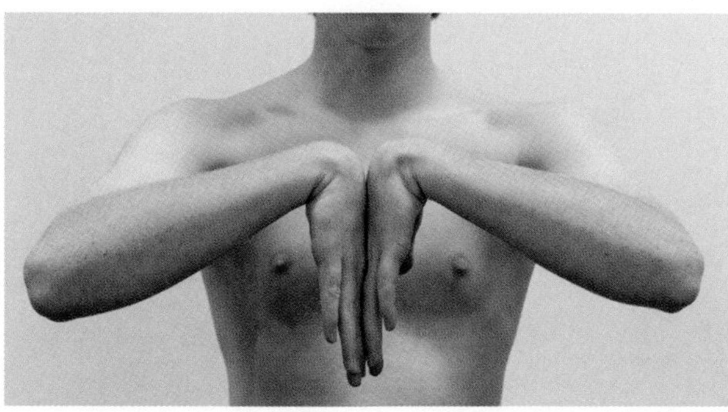

FIGURE 13-72 Phalen's test.

parallel to the floor (see **FIGURE 13-72**). The patient should be asked to hold the position and alert the provider when symptoms occur or for a maximum of 90 seconds. Reproduction of symptoms is a positive Phalen's.

Tinel's Sign

13-25 **Tinel's sign** is also a test that attempts to reproduce the symptoms the patient is experiencing. The provider elevates the forearm just behind the wrist, allowing the hand to extend. Using one finger, the provider percusses over the median nerve at the carpal tunnel (see **FIGURE 13-73**). Reproduction of symptoms is a positive Tinel's.

DOCUMENTATION

- Negative Phalen's and Tinel's signs.

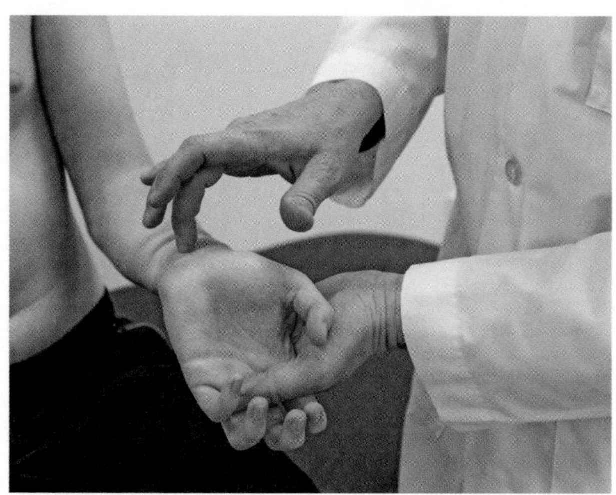

FIGURE 13-73 Tinel's sign.

SHOULDER PAIN OR INJURY

Examination of shoulder pain or injury begins with almost incidental inspection, which can begin with observation of shoulder movement with an introductory handshake, the laying-down of a magazine, or the removal of a shirt or gown.

A patient with shoulder pain presents for a disability examination. Upon introduction he is unable to lift his right arm independently to shake hands, instead using his left arm to lift his right. After completing 15 minutes of history taking, he is asked to remove his shirt for the examination, which he does fluidly, crossing his arms to grab his shirt at the waist and stripping off the shirt over his head with both arms, a most rapid cure.

History taking presents an opportunity to observe restrictions or favoring of an arm, as well as to help the patient relax so that natural motions can also be assessed. Inspection, range-of-motion assessment, and palpation should be compared bilaterally.

Palpating in the manner described previously, note step deformity of the clavicle. A cephalad AC joint with tenderness may reflect AC separation. Assure correct positioning of the humeral head with anterior and posterior prominence, suggesting correlating dislocations.

Phalen's sign: reproduction of pain or numbness of the hand in the distribution of the median nerve as the patient holds the dorsal aspects of the hands together with the wrists flexed at 90 degrees, suggesting the presence of carpal tunnel syndrome

Tinel's sign: reproduction of pain or numbness of the hand in the distribution of the median nerve as the provider percusses the extended wrist over the carpal tunnel, suggesting the presence of carpal tunnel syndrome

Rotator cuff: complex of tendinous insertions of the supraspinatus, infraspinatus, teres minor, and subscapularis muscles of the shoulder and site of common shoulder injuries

Rotator Cuff Injury

Injury or impingement of the **rotator cuff** is a common injury, especially in occupations where use of the arms in a position over the head is required.

SUPRASPINATUS.

The supraspinatus aids in abduction of the arm at the shoulder, with the majority of its action through 30 degrees but assisting through 90 degrees.

13-26 ***Painful Arc Test.*** To assess integrity of the supraspinatus, the patient is asked to abduct the arms with elbows straight and indicate if pain is experienced during the motion (see **FIGURES 13-74A**, **13-74B**, and **13-74C**). Pain after 90 degrees is considered a positive painful arc test.

13-27 ***Arm-Drop Test.*** The arm-drop test assesses possible tears of the supraspinatus tendon and can be combined with the painful arc test. After abduction has been completed, the patient is asked to begin lowering the arms but to briefly hold them at about 120 degrees of abduction (see **FIGURE 13-75**). The patient is then advised to drop the arm slowly as the provider watches for fluidity in movement. A positive arm-drop test is noted if fluidity is not maintained.

13-28 ***Empty Can Test.*** The empty can test also evaluates supraspinatus integrity. As if holding a can, the patient abducts the arm to 90 degrees, keeping the elbow straight, and then internally rotates the arm as if emptying the can. The provider then presses down on the arm as the patient resists (see **FIGURE 13-76**). If weakness is demonstrated, a tear of the supraspinatus should be suspected and investigated.

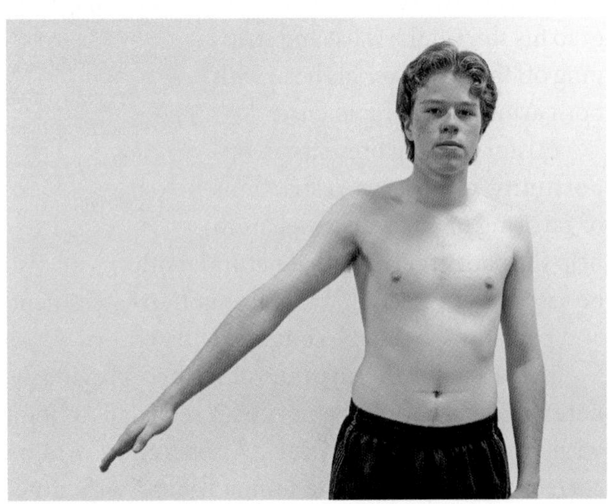

FIGURE 13-74A Painful arc test at 45 degrees.

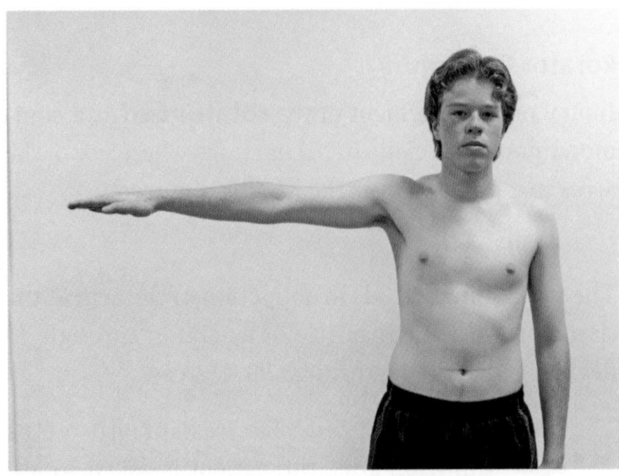

FIGURE 13-74B Painful arc test at 90 degrees.

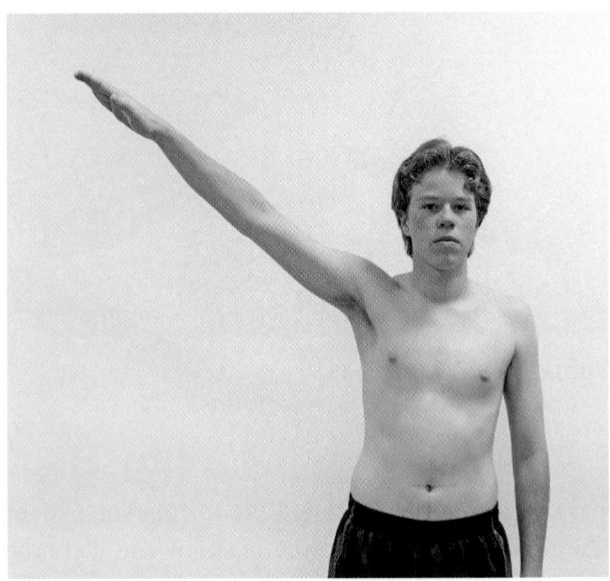

FIGURE 13-74C Painful arc test at 120 degress.

Infraspinatus.

13-29 The primary action of the infraspinatus is external rotation. To assess integrity of the infraspinatus, the provider has the patient hold the

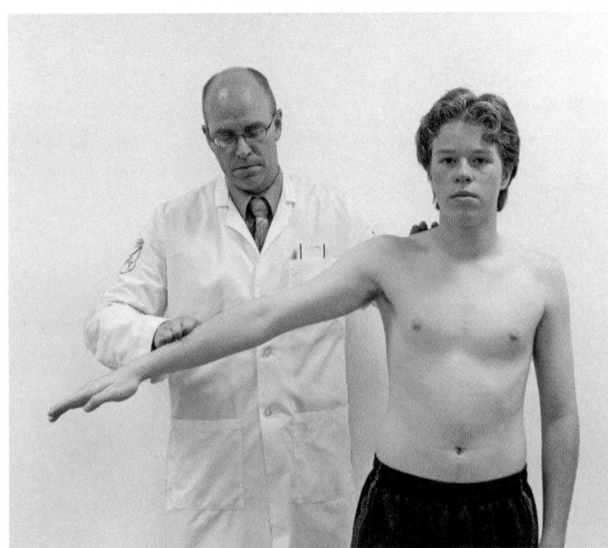

FIGURE 13-75 The arm-drop test starts at 120 degrees, with the provider then pushing the arm downward.

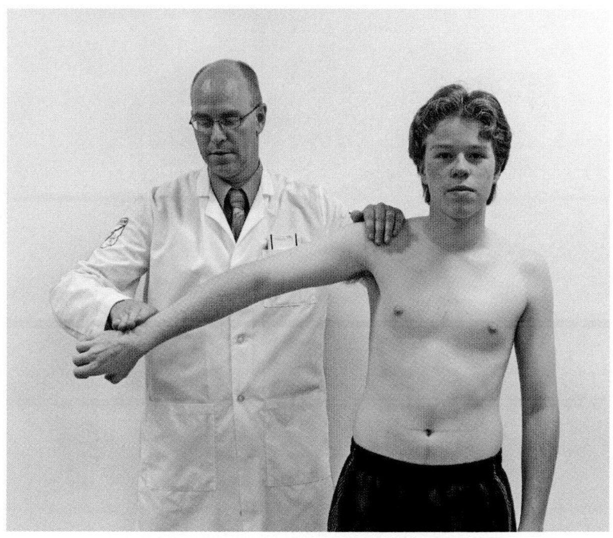

FIGURE 13-76 Empty can test with abduction and pronation.

arm at the side with the elbow bent at 90 degrees. The provider holds the elbow with one hand and the wrist with the other (see FIGURE 13-77). The patient is then asked to externally rotate the arm while the provider resists. Pain or weakness indicates injury.

Subscapularis.

The primary action of the subscapularis is internal rotation.

Push-Off Test. To test integrity of the subscapularis, ask the patient to put the hand of the affected side behind the back. Then provide resistance as the patient is asked to push off the hand from the back (see FIGURE 13-78). Pain or weakness indicates injury.

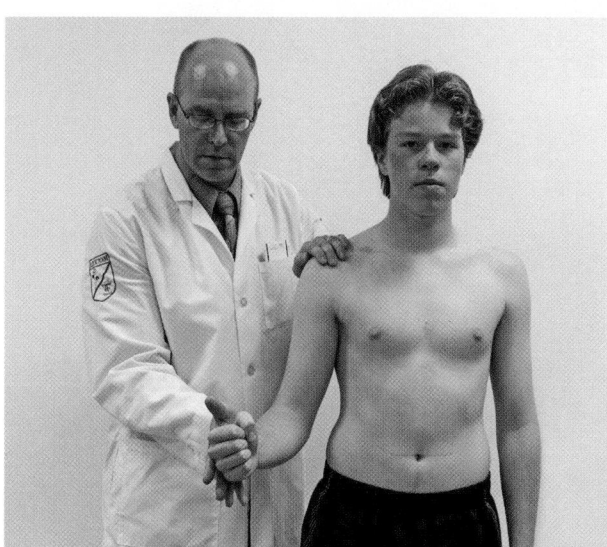

FIGURE 13-77 Infraspinatus testing with the arm flexed at the elbow to 90-degrees, the provider provides resistance against external rotation.

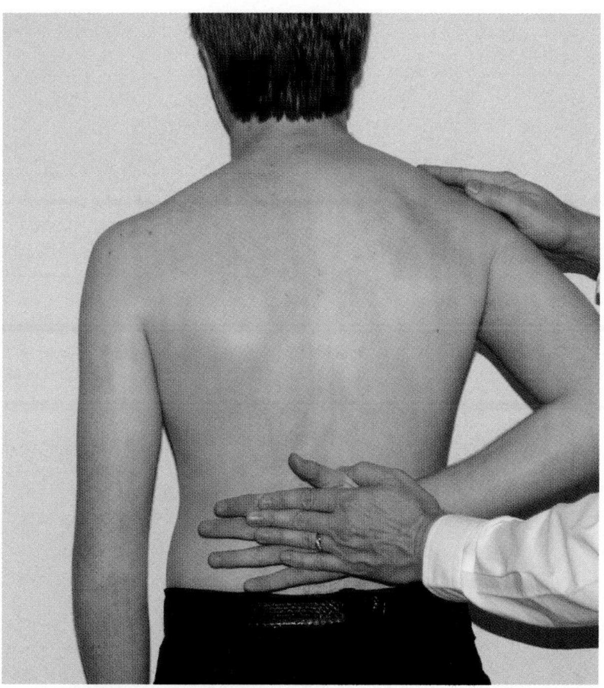

FIGURE 13-78 Push-off test.

Shoulder Impingement

Shoulder impingement syndrome is a general term referring to compression of anatomic structures that occurs when lifting the arm, rather than identifying which exact structure has been impinged. Several tests can be used to diagnose impingement.

Passive Painful Arc Test.

13-31 The passive painful arc test can be used to assess the degree of impingement. In this test, the provider stands behind the patient on the side of concern. The patient is instructed to keep the arm completely relaxed, allowing the provider to move the arm through a range of motion. The provider places one hand on the patient's shoulder to stabilize and takes the patient's wrist in the other (see FIGURE 13-79A). Keeping the elbow straight, the provider moves the arm through the full flexion range of motion (see FIGURES 13-79B and 13-79C). The farther the arm can be moved through PROM until pain is experienced, the less the degree of impingement.

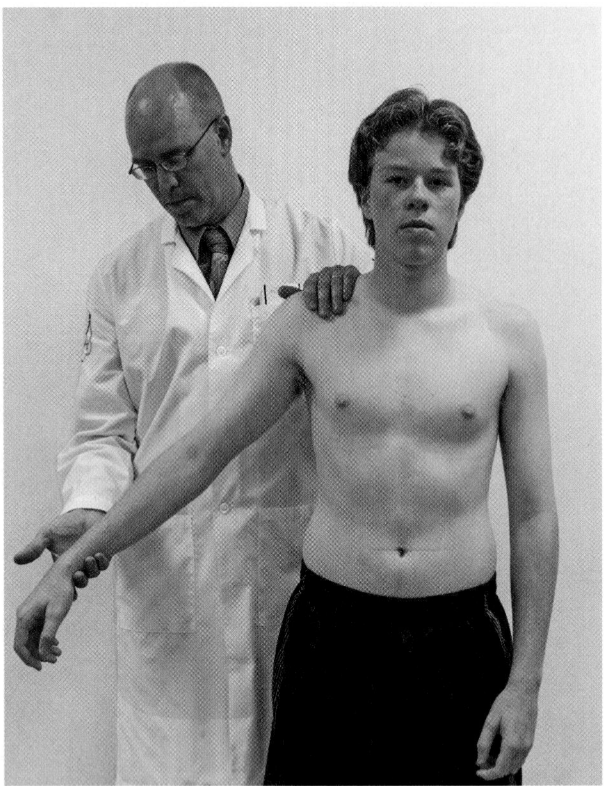

FIGURE 13-79A Passive painful arc test at 45 degrees.

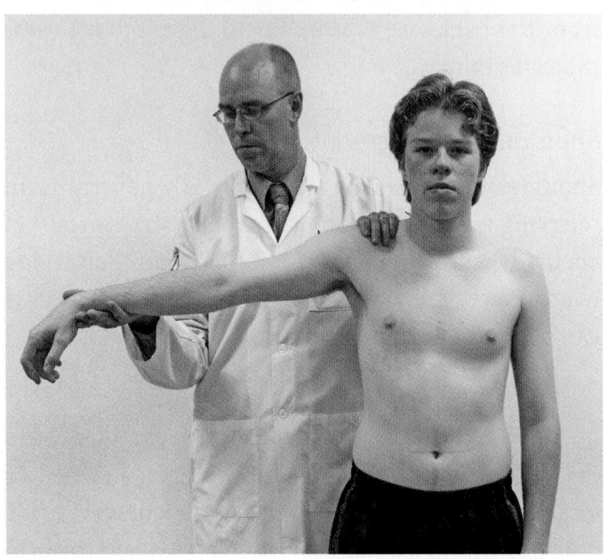

FIGURE 13-79B Passive painful arc test nearing 90 degrees.

Shoulder Instability and Dislocation

The structure of the shoulder joint allows for great range of motion but requires complex structural integrity to do so. Dysfunction may result in shoulder instability and even dislocation.

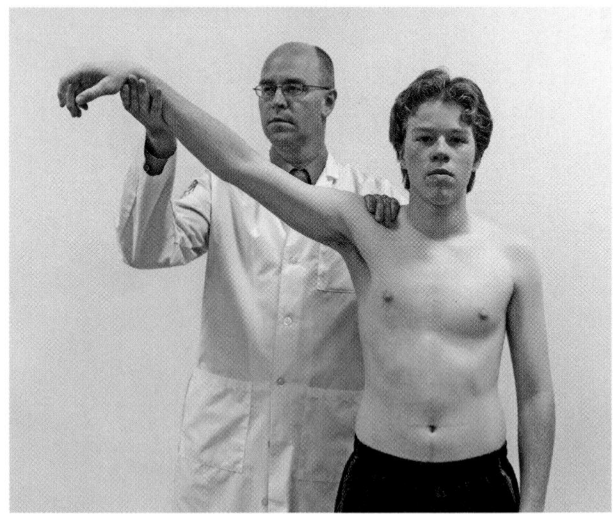

FIGURE 13-79C Passive painful arc test at 120 degrees.

Sulcus Sign.

13-32 Begin testing the integrity of the shoulder joint with assessment of the sulcus sign. For this test the provider stands beside the patient with the patient's arm hanging at the side. A stabilizing hand is placed on top of the shoulder palpating the humeral head, and the other hand grasps above the patient's elbow (see **FIGURE 13-80**). The arm is pulled

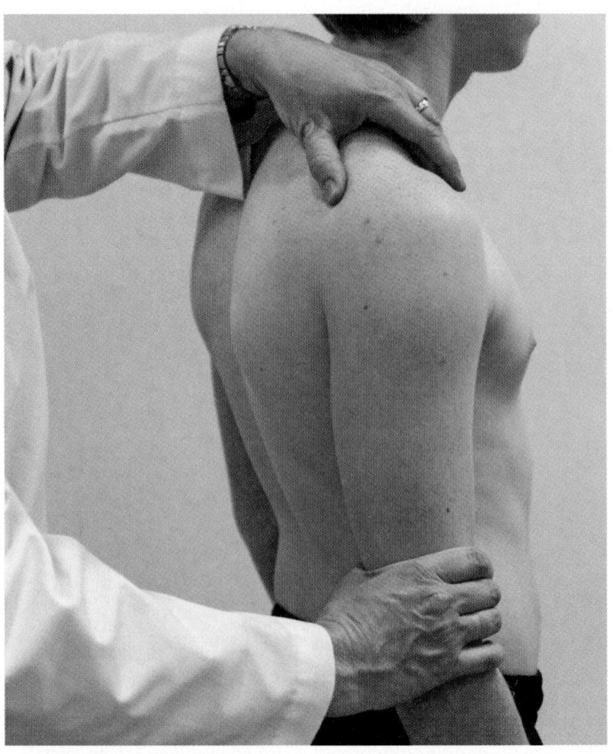

FIGURE 13-80 Sulcus sign.

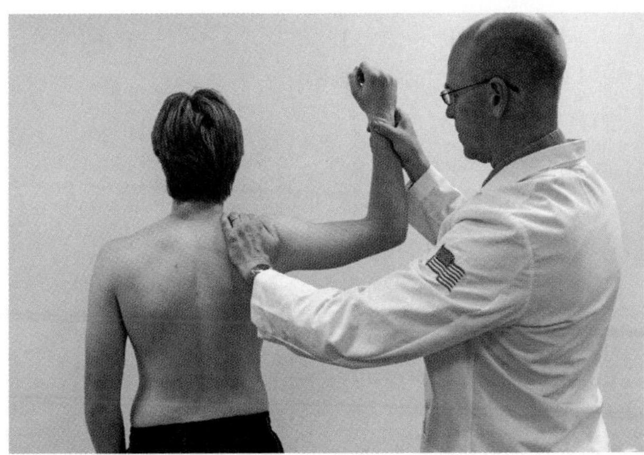

FIGURE 13-81 Apprehension test.

downward to assess laxity of the joint. More than 2 cm of movement is considered abnormal glenohumeral subluxation. However, comparison must be made with the other side, as bilateral hypermotility may suggest congenital disorder.

Apprehension Test.

13-33 The apprehension test assesses the patient's apprehension that the shoulder is about to dislocate or experience pain. The patient is asked to hold the arm at 90 degrees abduction with the elbow at 90 degrees of flexion, resulting in external rotation of the shoulder. The provider stands behind the patient stabilizing the posterior shoulder with one hand and holding the wrist with the other (see **FIGURE 13-81**). The patient is then asked to resist posterior motion of the wrist as the provider pushes backward, increasing external rotation, and to advise the provider if it is felt that the shoulder is about to dislocate. A positive test is encountered if patient perception of impending dislocation is felt.

See **TABLE 13-2** for the muskuloskeltal flow.

TABLE 13-2 Musculoskeletal Flow

Introduces self and explains that physical exam will now be performed		
Washes hands for 15 seconds, turning off water with towel		
General inspection—patient in seated position		
	Body symmetry—compare bilateral upper and lower extremity muscle mass	
	Head—normocephalic, microcephalic, hydrocephalic, syndromal appearance	
	Identify limb or bony deformity	
General considerations		
	Compare all joint exams bilaterally	
	State—passive ROM to be performed if limited AROM for any joint	
Temporomandibular joint (TMJ)		
	Visualize active ROM—assure midline movement	
	Palpation—place pad of index finger in conchal bowl, identify clicking	
Neck		
	Inspection—general symmetry, muscle mass, and alignment of the head	
	Range of motion	
		Flexion
		Extension
		Rotation
		Side bending
	Palpation—spinous and transverse processes, perivertebral muscle mass	
Shoulders		
	Bilateral inspection—symmetry, bony deformity, edema, ecchymosis	
	Bilateral active range of motion (AROM)	
		Abduction
		Adduction
		Flexion
		Extension
		Internal rotation
		External rotation
	Bilateral palpation	
		Joint structure—sternoclavicular, clavicle, acromioclavicular, scapulohumeral
		Rotator cuff muscles
		Bicipital groove with elbow bent at 90 degrees and external rotation
Elbows		
	Bilateral inspection—symmetry, bony deformity, masses	
	Bilateral AROM	
		Flexion
		Extension
		Supination
		Pronation
	Bilateral palpation	
		Joint structure—olecranon, epicondyles
		Bursa—olecranon

(continues)

TABLE 13-2 Musculoskeletal Flow *(Continued)*

Musculoskeletal Flow
Wrists
Bilateral inspection—symmetry, bony deformity
Bilateral AROM
Radial deviation
Ulnar deviation
Flexion
Extension
Bilateral palpation including anatomic snuff box
Fingers
Bilateral inspection—symmetry, bony deformity
Heberden's nodes—distal interphalangeal joint—osteoarthritis
Bouchard's nodes—proximal interphalangeal joint—osteoarthritis and rheumatoid arthritis
Bilateral AROM
Abduction
Adduction
Flexion
Extension
Bilateral palpation
Drape lower extremities with a sheet, lifting to examine the legs
Knees
Bilateral inspection—symmetry, bony deformity
Bilateral AROM
Flexion
Extension
Bilateral palpation
Peripatellar
Medial and lateral joint spaces
Tibial tubercle
Ankles/Feet
Bilateral inspection—symmetry, bony deformity
Bilateral AROM
Dorsiflexion
Plantarflexion
Inversion
Eversion
Internal rotation
External rotation
Bilateral palpation—medial and lateral malleoli, deltoid ligament, Achilles tendon
Patellar tracking
Assist patient to standing position
Thoracic and lumbar spine
Inspection
From side—note changes in lordosis and kyphosis
From behind—note rotoscoliosis (lateral curvature)
AROM
Flexion
Extension
Rotation
Side bending
Palpation—spinous and transverse processes, paravertebral musculature
Hips
Bilateral inspection—symmetry, bony deformity
AROM
Abduction
Adduction
Flexion
Extension
Internal rotation
External rotation
Bilateral palpation—bursa—greater trochanteric
Knees
Inspection—varus or valgus deviation
Palpation—popliteal fossa with patient standing—Baker's cyst
Feet—inspection for pes planus (flat feet)
CLINICAL SCENARIOS
KNEE PAIN OR INJURY
Ballottement—fluid in joint space
Varus and valgus stress—collateral ligament stability
Anterior drawer—anterior cruciate ligament (ACL) stability
Posterior drawer—posterior cruciate ligament (PCL) stability
Lachman test
McMurray's sign or Apley grind—meniscal tear
BACK PAIN
Straight leg raise (SLR)
Seated SLR
CARPAL TUNNEL SYNDROME
Phalen's sign

TABLE 13-2 Musculoskeletal Flow *(Continued)*

Tinel's sign
SHOULDER PAIN OR INJURY
Rotator cuff
Supraspinatus assessment
Painful arc test
Arm drop test
Empty can test
Infraspinatus—external rotation resistance
Subscapularis—push-off test
Shoulder impingement—passive painful arc test
Shoulder instability/dislocation
Sulcus sign
Apprehension test

CHAPTER 14

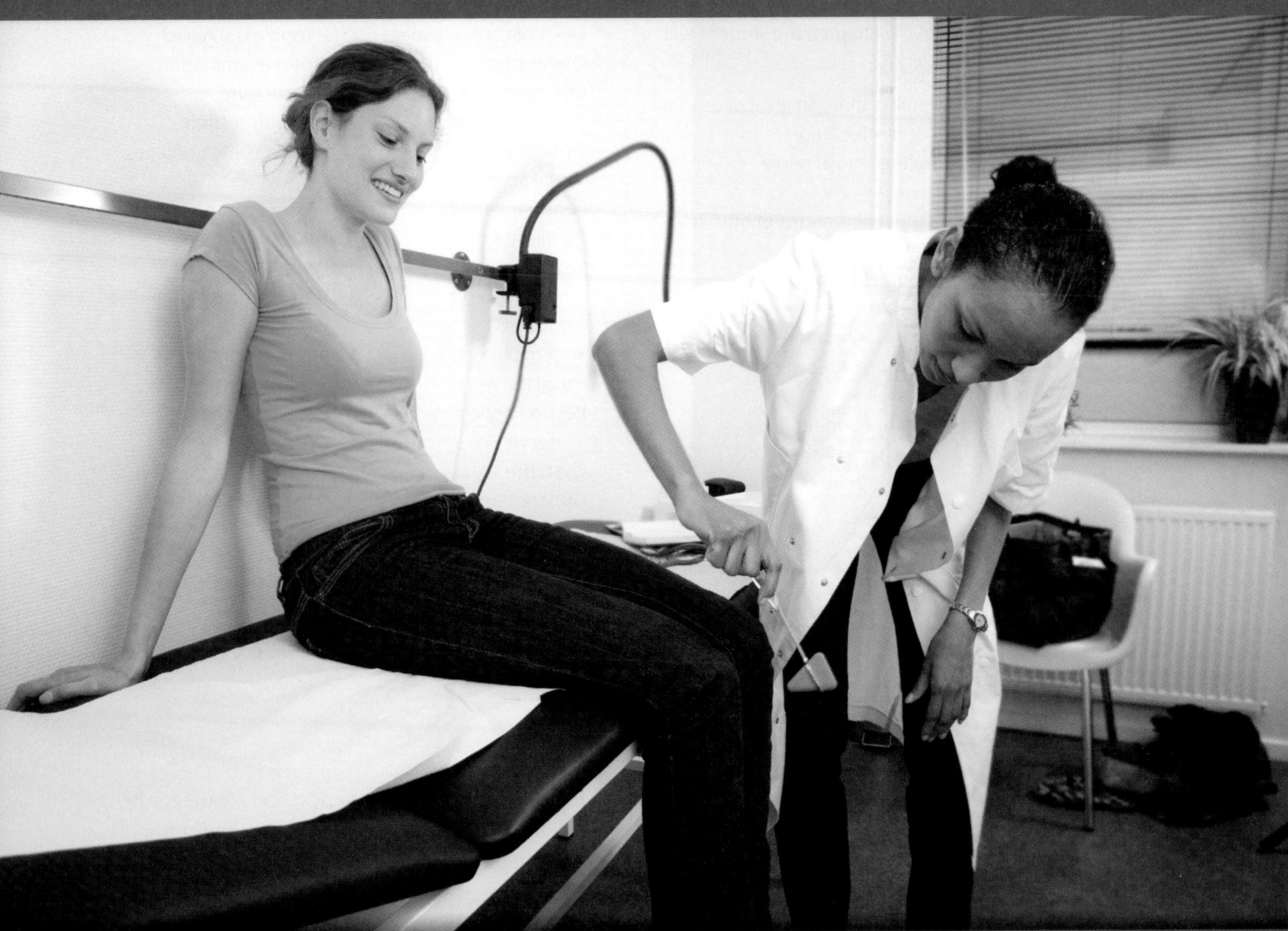

© Simone van den Berg/ShutterStock, Inc.

Neurologic Examination

Blake Hoppe, DO, MS (Med Ed)
Mark Kauffman, DO, MS (Med Ed), PA

OBJECTIVES

At the conclusion of the chapter, the student will be able to

1. Assess mental status through level of consciousness and orientation
2. Perform a complete cranial nerve examination
3. Describe and detect alterations of muscle tone, strength, and reflexes
4. Provide nerve roots responsible for innervation of the muscles being assessed
5. Associate sensory examination components with dermatomal innervation and responsible tracts
6. Assess cerebellar functioning

KEY TERMS

Level of consciousness
Orientation
Cranial nerves
Olfactory nerve
Optic nerve
Visual acuity
Peripheral fields
Pupillary reaction
Oculomotor nerve
Trochlear nerve
Abducens nerve
Trigeminal nerve
Facial nerve
Vestibulocochlear nerve
Nystagmus
Glossopharyngeal nerve
Vagus nerve
Spinal accessory nerve
Hypoglossal nerve
Motor examination
Muscle tone
Strength testing
Muscle stretch reflexes
Clonus
Sensory examination
Touch
Pain
Temperature
Vibratory sensation
Proprioception
Stereognosis
Graphesthesia
Extinction
Coordination
Romberg test
Gait

Where this icon appears, visit **go.jblearning.com/HPECWS** to view the video.

The neurologic examination is arguably one of the most interesting, fun, and exciting parts of the physical examination. Performance of a neurologic examination can be mastered with adequate tools and practice. As we review the various components of the neurologic exam, the focus should remain on the holistic approach, treating the patient as a whole, with clinical examples revealing its practicality and importance.

Mental Status

The first component of the neurologic examination is the mental status exam, which begins as soon as you walk into the patient's room.

Level of consciousness: awareness and cognitive function as assessed through behavior, arousability, and responses to stimuli

LEVEL OF CONSCIOUSNESS

Much confusion has been caused by improper use of terms employed to describe **level of consciousness**. Providers should strive to describe a patient's behavior, arousability, and responses to stimuli rather than attempt to use terminology that often lacks universal acceptance in definition. When assessing level of consciousness, approach the patient with heightening levels of stimuli, starting with verbal stimuli, then light touch, and finally painful or noxious stimuli such as the sternal rub, squeezing the trapezius or pinching the patient's thumb nail between the provider's thumb and index finger.

As standard definitions are often used inappropriately, the provider should instead observe and document eye-opening, verbal, and motor responses that occur. It is best to follow descriptives with responses to various stimuli such as, "drowsy but awakens to verbal stimulation, follows simple commands, and falls asleep within a few minutes." "Comatose" should be followed by "no response to verbal or noxious stimulation." Any rudimentary responses such as groaning should be documented.

ORIENTATION

Orientation requires that you ascertain specifically if the patient can identify (1) person (who he/she is), (2) place (where he/she is), and (3) time (what the date is). Do not assume that someone is oriented. For example, you may be hesitant to ask an elderly patient whom you've known for some time, "What is your name?" or "Can you tell me where you are?" knowing that the patient drives himself to his appointments. Yet if you advise the patient of the necessity and make orientation a part of the standard assessment, it will be accepted as routine and you will occasionally find that Mr. McGregor knows his name and where he is, but thinks it's 1980.

You may also employ the guise of rules, true or fictitious, to avoid putting your patient on guard. "Sorry, just the rules, can you tell me your full name?" or "Can you remind me of what today's date is?"

Generally the following three question assess orientation

1. Can you tell me your full name?
2. Can you tell me where we are?
3. Can you tell me what date it is today?

You can then expand into more detail as appropriate.

- Can you tell me where we are?
  - In a building
- Can you tell me what street this building is on?
  - Main Street?
- And the city?
  - Fayetteville
- The state?
  - Pennsylvania
- And the country
  - The United States

Likewise the date can be expanded to identify the time of day, day of the week, month, and year.

DOCUMENTATION

- Alert and oriented × 3.

General Observation

Speech is assessed continuously throughout the history and physical examination. Assess if speech is clear and fluent. Consider if the speech is slurred (dysarthric), nasal, or otherwise abnormal. Does the person have difficulty understanding what is said or difficulty finding words? In addition, assess whether a person is able to repeat something you say, and whether he/she can name objects that you point to.

As you talk to and begin to examine your patient, you should notice any obvious asymmetry or deformity. Sometimes in our efforts to document the details, the obvious is missed, such as failing to document a below-the-knee amputation. Note subtle findings such as position of comfort: for instance, a person holding an arm up against the body as if it's spastic or painful, or an arm hanging limply as if it's flaccid or neglected. Document involuntary movements: Does the patient have a resting tremor, chorea, myoclonic jerks, or tics?

While there is no required order of examination, the cranial nerve examination typically is next. No matter what order you use, be consistent to prevent forgetting a component of the examination. The standard head-to-toe approach can be used with the neurologic exam.

DOCUMENTATION

- Seated on the exam table with good posture. No obvious extremity weakness or asymmetry.

Cranial Nerve Examination

The **cranial nerve** examination should be completed in numerical order, utilizing memory tools such as On Old Olympus' Towering Top, A Finn and German Viewed Some Hops, until experience is gained.

CRANIAL NERVE I

Cranial nerve I (CNI), the **olfactory nerve**, is not routinely tested but can be used to assess an olfactory complaint or when a frontal lobe disorder is suspected. If testing is desired, two familiar yet distinctly different sources of smell, such as orange extract and coffee,

Orientation: a person's ability to identify (1) person (who he/she is), (2) place (where he/she is), and (3) time (what the date is)

Cranial nerve: a nerve that arises directly from the brain as opposed to the spinal column

Olfactory nerve: cranial nerve I, responsible for the sense of smell

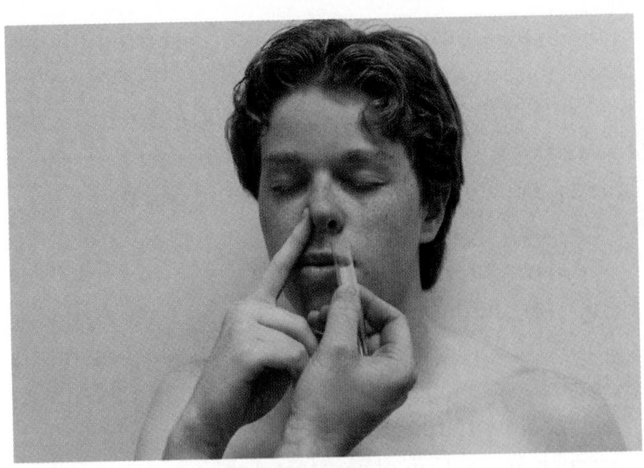

FIGURE 14-1 Olfactory testing with the patient closing one nares while assessing smell in the other.

must be available. Noxious stimuli should not be used as they do not test olfactory sensation. For example, ammonia stimulates pain endings of the trigeminal nerve.

14-1 Advise the patient that you will be assessing their sense of smell. Ask the patient to occlude one naris and close their eyes. Place a smell under the open naris and ask the patient to identify it (see **FIGURE 14-1**). Then repeat with the second source on the other side.

CRANIAL NERVE II

Assessment of CNII, the **optic nerve**, includes visual acuity, peripheral visual fields, and the sensory component of the pupillary reflex.

Visual Acuity

To assess **visual acuity**, each eye should be tested separately, using either a handheld chart or a wall visual acuity chart (see **FIGURE 14-2**). Visual acuity charts typically have the required distance from the patient printed on the chart. The distance can vary greatly, especially with the handheld charts. Each line on the chart will have an acuity measurement, such as 20/30.

Optic nerve: cranial nerve II, responsible for visual acuity, peripheral visual fields, and the sensory component of the pupillary reflex

Visual acuity: the ability to see clearly in the central line of vision

Peripheral fields: the areas of vision beyond a person's central vision

In this example, the reading means that the patient being tested must be 20 feet from the object to see it clearly, whereas a person with normal vision could see the same object clearly from a farther distance of 30 feet. In an extreme example, a reading of 20/800 would mean that what a person with normal vision clearly sees from 800 feet away could not be seen clearly by the patient until they were only 20 feet from the object.

14-2 To perform visual acuity, ask the patient to cover an eye with one hand. Position the chart correctly and instruct the patient to read the lowest line possible (see **FIGURE 14-3**). Note the level of acuity as printed on the card. Ask the patient to cover the opposite eye and read the lowest line possible backward.

DOCUMENTATION

- VA 20/20 OD, 20/30 OS

OD stands for right eye—think "DR" as in "doctor." OS stands for left eye. OU stands for bilateral eyes.

Peripheral Fields

8-4 **Peripheral fields** of vision are divided into four quadrants: upper medial, upper lateral, lower medial, and lower lateral. Each quadrant must be assessed individually.

To test peripheral fields:

1. Position yourself approximately 3 feet directly in front of the patient, making sure that you are on the same eye level.
2. Have the patient cover the left eye with the left hand while you close your right eye. This allows you to use your field of view as a reference.
3. Ask the patient to fixate on your left eye.
4. Position your hands equidistant between yourself and the patient. Test each quadrant by holding up either one, two, or five fingers (see **FIGURE 14-4**). Be sure that the patient does not look directly at your fingers.
5. Repeat the procedure for the other eye by having the patient cover the right eye while you close your left eye.

Case Example

A middle-aged gentleman was being seen for confusion. Upon entering the room, he was found to be awake, alert, and oriented × 3. His wife related a history of his running into mailboxes when driving. A

© Alexander Kaludov/ShutterStock, Inc.

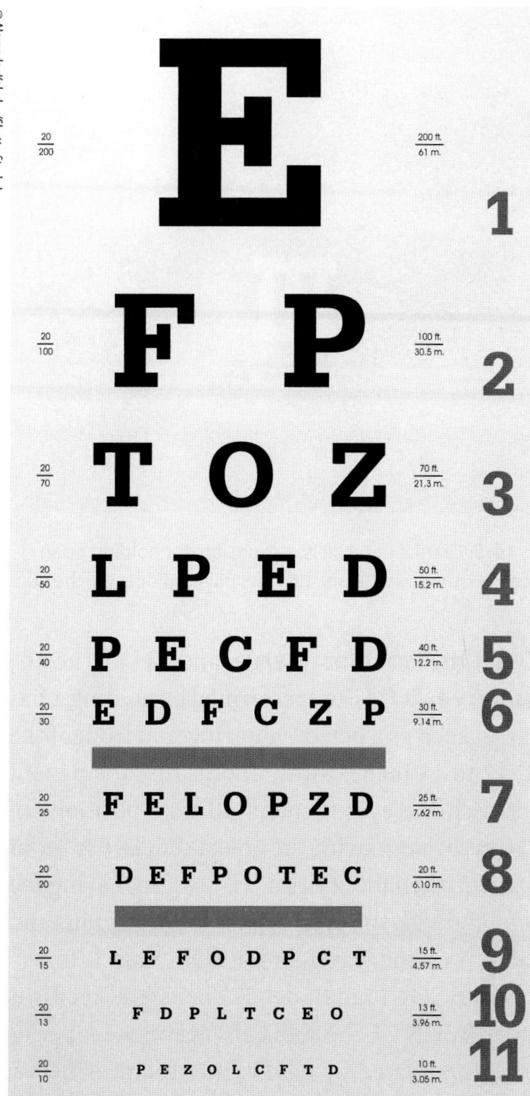

FIGURE 14-2 Visual acuity chart.

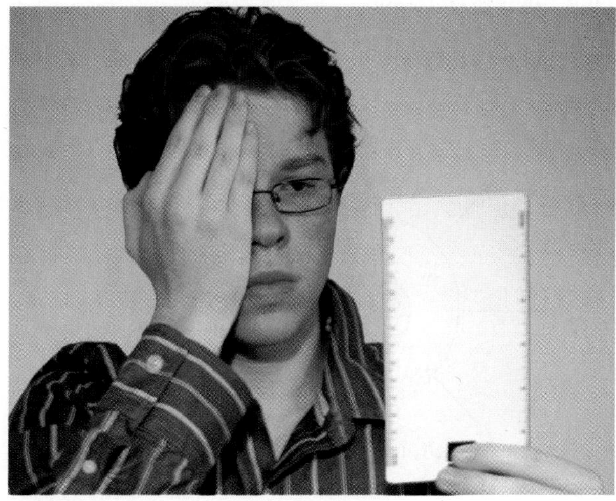

FIGURE 14-3 Visual acuity testing with a handheld chart.

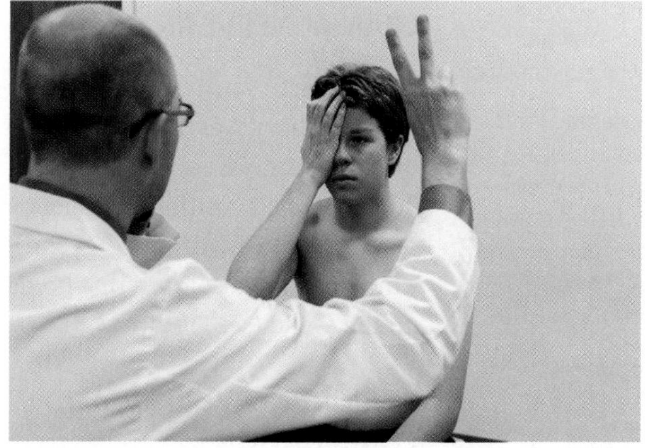

FIGURE 14-4 Peripheral field exam with provider on the same eye level as the patient and the hand placed halfway between the provider and the patient.

thorough neurologic examination revealed a right visual field cut (a right homonymous hemianopsia). He simply couldn't see the mailboxes, or, scarier yet, pedestrians along the right side of the road. His brain scan revealed a large posterior cerebral artery stroke.

Ophthalmoscopy

Finally, perform the ophthalmoscopic exam to directly visualize the optic disc, retina, fovea, and macula.

CRANIAL NERVE II AND III COMBINATION

8-6 The pupils should be examined for size, shape, and symmetry. Test direct and consensual **pupillary reaction**. Light stimulus is perceived by CNII (sensory) but the pupil constricts by CNIII (motor). Direct pupillary reaction is performed by having the patient look at a distant object and then shining the light in the right eye, which should result in constriction of the pupil. The light is then shown into the left eye. The consensual response is performed by shining the light in the right eye while watching the left pupil for constriction. Again repeat in the left eye while watching the right. The pupils should constrict, both direct and consensually, to equal degrees.

Pupillary reaction: constriction of the pupil as light is shown into the eye being examined (direct) and into the opposite eye (consensual)

Oculomotor nerve: cranial nerve III, responsible for constricting the pupil with pupillary reaction, keeping the eyelid in the open position, and extraocular movements through all positions of gaze except lateral and inferior, lateral movements

Trochlear nerve: cranial nerve IV, responsible for movement of the eye in the inferior, lateral (down and out) direction through the innervation of the superior oblique muscle

Abducens nerve: cranial nerve VI, responsible for the movement of the eye in the lateral direction through the innervation of the lateral rectus muscle

DOCUMENTATION

- "PERRL" (pupils equally round and reactive to light)

CRANIAL NERVE III

In addition to constricting the pupil with pupillary reaction, CNIII, the **oculomotor nerve**, keeps the eyelid in the open position. Deficiency results in ptosis (drooped eyelid). Think of III as a column that holds up the eyelid (see **FIGURE 14-5**).

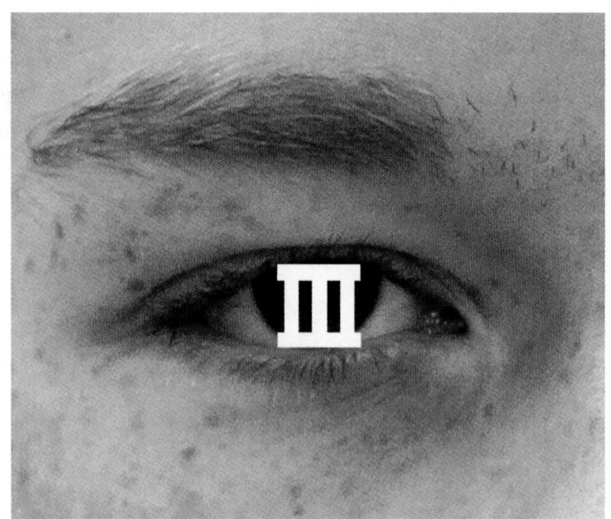

FIGURE 14-5 Cranial nerve III is responsible for holding open the eye can be remembered as the CNIII pillar holding up the lid.

CRANIAL NERVE III, IV, AND VI COMBINATIONS

CNIII is also involved in the extraocular movements (EOM) along with CNIV, the **trochlear nerve**, and CNVI, the **abducens nerve**. EOMs are performed by holding a fixation target such as a pen or your finger in front of the patient, 12 to 14 inches away, and having the patient follow it with the eyes through all nine positions of gaze. To do so, begin with the object centered in front of the patient, then move in an "H" pattern, having the patient follow with the eyes. Assess for nystagmus and gaze palsy. A memory trigger for EOM muscle innervation is LR6 SO4 Remainder 3. The lateral rectus is innervated by CNVI, the abducens nerve; the superior oblique is innervated by CNIV, the trochlear nerve; and all the other movements are innervated by CNIII, the oculomotor nerve (see **FIGURE 14-6**).

DOCUMENTATION

- "EOMI" (extraocular movements intact)

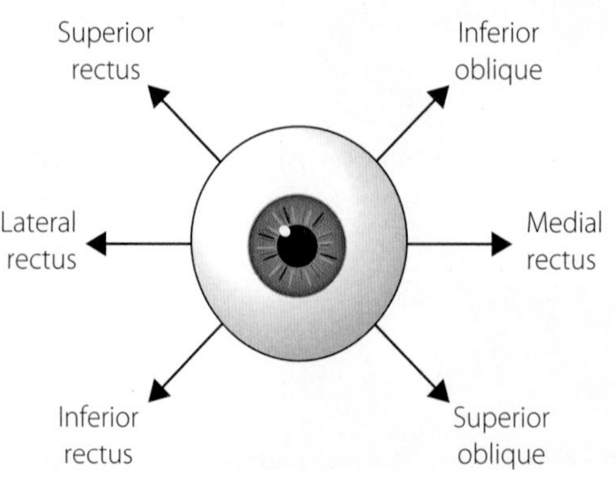

FIGURE 14-6 EOM innervation of the right eye.

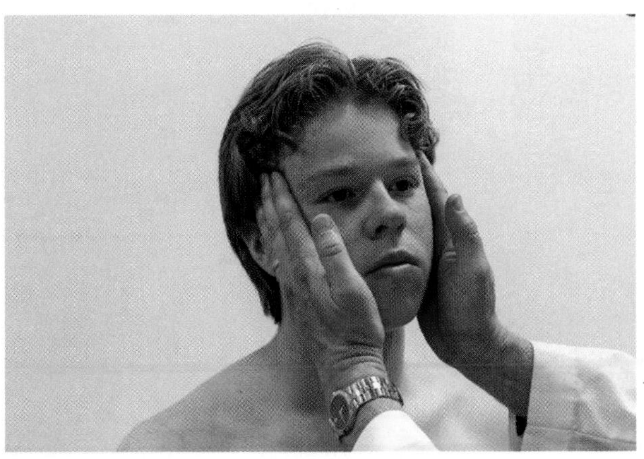

FIGURE 14-7 Palpation of the muscles of mastication.

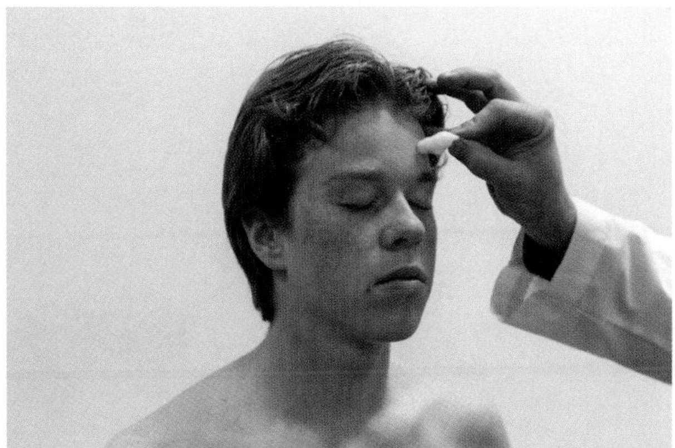

FIGURE 14-8A Soft touch of the superior branch of the trigeminal.

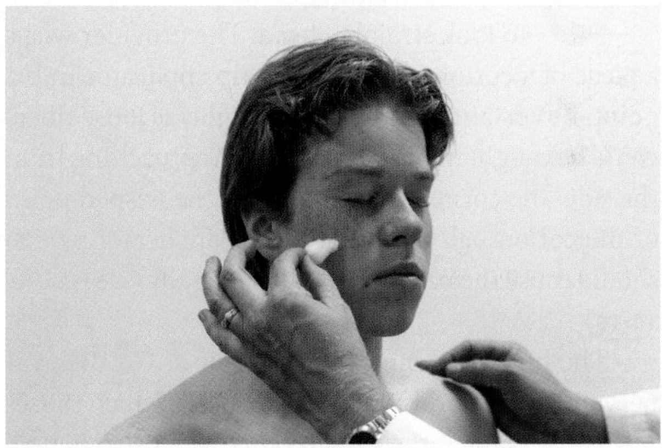

FIGURE 14-8B Soft touch of the middle branch of the trigeminal.

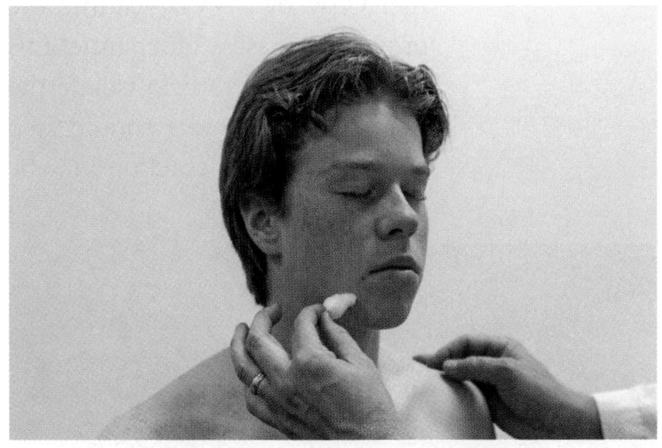

FIGURE 14-8C Soft touch of the inferior branch of the trigeminal.

CRANIAL NERVE V

The motor branch of CNV, the **trigeminal nerve**, innervates the muscles of mastication. To examine these, have the patient clench the teeth while you palpate the muscles of mastication (see **FIGURE 14-7**). Also, have the patient open the mouth to look for symmetry. The sensory branch of CNV supplies sensation to the face by branches to the forehead, cheek, and jaw. Use soft touch or a sharp object to test both sides of the face. This can be done simultaneously, side to side looking for symmetry, or it can be tested separately on all three areas (see **FIGURES 14-8A**, **14-8B**, and **14-8C**). Do not test at the angle of jaw, as this is innervated by the great auricular nerve.

14-3 A less commonly performed test for CNV is the jaw jerk. The jaw jerk is normally absent or only weakly present. If it is exaggerated and brisk, lesions affecting the descending motor tracts above the CNV's motor nucleus should be suspected, especially if there are bilateral lesions. To perform this test, the examiner places the index finger or thumb over the middle of the patient's chin, with the patient's mouth slightly open and the jaw relaxed. The finger or thumb is then tapped with a reflex hammer, delivering a downward stroke (see **FIGURE 14-9**). The normal response is that the jaw should not deviate to either side.

CRANIAL NERVE V AND VII COMBINATION

CNV is also involved in the corneal reflex as the afferent sensory component. This is not routinely tested in an awake patient, but it is employed in patients with a suspected facial nerve, CNVII, deficit and decreased levels of consciousness, such as with coma or brain death exams.

Trigeminal nerve: cranial nerve V, responsible for the motor action of the muscles of mastication and sensation to the forehead, cheek, and jaw

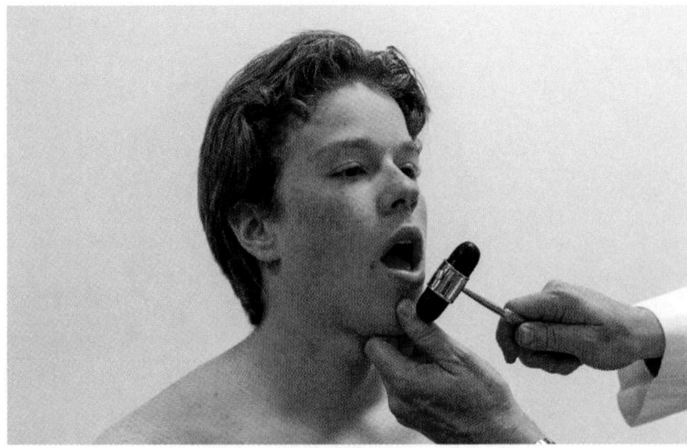

FIGURE 14-9 Jaw jerk.

14-4 To perform the test, the patient is advised to look straight ahead. The provider wisps a piece of a cotton ball or cotton tip applicator into a point. Be certain that the point is tight, as loose fibers could be caught in the patient's eye. Approaching from the side, the cornea is touched with the wisped point of the cotton ball or cotton-tipped applicator, which should cause the patient to blink bilaterally (see **FIGURE 14-10**).

The blink is a motor component of CNVII's innervation of the orbicularis oculi muscle, which causes the eyes to blink when stimulated. A diminished corneal reflex can therefore reflect pathology of either CNV or CNVII, leading the provider to assess other functions of these nerves to help isolate the lesions. The provider should also be aware that the reaction may be diminished in contact-lens wearers who have essentially learned to inhibit the blink response by repeatedly touching the cornea as they insert their lenses.

Facial nerve: cranial nerve VII, responsible for innervation of the muscles of facial expression, the ability to close the eyes, and taste sensation of the anterior two-thirds of the tongue

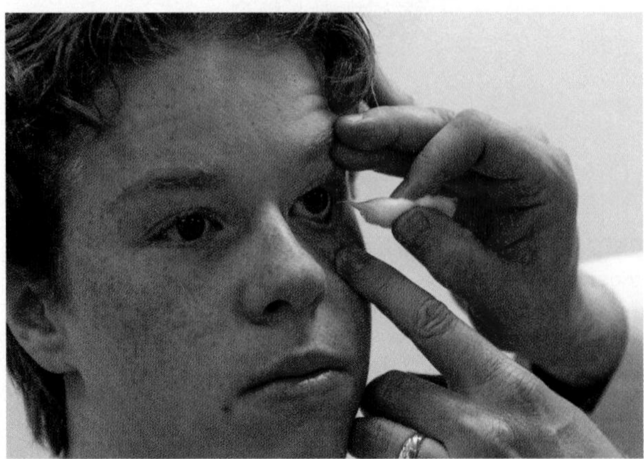

FIGURE 14-10 Corneal reflex test.

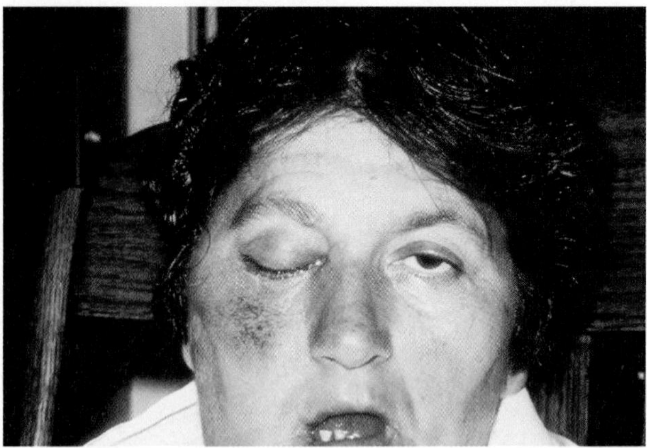

FIGURE 14-11 Facial droop.

CRANIAL NERVE VII

CNVII, the **facial nerve**, has a motor branch that innervates the facial muscles and can be assessed by observing facial symmetry, both when the patient is at rest and when he/she is making facial expressions.

14-5 Disruption of the innervation to the facial nerve can result in weakness of facial muscles and can be seen as flattening of the forehead wrinkles, loss of the nasolabial fold, drooping of the corner of the mouth, and inability to close the eye fully (see **FIGURE 14-11**). Assess the face at rest by observing the nasolabial folds and corners of the mouth for symmetry. Is one side flattened or drooping? Then ask the patient to complete a series of facial expression motions, comparing symmetry during movement:

- Please raise your eyebrows.
- Puff out your cheeks.
- Show me your teeth.
- Frown.

If the disruption to the facial nerve is peripheral or a lower motor neuron lesion, deficits will be found throughout the entire side of the face, with lower facial droop and loss of forehead wrinkling. In an upper motor neuron lesion, the forehead wrinkling is preserved through bilateral innervation from the cerebral cortex.

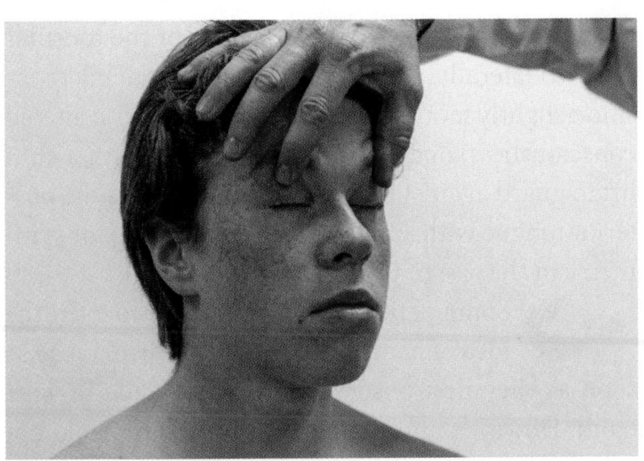

FIGURE 14-12 The patient closes the eyes and resists as the provider attempts to open them in assessment of CNVII.

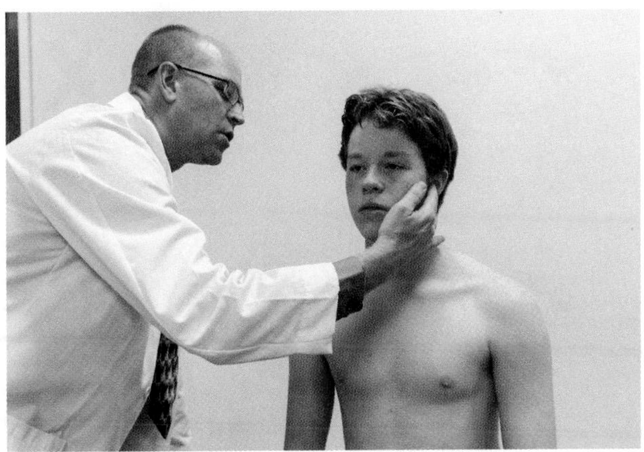

FIGURE 14-13 Whispered word with the provider occluding the opposite ear.

14-6 CNVII innervates the orbicularis oculi muscle, which allows the eyes to be forceably closed, a memory tool being the hooklike shape of a "7," pulling the eyelid down. To test, the patient is asked to hold the eyes closed tightly while the provider places a thumb and finger between the upper lids and eyebrows and tries to raise the lids against resistance (see **FIGURE 14-12**).

The facial nerve also has a sensory branch that allows for taste to the anterior two-thirds of the tongue, but taste is not routinely tested.

Other signs of CNVII injury are dry mouth, dry eye, and hyperacusis.

CRANIAL NERVE VIII

14-7 CNVIII, the **vestibulocochlear nerve**, also known as the acoustic nerve, is responsible for balance (vestibular) and hearing (cochlear). To assess proper functioning, a general screening examination should be completed, such as with the whispered word test or finger rub. To assess by whispered word, the provider occludes the opposite ear being tested and whispers a word at a distance of 24 inches from the ear, asking the patient to repeat the word (see **FIGURE 14-13**). The other ear is then tested.

Alternately, the examiner can ask the patient to close the eyes and identify through which ear he/she hears the fingers and thumb rub together. The provider then alternates from right to left, or both simultaneously, as the patient identifies which ear the sound is heard in.

8-10 If a deficit is found, the Weber and Rinne tests can be performed to distinguish between sensorineural and conductive hearing loss.

8-11 The vestibular component of CNVIII can be assessed by looking for **nystagmus**, involuntary beating movements of the eyes in horizontal, vertical, or circular motions (see **FIGURE 14-14**). Nystagmus can be induced in normal patients with extreme lateral gaze. Benign nystagmus typically demonstrates horizontal beats.

Pathologic nystagmus may have two phases—a slow movement in one direction and a fast movement in the opposite direction—and can suggest vestibular dysfunction. Vertical nystagmus should always prompt evaluation for pathologic conditions such as lesions of the cerebellum, stroke, tumors, and multiple sclerosis. Nystagmus is also a finding in many drug ingestions, such as alcohol, phenytoin, and benzodiazepines.

Assess the eyes for nystagmus with the patient focusing on a fixed object and observer, as well as while EOM testing is being performed.

CRANIAL NERVE IX

One major function of CNIX, the **glossopharyngeal nerve**, is taste sensation to the posterior one-third

Vestibulocochlear nerve: cranial nerve VIII, also known as the acoustic nerve, responsible for balance (vestibular) and hearing (cochlear)

Nystagmus: involuntary beating movements of the eyes in horizontal, vertical, or circular motions

Glossopharyngeal nerve: cranial nerve IX, responsible for taste sensation to the posterior one-third of the tongue and the sensory component of the gag reflex

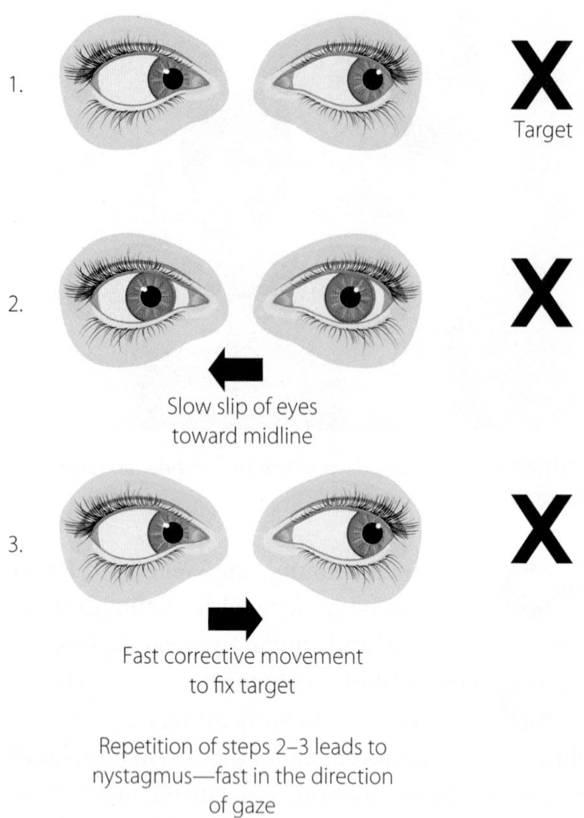
1.
Target
2.
Slow slip of eyes toward midline
3.
Fast corrective movement to fix target
Repetition of steps 2–3 leads to nystagmus—fast in the direction of gaze

FIGURE 14-14 Nystagmus.

Vagus nerve: cranial nerve X, responsible for the motor component of the pharynx (gag reflex), larynx, and esophagus; sensation to the ear, tongue, pharynx, and larynx, and providing parasympathetic innervation to thoracic and abdominal organs

Spinal accessory nerve: cranial nerve XI, responsible for the motor action of the sternocleidomastoid and trapezius muscles

of the tongue, but again, this is not tested routinely.

Signs of CNIX injury include dry mouth and dysphagia.

CRANIAL NERVE IX AND X COMBINATION

The gag reflex is not routinely tested in awake patients during neurologic exams unless the patient has a complaint, such as difficulty swallowing. CNIX provides the sensory component of the gag reflex while CNX, the **vagus nerve**, provides the motor reaction.

If the test is to be performed in a patient, advise the patient that you will be testing the gag reflex and ask him/her to open the mouth. Using a light source, touch a tongue blade firmly to the posterior tongue and observe for the spontaneous rise of the tonsillar pillars bilaterally. If a gag reflex is not obtained, reposition slightly more posterior. In a patient with altered consciousness, open the patient's mouth with a chin lift to guard against being bitten and depress the posterior tongue with a tongue blade, observing for symmetry in the rise of the tonsillar pillars.

14-8 Some patients are so sensitive to even the idea of being gagged that they will do so as soon as they first observe the tongue blade in your hand. However, approximately 20% of people do not have a gag reflex. Asymmetric findings are particularly indicative of pathology.

CRANIAL NERVE X

14-9 To further assess CNX, ask the patient to open the mouth and say "Ahh." Observe the soft palate for symmetrical elevation. The uvula should remain in midline. If the uvula deviates to either side, a dysfunction of the vagus nerve should be considered with the uvula deviating away from the side of the lesion.

The recurrent laryngeal branch of the vagus innervates the vocal cords, which can be assessed by listening for dysphonia as the patient talks, another indication of CNX dysfunction. This is easy enough to recognize in an established patient, but if a new patient presents with a deep, rough voice, do not assume it is the person's normal voice pattern. Further inquiry into changes in the character or volume of the voice is warranted.

CRANIAL NERVE XI

CNXI, the **spinal accessory nerve**, innervates the sternocleidomastoid (SCM) and trapezius muscles. To assess the SCM muscle, have the patient rotate the head to one side. The provider places a hand against the side of the exposed face (see **FIGURE 14-15**). The patient is then asked to rotate the head to midline, and "look forward" while resistance is provided. Compare to the opposite side.

14-10 To assess the trapezius muscle, have the patient shrug the shoulders against resistance (see **FIGURE 14-16**).

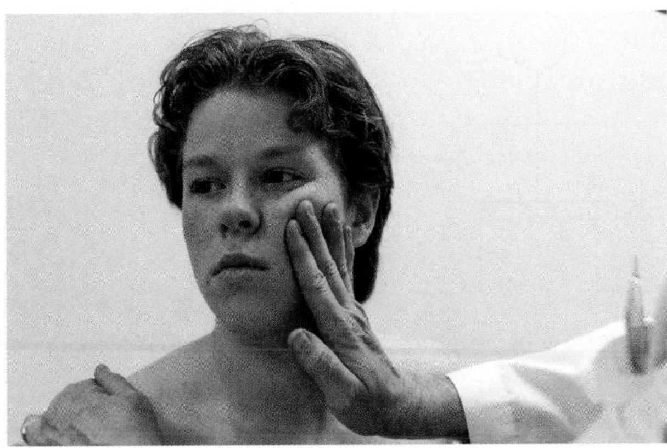

FIGURE 14-15 CNXI assessment of the SCM muscle with the patient attempting to rotate the head to midline against resistance.

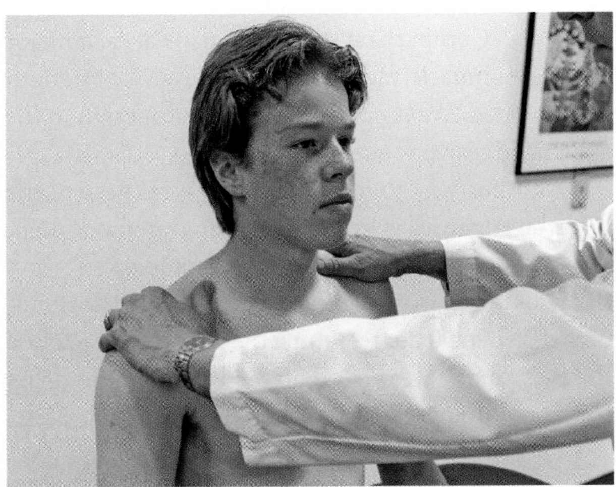

FIGURE 14-16 Trapezius test.

CRANIAL NERVE XII

14-11 CNXII, the **hypoglossal nerve**, provides motor innervation to the tongue. Ask your patient to stick the tongue straight out (see FIGURE 14-17). The tongue should protrude in midline. Deviation to one side suggests a lesion on the same side in lower motor neuron lesions or the opposite side in upper motor neuron lesions. Tongue atrophy and fasciculations occur only in lower motor neuron lesions, helping to differentiate them from upper motor neuron lesions.

DOCUMENTATION

- CN II–XII intact except CNVI with loss of lateral gaze in the right eye with EOM.

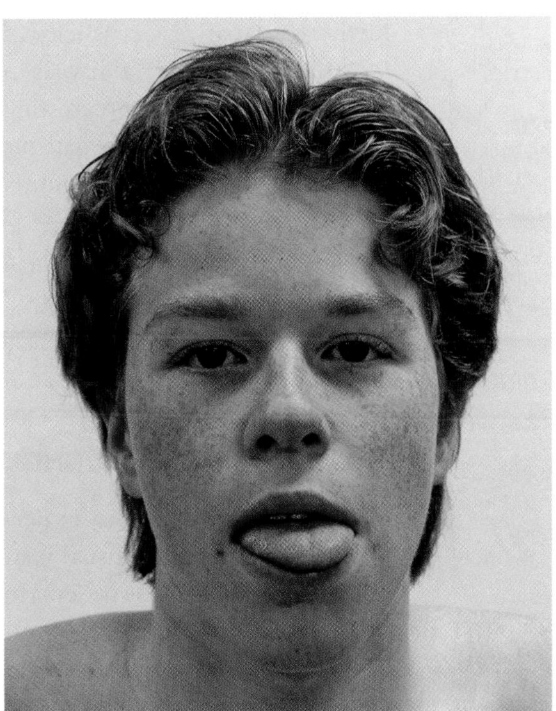

FIGURE 14-17 Tongue deviation occurs toward the side of the lesion of the hypoglossal nerve. In this picture, the lesion would be on the left.

Motor Examination

Completion of the cranial nerve examination with assessment of muscle strength of the SCM and trapezius may naturally lead the provider into the **motor examination** and the assessment of muscle strength testing throughout the rest of the body.

The motor examination consists first of a general inspection of the muscles, looking for atrophy or fasciculations. As with any other examination, proper exposure is essential.

MUSCLE TONE

14-12 **Muscle tone** is assessed by asking your patient to relax. The examiner then passively moves the patient's extremities, checking for hypotonia or hypertonia. Hypertonia (increased muscle tension or resistance) is indicative of upper motor neuron lesions and is marked by the decreased ability of the muscle to stretch. Hypertonia can

Hypoglossal nerve: cranial nerve XII, responsible for the motor movement of the tongue

Motor examination: component of the neurologic examination that assesses muscle tone, strength, and reflexes

Muscle tone: state of tension of the muscles

Strength testing: assessment of the ability to move a joint against gravity and resistance using a scale ranging from 0 (no movement) to 5 (movement against full resistance)

Muscle stretch reflex: assessment of upper and lower motor neuron lesions accomplished by the provider striking a muscle with a reflex hammer, activating the stretch receptor that communicates with lower motor neurons in the anterior horn, resulting in a reflex contraction of the muscle, which is graded by the provider on a scale from 0 (no reflex) to 4 (hyperreflexia)

further be classified as spasticity, as in chronic stroke, or rigidity, as in Parkinson's disease. An interesting example is seen with stroke patients who acutely may have hypotonia but later develop hypertonia.

DOCUMENTATION

- Hypertonicity of the left upper extremity.

MUSCLE STRENGTH TESTING

Muscle **strength testing** is performed symmetrically, usually simultaneously asking the patients to resist your strength. This is typically performed from proximally to distally in the arms and then the legs.

A scale is used for documenting muscle strength:

- 0/5 = No muscle twitch with attempted movement.
- 1/5 = The muscle can be seen to twitch but no movement at the joint is seen.

TABLE 14-1 Muscle Action and Innervations

Motion	Nerve	Root
Shoulder abduction	Axillary	C5–6
Elbow flexion	Musculocutaneous	C5–6
Elbow extension	Radial	C6, C7, C8
Wrist flexion	Median	C6, C7, C8
Wrist extension	Radial	C6, C7, C8
Finger adduction	Ulnar	C8, T1
Finger abduction	Ulnar	C8–T1
Thumb abduction (perpendicular to plane of hand)	Median	C8–T1
Hip adduction	Obturator	L2, L3, L4
Hip abduction	Superior gluteal	L4, L5, S1
Knee extension	Femoral	L2, L3, L4
Knee flexion	Sciatic	L5, S1, S2
Dorsiflexion	Deep fibular	L4–L5
Plantarflexion	Tibial	L5, S1, S2

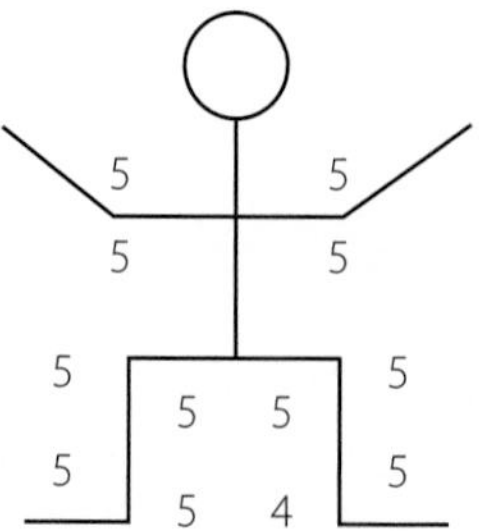

FIGURE 14-18 Figure for documentation of muscle strength.

- 2/5 = Movement occurs in the horizontal plane but not against gravity.
- 3/5 = Movement against gravity but not resistance.
- 4/5 = Movement against some resistance.
- 5/5 = Movement against full resistance.

14-13 Comparison should be made at each major muscle movement, with levels of strength documented. Weaknesses indicate dysfunction in the associated nerve roots (see **TABLE 14-1**).

Another way to look for subtle weakness of the upper extremities is by assessing for a pronator drift. To assess for pronator drift, the patient is asked to put the arms out in front of himself/herself with the shoulders flexed to 90 degrees, turn the palms up, and close the eyes. Subtle weakness can be seen if an arm drifts from the 90-degree position or if the hand pronates.

DOCUMENTATION

- The use of this graphic (see **FIGURE 14-18**) shows that muscle strength is graded at 4/5, with some weakness to resistance in left plantar and dorsiflexion.

Muscle Stretch Reflexes

Muscle stretch reflex testing is accomplished by the provider striking a muscle with a reflex hammer, activating the stretch receptor, which communicates with lower motor neurons in the anterior horn. The result is a reflex contraction of the muscle, which is graded by the provider.

Reflexes are graded on a on a scale from 0 to 4:

- 0/4 = no response
- 1/4 = diminished response
- 2/4 = normal

- 3/4 = somewhat increased
- 4/4 = greatly increased, clonus

The presence of hyporeflexia classically indicates lower motor neuron lesions. Hyperreflexia refers to an increase in contraction and classically indicates a lesion of upper motor neurons. The greatest degree of hyperreflexia is termed "clonus," which is seen as a series of pulsing muscular contractions, most commonly while performing reflex testing. Typically when performing a muscle stretch reflex, only a single response is elicited. With clonus, the contractions continue in a series lasting from a few seconds to several minutes. Clonus can be found in patients with multiple sclerosis and end-stage liver disease with encephalopathy, or in patients who have suffered spinal cord damage or stroke.

Muscle stretch reflex testing is a skill that can easily be mastered. In order to get the best results, the patient should be relaxed. If the patient is tensing the muscle being tested, the reflex will be muted. Reflex testing is most commonly performed with the patient in a seated position, though supine testing is often utilized in patients with altered consciousness. The reflex hammer should be held firmly at the end with the wrist swung loosely. Heavier hammers assist in eliciting reflexes. Bilateral comparison is essential, as asymmetry is always abnormal.

When testing reflexes, the provider should recall the level of innervation (see **TABLE 14-2**).

If a patient has depressed muscle stretch reflexes or has a difficult time relaxing the muscle, then distraction maneuvers can be utilized. When testing the upper extremity reflexes, ask the patient to clench the teeth. To test the lower extremity reflexes, ask the patient to grasp his/her fingers and pull apart while looking upward (see **FIGURE 14-19**).

TABLE 14-2 Muscle Stretch Reflexes and Nerve Root Innervation

Reflex	Nerve Root
Biceps	C5–6
Brachioradialis	C5–6
Triceps	C6–7
Patellar	L2–L4
Achilles	S1–S2

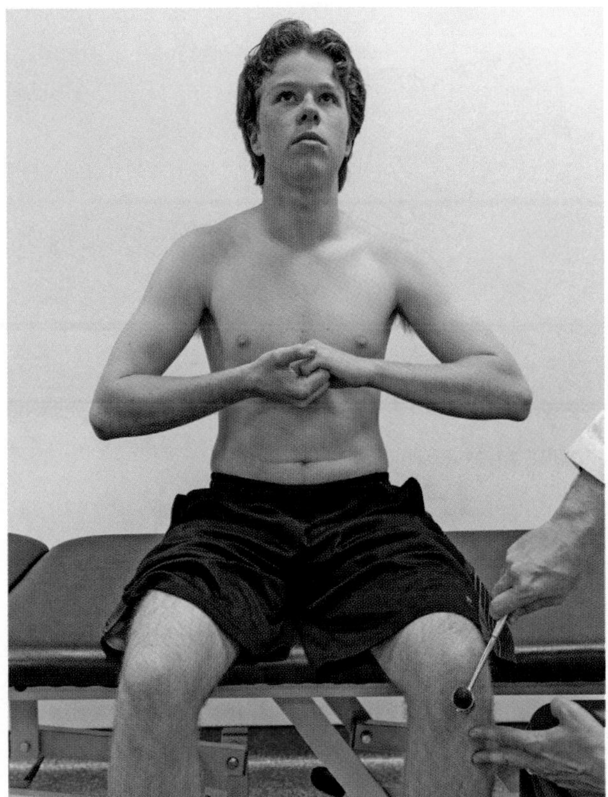

FIGURE 14-19 Lower extremity reflex distraction.

BICEPS REFLEX

14-14 Biceps reflex testing assesses the C5–6 nerve roots. With the patient in the seated position, rest the medial side of the forearms on the patient's upper thighs with the elbow extended to approximately 60 degrees. The provider places a hand behind the elbow with the thumb resting on the biceps tendon and then strikes the thumb, resulting in contraction of the biceps muscle (see **FIGURE 14-20**). Compare bilaterally.

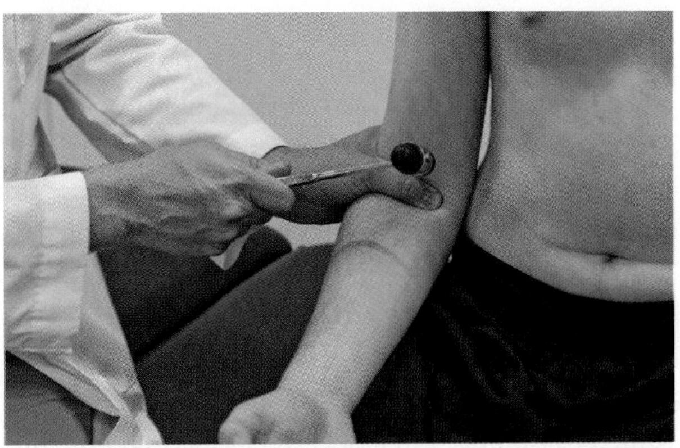

FIGURE 14-20 Biceps reflex.

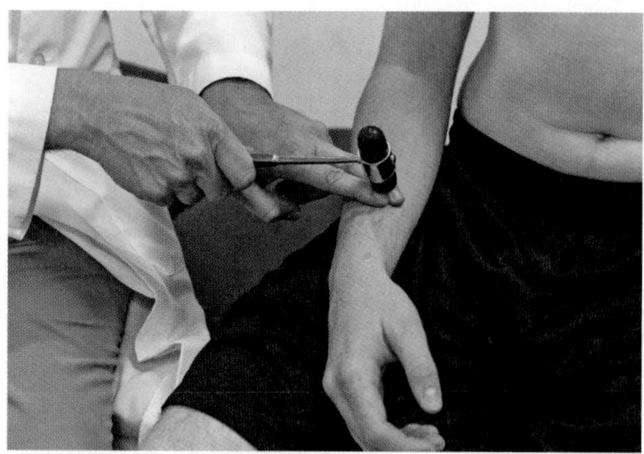

FIGURE 14-21 Brachioradialis reflex.

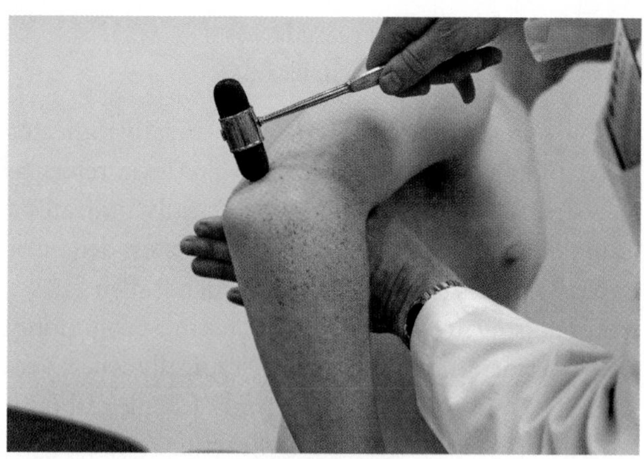

FIGURE 14-22 Triceps reflex.

BRACHIORADIALIS REFLEX

The brachioradialis is also innervated by the C5–6 nerve root. Assessment can immediately follow the biceps reflex with the patient in the same position. The provider strikes the brachioradialis tendon on the lateral side of the forearm approximately 5 inches proximal to the base of the thumb. The tendon can be struck directly; however, because of the thin layer of muscle overlying the radius, it may cause pain. The provider can lay a finger over the tendon and strike the finger instead (see **FIGURE 14-21**).

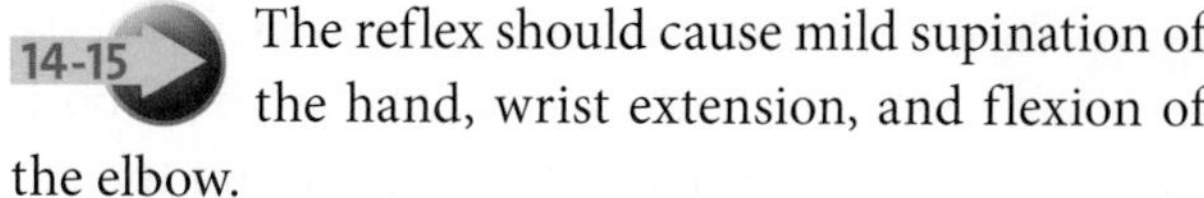

14-15 The reflex should cause mild supination of the hand, wrist extension, and flexion of the elbow.

TRICEPS REFLEX

14-16 To assess the triceps reflex, hold the patient's arm up with the shoulder at 90 degrees and the forearm hanging down with the elbow bent at 90 degrees (scarecrow position). Ask the patient to completely relax the arm, or say, "Let me hold up your arm," then let the arm drop slightly. The patient who is not completely relaxed will hold the arm up. Once you have patient compliance, palpate the triceps tendon to the insertion of the olecranon process and strike the tendon 1 to 2 inches proximal to the olecranon (see **FIGURE 14-22**). Observe for extension at the elbow.

If the patient cannot relax the arm, the triceps reflex can be assessed with the patient's arms in the same position used to assess the biceps and brachioradialis reflexes.

PATELLAR REFLEX

14-17 The patellar reflex assesses primarily the L4 nerve root. Ask the patient to slide backward so that the knees are just off the exam table. The provider should be positioned to the side of the patient to allow unimpeded extension of the lower leg. Palpate the patella, the patellar tendon, and the insertion into the tibial tuberosity. Strike the tendon halfway between the patella and the tuberosity (see **FIGURE 14-23**).

ACHILLES REFLEX (CALCANEAL)

14-18 Moving downward, assess the Achilles reflex, primarily the S1 nerve root, by holding the patient's foot in dorsiflexion. This is another exam that is sometimes difficult to get complete relaxation of the muscle before testing. Lift the forefoot in dorsiflexion and ask the patient to relax then let the foot

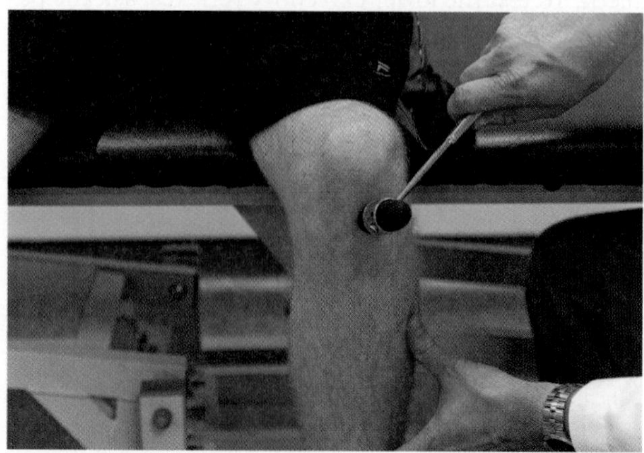

FIGURE 14-23 Patellar reflex.

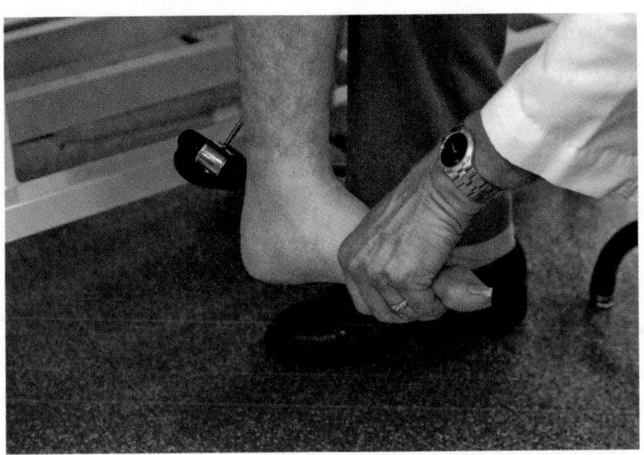

FIGURE 14-24 Achilles reflex.

drop. If the patient holds the foot up, repeat the lift and drop several times, advising the patient to "Let me do all the work." When the foot drops easily, lift once more and strike the Achilles tendon, looking and feeling for the foot to plantarflex (see **FIGURE 14-24**).

DOCUMENTATION

- The use of this graphic (see **FIGURE 14-25**) shows that all reflexes are intact but with hyperreflexia of the left patellar and Achilles reflexes.

CLONUS

Clonus is seen as a series of involuntary contractions and relaxations of a muscle when a reflex is assessed either by reflex hammer or by rapid stretching of the muscle.

14-19 Assess for clonus by rapidly dorsiflexing the foot at the ankle and maintaining a light upward pressure on the sole. Clonus—repeated downward, rhythmic contractions into the examiner's hand—is abnormal and is a sign of upper motor neuron lesions involving descending motor pathways.

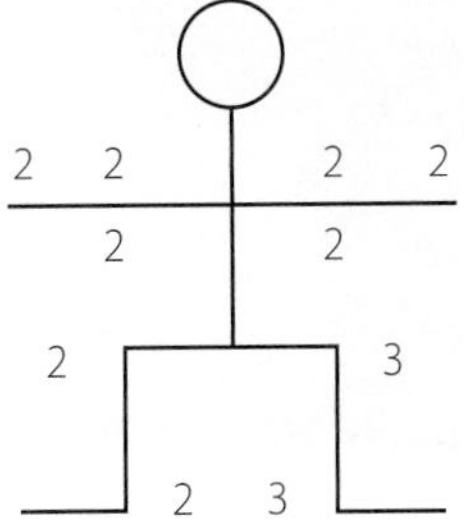

FIGURE 14-25 Figure for documentation of stretch reflexes.

PLANTAR REFLEX

Clonus: a sign of upper motor neuron lesions involving descending motor pathways, seen as a series of involuntary contractions and relaxations of a muscle when a reflex is assessed either by reflex hammer or by rapid stretching of the muscles

14-20 The next reflex in our head-to-toe approach is the plantar or flexor plantar reflex, or Babinski response. To perform this examination, a firm, but not sharp object such as a tongue blade, handle end of a tomahawk hammer, or the provider's thumb nail is used to stroke the lateral plantar surface of the foot from the heel anteriorly, crossing medially at the ball of the foot (see **FIGURES 14-26A**, **14-26B**, and **14-26C**). The examination should be explained and permission to perform received prior to performing, as some patients are anxious or severely ticklish when their feet are touched. A firm pressure should be used so as not to tickle the patient, but not so firm as to cause pain. Sharp objects are never used as they could damage the skin, especially in patients with peripheral

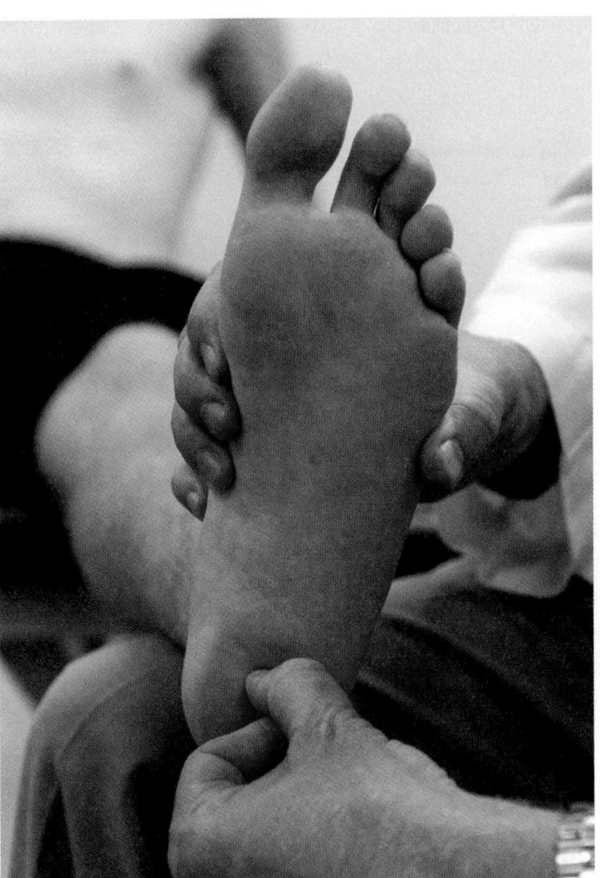

FIGURE 14-26A Begin assessment of the plantar reflex by forcefully pressing in on the heel of the foot.

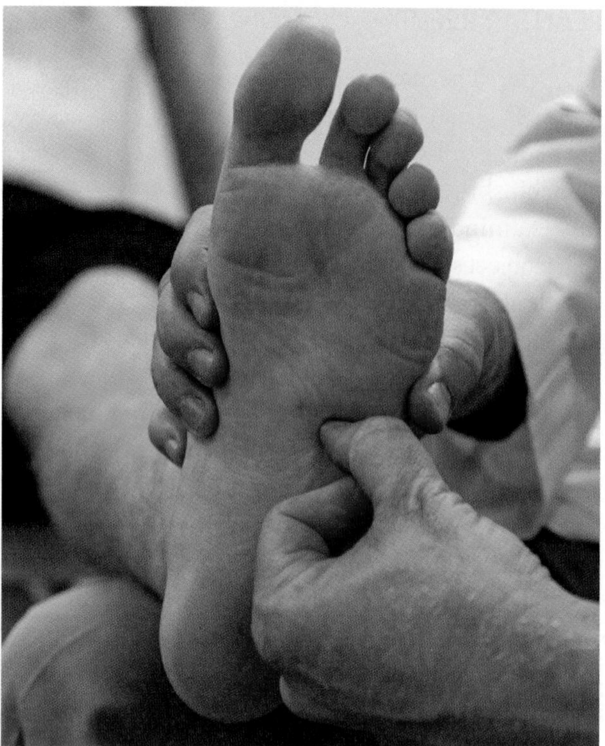

FIGURE 14-26B Drag the point of pressure along the lateral aspect of the foot while.

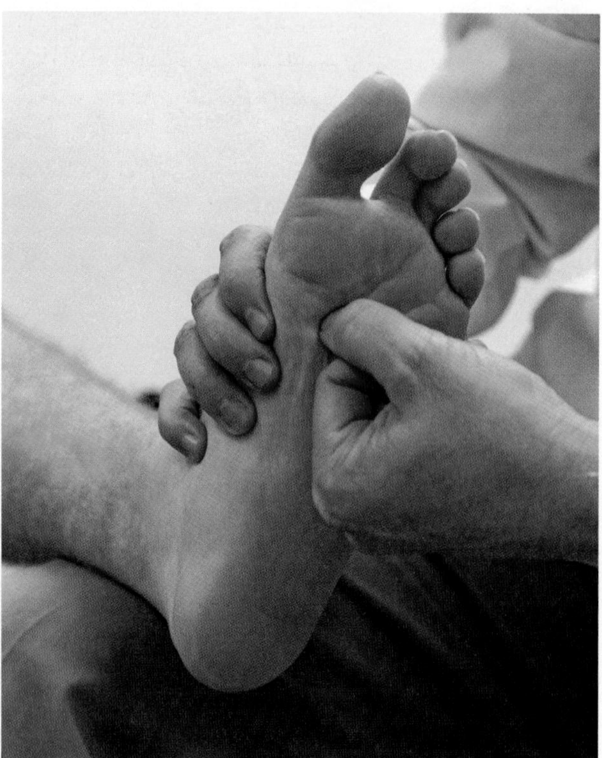

FIGURE 14-26C Continue dragging the point of pressure across the ball of the foot from the lateral to the medial aspect while watching the toes.

neuropathy who may not feel pain, which would cause patients with intact sensation to withdraw the foot.

The normal response is plantarflexion of the first digit, documented as "downgoing," "negative Babinski," or "flexor plantar response." Dorsiflexion of the first digit is always an abnormal response except in children younger than 2 years of age. This is documented as "upgoing," "positive Babinski," or "extensor plantar response," and indicates an upper motor neuron problem.

HOFFMAN REFLEX

14-21 The Hoffman or finger flexor reflex may also be a sign of an upper motor neuron problem. The test is performed by grasping the patient's hand and extending the wrist and middle finger. The provider then flicks the nail of the terminal phalanx downward. If the thumb or other digits flex, a positive response, or positive Hoffman sign, is documented (see FIGURE 14-27). Compare to the opposite extremity.

Case Example

Abnormalities in reflexes can be a powerful tool for diagnosis. A middle-aged man presented to the

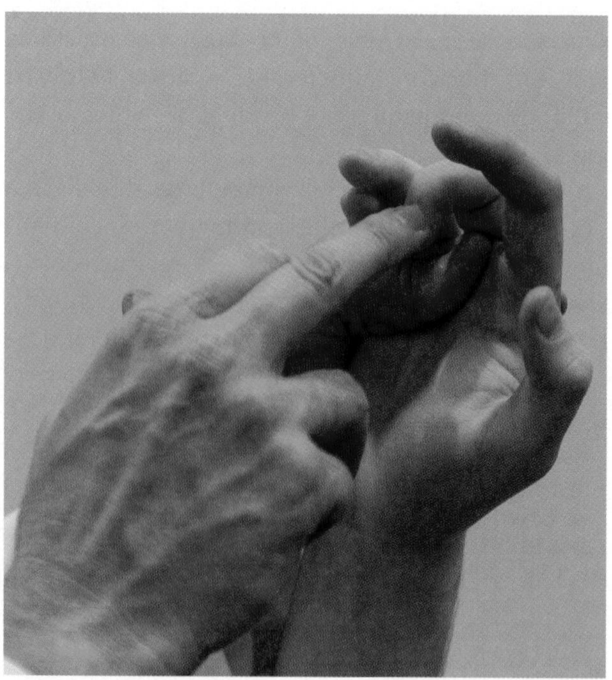

FIGURE 14-27 Hoffman reflex.

emergency room with unsteady gait, falls, and low back pain. He had been to numerous other emergency rooms and was discharged after having his low back scanned. On examination, his cranial nerves were intact, but he was diffusely hyperreflexic with clonus in all four extremities. A stat MRI of his cervical spine was ordered. When he reached the scanner, the technician called the ordering physician to ask if she wanted the lumbar spine scanned instead of the neck, saying that the patient was complaining of low back pain. After the doctor insisted on the cervical spine scan, a cervical cord compression was found. The patient successfully underwent neck surgery. The diagnostic clues from assessment of the reflexes led to a good outcome after a nearly disastrous start.

DOCUMENTATION

- No clonus. Downgoing plantar reflex. Negative Hoffman.

Sensory Examination

The **sensory examinations** consist of a symmetrical assessment of the patient's perception of light touch, pain, temperature (hot or cold), proprioception (position sense), and vibratory sensation. In addition, stereognosis, graphesthesia, and extinction can be tested.

TABLE 14-3 Sensory Examination Screening Dermatome Levels

Area of Examination	Dermatome Level
Lateral shoulder	C4
Lateral forearm	C5
Thumb	C6
Middle finger	C7
Fifth finger	C8
Medial forearm	T1
Nipple line	T4
Umbilical line	T10
Anterior thigh	L2
Medial calf	L4
Lateral calf	L5
Fifth toe	S1

Screening examinations for light touch and pain are conducted at representative dermatome levels to detect deficiencies deficiencies (see **TABLE 14-3**).

If a deficiency is found at any of the screening levels, sequential dermatomal levels should be examined to define precise mapping of deficiencies.

Vibratory assessment is performed at distal joints first, working proximally as deficiencies are observed.

TOUCH

Touch is perceived through a combination of the posterior column/medial lemniscus and spinothalamic tracts. The posterior column transmits fine-touch sensation and, as such, a cotton ball can be used to test this sensory pathway. Because the spinothalamic tract transmits crude-touch sensation, the fingers can be used for this assessment.

14-22 With the patient watching, lightly touch the open palm and confirm that the patient can feel it. Then ask the patient to close his/her eyes and tell you which side you touch him/her on. Typically the upper extremities are tested as a group, then the thorax, followed by the lower extremities. Be sure to expose the entire area being examined so that you don't have to push up a sleeve before testing the area, as the patient will be alerted as to the intended target.

When testing an area, avoid testing dermatomal levels in an exact pattern—that is, right shoulder, left shoulder, right lateral forearm, left lateral forearm, right thumb, left thumb, etc. Instead, vary the approach: right lateral shoulder, left fifth finger, right thumb, right medial forearm, left shoulder, left medial forearm, and so on, being sure to cover all dermatome levels. Then move to the thorax and finally the lower extremities.

Some providers prefer to examine symmetrically by simultaneously touching the patient on both sides at a dermatome level and asking the patient to report whether the touches feel the same on both sides or whether they are different. Again, light touch is perceived

Sensory examinations: component of the neurologic examination that assesses touch, pain, temperature (hot or cold), proprioception (position sense), and vibratory sensation

Touch: sensory perception transmitted through a combination of the posterior column/medial lemniscus and spinothalamic tracts, assessed through fine touch

Pain: sensory perception transmitted through the spinothalamic tract

Temperature: sensory perception transmitted through the spinothalamic tract, assessed through the distinction of hot verses cold

Vibratory sensation: sensory perception transmitted through the posterior columns/medial lemniscus, assessed through the ability to sense vibrations

through the posterior column/medial lemniscus pathway. If heavier pressure (crude touch) is used, perception is occurring through the spinothalamic tract.

PAIN

Sensory perception of **pain** is also transmitted through the spinothalamic tract. Pain is assessed through sharp sensory testing and can be performed using a cotton-tipped applicator broken in half or a tongue blade snapped in half lengthwise (see **FIGURES 14-28A** and **14-28B**). A safety pin can also be used. All of these are to be disposed of after use on a single patient to prevent possible transfer of infection from patient to patient.

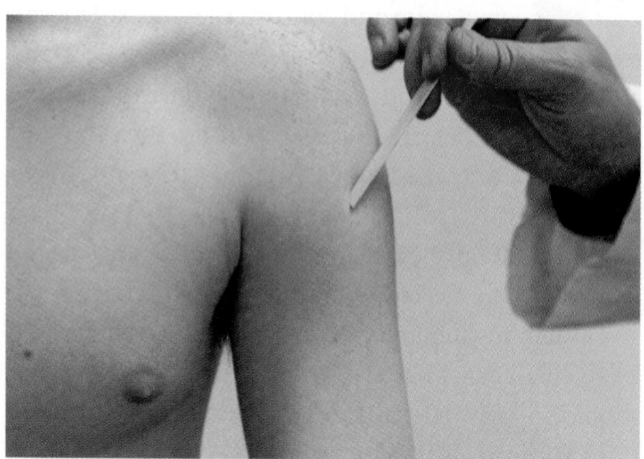

FIGURE 14-28A A tongue blade can be split lengthwise using the blunt side to assess the perception of dullness.

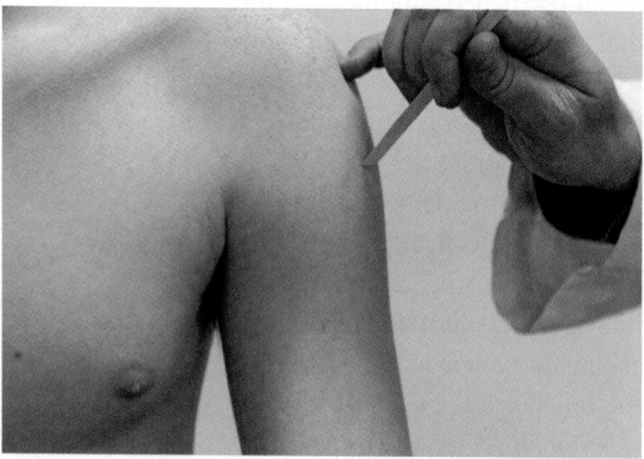

FIGURE 14-28B The pointed side is then used to assess perception of sharpness.

14-23 Allow patients to see the object you will be testing with and either allow them to touch the sharp end or touch them with it to demonstrate sharp sensation. Ask patients to close their eyes and instruct them to tell you if the sensation feels sharp at each screening area. Perform screening at the same levels as soft touch.

It is also important to note if the patient has a gradient to sharp sensation. To do this, test sharp sensation distally in the feet and compare to sensation in the legs. The patient should be able to feel more sharpness in the feet. This can also be done by comparing the hands to the arms, with more sharpness normally in the hands. Patients with peripheral polyneuropathies (for example from diabetes) often have decreased sensation in their distal extremities.

TEMPERATURE

Assessment of **temperature** sensation is less frequently used for testing in clinical practice but should be employed especially in those patients who show deficiency in other sensory modalities, as it is also an assessment of the spinothalamic tract.

To assess temperature sensation, use the cold handle of a tuning fork or reflex hammer to touch the patient at the perceived sites of deficiency. Ask patients to close their eyes and tell you if they perceive hot or cold.

VIBRATION

A vibratory 128-Hz tuning fork is used to test **vibratory sensation** which is transmitted through the posterior columns/medial lemniscus. This tuning fork should be hit lightly enough that there is no audible sound. Loss of vibratory sensation occurs from distal to proximal, so testing can be approached by testing the distal joints first and moving proximally only if a deficit is encountered.

14-24 Advise the patient that you will be striking a tuning fork and placing it on a joint. Ask the patient to close the eyes, then strike and place the tuning fork firmly on the distal interphalangeal joint of one hand (see **FIGURE 14-29**). Be careful to hold the tuning fork by the handle so as to avoid dampening the vibration. Ask the patient if he/she can feel the vibration. If so, ask the patient to say "stop" when the vibration stops. Wait a few seconds and then stop the

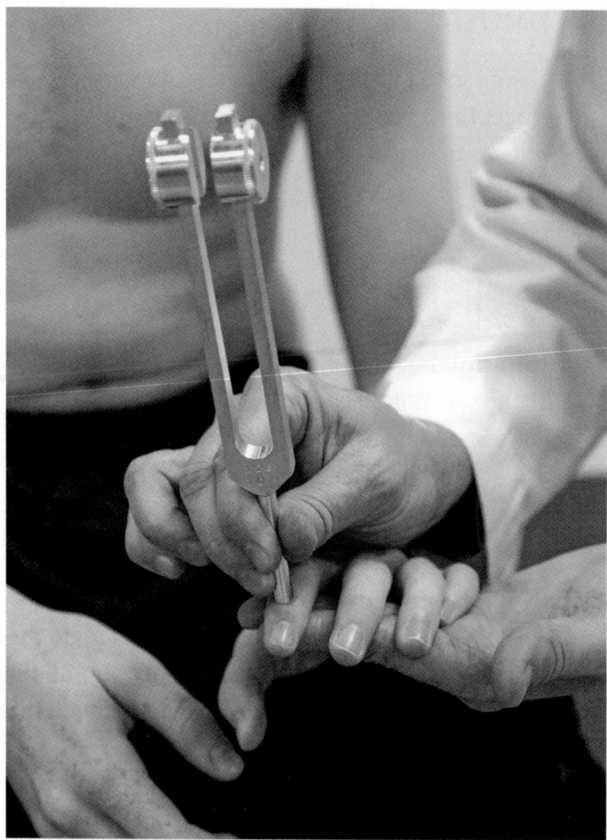

FIGURE 14-29 Vibratory sensation.

vibration briskly by dampening the tines with the other hand.

If a patient has decreased vibratory sense, being unable to feel the vibration or its suddenly stopping, the examiner should progress proximally one joint at a time until the vibration is felt.

During testing, instead of briskly halting the vibration, the provider may choose to slowly slide a finger up the tuning fork, asking the patient to identify when the vibration stops, so that both the provider and the patient should feel the halt in vibration simultaneously.

PROPRIOCEPTION

Conscious **proprioception** refers to the ability to sense the position of one body part in relation to others. Testing proprioception is another assessment technique for evaluating the posterior columns.

14-25 Advise the patient that you will be testing their ability to tell whether their finger is placed in an up or down position, and ask them to close their eyes. Hold the sides of a finger distally, then move it up and down a few degrees (see **FIGURE 14-30**). Then ask the patient to determine if the finger is in the up or down position. The test should be repeated several times on the same digit. It can then be repeated in the other extremities.

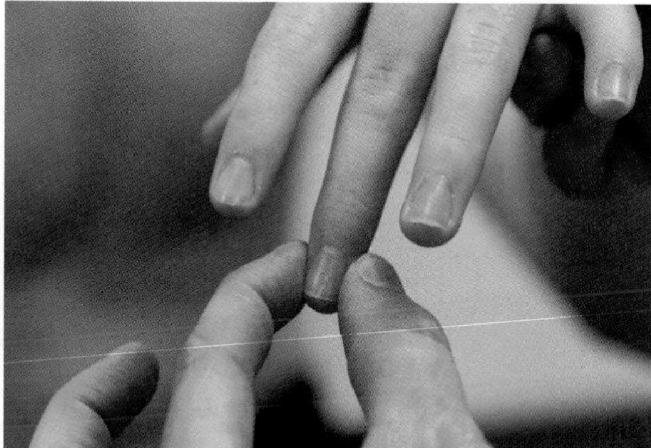

FIGURE 14-30 Proprioception.

Inaccuracies indicate dysfunction of the posterior column/medial lemniscus pathway.

The sensory examination should also include assessment of cortical functioning. Please note that primary sensation must be intact to assess cortical function. Functions include:

- Stereognosis: ability to identify a familiar object in the hand
- Graphesthesia: ability to identify a tracing on the palm
- Extinction: ability to identify which side of the body is touched

STEREOGNOSIS

Stereognosis is the ability to recognize common objects by touch. To assess, advise patients that you will be placing a small object in their hand and that you want them to identify it with their eyes closed. Ask patients to close their eyes and place a common object in their hand, such as a key, coin, or paper clip. Assess bilaterally. Deficiency reflects parietal lobe pathology.

Proprioception: sensory perception transmitted through the posterior columns, referring to the ability to sense the position of one body part in relation to others

Stereognosis: the ability to recognize common objects by touch as a function of the parietal lobe

Graphesthesia: the ability to recognize numbers, letters, or symbols traced on the palm as a function of the parietal lobe

Extinction: the inability to appreciate touch in an area on one side of the body as a function of the parietal cortex

Coordination: the interaction between the cerebellum and the motor, vestibular, and sensory systems that may be assessed through techniques of examination such as finger-to-nose, rapid alternating movements, and heel-to-shin testing

GRAPHESTHESIA

Graphesthesia is the ability to recognize numbers, letters, or symbols traced on the palm. Numbers are most frequently used. To perform number identification, advise patients that you will be drawing a number on their palm with their eyes closed and that you would like them to identify the number. Ask them to close their eyes and open their palm. Draw a number, standing beside patients so that the number is facing them rather than upside-down (see **FIGURE 14-31**). Ask the patient what number was drawn. Repeat in the other hand. Deficiency indicates parietal lobe pathology.

EXTINCTION

Finally, also test for **extinction**—the inability to appreciate touch in an area on one side of the body—in order to test for parietal cortex dysfunction. In this test, advise patients that you want them to identify if they are being touched on the right side, left side, or both sides simultaneously when their eyes are closed. Ask patients to close their eyes, then touch them, varying among right side only, left side only, or both. Repeat for consistency. Extinction occurs when the patient cannot identify touch on one side, indicating the presence of pathology.

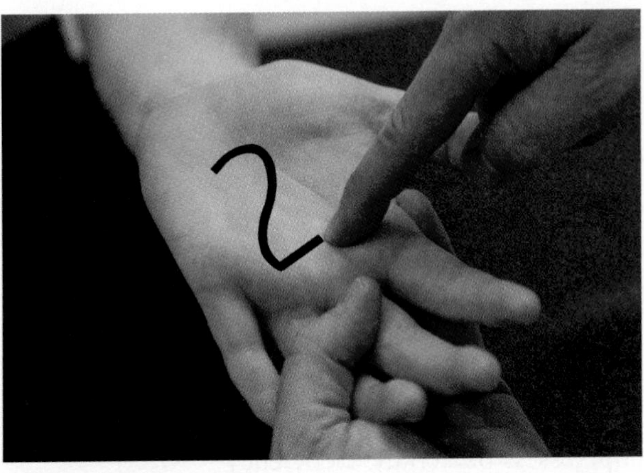

FIGURE 14-31 Graphesthesia.

DOCUMENTATION

- Sensory intact to light touch, sharp, vibration, proprioception, and temperature throughout. Stereognosis and graphesthesia are intact. There is no extinction.

Cerebellar Functioning

Coordination involves interactions between the cerebellum and the motor, vestibular, and sensory systems. Multiple tests assess this interaction, with deficiencies indicating possible cerebellar pathology.

FINGER TO NOSE

14-26 The provider demonstrates touching his/her own nose and asks the patient to do the same. The provider then points to a location about halfway to the patient and asks the patient to touch the tip of his/her finger. Each touches his/her own nose again, then the provider picks other random areas, assessing the ability of the patient to touch the proffered fingertip accurately (see **FIGURES 14-32A** and **14-32B**).

RAPID ALTERNATING MOVEMENTS

A dysfunction in the performance of rapid alternating movements (RAMs) is known as dysdiadochokinesia. To perform RAM testing, ask the patient to quickly tap his/her index fingers and thumbs.

14-27 RAM can also be assessed by having the seated patient put his/her hands against the thighs, then quickly alternate flipping the hands back

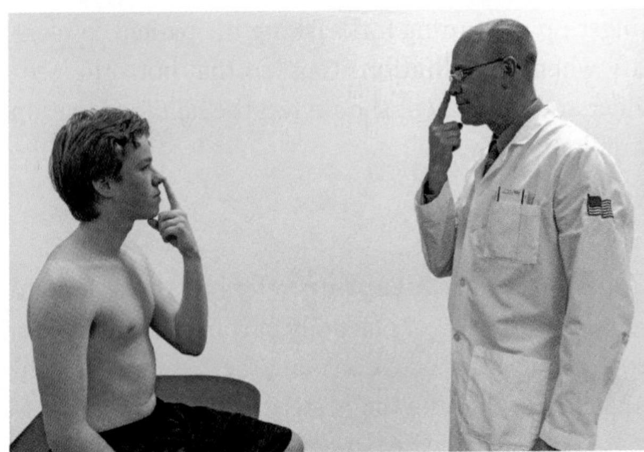

FIGURE 14-32A Finger-to-nose testing begins with the provider and patient touching their own noses.

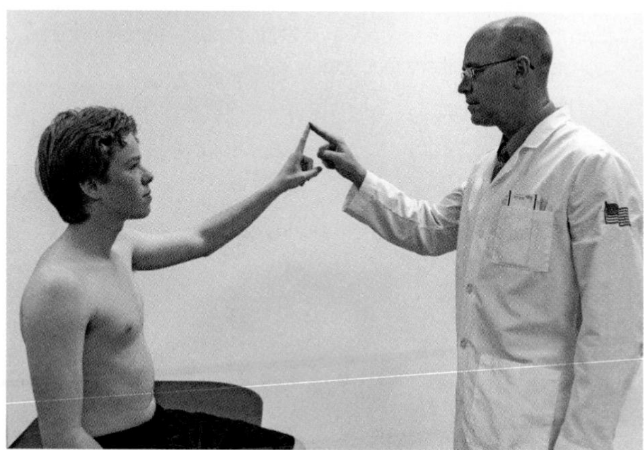

FIGURE 14-32B The provider then randomly places his/her finger halfway toward the patient, who is asked to touch it. The sequence is then repeated.

and forth, striking the palmar then dorsal surface of the hands.

HEEL TO SHIN

14-28 The heel-to-shin test assesses the patient's ability to move the heel smoothly down the shin. With the patient seated, ask the patient to place the heel of one foot on the shin of the opposite leg, just below the knee, and then drag the heel down the shin to the ankle (see **FIGURES 14-33A** and **14-33B**). The patient should be able to do so in a nearly linear path. Significant deviation may indicate cerebellar dysfunction.

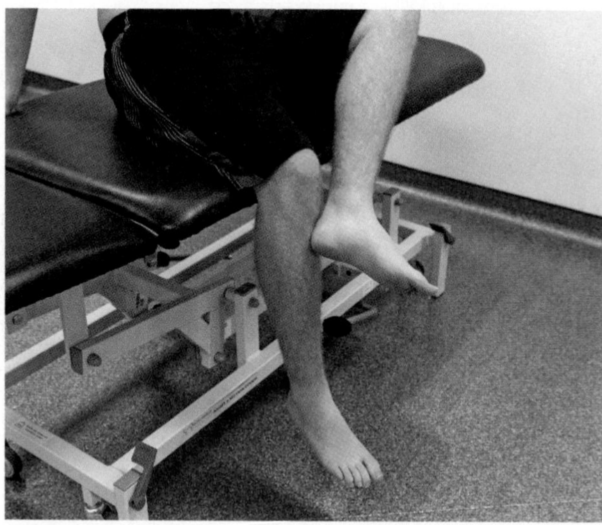

FIGURE 14-33A Heel-to-shin testing begins with the patient placing the heel superiorly on the shin.

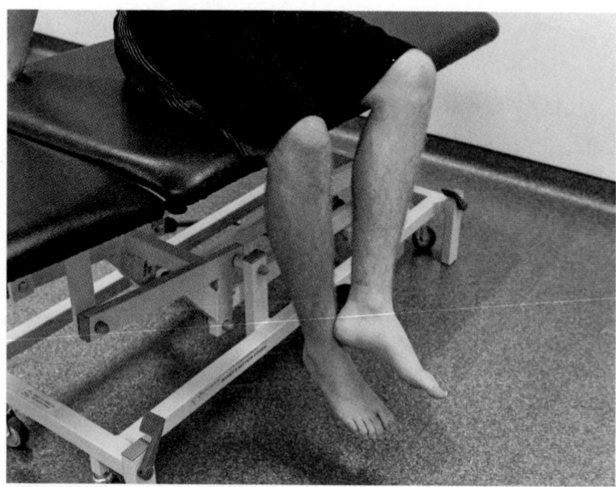

FIGURE 14-33B The heel is then dragged downward along the shin as the provider assesses the ability of the patient to keep the heel in midline.

ROMBERG TEST

The **Romberg test** assesses the patient's ability to maintain balance when standing with eyes closed, removing the sensory component of stability.

14-29 Assist the patient to the standing position and advise him/her that you will be testing his/her balance. Ask the patient to stand with the feet together and to close the eyes. Advise the patient that you will not let him/her fall, and position yourself so that you are at the patient's side. This provides the patient with assurance and allows you to easily assist the patient should the patient lose his/her balance.

Minimal swaying may occur, but should the patient sway or adjust the feet to regain balance, the Romberg test is positive, indicating posterior column or vestibular dysfunction.

Patients with severe proprioceptive deficits or midline cerebellar lesions may not be able to stand upright with their eyes open, and performing the Romberg test may not be necessary or safe.

GAIT

Lastly, the complex interaction of cerebellum, vestibular, motor, and sensory functioning is evaluated through observation of the patient's **gait**.

Romberg test: evaluation of cerebellar functioning where the patient's ability to maintain balance is assessed as he/she stands with eyes closed, removing the sensory component of stability

Gait: pattern of walking requiring interaction of cerebellar, vestibular, motor, and sensory functioning

14-30 Advise the patient that you will be observing his/her gait. First ask the patient to walk normally across the room or down a hallway. After a sufficient length, ask the patient to turn around, as you observe his/her coordination, and walk back toward you on the toes. Ask the patient to turn again and walk away on the heels. And finally, have the patient turn and walk toward you once more heel-to-toe (tandem gait).

The provider should be acutely observant for fall risk, especially in the elderly, and either ask trained staff to accompany the patient to allow the provider to observe appropriately or be prepared to assist the patient immediately if necessary.

DOCUMENTATION

- Cerebellar functioning intact to finger/nose, RAM, and heel to shin. Negative Romberg, stable gait.

The basic adult neurologic examination has been completed. While other tests can be performed, such as primitive reflexes, these are not performed on every patient and have not been covered in this chapter. In addition, for the pediatric patient a variety of other neurologic tests must be performed.

See **TABLE 14-4** for the neurologic flow.

Special thanks to Dr. Randy Kulesza, PhD, Neuroanatomist, for his review.

TABLE 14-4 Neurologic Flow

Introduces self and explains that physical exam will now be performed
Washes hands for 15 seconds, turning off water with towel
Level of consciousness—alert, drowsy, stuporous, comatose
Response to verbal, touch, or painful stimulation
Orientation—person, place, time (student must ask patient: name, date, and location)
General assessment—posture, obvious extremity weakness or asymmetry
CRANIAL NERVE (CN) EXAMINATION
CN II—optic
Assess visual acuity bilaterally
Assess peripheral fields bilaterally
Ophthalmoscopic examination
Combination CN II sensory and CN III motor—direct and consensual pupillary reaction
CN III—oculomotor—evaluate for ptosis
Combination CN III, IV, and VI—extraocular movements
CN V—trigeminal
Motor branch—palpate muscles of mastication with pt clenching teeth
Sensory branch—light touch in each branch of the trigeminal
CN V and VII—corneal reflex
CN VII—facial
Motor branch
Facial symmetry—nasolabial fold, facial range of motion
Hold eyes closed against resistance
Sensory branch—state tests for taste in anterior two-thirds of tongue
CN VIII—acoustic (vestibulocochlear)
Hearing—perform general screening hearing test bilaterally
Vestibular function—assess for nystagmus
CN IX—glossopharyngeal—state tests for taste to posterior one-third of tongue
Combination CN IX sensory and CN X motor—gag reflex
CN X—vagus
Assess symmetry in rise of uvula with patient saying "Ahh"
Assess for dysphonia—innervate the larynx
Identify deviation of uvula as away from side of neurologic lesion
CN XI—spinal accessory: motor
Sternocleidomastoid—patient rotates head from 90 degrees to midline against resistance
Trapezius—patient shrugs shoulders against resistance
CN XII—hypoglossal
Have patient protrude tongue
Observe tongue for fasciculations
Identify deviation of tongue
MOTOR
Inspection for involuntary movements, tone, and muscle atrophy
Strength testing
Explain each component of the scale, 0 to 5, as below
0 = no muscle twitch with attempted movement of muscle group
1 = twitch only of muscle with attempted movement

TABLE 14-4 Neurologic Flow *(Continued)*

2 = movement against horizontal plane only, not against gravity
3 = movement against gravity but not against resistance
4 = movement against gravity and some resistance
5 = movement against full resistance
Bilateral comparison—must state nerve root for each muscle
Shoulder abduction—axillary nerve C5–6
Elbow flexion—musculocutaneous nerve C5–6
Elbow extension—radial nerve C6, C7, C8
Wrist flexion—median nerve C6, C7, C8
Wrist extension—radial nerve C6, C7, C8
Finger adduction—ulnar nerve C8, T1
Finger abduction—ulnar nerve C8–T1
Thumb abduction perpendicular to the plane of hand—median nerve C8–T1
Hip adduction—obturator nerve L2, L3, L4
Hip abduction—superior gluteal nerve L4, L5, S1
Knee extension—femoral nerve L2, L3, L4
Knee flexion—sciatic nerve L5, S1, S2
Dorsiflexion—deep peroneal L4–L5
Plantarflexion—tibial L5, S1, S2
REFLEXES
Define each component of the scale, 0 to 4, as below
0 = no response
1 = diminished but present reflex
2 = normal reflex
3 = somewhat increased reflex
4 = greatly increased reflex
Facilitator prompts student to define motor neuron disease
Hyporeflexia suggests lower motor neuron disease
Hyperreflexia suggests upper motor neuron disease
Bilateral comparison, student must state innervation
Biceps—C5–6
Brachioradialis—C5–6
Triceps—C6–7
Patellar—L2–4
Achilles—S1–2
Clonus—rapid dorsiflexion of the foot
Babinski sign—stroke lateral plantar surface of foot and cross medially at the ball
Normal—state as first digit plantarflexes
Abnormal—state as first digit dorsiflexes—indicates upper motor neuron disease
Hoffman reflex—grasp hand and extend wrist and middle finger, flicking nail downward
SENSORY
Symmetrical: C4 (shoulder), C6 (thumb), C7 (middle finger), C8 (fifth finger), T1 (forearm), T4 (nipple line), T10 (umbilicus), L2 (anterior thigh), L4 (medial calf), L5 (lateral calf), and S1 (lateral foot)
Techniques
Light touch—cotton wisp—combination posterior column and spinothalamic tract
Sharp—spinothalamic
Temperature—state only, tests spinothalamic tract
Vibration—using 128-Hz tuning fork—posterior column, distal to proximal
Proprioception—posterior column
Cortical
Stereognosis—ability to identify a familiar object in the hand
Graphesthesia—ability to identify a tracing on the palm
Extinction—ability to identify which side of the body is touched
CEREBELLAR FUNCTION
Seated exam
Rapid alternating movements
Finger-to-nose testing—patient abducts arms to 90 degrees, touches nose with finger
Pronator drift—arms forward, palms up, eyes closed (patient seated)
Heel to shin—ask patient to touch the heel to the top of the shin and run down along shin
Gait
Tandem walk
On the toes
On the heels
Heel to toe
Romberg—feet together

CHAPTER 15

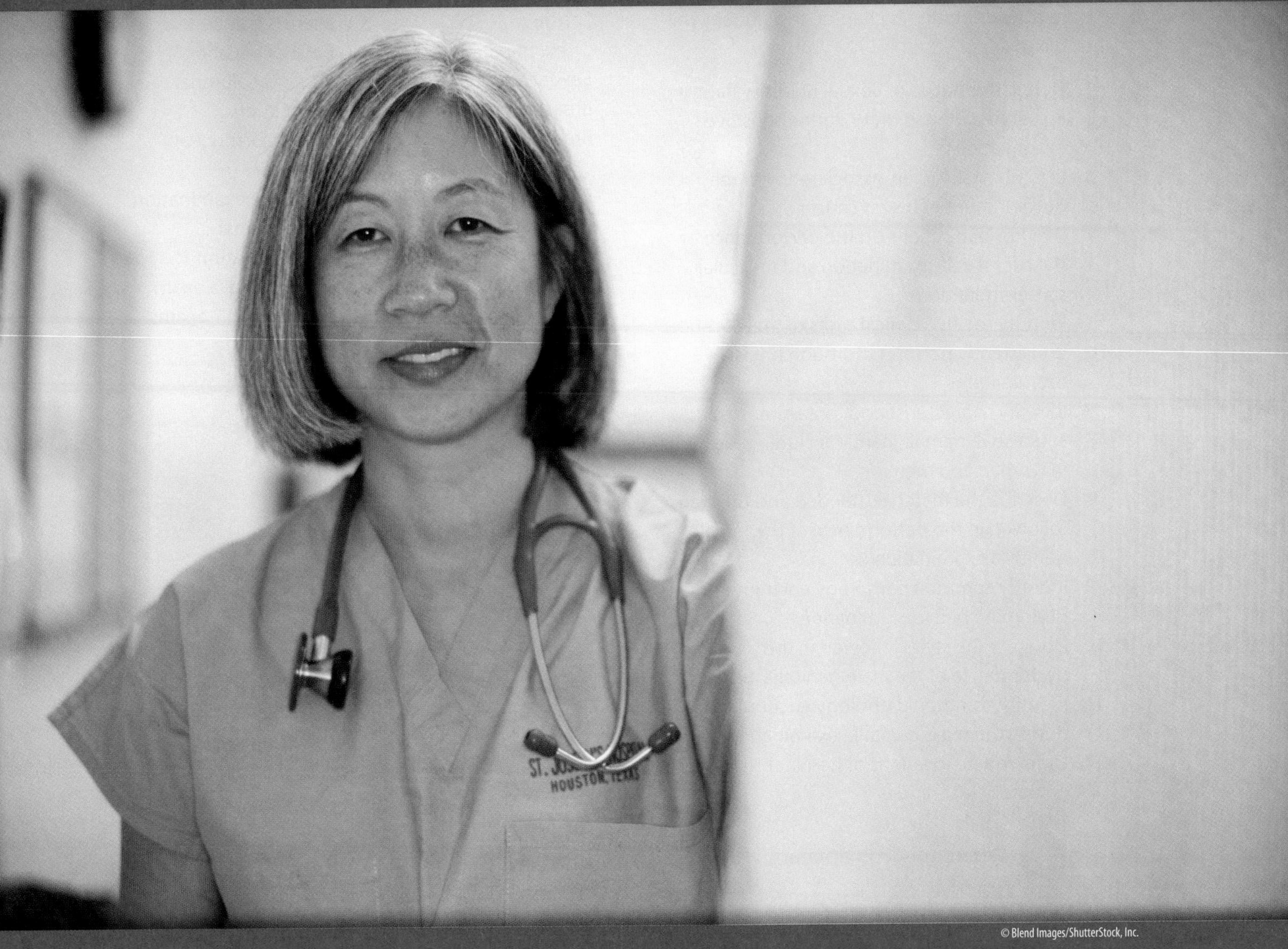

© Blend Images/ShutterStock, Inc.

Sensitive Examinations

Lynn McGrath, MSN, CRNP
Mark Kauffman, DO, MS (Med Ed), PA
Janet Newcamp, RNC, MN, CNS, CCE

OBJECTIVES

At the conclusion of this chapter, the student will be able to

1. Define the stages of Sexual Maturity Rating
2. Preserve patient dignity during sensitive examinations
3. Describe risk factors associated with the development of breast cancer
4. Provide instructions on the performance of the breast self-examination and testicular self-examination
5. Identify the five clinical signs of breast cancer
6. Consistently perform thorough breast examinations
7. Identify characteristics of breast masses suggestive of malignancy, including location in women and men
8. Describe the materials needed and the steps followed in the performance of the female genitalia examination
9. Identify common pathology encountered during the pelvic examination
10. Describe the steps followed in the performance of the male genitalia exam
11. Identify common pathology encountered during the male genitalia examination
12. Differentiate locations of hernia through palpatory techniques

KEY TERMS

Sensitive examinations
Sexual Maturity Rating
Breast cancer
Breast self-examination
Five signs of breast cancer
Lawnmower technique
Pelvic exam
Urethrocele
Cystocele
Skene's glands
Bartholin glands
Squamocolumnar junction
Papanicolaou (Pap) smear
Bimanual examination
Rectovaginal examination
Male genitalia exam
Testicular self-exams
Hernia
Rectal exam

Where this icon appears, visit **go.jblearning.com/HPECWS** to view the video.

Introduction

Sensitive examinations include female and male genitalia, breast, and rectal examinations. During the patient encounter, these examinations are typically performed after all other examinations required for the current visit have been completed. This allows the sensitive examination to be completed last, after which the patient can gown or dress, and discussion can occur while preserving dignity and demonstrating respect for the patient.

Sensitive examinations: female and male genitalia, breast, and rectal examinations

It is of the utmost importance to explain each part of the examination and obtain permission for it before performing the exam. This includes asking the patient to remove a gown or article of clothing to allow for proper inspection. It is not uncommon to see a student lift a patient's shirt, exposing the breasts, while attempting to auscultate heart sounds. Permission should be asked from both women and men for any examination where previously covered areas are now exposed: legs, arms, chest, back, and abdomen.

Though sometimes inconvenient, providers who are about to perform sensitive examinations in patients of the opposite sex should always have an assistant in the room who is the same sex as the patient. Though this is common practice in many offices, there are times when the provider may be tempted to forgo this advice in the name of expediency. Though we don't intend this to be cynical, should a provider perform an exam without an assistant in the room as a witness, the patient is at liberty to claim any occurrence of events that he/she sees fit. The provider has only his/her own testimony in rebuttal.

Sexual Maturity Rating

The **Sexual Maturity Rating** was devised by James Tanner to allow the staging of sexual development from puberty to adulthood in both females and males. Females are assessed by breast development while males are assessed through development of the testes, scrotum, and penis. Both females and males share maturation assessment through the development and distribution of pubic hair.

BREAST DEVELOPMENT

Breast development in the female is based on the size and shape of the breast and ranges from prepuberal stage 1 to mature adult stage 5 (see **FIGURE 15-1**). It is typically the first sign of sexual maturation.[1]

- Stage 1—Only the nipple is raised.
- Stage 2—Only the areola is raised (breast bud).
- Stage 3—Breast is raised beyond the areola but with a single, smooth contour.
- Stage 4—Breast forms a double mound, and the areola is raised above the surrounding breast tissue.
- Stage 5—Areola rejoins the surrounding breast tissue with single, smooth contour.

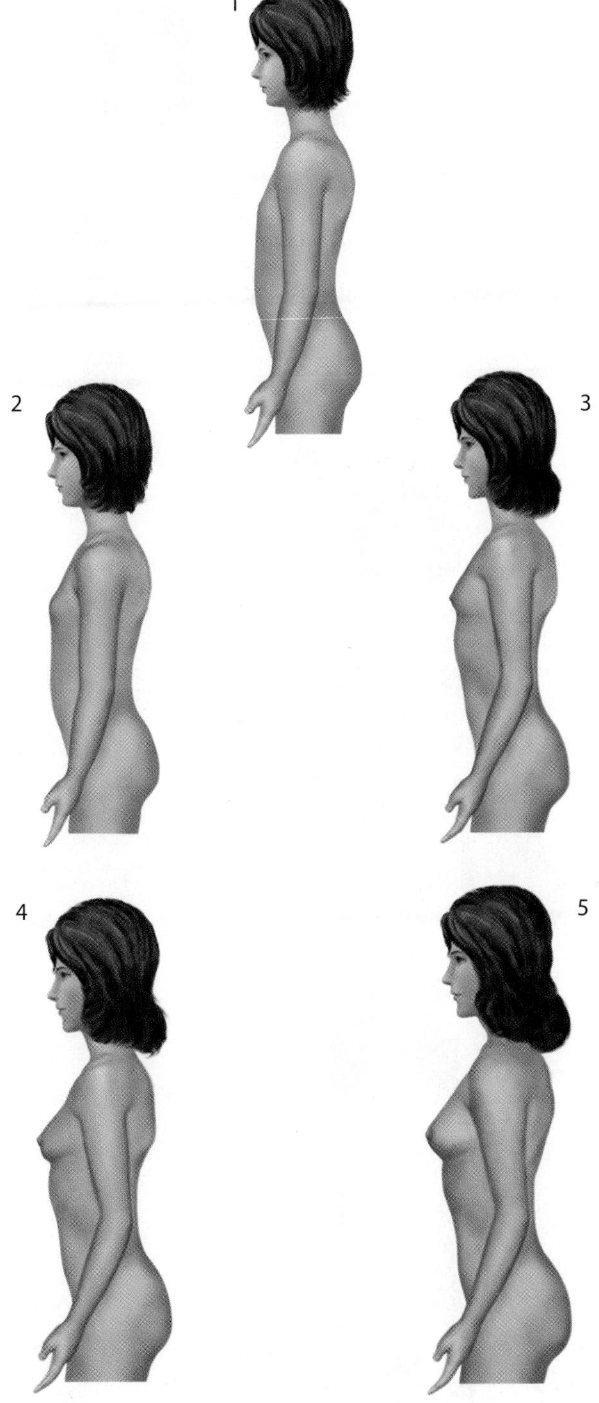

FIGURE 15-1 Tanner staging of breast development.

PUBIC HAIR DEVELOPMENT

Stages of pubic hair development are shared by both sexes (see **FIGURE 15-2**):

- Stage 1—No pubic hair.
- Stage 2—Scant, fine, midline hair growth.
- Stage 3—Hair becomes darker and coarse.
- Stage 4—Adult hair without spread to inner thighs.
- Stage 5—Spread of hair up the abdomen and to the inner thighs.

Sexual Maturity Rating: rating scale devised by James Tanner to define staging of sexual development from puberty to adulthood in both females and males

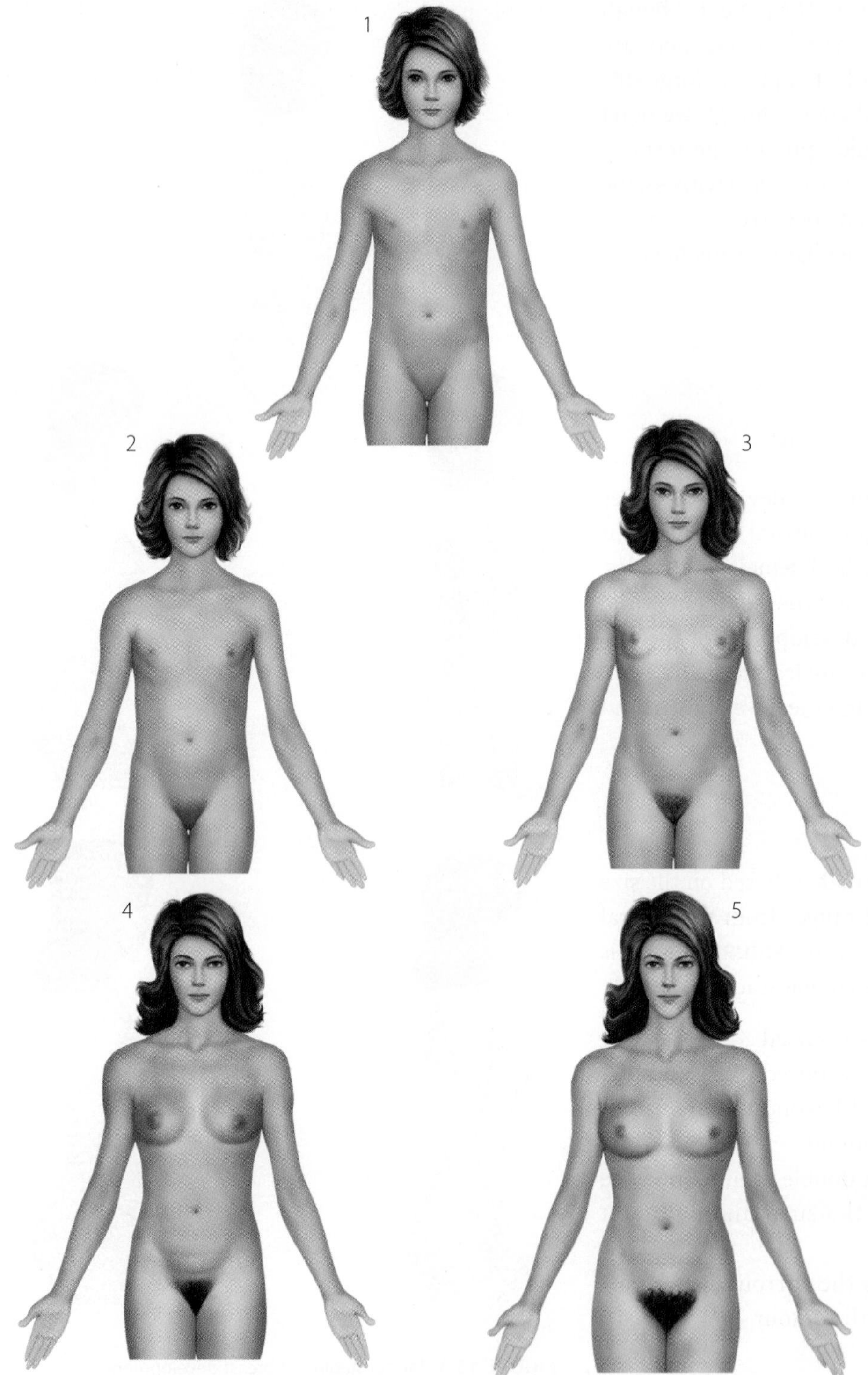

FIGURE 15-2 Tanner staging of pubic hair development.

MALE GENITALIA DEVELOPMENT

Stages of sexual maturation in males are based on the appearance of the scrotum and the size of the testes and penis (see **FIGURE 15-3**). Testicular growth is typically the first sign of sexual maturation.[1]

- Stage 1—Testes are small.

- Stage 2—Testes begin to enlarge, with scrotum becoming pendulous.
- Stage 3—Penis begins to lengthen, testes continue to enlarge, scrotum thickens.
- Stage 4—Penis begins to widen, testes continue to enlarge.
- Stage 5—Penis and testes attain mature adult size.

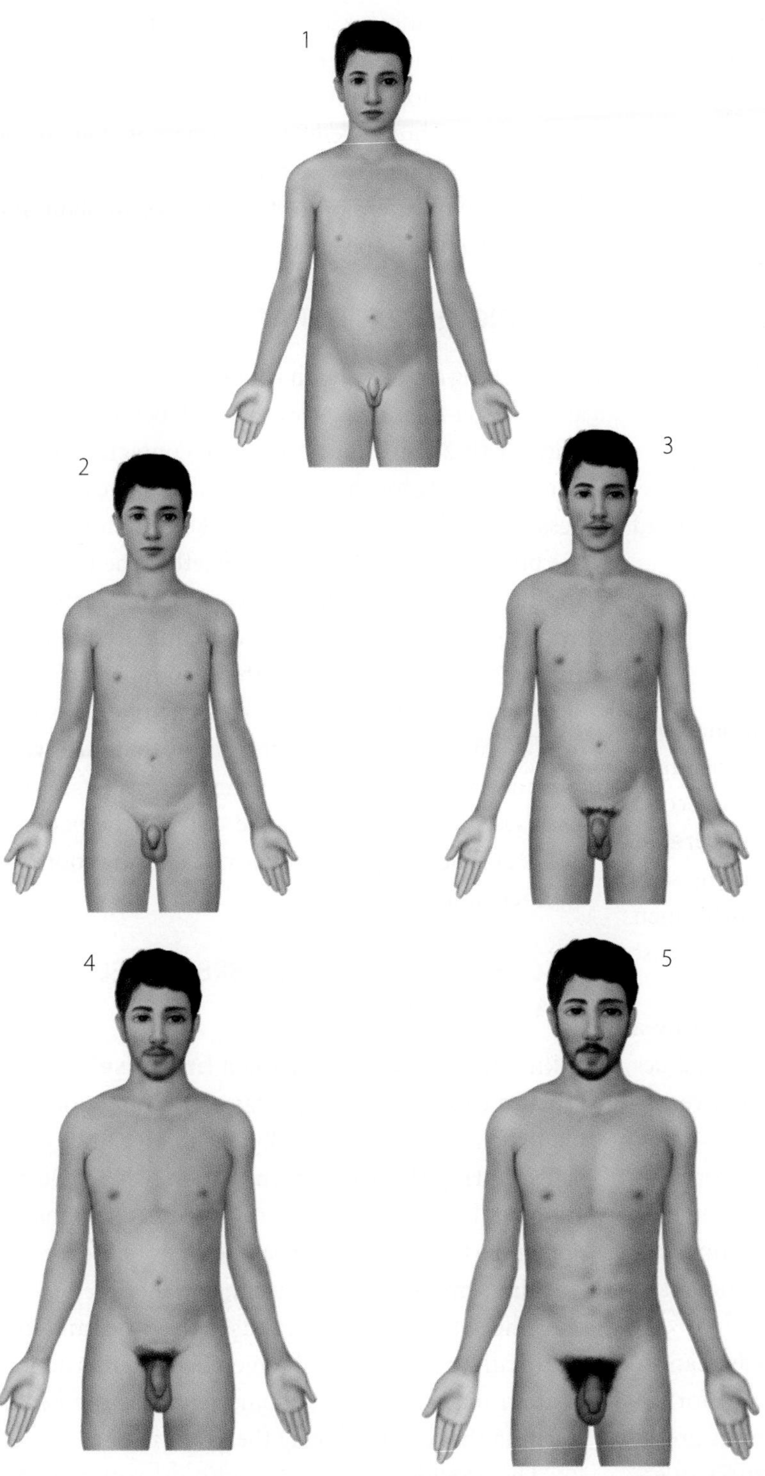

FIGURE 15-3 Tanner staging of male genitalia development.

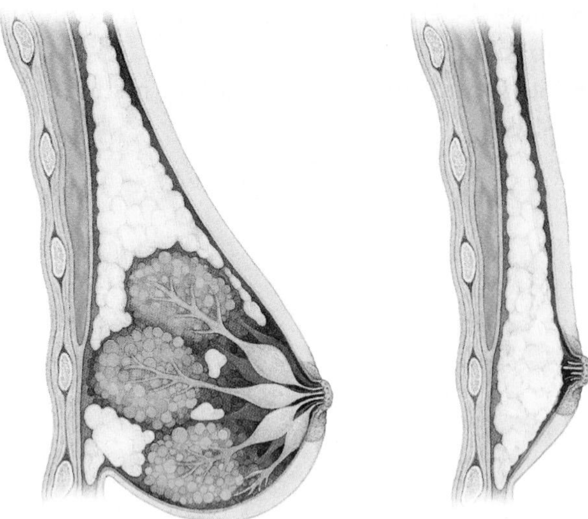

FIGURE 15-4 Female (left) and male breast anatomy.

Breast Anatomy

Review the female and male breast anatomy pictured in **FIGURE 15-4**.

Breast Examination

INTRODUCTION

The Centers for Disease Control and Prevention (CDC, 2012) reports cancer as the leading cause of death in women 35–65 years of age in the United States, second only to heart disease in women over 65,[2] with **breast cancer** being the most common type excluding skin cancer. Yet breast cancer is not a disease of women only. Approximately 2,200 men will develop breast cancer annually.[3]

A thorough breast examination performed by a skilled provider helps to ensure quality of life and decreased mortality by discovering masses earlier rather than later, helping to reduce the need for invasive treatment and overall heathcare costs.[4,5] Sensitive examinations require the examiner to have both skill and confidence.

Breast cancer: the second most common type of cancer in women, second only to skin cancer, which may also occur in men

Breast self-examination: process of inspecting and palpating the breast on a routine basis performed by the patient to identify signs of breast cancer

Risk factors for breast cancer include increasing age, a history of a first-degree relative with breast cancer, increased exposures to estrogen through early menarche, late menopause, nulliparity, or having a first child later in life. Advancing age is the greatest risk factor.

Develop an office routine to have staff that prescreens patients identify those who are to have a breast examination and ask if they are breastfeeding. If so, the patient should breastfeed or pump prior to the breast examination as it will empty the milk ducts and afford a more accurate examination.

Examination of breasts that have undergone augmentation or breast reduction surgery is done using the same technique as any breast examination, paying particular attention to the edges of implant and around the incisional area.

PUTTING THE PATIENT AT EASE

Establishing a rapport with your patient begins as soon as you enter the room. Always knock before entering. Enter with a smile and direct eye contact. The first nonthreatening touch is the handshake. Note the firmness or weakness of the handshake, which will give the provider some insight into whether the patient is confident, relaxed, apprehensive, or even fearful. Introduce yourself by giving your name, designation, and the role you will have in the encounter.

Commend the patient for coming in for this very important visit. You want her to know that she is your focus and you have genuine interest in her welfare. The assistant's focus should also be only on the patient's needs and not preparing other items in the room for another time.

DISCUSS IMPORTANCE OF BREAST SELF-EXAMINATION

Taking time to teach the patient **breast self-examination (BSE)** is also important. Teaching does not require a lot of extra time. BSE teaching can be completed during the actual examination, where you are afforded the opportunity to provide direct demonstration of the technique to the patient. This reinforces the teaching through tactile, visual, and auditory methods. The patient may be nervous in the office and find it difficult to attend to and remember the instruction. Written materials to take home reinforce the health teaching that occurs during the examination.

The provider should work with the patient to determine the best screening strategy based on individual risk and value. Guidelines from the American College of Obstetrics and Gynecology (ACOG) continue support of annual clinical breast examinations for all women beginning at age 40 and every one to three years for women ages 20 to 39.[6]

Finally ACOG encourages "breast self-awareness," including BSE, for all women beginning at age 20 years.[6] Women are encouraged to report any changes in their breast to their healthcare provider.

Although some agencies are advocating for women to have "breast self-awareness" and not do regular monthly BSE, we still recommend teaching patients to do monthly BSE after their menstrual periods, because of the percentage of breast masses initially found by the woman herself.

Advise the patient that the best time of the month to do a breast examination, whether by the medical provider or the patient, is one to two weeks *after* the menses. At this time, hormone levels have declined and the tissue is not as full and tender. Postmenopausal women should perform the BSE on the same date each month.

FIVE CLINICAL SIGNS

Another opportunity to provide distraction for patients during the breast examination is to ask them to name **five signs of breast cancer** that they should be examining themselves for. Allow patients time to identify as many as they can, elaborating on each offered response as appropriate. Discuss any remaining clinical signs that the patient did not identify. The signs are (1) change in nipple direction (see **FIGURE 15-5**): cancer tends to become fixed to the surrounding tissue. As a mass grows it may pull the tissue around the nipple, changing the direction of the nipple from midline or inverting it; (2) masses (see **FIGURE 15-6**): identify any lumps or obvious elevation of the breast tissue, noting any changes to the skin color or texture; (3) tenderness: note any areas of tenderness. Diffuse cyclic tenderness related to the menstrual cycle may not prompt a medical inquiry unless a change in pattern is detected: (4) dimpling of the skin (see **FIGURE 15-7**): dimpling can be subtle or pronounced. Skin that appears thickened and pitted, classically described as resembling the peel of an orange (peau d'orange), must have immediate attention; (5) discharge (see **FIGURE 15-8**): in the absence of lactation, discharge should prompt the patient to seek evaluation. Patients should be educated that there are many causes of breast discharge other than breast cancer; however, evaluation is essential. Cream-colored discharge in the pregnant or lactating woman is appropriate; otherwise color variation should also lead the patient to her provider for assessment.

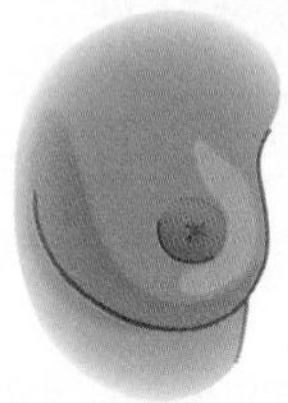

FIGURE 15-5 Change in nipple direction.

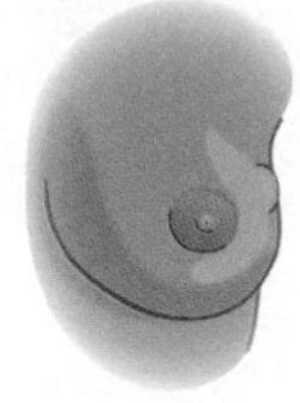

FIGURE 15-6 Mass.

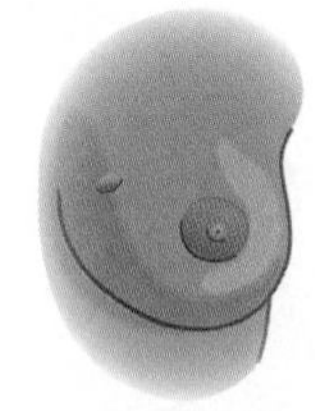

FIGURE 15-7 Dimpling of the skin.

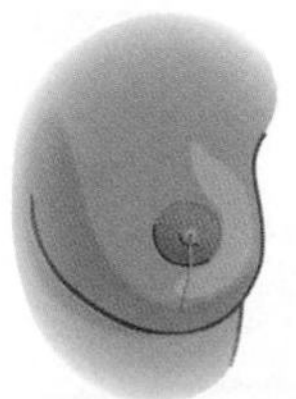

FIGURE 15-8 Discharge.

If any of the signs are found, the patient should seek evaluation from her provider.

EXPLAINING THE PROCEDURE

Advise the patient that the breast examination will involve examination in both the seated and supine positions and that you will need to inspect and compare her breasts to each other to aid in detection of masses. The breasts and the lymph nodes will then be palpated to assess for masses and discharge. Choose words that the individual will understand, avoiding medical terminology. Ask the patient if she has any questions before you begin and advise her to interrupt you at any time should she feel discomfort or have a question.

Five signs of breast cancer: signs of breast cancer that patients are advised to look for during the breast self-examination, which include change in nipple direction, masses, tenderness, dimpling of the skin, and discharge

INSPECTION

Beginning with the patient in a seated position, tell her that in order

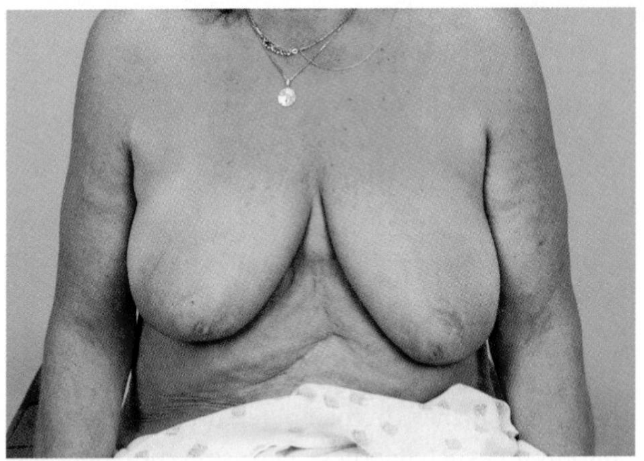

FIGURE 15-9 Inspection of the breasts begins in the seated position with the patient's arms relaxed at her sides.

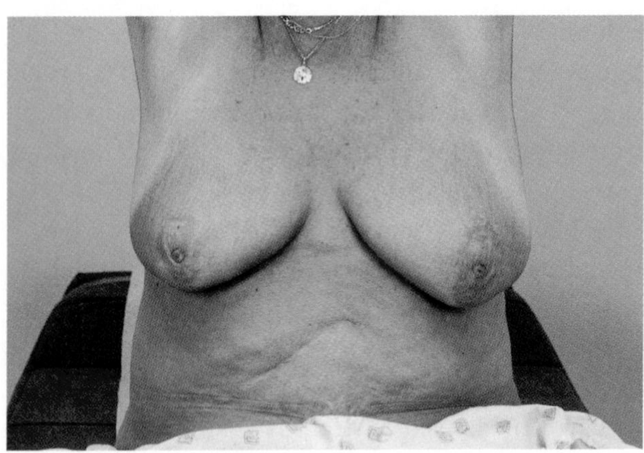

FIGURE 15-10 The second position for breast inspection is with the patient's hands over her head.

to detect masses you will be asking her to perform three maneuvers that help to stretch the breast tissues and reveal signs of underlying lesions. Ask her to lower the gown and relax her arms at her sides (see **FIGURE 15-9**). If the patient has poor posture with increased thoracic kyphosis, ask her to "please make yourself taller" instead of "sit up straight" or "stick out your chest."

Inspect the breasts bilaterally, noting symmetry. It is not uncommon for one breast to be noticeably larger than the other. If asymmetry is noted, ask the patient if she has ever thought that one breast is larger than the other and, if so, when she first noticed it. Ask about any recent changes in size or shape. Note the stage of sexual maturity and relate it to the reported age of the patient.

Inspect each quadrant in detail, avoiding a general scan over the entire breast. Identify nipple deviation, dimpling, masses, or obvious discharge. Note any skin changes, including erythema, rashes, or changes in pigmentation or texture, such as thickening or edema. Conditions such as Paget's disease of the breast and inflammatory carcinoma may manifest initially only as redness. If a lesion is encountered, evaluate for size, shape, color, consistency, and mobility.

Note the tissue around the areola where the Montgomery glands, or areolar glands, will appear as small bumps on the surface around the nipple. A cyst may appear in this area if a duct from the gland becomes obstructed. This finding does not increase the risk of cancer.

Now ask the patient to extend her arms overhead or place her hands behind her head (see **FIGURE 15-10**). This allows the tissues to be viewed while stretched over the rib cage, giving an optimal view of the skin contours. Repeat the detailed inspection.

Finally, ask the patient to place her hands on her hips and lean forward from the waist, allowing the breasts to hang freely (see **FIGURE 15-11**). Regown the patient.

Instruct her that when performing the SBE at home she should also examine herself in the same multiple positions while standing in front of a mirror.

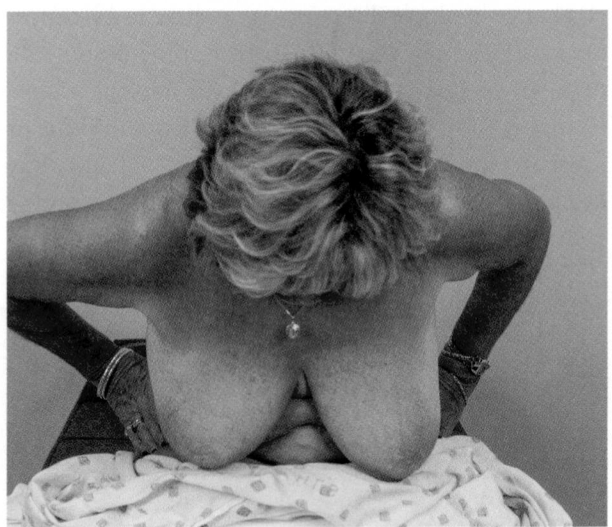

FIGURE 15-11 The third position for breast inspection is with the patient's hands on her hips, leaning forward.

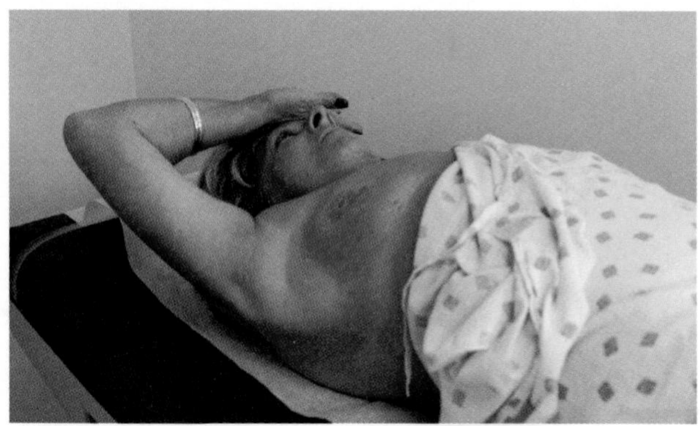

FIGURE 15-12 For palpation the patient is assisted to the supine position with her hip slightly rotated to the opposite side and her hand on her forehead.

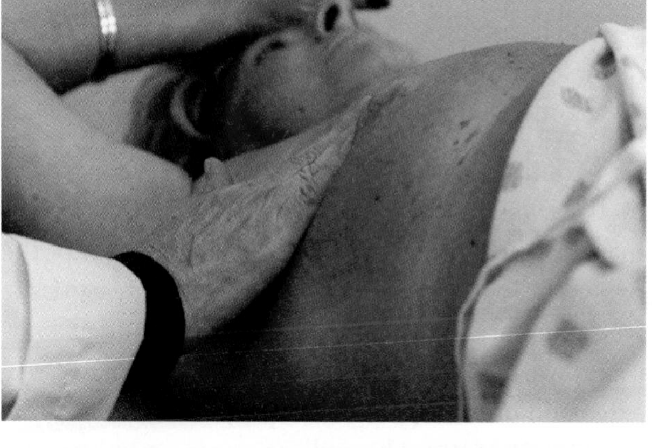

FIGURE 15-13 Palpation requires the provider to place the pads of his/her fingers flatly against the breast.

PALPATION

Assist the patient to the supine position. Ask the patient to slip her arms out of the gown, keeping it in place and covering the breasts. Ask her to raise the arm on the same side as the first breast to be examined, flexing it at the elbow and resting the hand palm up on the forehead (see **FIGURE 15-12**). The ipsilateral hip should also be slightly tilted away from the side being examined.

Some providers choose to place a rolled-up towel or pillow behind the shoulder of the side being examined, to stretch the breast tissue over the chest wall. This is no longer recommended.

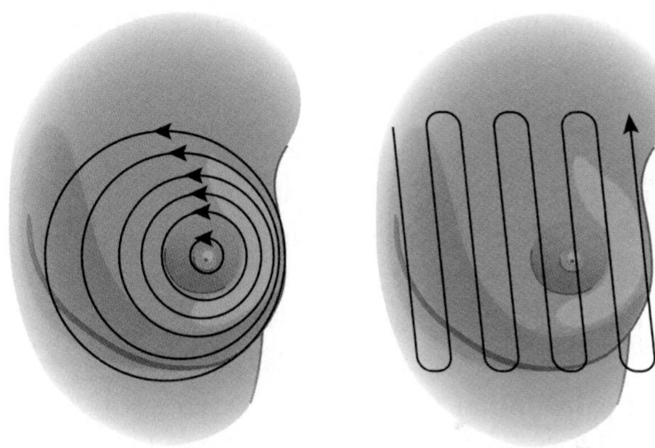

FIGURE 15-14 Circle and lawnmower palpatory techniques to assure no tissues are missed during the breast exam.

Technique

Advise the patient that you will now be touching the breast to look for masses or tenderness and ask for permission to expose one breast.

It is important to remain consistent with each examination. The pads of the three middle fingers of the dominant hand are used to palpate the breast tissue (see **FIGURE 15-13**). Using circular motions, mild pressure is applied first, then moderate, and then deep pressure, slightly overlapping each area examined until all tissues of the breast have been palpated, decreasing the possibility of missing any tissue.

Several methods of approach are used to assure all areas are examined. These include palpating in concentrically smaller circles from the outer margins of the breast (see **FIGURE 15-14**), and the checkerboard or **lawnmower technique**: moving horizontally along one line, dropping down, going back along the next line, and repeating until all tissues have been examined.

The National Cancer Institute provided funding for the University of Florida to perform a meta-analysis of 20 years of clinical research studies to determine which method of breast palpation offered a better examination. Their conclusion led to new guidelines for monthly BSE and annual clinical breast examinations after age 20 years.[4]

These guidelines include:

1. Always do the breast examination in the supine position, with arm flexed and palm up on forehead, and with hip tilted away from the examining side.

Lawnmower technique: also know as the checkerboard technique, method of palpating the breast during examination for breast cancer where slow, deliberate palpation occurs in a pattern of moving horizontally along one line, dropping down, going back along the next line, and repeating until all tissues have been examined

2. Use the lawnmower method to assure palpation of all tissues.
3. Use the pads of three fingers of the dominant hand, using three levels of pressure.

Examination of the breast with the lawnmower method was shown to be most effective for detecting masses, whether done by the medical examiner or the patient herself. Include the entire area of breast tissue from the sternum to the lateral chest wall and extending upward to the clavicle and the tail of Spence, the extension of breast tissue that projects into the axilla (see **FIGURE 15-15**). The axillary, supra-, and infraclavicular lymph nodes should also be palpated. About half of breast masses are found in the upper outer quadrant, highlighting the importance of including the tail of Spence.

Using three levels of pressure will help to express discharge from the nipple if present. Once the nipple is reached, it should also be gently pressed from either side in an effort to express discharge. The areola region is the second-most-frequent site of malignant lesions in the breast, accounting for 19% of breast masses.[3]

With the arm raised in this position, inspection and palpation of the axilla can be efficiently completed. Inspect the axilla and the lateral chest wall, looking for any changes in the contour or color of the skin, elevation of the tissue, or lymphadenopathy.

You may want to wear a glove for palpation of the axilla to avoid contact with perspiration. Palpate the axilla in sections: anterior axillary fold, posterior axillary fold, chest wall, and upper, inner arm. Methodically palpate the axillary, infraclavicular, and supraclavicular lymph nodes, as the amount of time spent on this examination directly corresponds to the effectiveness of finding an early mass.

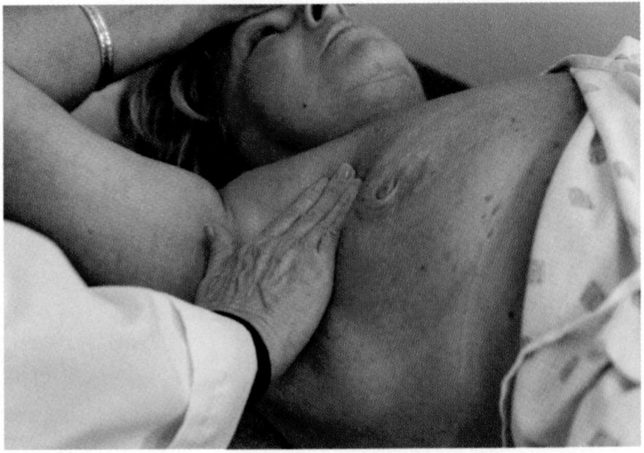

FIGURE 15-15 Palpation of the tail of Spence in the supine position.

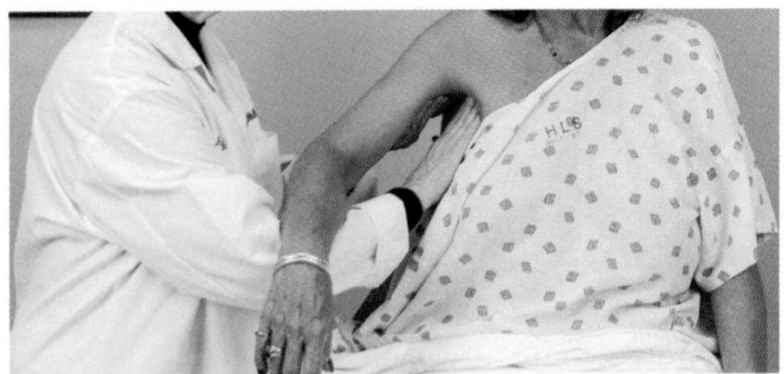

FIGURE 15-16 Palpation of the tail of Spence in the seated position.

Palpation of axillary nodes can also be accomplished with the patient in a seated position. If performed in this manner, ask the patient to relax the arm. The provider then slightly abducts the shoulder and palpates in sections as described (see **FIGURE 15-16**).

Findings

Assess the consistency of the tissue. Is it even, soft, firm, or cystic? Identify areas of tenderness. If tenderness is found, consider the timing of the menstrual cycle. If it is just prior to the patient's menstrual cycle, you may consider having her return a week after her menses for a repeat examination. However, if the patient admits to persistent tenderness throughout the month, immediate evaluation is appropriate.

Palpate for nodules or masses. Nodules that are soft and mobile are most likely of a benign or cystic nature but require evaluation until a definitive diagnosis is made. Firm or hard nodules that are fixed and nonpainful need expedient evaluation. Typically evaluation starts with mammography or ultrasonography. If the nodules are not seen on imaging but are still palpable, definitive diagnosis must be sought.

Cover the first breast and exam the other in similar fashion.

BREAST EXAMINATION IN THE MALE PATIENT

15-1 The majority of breast cancers in males are located behind the areola. The same approach for examination can be used in male patients as for females, with additional focus on the postareola area. See **TABLE 15-1** for the breast exam flow.

TABLE 15-1 Breast Flow

Introduces self by name and title, explaining role in the encounter
Asks for permission to begin the physical examination
Washes hands for 15 seconds before touching patient, turning off water with towel
GENERAL
Put the patient at ease
Explain the procedure to the patient before performing
Discuss importance of breast self-examination (BSE)
Educate the patient on five clinical signs of breast cancer
Change in nipple direction
Masses
Tenderness
Dimpling of the skin
Discharge
Discuss best time of month to perform (1 to 2 weeks after menses)
INSPECTION
Positions
Arms at sides
Arms overhead
Hands pressed on hips, leaning forward
Inspection
Symmetry
Tanner stage—explain stages
Skin appearance
Erythema
Lesions
Thickening/edema
Nipple deviation
Dimpling
PALPATION
Procedure
Patient supine
Tilt hip away from breast being examined
Ipsilateral arm bent at elbow with back of hand on forehead
Technique
Use finger pads
Circular motion
Systematic—e.g., circles, side to side
Include tail
Press on either side of the nipple and note discharge
Note
Consistency
Tenderness
Nodules
AXILLA
Inspection
Palpation of lymph nodes (best with patient seated)
Axillary
Infraclavicular
Supraclavicular

Female Genitalia Anatomy

Review the female genitalia anatomy pictured in **FIGURE 15-17.**

Pelvic Examination

APPROACH

Develop a routine that allows the patient to empty her bladder before the **pelvic exam**, as a full bladder will be uncomfortable for the patient during palpatory techniques. Have the patient change into a gown. If a breast examination will not be completed, allow the patient to keep her shirt on.

Assure that the room is properly set up and that all of your equipment is in place and within arm's reach of the seated provider so that the examination can be performed smoothly and without delay (see **FIGURE 15-18**).

Supplies that will be needed for the exam:

- Disposable gloves (nonlatex if allergy noted)
- Lubrication jelly
- Speculum
- Light source
- Pap spatula
- Pap endocervical brush
- Slides with fixative *or*
- Liquid media
- Labels completed with patient name, date of birth, date of FDLMP

Pelvis exam: examination of female genitalia including speculum and bimanual palpatory techniques

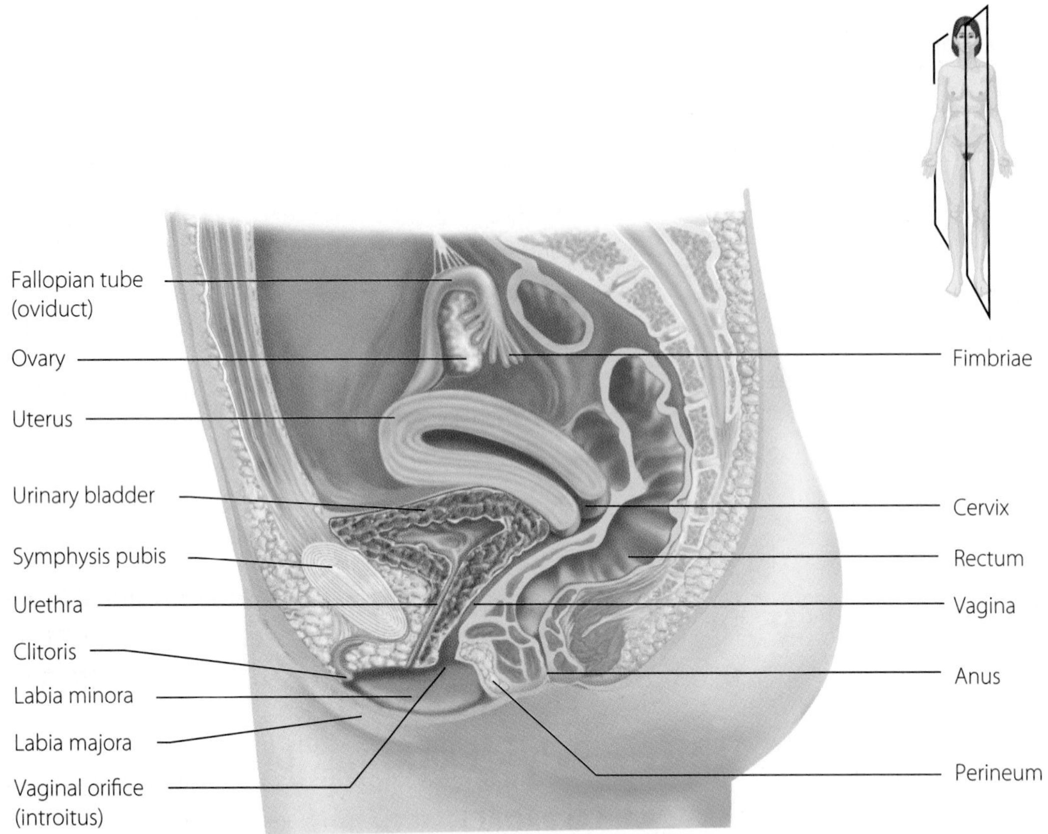

FIGURE 15-17 Cross-sectional view of female genitalia.

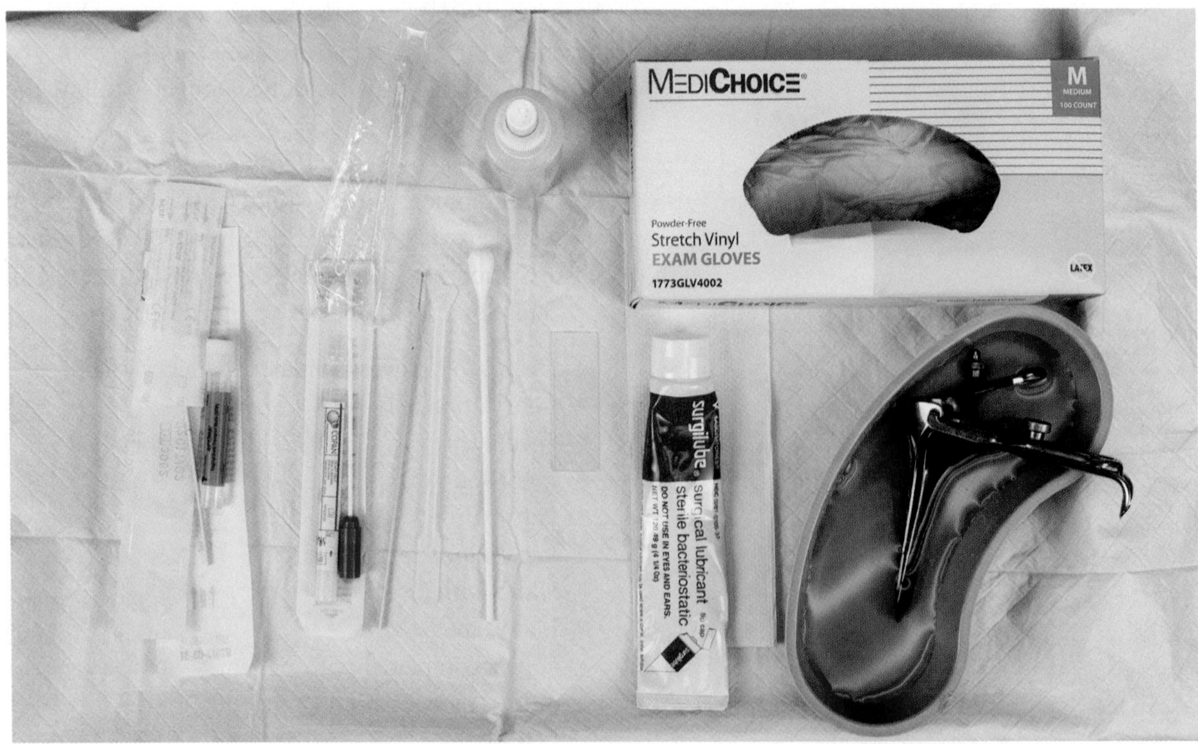

FIGURE 15-18 Supplies required for the pelvic exam.

Ask the patient if she has any questions before you begin and advise her to let you know if she has any concerns at any time. Explain each procedure and step as you are about to perform it so that the patient is fully aware and can anticipate what will occur, such as her being touched.

Conversation during the exam can add beneficial distraction. Medical history is typically sought; however, conversation unrelated to the examination, such as inquiries about the patient's family, can help to put the patient at ease.

PROCEDURE

Inform the patient that the pelvic examination is about to begin. Begin by positioning the patient properly. Proper positioning is important for both the ease of the examiner and the comfort of the patient. The head of the bed should be slightly elevated or a pillow should be available.

Cover the pelvis and lower extremities with a sheet and assist the patient into the supine position, putting her feet into the stirrups. Place a hand a couple centimeters off the bottom edge of the examination table and ask the patient to slide down until she touches your hand. The buttocks should align just over the edge of the table, which allows room for the handle of the speculum. Have the patient place her arms at her sides. The sheet should still be in place.

Position yourself on the examination stool at the end of the table. The patient will often have her knees together. Place a hand on top of the sheet above her knees and ask her to let her knees fall apart. As she does, press the sheet downward between the knees so that you gain a clear line of vision between yourself and the patient's face (see **FIGURE 15-19**). This will allow you to make periodic eye contact and watch her facial expressions during the examination for any signs of discomfort. Don gloves for the examination.

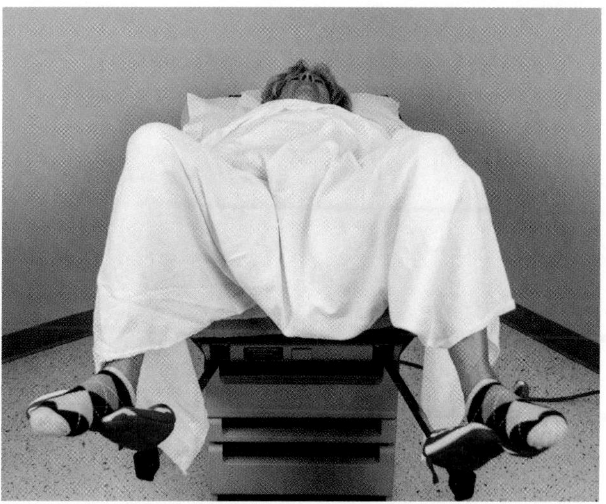

FIGURE 15-19 Sheet placement for pelvic exam.

EXTERNAL EXAM

Advise the patient that you are going to slide the sheet up. Do so, exposing the genital area but keeping the sheet on the legs (see **FIGURE 15-20**). Position the light to provide optimal inspection. Begin with observation of the mons pubis and the escutcheon (the hair pattern), noting thickness, texture, and distribution of hair. If the area is shaven, note any loss of the skin integrity. If noted, educate the patient about caring for small cuts with antibiotic cream and keeping the area clean and dry.

Continue inspection of the readily visible anatomy in an orderly manner from mons pubis downward. Inspect the vulva, labia majora, perineum, and anus without touching the patient. Identify any abnormalities, such as lesions, erythema, atrophy, or parasitic infections.

You will now need to touch the patient to continue the inspection. Place a glove on the hand you intend to use to perform the internal exam. Before touching the patient, advise her that you plan to do so—"I am going to touch you now. You will feel the back of my hand on your thigh"—and touch the patient. Touching in this less sensitive place introduces

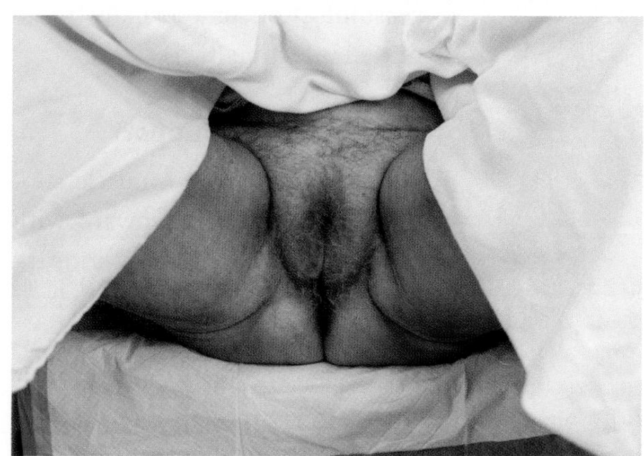

FIGURE 15-20 External genitalia inspection.

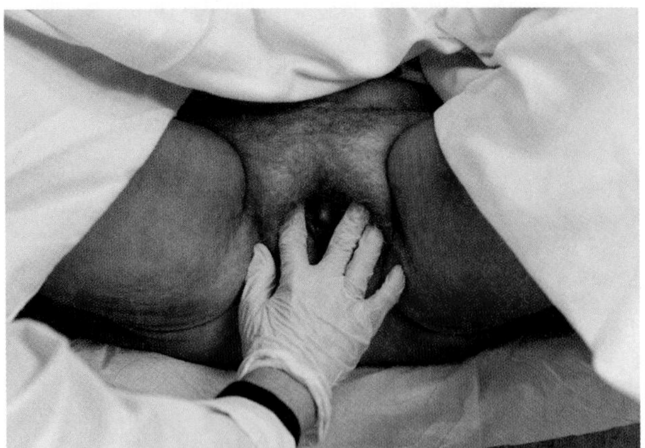

FIGURE 15-21 The labia majora are spread to inspect the underlying anatomy.

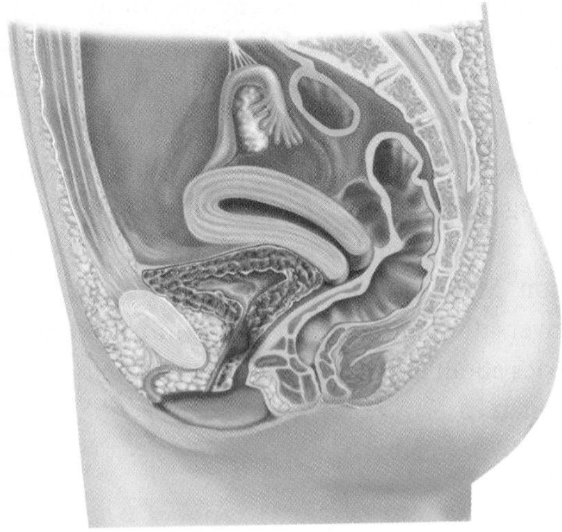

FIGURE 15-22 Cross section of urethrocele.

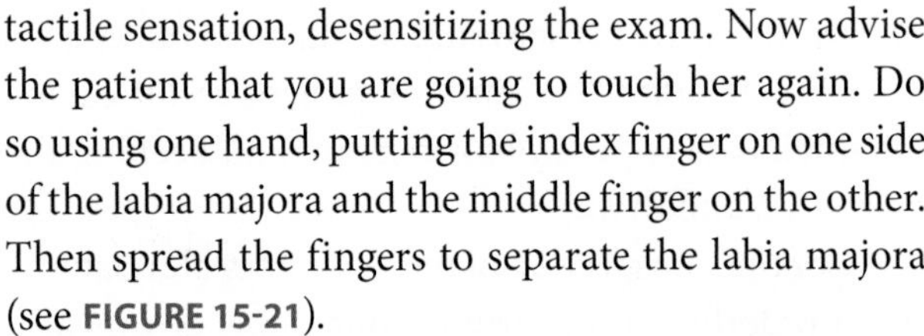

tactile sensation, desensitizing the exam. Now advise the patient that you are going to touch her again. Do so using one hand, putting the index finger on one side of the labia majora and the middle finger on the other. Then spread the fingers to separate the labia majora (see **FIGURE 15-21**).

Now inspect the clitoris by gently lifting the clitoral hood. Identify the urethral meatus, gently inspecting between all tissue folds, observing for erythema or discharge. Milk the urethra with one finger, noting tenderness or discharge, which would indicate urethritis.

Inspect the labia minora and the vaginal introitus, noting lesions or discharge. Thin, light, milky-white discharge may represent normal vaginal fluids. Heavier, darker, or malodorous discharge, or concurrent symptoms of irritation or itching, may signal bacterial vaginosis, yeast infection, or a sexually transmitted infection (STI).

Urethrocele: prolapse of the urethra into the vagina, seen as a bulge of the anterior vaginal wall

Cystocele: large weakening of the anterior wall that results in prolapse of the bladder into the vaginal space

Skene's glands: bilateral glands located lateral to the urethral meatus with ductal openings in the anterior vaginal introitus providing a source of lubrication for the vagina

Vaginal Muscle Support

To assess the vaginal muscle support, gently press downward with the two fingers in the posterior introitus and ask the patient to bear down. Examine for urethrocele, cystocele, and rectocele. A **urethrocele** is a prolapse of the urethra into the vagina and is seen as a bulge of the anterior vaginal wall (see **FIGURE 15-22**). A **cystocele** is a larger weakening of the anterior wall that results in prolapse of the bladder into the vaginal space (see **FIGURES 15-23A** and **15-23B**). Urethroceles and cystoceles often occur together; this is termed a cystourethrocele. A rectocele is the weakening of the floor of the vagina, allowing the rectal wall to prolapse into the posterior vaginal space (see **FIGURE 15-23B** and **FIGURE 15-24**).

Skene's and Bartholin Glands

The Skene's and Bartholin glands are the major source of lubrication for the vagina. The **Skene's glands** are located bilaterally lateral to the urethral meatus with ductal openings in the anterior vaginal introitus. The

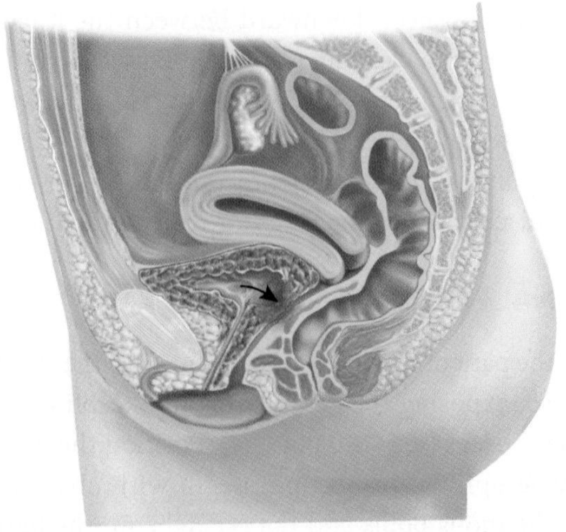

FIGURE 15-23A Cross section of cystocele.

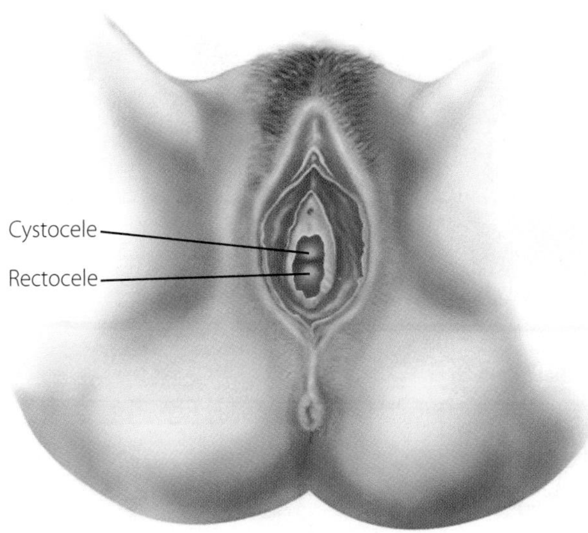

FIGURE 15-23B External inspection showing the anterior cystourethrocele and the posterior rectocele.

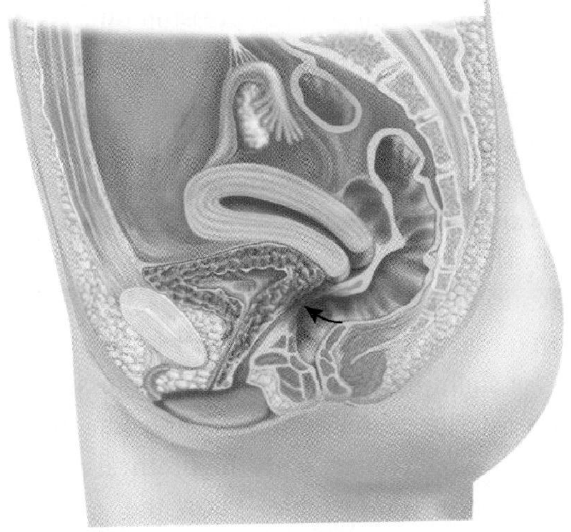

FIGURE 15-24 Cross section of rectocele.

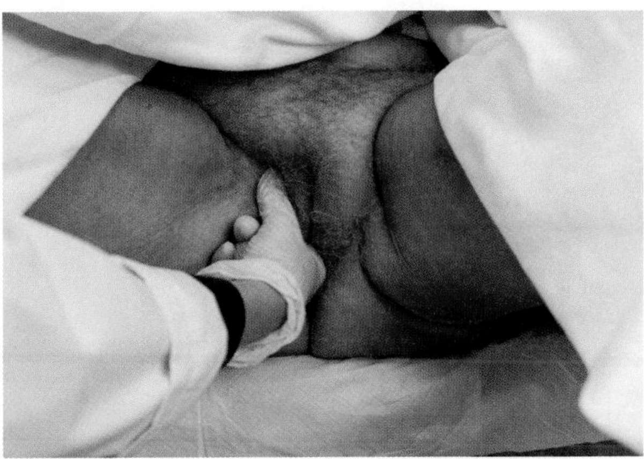

FIGURE 15-25 Anterolateral palpation of the Skene's glands.

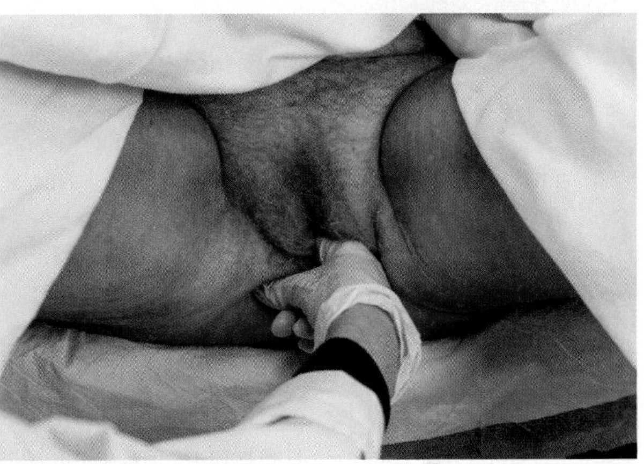

FIGURE 15-26 Posterolateral palpation of the Bartholin glands.

Bartholin glands and ducts are located at the posterior opening of the vaginal introitus.

Advise the patient that you will be touching the vaginal opening. Place two fingers along the posterior wall of the introitus. Inspect the glands for enlargement and the ductal openings for erythema or discharge. Then palpate each gland for enlargement or tenderness (see **FIGURES 15-25** and **15-26**).

15-2 As palpation has already been introduced, the provider can take the opportunity to note the position of the cervix. Advise the patient that you will be palpating her cervix and introduce one finger into the vagina. Noting the position of the cervix by palpation will help to locate it during the speculum exam. As providers gain experience and become adept at locating the cervix with the speculum alone, this step is often skipped.

SPECULUM EXAMINATION

Before beginning the internal examination, inspect the speculum to confirm understanding of its mechanics, as variability exists between instruments, and assure that it is in good working order.

Advise the patient that you will be starting the speculum exam. Place the speculum under warm water (see **FIGURE 15-27**). This serves two purposes: (1) the water warms the instrument, as a cold speculum is uncomfortable, and (2) the water acts as a lubricant on the moist vaginal membranes, allowing more comfortable insertion.

Bartholin glands: bilateral glands located at the posterior opening of the vaginal introitus providing a source of lubrication for the vagina

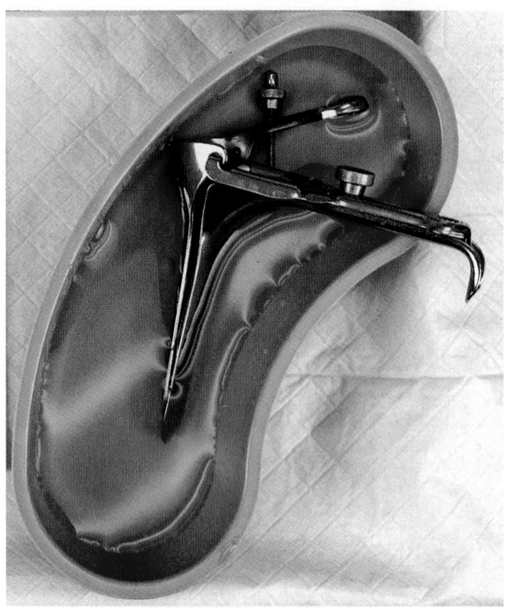

FIGURE 15-27 Speculum in warm water.

Lubricant has traditionally not been used prior to performing a Pap smear as it is thought to interfere with the reading of the cell sample. Several studies have shown that while the conservative use of water-based gel lubricant lessens discomfort during the exam, it does not increase the rate of unsatisfactory slides or inhibit the detection of abnormal cells.[7] If you choose to use water-based lubricant, apply only a small amount to the outside of the blades.

With the moist or lightly lubricated speculum in the closed position, keep it in a horizontal plane and turn the blades so that they are aligned in a nearly vertical position (see **FIGURE 15-28**). With the index finger

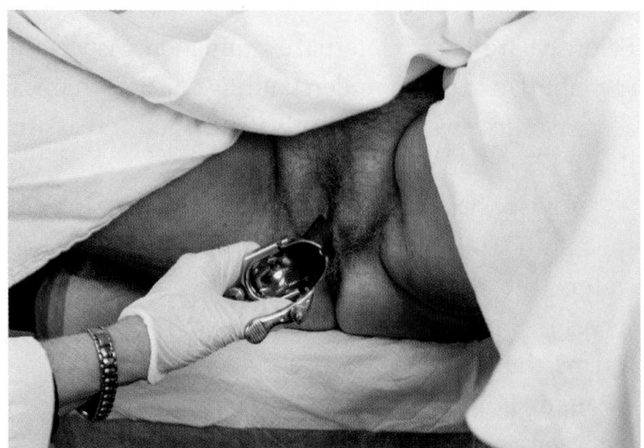

FIGURE 15-28 The speculum is held in the horizontal plane with the blades in the vertical position.

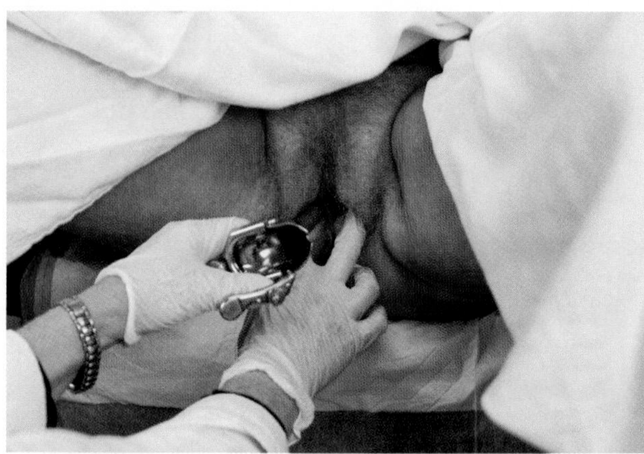

FIGURE 15-29 The labia are separated while providing posterior wall pressure.

and middle finger of the examining hand, gently open the labia and press the fingers downward on the posterior wall of the introitus (see **FIGURE 15-29**). Ask the patient to "relax the muscle I'm pressing on." As the patient does so, insert the speculum with a smooth motion, rotating the handle toward the floor while advancing to avoid catching any vaginal tissue between the blades. Insertion begins with the blades in the vertical position (see **FIGURE 15-30A**) rotating to about 45 degrees by the time half of the length of the blades has been advanced (see **FIGURE 15-30B**) and reaching the fully horizontal position at full insertion (see **FIGURE 15-31**). Use slight horizontal downward pressure toward the posterior vaginal wall while introducing the speculum to avoid contact with the urethral meatus, which may be uncomfortable. Allow the speculum to gently follow the contour of the vagina. Open the blades and visualize the cervix, then secure the blades

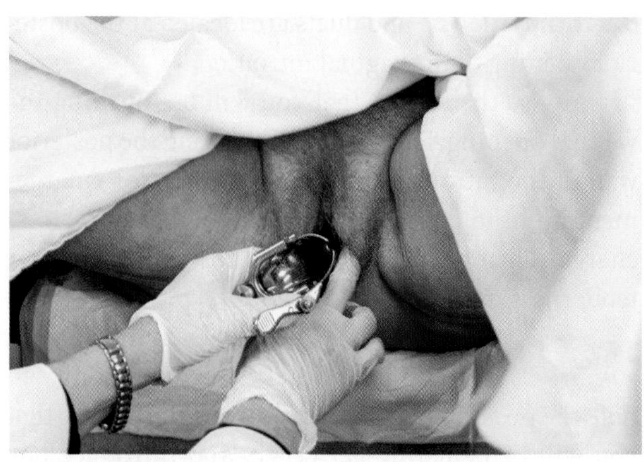

FIGURE 15-30A Early speculum insertion with vertical blades.

© Alex Luengo/ShutterStock, Inc.

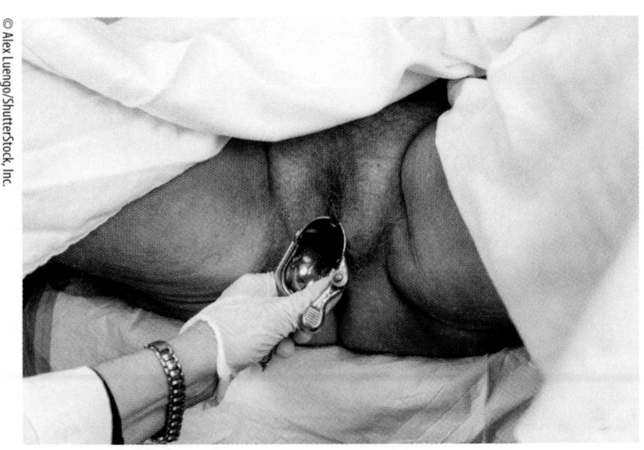

FIGURE 15-30B The blades are rotated to approximately 45 degrees when half the depth of insertion has been reached.

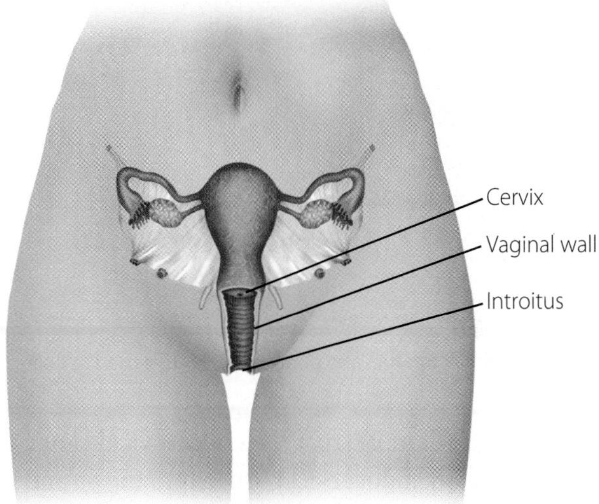

FIGURE 15-32 Anatomy demonstrating the typical location of the cervix.

in an open position. Occasionally a hooded effect from vaginal mucosa will drape over the anterior surface of the cervix. Carefully angle the speculum upward, stretching the anterior vaginal wall and allowing the cervix to come into view (see **FIGURE 15-32**).

15-3 Inspect the cervix, identifying the **squamocolumnar junction** and noting color and lesions (see **FIGURE 15-33**). Inspect the os for size and shape. A small round os may indicate nulliparity. A linear os is common following pregnancy. Inspect for erythema, lesions, or discharge. If discharge is present, a culture should be sent.

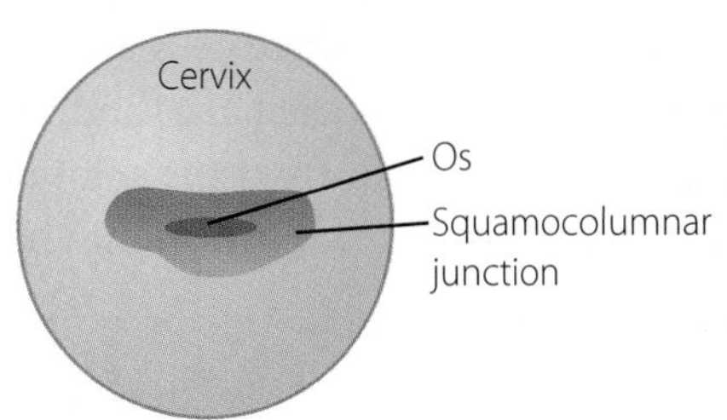

FIGURE 15-33 Cervix with squamocolumnar junction.

Papanicolaou Smear

The squamocolumnar junction (SCJ) is the area from which a sample of cells for the **Papanicolaou (Pap) smear** is obtained. The cells in this area are in "transition," and thus it is also called the transformation zone. Here, cells grow more rapidly, and like other areas where cell turnover has greater frequency, cancer cells are more likely to develop. This is most commonly associated with human papilloma virus (HPV). A second sample of endocervical cells from within the cervical os is also obtained. This technique was developed by Dr. Georgios Papanikolaou. To perform the Pap smear:

1. Assure that slides to be used for sample submission have been labeled with the patient's name, the date, and the date of the FDLNMP.
2. Obtain a sample of cells from the SCJ by scraping it with a spatula (see **FIGURE 15-34**).
3. Apply the sample to the slide and spray with fixative solution.

Squamocolumnar junction: zone of cell transition from squamous to columnar morphology where tissue samples are collected for identification of cervical cancer

Papanicolaou (Pap) smear: sample of cervical cells collected form the squamocolumnar junction and endocervix for identification of cervical cancer

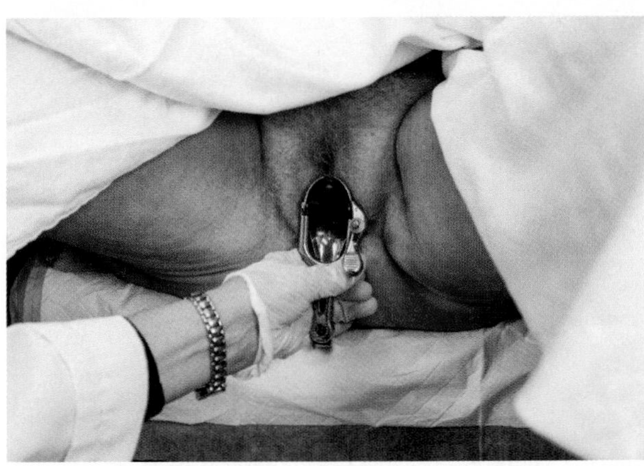

FIGURE 15-31 The blades rest horizontally when fully inserted.

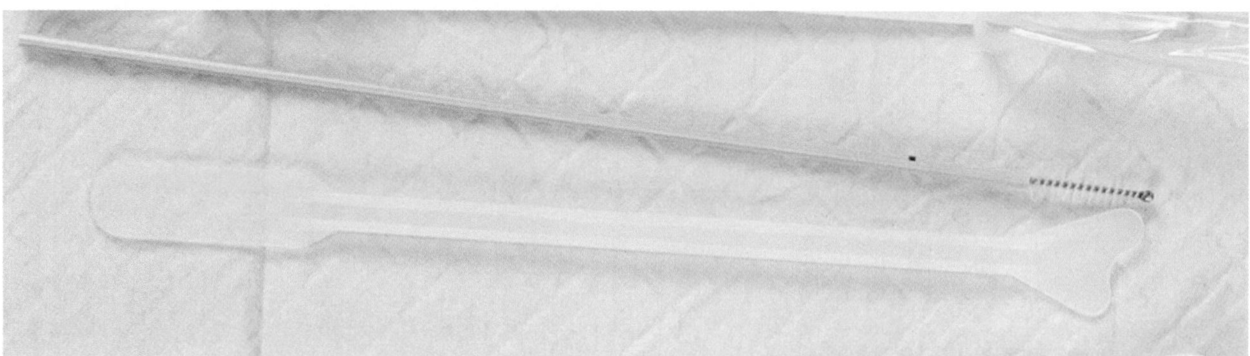

FIGURE 15-34 Spatula and endocervical brush used to collect cell samples.

4. Obtain a sample from the endocervical canal, inserting an endocervical brush into the os and rotating it.
5. Apply the sample to the slide and fixative solution.

15-4 A modified Pap test, called ThinPrep, uses liquid-based cytology, where cells are collected using a brush that is then washed in a fluid. An automated device then filters cells from the solution and plates them in a thin layer while removing contaminants.

Vaginal Walls

From the 1940s through the 1960s, pregnant women who were in danger of miscarriage were given diethylstilbestrol. This potent estrogen compound caused the daughters of these women to have a greater risk of developing tumors of the vagina and cervix.

Unlock the speculum but apply pressure on the handle to keep the blades open. As you begin to withdraw the speculum, examine the vaginal walls. As the speculum is withdrawn, narrowing of the introitus will cause the speculum to begin to close on its own; allow it to do so slowly. Two things very uncomfortable for the patient are clamping the blades of the speculum on the cervix and bringing the speculum out of the vagina in a forced, open position. Avoid both.

BIMANUAL EXAMINATION

The **bimanual examination** is so named because both hands are used, one for the internal vaginal examination and one on the surface of the abdomen.

Bimanual examination: internal palpatory technique of the female genitalia exam

The examination is performed with the provider in the standing position. To perform the examination, liberally lubricate the index and middle fingers of one hand. Advise the patient that you will be performing the internal exam. Bend the elbow to 90 degrees, keeping the wrist straight, the hand vertical, and the middle and index fingers extended. Anchor the elbow into the hip so that the arm, hand, and wrist move as a single unit as the two fingers are inserted into the vagina.

Palpate the vaginal wall for masses, gland enlargement, or tenderness. Palpate fornices, sweeping around the cervical neck and posterior fornices for masses. Then palpate the cervix, inducing motion to assess for cervical motion tenderness.

Place the ungloved hand on the abdomen 3 to 4 cm below the umbilicus and press downward as the internal fingers lift upward, in effect capturing the uterus between the two hands (see **FIGURE 15-35**). This enables the provider to palpate the size, shape, position, and character of the uterus.

Move the internal fingers laterally to one side of the cervix to examine the adnexa, with the ovaries,

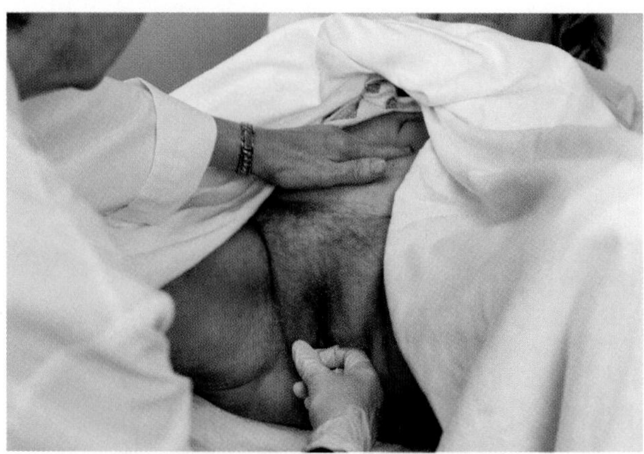

FIGURE 15-35 The bimanual examination with one hand placed on abdomen above the pubis and the other within the vagina.

fallopian tubes, and supporting ligaments. With the abdominal hand, find the anterior superior illiac spine and move your hand medially and down 3 to 4 cm. Press upward with the internal fingers and sweep down with the external hand, allowing the ovary to slip through your fingers. You do not want to attempt to palpate the ovary with direct pressure, as this would be painful. The same pressure should be applied to palpate the ovary as would be used to palpate a testicle. Palpate bilaterally for masses or tenderness.

15-5 Withdraw your vaginal fingers, keeping the glove low and away from the patient's view. Be aware of the likelihood of secretions, removing gloves in a direction away from yourself to avoid accidental contact with the fluids.

RECTOVAGINAL EXAMINATION

Replace your glove for the next exam. The **rectovaginal examination** is done routinely beginning at 50 years of age as part of the screening for colorectal cancer and to aid in palpation of the posterior cul-de-sac, uterus, adnexa, and supporting ligaments. If the patient has a first-degree relative with a history of colorectal cancer or advanced colonic polyps described as greater than 1 cm, villous, or with high-grade dysplasia, rectal examinations should begin at age 40 or at 10 years before the age of onset in the relative. Adequate explanation should be given to the patient as to the indications and need for the exam, as it is often cited as the most unwanted part of the examination.

15-6 Since you have just completed the vaginal examination, let the patient know that she will feel pressure in the vagina once again and you will be performing a rectal examination at the same time.

Rectovaginal examination: technique performed during the female genitalia exam where the provider simultaneous introduces one finger into the rectum and one into the vagina

15-7 Bring the pad of your middle finger to rest on the edge of the rectum. Ask the patient to bear down and wait for the sphincter to tighten. Then ask the patient to relax, and as the muscle relaxes advance both the vaginal finger and the rectal finger with an even motion (see **FIGURE 15-36**). Palpate the walls of the rectum, the septum between the vagina and rectum, and surrounding structures. The fundus of the uterus may be palpable if the uterus is in a retroverted position. Remove your fingers with an even motion and check the secretions from the rectal examination for occult blood.

See **TABLE 15-2** for the female genitalia exam flow.

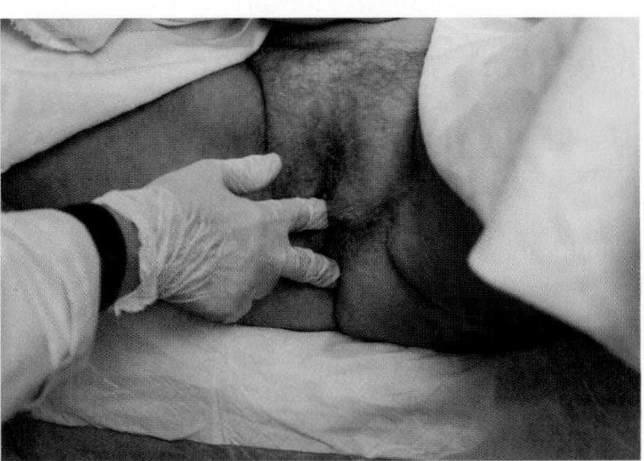

FIGURE 15-36 Rectovaginal exam with one finger placed in the vagina and one within the rectum.

TABLE 15-2 Female Genitalia Flow

Introduces self by name and title, explaining role in the encounter
Asks for permission to begin the physical examination
Washes hands for 15 seconds before touching patient, turning off water with towel
Ensures assistant is in the room if appropriate
Preparation
Ensure female attendant is in room
Position patient in lithotomy position with drape covering legs
Advise patient of each step of the exam so that she knows what to expect
Have all equipment within arm's reach
INSPECTION
Ask the patient to allow her knees to fall out to side.
Depress drape toward the abdomen so that you can see the patient's face
Position light source to illuminate the genitalia
External genitalia
Note sexual maturity rating
Stage 1—no pubic hair
Stage 2—scant fine hair growth
Stage 3—hair becomes darker and coarse
Stage 4—adult hair without spread to inner thighs
Stage 5—hair spread to inner thighs
Identify structures for lesions, rashes, atrophy, parasites

(continues)

TABLE 15-2 Female Genitalia Flow *(Continued)*

Mons pubis
Vulva
Labia majora
Perineum
Anus—identify
Advise patient you are going to touch her, and touch the thigh with back of hand
Advise that you are going to touch the labia and separate them
Indentify structures for lesions, discharge, erythema
Clitoris
Urethral meatus
Introitus
Labia minor
Advise patient you will be touching the vaginal opening
Place two fingers at the posterior introitus
Have the patient bear down
Examine for urethrocele, rectocele, glandular enlargement
PALPATION
Milk urethra for discharge
Palpate secretory glands for enlargement or tenderness
Bartholin
Skene's
Place one finger into the vagina and note position of the cervix
SPECULUM EXAMINATION
Advise patient that you are now going to place a speculum into the vagina
Prepare speculum by testing function and warming with warm water
OR consider applying small amount of lubricant to outside of blades
Place two fingers in the posterior introitus and press downward
Introduce speculum
Blades closed
Vertically oriented
45-degree downward angle
Rotate to horizontal while inserting
Inspection
Bring cervix into view and lock speculum in place
Note squamocolumnar junction, shape of os, color
Indentify lesions, discharge
Obtain cultures if discharge apparent
Perform Pap smear at SCJ
Obtain endocervical sample
Unlock blades
Remove speculum slowly while closing blades slowly
Inspect vaginal walls for lesions, discharge
BIMANUAL EXAMINATION
Stand at end of bed
Advise that you will be inserting two fingers into the vagina
Lubricate fingers
Insert fingers with thumb retracted to avoid contact with the urethra and clitoris
Palpate cervix and assess for cervical motion tenderness
Palpate fornices and vaginal walls
Assess height and position of the uterus with free hand depressing the abdomen
Palpate the adnexa for masses, tenderness
Perform rectovaginal exam
Change gloves
Advise patient rectal examination will now be performed
Ask the patient to bear down then relax
Insert one lubricated finger into rectum and one finger intervaginally
Palpate the posterior vaginal wall
Remove vaginal finger, palpate the rectal wall in 360 degrees for masses
Remove finger and perform fecal occult blood testing

Male Anatomy

Review the male genitalia pictured in **FIGURE 15-37A** and **15-37B**.

Male Genitalia and Rectal Exam

The **male genitalia exam** should be performed with as much preservation of dignity and respect as afforded the female patient. The male examination focuses on identification of hernias, testicular carcinoma, and STIs.

Just as male providers should have a female assistant in the room during female sensitive exams, the female provider should have an assistant in the room when performing a male genitalia exam; however, staffing limitations may prevent the assistant from being male. Permission to have an assistant in the room should always be sought.

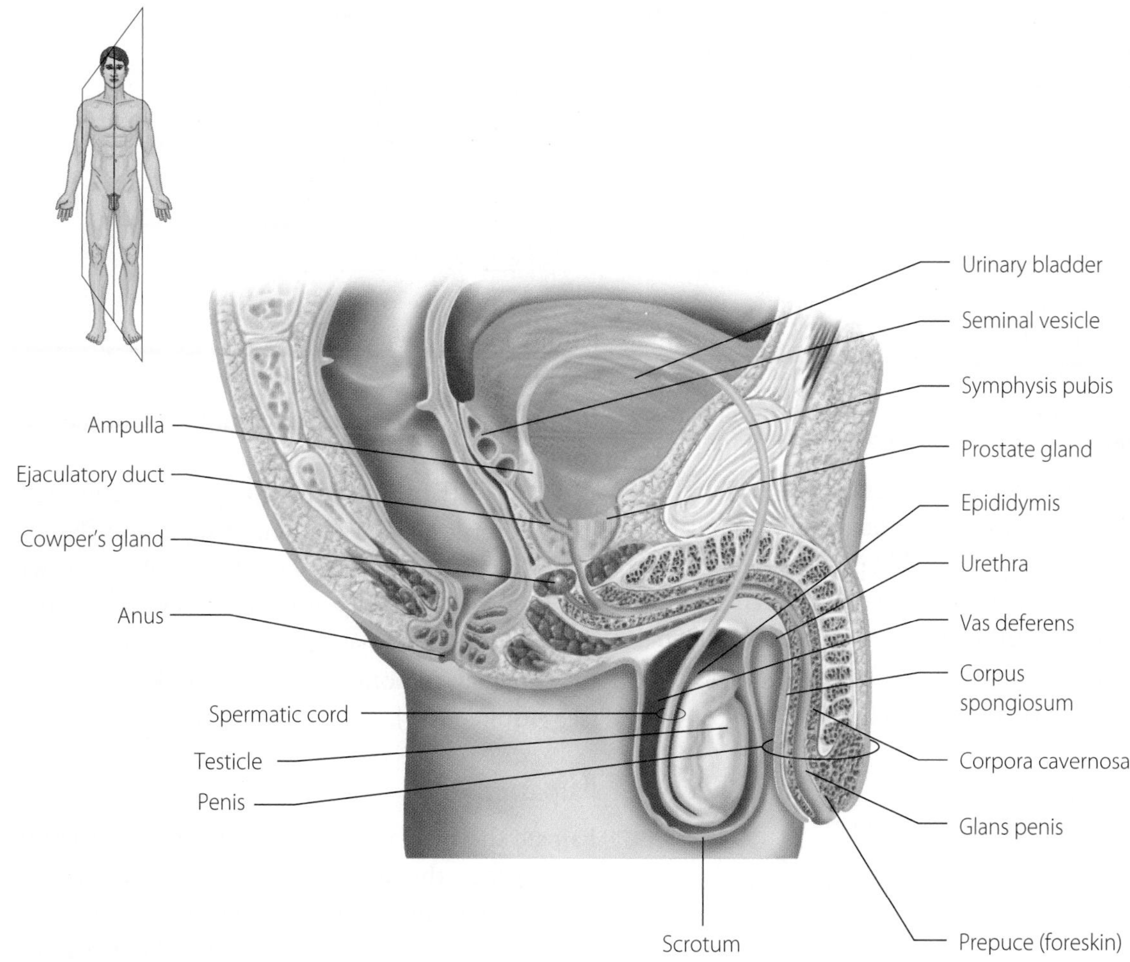

FIGURE 15-37A Cross-sectional view of male genitalia.

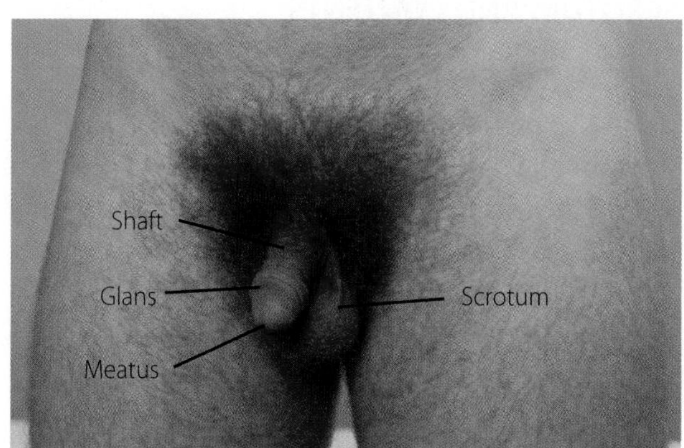

FIGURE 15-37B External male genitalia.

TESTICULAR SELF-EXAM

Men should be instructed to perform **testicular self-exams** on a monthly basis. The patient should pick a time of month that they can easily remember, such as the first day of the month or when a recurrent monthly bill is due. Instruct the patient to gently palpate the testicles for nodules. Nodules from testicular carcinoma are palpated as firm irregularities on an otherwise smooth testicular surface and are typically nontender. Posteriorly the epididymis may be palpated as a cord-like structure and should not be confused with testicular nodules. If a nodule is found, the patient should bring it to the attention of his provider immediately.

PREPARATION

For optimal examination the patient should be in a gown with underwear removed. This allows the patient to spread the legs for examination of the scrotum and testicles. Ask the patient to stand, as this position helps to identify hernias by increasing intra-abdominal

Male genitalia exam: inspection and palpation of the penis, scrotum, and inguinal areas

Testicular self-exams: process of palpating the testes on a routine basis performed by the patient to identify signs of testicular cancer

pressure. Don gloves and ask the patient for permission to begin the examination. With permission granted, ask the patient to hold the gown up at his waist.

PENIS

Inspection

Begin with inspection of the penis. Identify the presence or absence of the prepuce. If the prepuce is present, gently retract to examine the glans, noting any lesions or erythema or discharge. Note the location of the urethral meatus, normally at the tip of the glans. Surfaces of the penis are described in anatomical position with the penis in an erect state. Malpositioning of the urethral opening occurs congenitally. A meatus on the ventral surface is called hypospadias and typically is not associated with other abnormalities (see **FIGURE 15-38**). A urethral meatus on the dorsal surface is called epispadius and is commonly associated with bladder abnormalities (see **FIGURE 15-39**). Replace

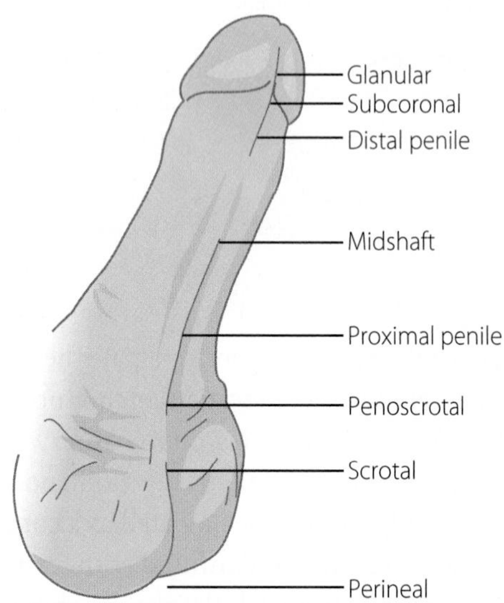

FIGURE 15-38 Hypospadias with the urethral meatus opening on the ventral surface of the penis.

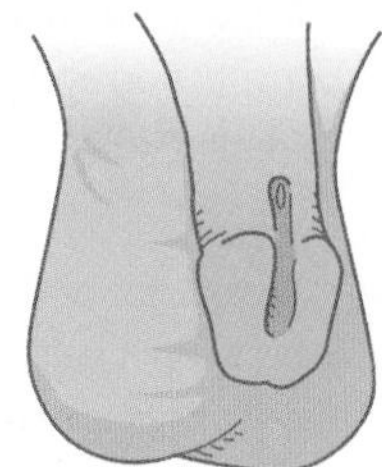

FIGURE 15-39 Epispadius with the urethral meatus opening on the dorsal surface of the penis.

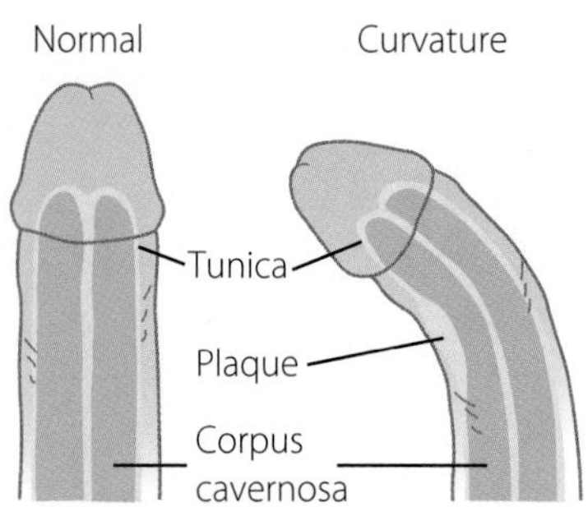

FIGURE 15-40 Peyronie's disease.

the prepuce when examination of the glans has been completed.

Inspect the skin of the shaft of the penis, again looking for lesions, deviation, or signs of inflammation. If the patient relates curvature of the penis with erection, Peyronie's disease—scar tissue from chronic inflammation of the sheath, the tunica albuginea, surrounding the corpora cavernosa—should be suspected (see **FIGURE 15-40**).

Palpation

Palpate the two lateral corpus cavernosa for lesions. Then palpate the central corpus spongiosum from the base of the penis toward the glans. Palpate and compress the glans, looking for discharge at the meatus. If found, culture the fluids.

SCROTUM AND CONTENTS

Inspection

Inspect the scrotum for general appearance. The left scrotum and testicle hangs lower than the right, allowing the legs to be adducted without compressing the testicles together. Note any rashes, lesions, masses, swelling, or inflammation (see **FIGURE 15-41**). Be certain to inspect the posterior surface.

Palpation

Advise the patient that you will now be touching him and to let you know if he experiences any tenderness. Using the thumb and first two fingers, gently palpate the testes' size, shape, and consistency, comparing bilaterally. The testes are typically oriented with the long axis vertically. The surface should be smooth without nodules or tenderness. If a mass is felt, evaluation for definitive diagnosis is imperative. Palpate the

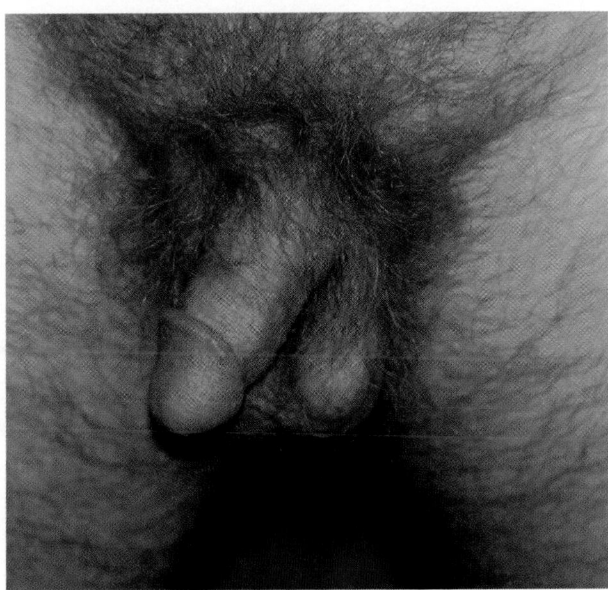

FIGURE 15-41 Spermatocele seen as a scrotal mass on inspection.

epididymis posteriorly for tenderness. Acute epididymitis is exquisitely tender and palpation should be performed with great care.

Patients with acute, intense testicular pain should be suspected of having testicular torsion. A history of trauma is not necessary. Palpation of the testes will reveal the long axis of the testes to be horizontal with the testicle high up in the scrotum. Testicular torsion is a medical emergency, as the testicle may become ischemic from compromised blood flow.

Palpate the spermatic cord, which is felt as a thin, firm, round cord along with the vas deferens. Follow these superiorly to the inguinal canal. Dilation of the cord may represent a spermatocele.

Palpate the scrotum for masses. A mass with the characteristic feel of a "sac of worms" is indicative of scrotal varicosities, a varicocele. If a scrotal mass is found, transilluminate it by darkening the room and placing a light source behind the mass. Even transillumination suggests the presence of fluid, as found with a hydrocele. Dullness to transillumination may indicate the presence of a **hernia** with bowel protruding into the scrotum (see **FIGURE 15-42**). Auscultate the mass for bowel sounds by placing a glove over the head of the stethoscope.

If a hydrocele or hernia is suspected, attempt to reduce it by applying gentle pressure. Any mass detected

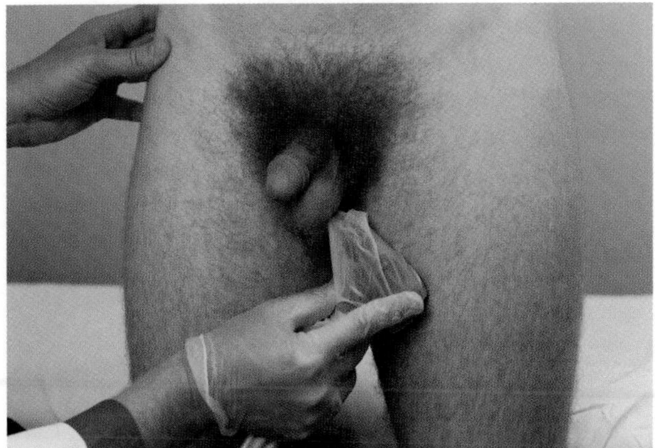

FIGURE 15-42 Scrotal transillumination.

will also need to be rechecked in the supine position to see if reduction occurs.

Finally, palpate for inguinal lymphadenopathy.

HERNIAS

Inspection

Hernias may be present without large scrotal masses. Every patient should be checked for the presence of a hernia. With the patient in the standing position, inspect along the inguinal canal and upper scrotum for bulges. Ask the patient to perform a Valsalva maneuver (bearing down to increase intra-abdominal pressure) while watching the same areas for the appearance of a bulge.

Palpation

Femoral Hernias.

Place the hands flatly over the femoral canals on each side. Ask the patient to bear down once again, palpating for enlarging bulges during Valsalva (see **FIGURE 15-43**). A bulge of the femoral canal suggests a femoral hernia. Femoral hernias are the most frequent type of hernias found in female patients.

Inguinal Hernias.

To assess for inguinal hernias, the provider should use the right hand to examine the right side for inguinal hernias and the left hand to examine the patient's left side. Using the index finger, invaginate the

Hernia: in relation to the genitalia examination, weakness in the abdominal wall often allowing protrusion of abdominal contents into the inguinal or femoral canals

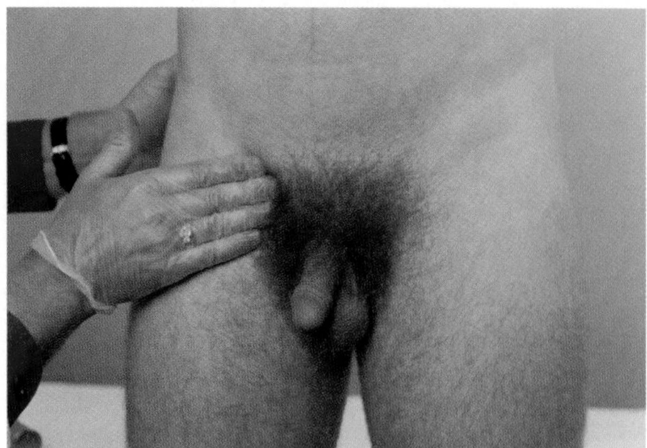

FIGURE 15-43 Femoral hernia palpation.

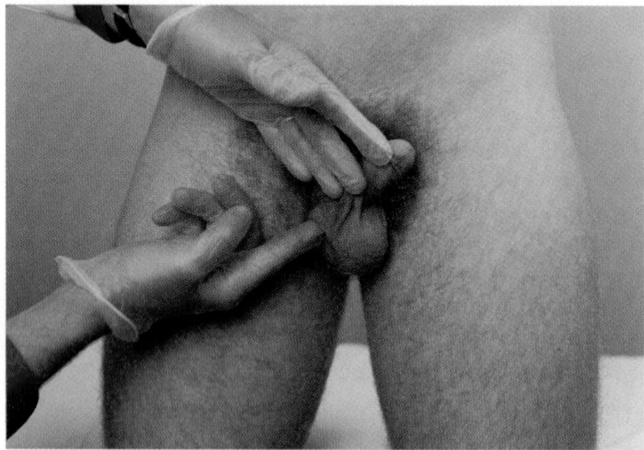

FIGURE 15-44 Inguinal hernia palpation invaginating the skin of the scrotum in order to palpate the inguinal ring.

scrotal skin to place the finger in the superficial inguinal ring into the inguinal canal (see **FIGURE 15-44**). Ask the patient to turn his head and then cough. The patient is asked to turn his head only to avoid coughing directly on the provider.

See **TABLE 15-3** for the male genitalia exam flow.

If a tap is felt at the tip of the finger, an indirect inguinal hernia is suspected, meaning the abdominal contents are protruding through the deep inguinal ring and into the canal. If a tap is felt along the side of the finger, a hernia is suspected through the posterior

TABLE 15-3 Male Genital Exam Flow

Introduces self by name and title, explaining role in the encounter
Asks for permission to begin the physical examination
Washes hands for 15 seconds before touching patient, turning off water with towel
Ensures assistant is in the room if appropriate
EDUCATION—instruct patient on need for monthly TSE
PENIS
Inspection
Prepuce (retract if present, replace when done)
Glans—lesions
Skin—lesions, inflammation, parasites
Urethral meatus—note location
Palpation
Glans
Shaft
SCROTUM AND CONTENTS
Inspection
Skin—rashes, lesions, inflammation
Posterior surface
Scrotal contour—lumps, swelling
Palpation
Use thumb and first two fingers
Testes and epididymis
Size, shape, consistency
Nodules
Tenderness
Spermatic cord with vas deferens—follow superiorly
Scrotal mass—if present
Have patient lie down to check for reduction
Auscultate for bowel sounds
Transilluminate
Inguinal lymph nodes
HERNIAS
Inspection
Patient standing
Bulges—inguinal, femoral
With Valsalva
Palpation
Inguinal
Right hand for patient's right side
Left hand for patient's left side
Invaginate scrotal skin with index finger to external ring
Have patient cough or strain
Femoral
Palpate anterior femoral canal
Have patient cough or strain

wall in the inguinal canal and is termed a direct inguinal hernia. To remember this, think of the abdominal contents as herniating "directly through the wall" of the canal.

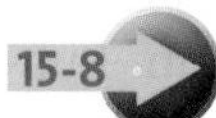

Assist the patient into the supine position and recheck any masses for reducibility.

RECTAL EXAM

To perform the **rectal exam**, first explain the procedure to the patient, including indications for its performance. Ask the patient to lie on his left side, assisting him with position change as necessary and covering him with a sheet (see **FIGURE 15-45**). Another common position in which the rectal exam can be completed is to have the patient stand and bend over the examination table.

Inspection

Don gloves. Ask the patient for permission to expose the area. Inspect the sacrococcygeal and perianal areas for lesions, inflammation, evidence of fistulas, and hemorrhoids.

Palpation

Advise the patient that you will be touching him, and gently palpate the perianal area for masses or tenderness. Now apply lubrication to the index finger. Explain that you are going to insert your finger into the rectum and that he will feel some pressure. Place the pad of your index finger just at the edge of the anus (see **FIGURE 15-46**). Ask the patient to bear down and observe for relaxation of sphincter. Note any lesions

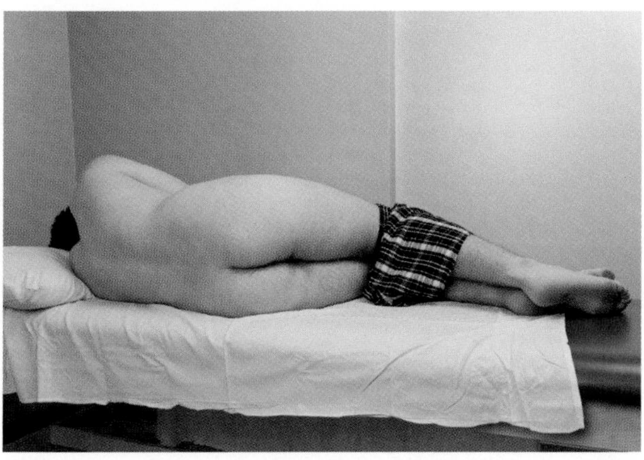

FIGURE 15-45 Lateral decubitus positioning for the rectal exam.

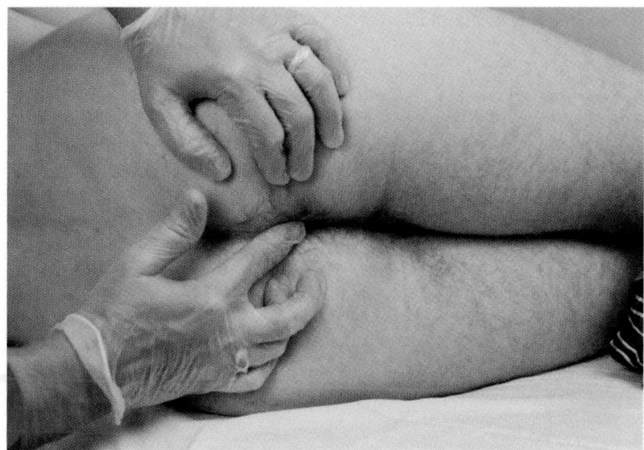

FIGURE 15-46 The finger is placed on the perianal verge. The patient is asked to bear down and then relax, after which the finger is inserted.

or protrusion of hemorrhoids with the Valsalva maneuver. Now advise the patient to relax, and as he does so, gently insert the length of the finger in the direction of the umbilicus.

Rectal exam: external inspection and internal palpation of the rectum

Note sphincter tone. Palpate the rectal wall, rotating the finger a full 360 degrees while identifying masses or tenderness. Palpate the prostate with the pad of your finger and identify the lobes, median sulcus, size, shape, and consistency. Note any nodules or tenderness.

Withdraw finger gently, continuing to rotate 360 degrees so that the pad assesses all walls of the rectum between the internal and external anal sphincters. Once the finger has been removed, note any fecal material and test for occult blood.

15-9 Advise the patient to wait just a minute ("Just let me wipe the jelly off") and use a tissue to clean him. Extra tissues may be offered.

See **TABLE 15-4** for the rectal exam flow.

TABLE 15-4 Rectal Exam Flow

Introduces self by name and title, explaining role in the encounter
Asks for permission to begin the physical examination
Washes hands for 15 seconds before touching patient, turning off water with towel
Ensures assistant is in the room if appropriate
APPROACH
Explain the procedure to the patient

(continues)

TABLE 15-4 Rectal Exam Flow *(Continued)*

Drape patient
Position the patient
Left side with hips and knees bent
Standing, bending over
INSPECTION—sacrococcygeal and perianal areas
Lesions
Inflammation
PALPATION
External examination
Masses
Tenderness
Lubricate gloved index finger
Explain that you are going to do the rectal exam
Ask patient to bear down and observe for
Relaxation of sphincter
Lesions
Hemorrhoids
Place pad of index finger on anus
Gently insert finger toward umbilicus
Note sphincter tone
Palpate rectal wall, rotating finger full 360 degrees
Masses
Tenderness
Palpate the prostate anteriorly with pad of finger and identify
Lobes
Median sulcus
Size
Shape
Consistency
Nodules
Tenderness
Withdraw finger gently
Note fecal material and test for occult blood
Clean patient or offer tissues

References

1. Rupp R. Adolescent medicine. *Core Concepts of Pediatrics e-Book*. http://www.utmb.edu/pedi_ed/CORE/AdolescentMedicine/page_03.htm. Published 2008. Accessed May 25, 2012.
2. Centers for Disease Control and Prevention. Leading Causes of Death by Age Group, All Females-United States, 2007. http://www.cdc.gov/women/lcod/07_all_females.pdf. Published 2012. Accessed May 30, 2012.
3. National Cancer Institute. Breast Cancer. http://www.cancer.gov/cancertopics/types/breast. Accessed May 30, 2012.
4. National Cancer Institute. Breast Cancer Screening (PDQ). http://www.cancer.gov/cancertopics/pdq/screening/breast/healthprofessional#Section_182. Accessed May 30, 2012.
5. Barton MB, Harris R, Fletcher SW. The rational clinical examination. Does this patient have breast cancer? The screening clinical breast examination: should it be done? How? *JAMA*. 1999;282:1270–1280.
6. American College of Obstetricians-Gynecologists, Committee on Practice Bulletins. Breast cancer screening. *Obstet Gynecol*. 2011;118:372–382.
7. Wright JL. The effect of using water-based gel lubricant during a speculum exam on Pap smear results. Pacific University Oregon, School of Physician Assistant Studies, Paper 190. http://commons.pacificu.edu/pa/190. Published 2010. Accessed May 30, 2012.

CHAPTER 16

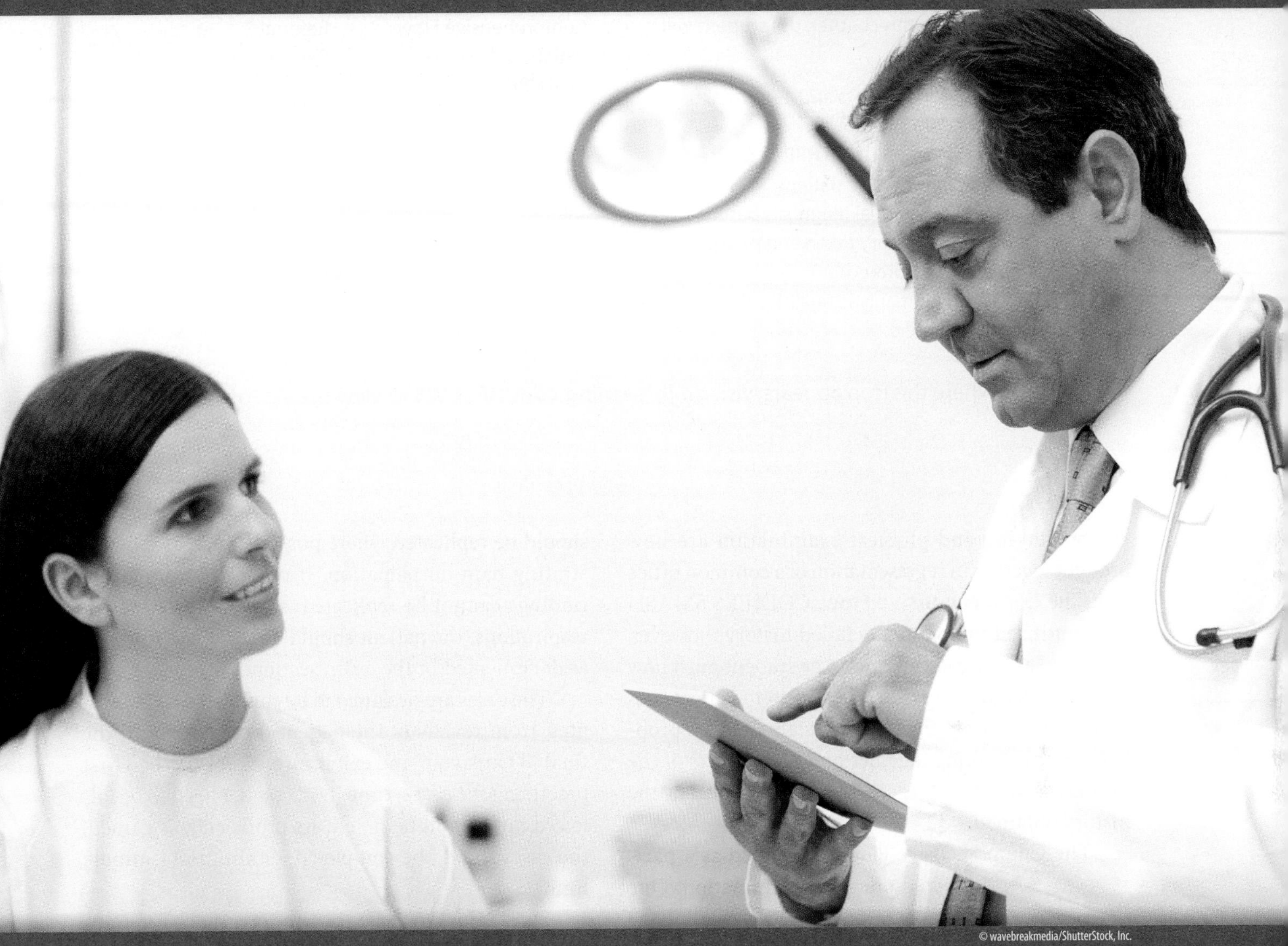
© wavebreakmedia/ShutterStock, Inc.

Comprehensive Flows

OBJECTIVES

At the conclusion of this chapter, the student will be able to

1. Identify the components and abnormalities of a patient data sheet
2. Utilize the mnemonic MOTHRR to devise a treatment plan with the patient
3. Construct a differential diagnosis based on the medical history taken and physical examination performed
4. Demonstrate humanistic qualities during patient encounters

KEY TERMS

Comprehensive Flow
Patient data sheet
MOTHRR
Referral
Return plan

Where this icon appears, visit **go.jblearning.com/HPECWS** to view the video.

History taking and physical examination are now brought together in representation of a common office visit, the **Comprehensive Flow**. CODIERS SMASH FM is utilized to obtain a detailed history; however, instead of asking each question, the student must now begin to ask if the question is pertinent to patient presentation. Likewise, the physical exam must be problem-specific, pulling together only those parts of the exam related to the chief complaint and guided by the history obtained.

The Comprehensive Flow is designed as a partnered practical examination. One student is the provider, eliciting the history and performing the physical examination, while the other is the patient.

Comprehensive Flow: clinical case presentations requiring the student to obtain a thorough medical history, perform a problem-specific examination, and develop a differential diagnosis and treatment plan while exhibiting humanistic traits

Patient data sheet: introductory information about the patient who is about to be encountered providing the patient's name, office setting, reason for visit, demographics, and screening vital signs

Each case starts with the provider's review of the patient data sheet. This sheet contains the patient's name, clinical setting, chief complaint, and vital signs, and simulates typical pre-visit screening performed by ancillary office staff.

The student in the role of the patient should review the historical questions and answers to become familiar with the clinical scenario. Physical examination findings should be replicated where possible, such as demonstrating pain on palpation. If physical examination findings cannot be replicated, such as wheezes with respirations, the patient should describe the findings as documented in the exam section.

The cases are designed to be completed in 14 minutes, from review of the patient data sheet until the final "Thank you" and exit from the room. When first practicing the cases, time limits do not need to be followed but should be noted. As proficiency is gained, the cases should be completed within the 14-minute limit.

Start a timer or note the time on a clock. The student in the role of the provider may then begin to review the **patient data sheet**.

Review of the Patient Data Sheet

- Patient's Name—Use the patient's title and last name when greeting the patient
- Office setting—To be utilized when developing the treatment plan
- Reason for the visit—Reason given to staff by the patient as to why he/she is seeking care
- Demographics—Age, sex, and race, allowing narrowing of the differential based on epidemiology

- Screening vital signs—Blood pressure, pulse, respirations, temperature, height, and weight of the patient

Abnormal vital signs should be circled during the review in order to prompt repeating abnormal vitals when beginning the physical examination.

The provider should then write the CODIERS SMASH FM mnemonic on the patient data sheet or other paper to help guide the history taking. In addition, "DDx" should be written in the right upper corner, where the provider can write possible diagnoses as they present themselves.

Finally, the provider should write the mnemonic **MOTHRR** vertically in the bottom right corner to guide the development of the treatment plan.

The Encounter

Once the provider has reviewed the patient data sheet and the patient is prepared, the provider should knock, enter the room, and provide introductions as he/she would in a clinical setting and as previously described in the section on history taking. The provider should then obtain the history and perform the physical examination. Once these are completed, two tasks remain: advising the patient of the diagnosis and developing a treatment plan.

Differential Diagnosis

The differential diagnosis is fluid, with potential diagnoses rising and falling in likelihood as the history is revealed and exam performed. Anytime a possible diagnosis is considered, it should be noted under the "DDx" written in the right upper corner.

By the end of the physical exam, some possible diagnoses may have been completely eliminated. For those that remain, the provider must rank them in order of likelihood. The patient should then be presented with the primary diagnosis. Less likely diagnoses should also be shared if testing is to be performed. Presenting all possible diagnoses on the differential is rarely appropriate; however, they would be documented in the SOAP note.

The Treatment Plan: MOTHRR

MOTHRR: mnemonic used to guide the student in developing a treatment plan, representing **M**edication, **O**steopathic Manipulative Medicine, **T**esting, **H**umanistic domain, **R**eferrals, and **R**eturn plan

After sharing the diagnosis with the patient, the provider uses the mnemonic MOTHRR to cover the basic elements needed to construct a complete plan for the patient. MOTHRR stands for:

- Medicines
- Osteopathic manipulative medicine
- Testing
- Holistic/Humanistic items
- Referrals
- Return plan

Not every aspect of this mnemonic is required for every case, but each category should be considered in the treatment of the patient. As development of the plan begins, the provider should look at each letter, then consider or reject it.

For example, a patient has epicondylitis. Using the mnemonic, the provider would first consider "M" for medications, and then ask, "Are any medications appropriate?" If so, the provider would make a recommendation, in this case, anti-inflammatories. If not, the category is skipped after having been considered.

The development of the treatment plan should include the patient. When a patient actively participates in the decision making, successful compliance is more likely, as the patient has invested in the process.

MEDICATIONS

Document the drug name, dose, frequency, amount dispensed, number of refills, and specific instructions that were shared with the patient.

- Ibuprofen 600 mg PO three times a day with food, Disp #30, 1 refill.

In addition, consider if the patient is on any medications, the dosages of which should be reduced or the medication should be completely removed.

OSTEOPATHIC MANIPULATIVE MEDICINE

For each diagnosis, consider if osteopathic manipulation is appropriate. If so, the patient should be educated

Referral: component of the treatment plan where the patient is referred to another provider or service

Return plan: component of the treatment plan defining the timing and instructions for follow-up intervention with the patient

about the appropriateness and benefits of manipulation and offered the intervention.

TESTING

Testing includes those tests required to confirm the diagnosis, rule out less likely diagnoses, and guide the treatment plan. This includes such things as blood work, radiological studies, and specialized tests performed by other providers.

HOLISTIC/HUMANISTIC

The holistic/humanistic category addresses concerns for the patient beyond basic medical needs and includes support in relation to social and emotional needs and activities of daily living, such as work and school restrictions.

Classic examples include asking if the patient would like to include a relative, friend, or other support person in the discussion of diagnosis and building of a treatment plan. Exploring how the diagnosis may interfere with work or activities of daily living also demonstrates humanistic qualities and should be asked of every patient.

Humanistic Domain Opportunity (HDO)

Within the Comprehensive Flows, opportunities for demonstration of humanistic qualities are noted as HDO. These are associated with patient responses that naturally allow the provider to demonstrate empathy, respect, reassurance, or professionalism.

REFERRAL

If a **referral** is appropriate to the plan, it should be discussed with the patient. In some cases a referral may not seem immediately necessary but would be considered if improvement does not occur. For example, a patient has an ankle injury. The provider may decide to prescribe anti-inflammatories, wrap the ankle, and perform home range-of-motion exercises. However, due to the severity of the injury, she anticipates that the patient may need a referral to physical therapy if improvement does not occur. This possibility for a possible future referral should be briefly discussed.

RETURN PLAN

The **return plan** is the last thing to address. If the patient is currently being evaluated in the emergency room or is to be admitted to the hospital, a return plan may not be appropriate until the outcome of the evaluation and admission is known. In all other instances, a follow-up plan to see the patient should be defined.

Ending the Encounter

Once the treatment plan has been reviewed, the patient should be asked if there are any questions. If there are, these should be addressed. Finally the provider should thank the patient, shake hands, and exit the room.

Hand washing is advocated both prior to seeing the patient and at the conclusion of the visit. The potential to offend the patient exists should the provider shake the patient's hand and then walk to the sink to wash. One alternative is to conclude the visit, exit the room, and use hand sanitizer located outside the room.

Documentation of the Encounter

The provider should now document the encounter using the standard SOAP note format. The advancement of electronic records has eased the burden of the handwritten note, but implementation is far from universal. The ability to accurately and efficiently document the encounter in handwritten form should be attained by every provider.

For practice purposes, attempt to document the complete encounter in written SOAP note format within a nine-minute time limit.

Comprehensive Flow Summary

1. Pair into partners, with one provider and one patient.
2. The patient reads the flow to become familiar with answers and portray pertinent findings during the examination.
3. Start a countdown timer set at 14 minutes or note the time.

4. The provider reviews the patient data sheet, then enters the room and makes introductions.
5. The history is obtained utilizing CODIERS SMASH FM.
6. A problem-specific examination is performed.
7. The patient is educated about the likely diagnosis.
8. A plan for evaluation and treatment is built with the patient, utilizing MOTHRR.
9. Conclude the encounter, asking for questions from and thanking the patient.
10. Document the encounter in SOAP note format (see **FIGURE 16-1**) within a nine-minute time limit.

Subjective (S):
Objective (O):
Assessment (A):
Plan (P):

FIGURE 16-1 SOAP note template.

CASE 1

Clinical Setting: Emergency Room
Gail Pebbles—43-year-old female
CC: Abdominal pain

Vital Signs

Blood pressure: 112/58

Respirations: 22 per minute

Pulse: 108 bpm

Temperature: 101.9 degrees F

Weight: 152 lbs

Height: 5′4″

CASE 1

Gail Pebbles
43-year-old female
CC: Abdominal pain

___ Addresses patient by name	
___ Introduces self and explains role	
___ Properly washes hands prior to touching patient	
___ What brings you in today?	I have really bad pain in my stomach.
Chronology/Onset	
___ When did it **start**?	Last night.
___ What were you **doing when it started**?	Having dinner.
___ Have you ever **had this before**?	Yes, on and off for a year or so.
___ What have you **done for it** in the past?	Nothing, it would go away in an hour or so.
___ **How often** do you get it?	Lately, it seems every couple of weeks.
___ Has it **changed** in any way?	It just isn't going away this time.
Description/Duration	
___ Can you **describe** the pain?	It's really crampy.
___ **Where** is it?	(Holds right epigastrium.)
___ Does it **radiate** [go] anywhere?	To my back (touches right scapula).
___ **Constant or come-and-go**?	Constant but gets better, then worse.
Intensity	
___ How **severe** is it, on a scale from 1 to 10?	Right now, a 9.
___ Define "better, then worse."	It goes to 4, then up to 9, then back down. (HDO)
Exacerbation	
___ Does anything **make it worse**?	Certain meals used to.
___ What kind of meals?	Fried foods get me a lot.

Remission	
___ Does anything **make it better**?	It always went away on its own before.
Symptoms Associated	
___ **Fever or chills**?	I think I have a fever.
___ **Yellowness** to your eyes?	No.
___ **Heartburn**?	No.
___ **Nausea or vomiting**?	I vomited once last night and this morning.
___ What did it look like?	I don't know. I just flushed it.
___ **Diarrhea or constipation**?	It was just a little loose this morning.
___ **Dark or bloody stools**?	No.
SMASH FM	
Social History (FED TACOS)	
___ Could you describe your **diet**?	I don't like to cook. We eat out a lot.
___ How much **caffeine** in your diet?	Just a cup of tea or two a day.
___ Have you ever used **tobacco**?	No.
___ Do you drink **alcohol**?	Yes.
___ **How much a day**?	My husband and I share a bottle of wine after dinner.
___ What is your **occupation**?	I'm an administrative assistant.
___ When was the **FDLNMP**?	About a week ago.
___ Do you have any **medical** conditions?	I have hypothyroidism.
___ Do you have any **allergies**?	No.
___ Any prior **surgeries**?	I had a C-section 10 years ago.
___ Any prior **hospitalizations**?	Just for the C-section.
___ **Medical conditions** that run in the **family**?	Just blood pressure.
___ Anyone with gallstones?	Not that I know of.

___ Are you on any other **medications**?	Synthroid.
___ Do you know the **dose**?	0.125.
___ **How many times** a day?	Just once.
Physical Examination	
___ Informs patient that the physical exam is to begin and asks permission.	
General	
___ Assess for distress	Holding RUQ/epigastrium
___ Position of comfort	Seated, slight thoracic kyphosis
HEENT	
___ Inspection for icterus	No icterus
Respiratory	
___ Auscultation performed on bare skin	Clear to auscultation
___ Complete inspiration and expiration	Shallow inspiration
___ Symmetrically	
___ Minimally 3 anterior, 2 lateral, and 3 posterior	
Cardiac	
___ Auscultation performed on bare skin	Regular rhythm without rub or gallop
___ Aortic, pulmonic, tricuspid, and mitral	No murmur
Abdominal	
___ Helps patient to supine position	
___ Drapes lower extremities with sheet	
___ Inspection: properly exposes the abdomen	Rounded without masses
___ Auscultation prior to palpation	Normoactive bowel sounds throughout
___ Palpation watching facial expression	Tenderness greatest in the RUQ
___ Percussion: four quadrants	Tympanic gastric bubble and LLQ

Special Testing	
___ Rebound, Rigidity, Guarding	Guarding RUQ
___ Murphy's sign: arrest of inspiration	Positive with deep palpation of RUQ
Rectal	
___ Offers rectal exam (does not perform)	Heme negative
___ Helps patient to seated position	
Assessment	
___ Presents patient with a proposed diagnosis	Acute cholecystitis
Plan/MOTHRR	
___ Medications	Antibiotics, pain control, IV fluids
___ Testing	Imaging
___ Humanistic/Holistic	Offers contact with family (HDO)
___ Referral	Surgical evaluation
___ Return	Consider admission to the hospital
Patient now completes the Humanistic Domain Assessment.	

Case 1 Review

The patient has acute abdominal pain. In exploring onset, we learn that it began while eating dinner the night before. At this point the provider should consider what causes of abdominal pain are related to eating. These may include esophagitis, gastroenteritis, gastric or duodenal ulceration, and cholelithiasis.

Chronology further reveals intermittent episodes of similar, self-resolving symptoms over the last year with increasing frequency. Looking at the differential, which is less likely and should move down in order of probability? Gastroenteritis does not typically present with increasing frequency.

The pain is described as colicky, being crampy and constant but with waxing and waning intensity varying from a 4 to a 9 out of 10 and currently at a 9, suggesting urgency in treatment. Whenever pain is noted, especially with increasing severity, the provider is presented with an opportunity to express empathy and offer reassurance and should do so before moving on to the next question.

It is located a little to the right of the epigastrium. Which organ systems are found in this area? Pathology of the stomach, small bowel, liver, gallbladder, head of the pancreas, and transverse colon could account for pain in this area. Of these, we have not included pathology of the liver or pancreas in the differential. The provider could consider adding hepatitis and tumor of the pancreas. Description includes the primary location and radiation. When the patient admits radiation to the right scapula, cholelithiasis rises rapidly to the top of the differential.

When asked about exacerbating factors, the patient replies "certain meals." This is a clue that the provider must follow by having the patient define which "certain meals" she means. Fried foods are fatty, again corresponding with cholelithiasis.

Symptoms associated reveals positives for fever, corroborated by the patient data sheet showing a temperature of 101.9, vomiting, and slight diarrhea. Remember the rule: When anything comes out of the body, you must get descriptions. Little was obtained here as the emesis was not observed by the patient. Lack of dark stools decreases the likelihood of a bleeding ulcer, as a single loose stool would decrease the likelihood of gastroenteritis. A lack of dyspepsia pushes esophagitis down on the differential as well, demonstrating that the negative symptoms associated are as important as the positives.

The social history contributes through identification of the patient eating out a lot, with restaurant foods commonly being higher in fat content, which corresponds with cholelithiasis. Frequent alcohol use could result in gastritis and esophagitis, though they would remain lower on the differential as other associated symptoms are lacking. Other SMASH FM history appears noncontributory.

The physical examination begins with review of the vital signs showing elevated pulse, respirations, and temperature. Pain alone can elevate the pulse and respirations; however, elevation of temperature should prompt the provider to consider infectious causes. Her BMI is also elevated, which is a risk factor for cholelithiasis.

Working head to toe, consideration of hepatitis or biliary duct obstruction would lead the provider to inspect the conjunctiva for icterus, the first place that hyperbilirubinemia presents.

The abdomen is the primary area of concern. Each technique of examination should be performed. Tenderness is noted in the right upper quadrant. Considering acute pathology of the abdomen, special testing should be performed for perforated viscous. Guarding is evident but no rigidity or rebound, making peritonitis less likely. Murphy's sign is positive, pointing toward cholecystitis as the primary diagnosis

A rectal exam would be indicated and offered. The student portraying the patient should offer the results of the examination, which in this case is Hemoccult negative, making an upper gastrointestinal bleed less likely.

Cholecystitis should be considered the primary diagnosis. For practice purposes the expanded differential diagnosis could include others such as esophagitis, gastritis, or gastric or duodenal ulceration.

CASE 2

Clinical Setting: Emergency Room
Arthur Scerro—59-year-old male
CC: Chest pain

Vital Signs

Blood pressure: 160/100

Respirations: 24 per minute

Pulse: 120 bpm

Temperature: 98.3 degrees F

Weight: 230 lbs

Height: 6′1″

CASE 2	
Arthur Scerro **59-year-old male** **CC: Chest pain**	
___ Addresses patient by name	
___ Introduces self and explains role	
___ Properly washes hands prior to touching patient	
___ What brings you in today?	I have chest pain.
Chronology/Onset	
___ When did it **start**?	Two hours ago.
___ What were you **doing when it started**?	Mowing the grass.
___ Have you ever **had this before**?	Yes.
___ When was that?	For the last month, it's every time I mow the lawn.
___ Did it come on **suddenly or gradually**?	It sneaks up on me.
___ What have you **done for it** in the past?	I just stop and it goes away in a couple minutes.
___ Has it **changed** in any way?	It just isn't going away this time.
Description/Duration	
___ Can you **describe** the pain?	It's like a heaviness in my chest.
___ **Where** is it?	(Holds hand over left sternal border.)
___ Does it **radiate** [go] anywhere?	Up into the left side of my neck and arm.
Intensity	
___ How **severe** is it, on a scale from 1 to 10?	An 8. (HDO)
Exacerbation	
___ Does anything **make it worse**?	Walking in from the parking lot. (HDO)
Remission	
___ Does anything **make it better**?	Not exerting myself helps a bit.

Symptoms Associated	
___ **Fever or chills**?	No fever but I feel cold and clammy.
___ **Sweating**?	Yes.
___ **Heartburn**?	Maybe a little.
___ **Nausea or vomiting**?	I'm a little nauseated. (HDO)
___ **Cough**?	No.
___ **Numbness or tingling**?	My left hand feels a bit dull.
SMASH FM	
Social History (FED TACOS)	
___ Could you describe your **diet**?	Meat and potatoes
___ Do you **exercise** routinely?	No. I know I should. (HDO)
___ How much **caffeine** in your diet?	About a pot of coffee a day.
___ Have you ever used **tobacco**?	Yes, I smoke.
___ How much a day?	2 packs.
___ How long have you been smoking?	40 years.
___ Do you drink **alcohol**?	No.
___ Do you use **recreational drugs**?	No.
___ What is your **occupation**?	I'm a machinist.
___ Are you **sexually active**?	Yes.
___ Have you gotten any chest pain then?	A couple of times.
___ Do you have any **medical** conditions?	My blood pressure's high.
___ Do you have any **allergies**?	No.
___ Any prior **surgeries**?	No.
___ Any prior **hospitalizations**?	No.
___ **Medical conditions** that run in the **family**?	Heart troubles.

___ Do you know what kind of troubles?	My dad and brother died of heart attacks.
___ How old were they?	Dad was 50 and my brother was 52. (HDO)
___ Are you on any other **medications**?	Hydrochlorothiazide.
___ How many **milligrams**?	50.
___ **How many times** a day?	In the morning.
Physical Examination	
___ Informs patient that the physical exam is to begin and asks permission	
General	
___ Assess for distress	Appears in moderate distress
___ Position of comfort	Reclined on stretcher
Vitals	
___ Repeats blood pressure with correct technique	160/90 right arm
___ Both arms	160/92 left arm
___ Repeats pulse	100 bpm, irregularly irregular
Neck	
___ Inspection JVD	No JVD
___ Auscultation of carotids	No bruits
Cardiac	
___ Inspection: properly exposes patient	
___ Heave/PMI	No visible heave or PMI
___ Auscultation performed on bare skin	Irregularly irregular rhythm without rub
___ Aortic, pulmonic, tricuspid and mitral	No murmur
___ Palpation for reproducibility of pain	Nontender to palpation
Respiratory	
___ Inspection: signs of distress	No cyanosis or accessory muscle use

___ AP:Lateral ratio	1.5:1
___ Auscultation performed on bare skin	Distant breath sounds without wheezes
___ Complete inspiration and expiration	
___ Symmetrically	
___ Minimally 3 anterior, 2 lateral, and 3 posterior	
Abdominal	
___ Helps patient to supine position	
___ Drapes lower extremities with sheet	
___ Inspection: properly exposes the abdomen	Rounded without masses
___ Auscultation prior to palpation	NABS × 4, no bruits
___ Palpation watching facial expression	Nontender without pulsatile masses
Extremities	
___ Inspection	No edema
___ Palpation of distal pulses	Dorsalis pedis/posterior tibialis 1/4 b/l
Assessment	
___ Presents patient with a proposed diagnosis	Acute coronary syndrome
Plan/MOTHRR	
___ Medications	Acute coronary syndrome protocol such as IV, O2, ASA, morphine
___ Testing	Stat ECG, chest x-ray, cardiac profile
___ Humanistic/Holistic	Offers to contact family (HDO)
___ Referral	Cardiology consult
___ Return plan	Advises admission
Patient now completes Humanistic Domain Evaluation.	

Case 2 Review

From the patient data sheet, we know that Mr. Scerro is a 59-year-old male presenting to the ER with chest pain and elevated blood pressure, respirations, and pulse. Acute coronary syndrome should be expected immediately prompting urgent intervention with this patient. His elevated BMI increases his risk.

The pain began while he was mowing the lawn two hours prior. The patient describes the pain as heaviness in his chest and visceral pain over the precordium, with radiation into the neck and arm. It has been occurring every time he mows his grass for the last month, which is consistent with angina and coronary artery disease. By asking how it has changed since onset, the provider determines that, having as opposed to prior events that resolved spontaneously with rest, on this occasion it has not.

The pain is worse upon exertion and improves with rest, typical of ischemic pain. Exploration of symptoms associated reveals classic findings of cardiac ischemia including diaphoresis, nausea, and paresthesia.

It is important to determine the patient's risk for coronary artery disease through historical questions. This male patient admits a diet high in meats and carbohydrates, does not exercise, smokes, has high blood pressure, and has a strong family history of heart attack. Recreational drug use should always be questioned in the presence of cardiac ischemia. Exploring his sexual history reveals chest pain with this exertional activity.

Though his medication list includes only HCTZ and he admits only to having hypertension, asking specifically about a history of hyperlipidemia would be appropriate.

Multiple opportunities to demonstrate humanistic qualities of empathy, respect, and professionalism present themselves.

When performing the examination, the general assessment should note any distress. The patient's vital signs should be repeated to ensure accuracy. As the blood pressure is elevated, repeating in both arms is indicated not only for blood pressure accuracy but also to assess for a possible dissecting thoracic aorta, which must be included in the differential diagnosis. The pulse is noted to be irregularly irregular prompting the provider to add atrial fibrillation to the differential and ordering an ECG and telemetry. In clinical practice, these measures are occurring simultaneously with the patient assessment.

The patient should be assessed for signs of heart failure such as JVD, an S3, crackles in the lungs, and edema. The provider should also assess for an enlarged heart by examining for a displaced point of maximal impulse (PMI). The cardiac system represents the primary area of concern. Both it and the respiratory system require deliberate, detailed examination utilizing all appropriate examination techniques.

A decreasing AP:lateral ratio suggests COPD, which would align with the patient's tobacco use history. In all chest pain cases, reproducibility of the pain should be sought to rule out musculoskeletal origin.

Signs of atherosclerosis in other vessels should be assessed, including listening for bruits in the carotids and abdominal aorta. Palpation should include assessment of the abdominal aorta for aneurysm and peripheral pulses for asymmetry and diminished lower extremity pulses, associated with thoracic aneurysm and peripheral arterial disease.

This patient's historical and physical findings point to pain of a cardiac origin. This patient should be treated following acute coronary syndrome protocols. The patient should have a stat chest x-ray to rule out thoracic aortic aneurysm and be evaluated for possible emergent intervention such as cardiac catheterization.

CASE 3

Clinical Setting: Family Practice Office
Seth Falga—22-year-old male
CC: Headache

Vital Signs

Blood pressure: 114/60

Respirations: 16 per minute

Pulse: 72 bpm

Temperature: 98.5 degrees F

Weight: 128 lbs

Height: 5′4″

CASE 3	
Seth Falga **22-year-old male** **CC: Headache**	
___ Addresses patient by name	
___ Introduces self and explains role	
___ Properly washes hands prior to touching patient	
___ What brings you in today?	I have a headache.
Chronology/Onset	
___ When did it **start**?	Yesterday morning.
___ What were you **doing when it started**?	They can happen at any time.
___ Did it come on **suddenly or gradually**?	Gradually. I know when one's coming.
___ How you do you know?	I can't focus on what I'm looking at.
___ **How often** do you have one?	About once a month.
___ When did they **first start**?	About two years ago.
___ What do you do when you get one?	I take ibuprofen when I know it's coming
___ How many at a time?	Three.
___ How many milligrams?	200 each.
___ Has it **changed** in any way?	Not that I can think of.
Description/Duration	
___ Can you **describe** the pain?	Like a drum in my head.
___ **Which part** of your head?	(Places hand over right occipitoparietal area.)
___ Does it **radiate** [go] anywhere?	No.
Intensity	
___ How **severe** is it, on a scale from 1 to 10?	A 6 or 7. (HDO)

Exacerbation	
___ Does anything **make it worse**?	I can't pinpoint anything.
Remission	
___ Does anything **make it better**?	Sometimes I'll take a nap.
Symptoms Associated	
___ **Fever or chills**?	No.
___ **Stiff neck**?	No.
___ **Lights bother your eyes**?	Yeah, I think so.
___ **Nausea or vomiting**?	I get nauseated after the headache starts.
___ **Stress or anxiety**?	I never thought about it. I don't think so.
___ **Numbness or tingling**?	No.
SMASH FM	
Social History (FED TACOS)	
___ Could you describe your **diet**?	I avoid fats and carbs.
___ Do you **exercise** routinely?	Definitely—I lift and run. (HDO)
___ How much **caffeine** in your diet?	Those caffeine drinks help me lift and run.
___ How many do you drink a day?	Two. Three if I lift.
___ Have you ever used **tobacco**?	No.
___ Do you drink **alcohol**?	No.
___ Do you use **recreational drugs**?	No.
___ What is your **occupation**?	I'm in college. Physical therapy.
___ Do you have any **medical** conditions?	No.
___ History of head trauma?	No.
___ Do you have any **allergies**?	No.
___ Any prior **surgeries**?	No.

___ Any prior **hospitalizations**?	No.
___ **Medical conditions** that run in the **family**?	No.
___ Are you on any other **medications**?	No.
Physical Examination	
___ Informs patient that the physical exam is to begin and asks permission	
General	
___ Assess for distress	No apparent distress
___ Position of comfort	Seated on side of exam table
Head	
___ Inspection	NCAT
___ Palpation	Without tenderness
Eyes	
___ Ophthalmoscopic examination	Cup:disc ratio 1:2 with sharp margins
Neck	
___ Inspection	Symmetrical
___ Range of motion	Full AROM
___ Auscultation of carotids	No bruits
___ Palpation	Tissue texture changes T1–4 right
Cardiac	
___ Auscultation performed on bare skin	Regular rhythm without rub
___ Aortic, pulmonic, tricuspid, and mitral	Without murmur
Respiratory	
___ Auscultation performed on bare skin	Clear to auscultation
___ Complete inspiration and expiration	

____ Symmetrically	
____ Minimally 3 anterior, 2 lateral, and 3 posterior	
Neurologic	
____ Cranial nerve testing	CNII through XII intact
____ Motor strength testing—bilateral comparison	5/5 throughout
____ Reflexes	2/4 throughout
Assessment	
____ Presents patient with a proposed diagnosis	Migraine
Plan/MOTHRR	
____ Medications	Triptans
____ OMM	Myofascial release, cranial techniques
____ Testing	Consider imaging
____ Humanistic/Holistic	Headache log for trigger identification
	Offers to contact family (HDO)
	Lifestyle modification
____ Return plan	Early follow-up
Patient now completes Humanistic Domain Evaluation.	

Case 3 Review

Seth is a 22-year-old male who presents to the office with a headache. With this information alone, the provider should consider common causes of headache such as migraine, tension, and cluster headaches as well as meningitis. Review of the patient data sheet shows that his vital signs are stable, including the temperature, which lessens the likelihood of meningitis.

Though headaches are most commonly benign, it is important to rule out a secondary cause of headache that could be life-threatening, such as aneurysm or increased intracranial pressure from a mass.

We quickly learn that these headaches are recurrent in nature for the past two years, nearly removing meningitis as a possible cause. Exploring the onset reveals the inability to focus, which likely reflects an aura consistent with migraine headache. The description with drumlike quality further increases the likelihood of migraine, though cluster headaches can share this characteristic. Unilaterally also suggests these two diagnoses as opposed to tension headaches.

Some relief is suggested in regard to taking a nap, and symptoms associated confirms nausea while hinting at photophobia, both commonly associated with the diagnosis of migraine.

Social history should be explored: Both alcohol, which often triggers cluster headaches, and drug use are negative. Weightlifting increases blood pressure, as does caffeine use, which might make the provider concerned about intracranial aneurysm. Interestingly, caffeine is often advocated for use in migraine treatment and is contained in many over-the-counter preparations.

The location of the headache makes referred pain less likely, though a history of head trauma should be sought.

The majority of headaches are diagnosed through historical data because most patients do not have any physical findings. A funduscopic exam should be performed to rule out papilledema. If a patient has papilledema, nuchal rigidity, or a focal defect on cranial nerve exam, a CT scan should be performed immediately. These findings point to a secondary cause of the headache. If there is no papilledema, nuchal rigidity, or focal defects on neurologic exam, then the decision to order a CT is made based on clinical judgment.

Neck examination should be performed to rule out meningitis. Palpation demonstrates viscerosomatic tissue texture changes. A neurologic exam should also be performed. No deficits are noted.

The most likely diagnosis in this patient is migraine. The treatment plan should be built around this; however, the provider should also keep other etiologies in mind should initial treatment be unsuccessful. Treatment options for this patient would include triptans, with consideration for starting daily medication as prophylaxis should they be unsuccessful.

Patient education is paramount and should include exploration for triggers and behavioral modification, such as lessening caffeine intake, which may be directly related to the headaches. Manipulation can also be performed. The provider should schedule a follow-up within the next several weeks.

CASE 4

Clinical Setting: Internal Medicine Office
Hiram Tensen—51-year-old male
CC: Elevated blood pressure

Vital Signs

Blood pressure: 182/69

Respirations: 16 per minute

Pulse: 72 bpm

Temperature: 98.6 degrees F

Weight: 242 lbs

Height: 6′4″

CASE 4

Hiram Tensen
51-year-old male
CC: Elevated blood pressure

___ Addresses patient by name	
___ Introduces self and explains role	
___ Properly washes hands prior to touching patient	
___ What brings you in today?	I was told my blood pressure was up **again**.
Chronology/Onset	
___ **When** were you told that?	Last week.
___ Who told you it was elevated?	They were doing blood pressures at the mall.
___ You said "again." It's been high before?	Yes.
___ When were you **first told**?	Oh, a couple of years ago.
___ How was it treated?	I was given a pill to take.
___ Are you still taking it?	No.
___ When did you stop it?	About a year ago.
___ Why did you stop it?	I was up all night peeing. (HDO)
___ Do you remember the **name** of it?	No. Some big long word.
___ Hydrochlorothiazide?	Might have been.
___ How many milligrams?	No idea.
___ How many times a day?	Twice.
Exacerbation	
___ Does anything **make your BP go up**?	Not that I know of.
Remission	
___ Did the medication make it better?	They told me it was where it needed to be.

Symptoms Associated	
___ **Headaches**?	No.
___ **Heart racing or sweating**?	Only if I'm **working out**.
___ What kind of "workout" do you do?	I mean like working out in the yard.
___ **Weakness or urinating a lot**?	Not since I stopped that pill.
___ **Pain in your legs when you walk**?	No.
___ **Chest pain/shortness of breath on exertion**?	No.
___ **Visual changes**?	No.
___ **Stress or anxiety**?	My job keeps me running.
___ What do you do?	I'm an editor at the newspaper. (HDO)
SMASH FM	
Social History (FED TACOS)	
___ Could you describe your **diet**?	I eat on the run a lot.
___ Do you limit **salt** in your diet?	Food tastes better with salt.
___ Do you **exercise** routinely?	No time for that.
___ How much **caffeine** in your diet?	Five or six cups of coffee a day.
___ Have you ever used **tobacco**?	Yes, I smoke.
___ How much a day?	Half a pack. I'm trying to quit. (HDO)
___ How many years?	30 or so.
___ Do you drink **alcohol**?	A beer every couple of weeks.
___ Do you use **recreational drugs**?	No.
___ Do you have any **medical** conditions?	No.
___ Do you have any **allergies**?	Just some seasonal allergies.
___ Any prior **surgeries**?	No.
___ Any prior **hospitalizations**?	No.

___ **Medical conditions** that run in the **family**?	Blood pressure and cholesterol mostly.
___ **Medications**?	Sudafed for the allergies.
___ How many milligrams?	I don't know. Two tablets at a time.
___ How many times a day?	Two or three when the pollens are bad.
Physical Examination	
___ Informs patient that the physical exam is to begin and asks permission	
Vitals	
___ Repeats blood pressure with correct technique	176/96 right arm
___ Both arms	178/92 left arm
Eyes	
___ Ophthalmoscopic examination	No papilledema or hypertensive retinopathy
Neck	
___ Auscultation of carotids	No bruits
___ Palpation	No masses or thyromegaly
Cardiac	
___ Inspection: properly exposes patient	
___ Heave/PMI	No visible heave or PMI
___ Auscultation performed on bare skin	Regular rhythm without rub or gallop
___ Aortic, pulmonic, tricuspid, and mitral	No murmur
___ Palpation	Anterior axillary line 5th ICS
Respiratory	
___ Inspection	AP:lateral ratio 2:1
___ Auscultation performed on bare skin	Clear to auscultation
___ Complete inspiration and expiration	

___ Symmetrically	
___ Minimally 3 anterior, 2 lateral, and 3 posterior	
Abdominal	
___ Helps patient to supine position	
___ Drapes lower extremities with sheet	
___ Inspection: properly exposes the abdomen	Rounded without masses
___ Auscultation prior to palpation	Normoactive bowel sounds
___ Aorta and renal arteries	No bruits
___ Palpation including size of aorta	Nontender without masses
Peripheral Vascular	
___ Palpation for peripheral pulses	2/4 throughout
Assessment	
___ Presents patient with a proposed diagnosis	Hypertension
Plan/MOTHRR	
___ Medications	Antihypertensive; education on discontinue OTC Sudafed; seasonal allergy prescription
___ Testing	Laboratory assessment, possible imaging
___ Humanistic/Holistic	Patient education on past medication side effects and choice of other class.
	Offers to contact family (HDO)
	Lifestyle modification—salt avoidance, assistance with smoking cessation
	Blood pressure monitoring at home
___ Return plan	Early follow-up
Patient now completes Humanistic Domain Evaluation.	

Case 4 Review

Review of the patient data sheet shows a 51-year-old male with elevated blood pressure and BMI.

When we ask, "What brings you in today," we get our first clue that the patient has a prior history of the same, as he says his blood pressure is up "again." The provider should immediately note that he has been told this before and explore chronology to review when and how it was treated. We quickly learn that the patient was diagnosed with high blood pressure several years prior and was treated with a medication that had side effects poorly tolerated by the patient—that of urinating frequently—and that were the likely cause of his discontinuing the medication.

The provider does not need to wait until M (medications) in SMASH FM to obtain related information, as the natural flow of questioning should be followed. Though he does not know the name, a diuretic should be expected, specifically HCTZ, which is commonly the first line of treatment. Interestingly, he took the pill twice a day and only complained of urinating too frequently at night, making the provider question if once-a-day dosing in the morning would have been better tolerated.

Symptoms associated are related to the consequences of elevated blood pressure, ruling out heart attack or stroke, as well as causes of secondary hypertension, tachycardia and sweating with pheochromocytoma, and renal disease.

Contributing factors from the patient's social history include use of salt in the diet, caffeine intake, tobacco use, and a high-stress occupation, all areas where humanistic domain principles should be employed. The patient also has a history of environmental allergies for which he takes Sudafed, another well-known cause of elevated blood pressure.

The physical examination should include repeating the blood pressure in both arms. Working head to toe, examine the eyes for evidence of hypertensive retinopathy, as it is quite likely the patient has had hypertension for many years, even prior to his initial diagnosis.

The primary system is cardiac, requiring proper exposure and detailed examination, which reveals a displaced PMI suggesting hypertrophy.

Also assess for signs of vascular disease, as the patient has a family history of hypertension and hyperlipemia. Assess the carotids for bruits, the aorta for aneurysm, and the renal and peripheral arteries for stenosis.

Treatment options should be explored with the patient. There are many lifestyle modifications that can occur, including discontinuation of Sudafed, salt restriction, exercise, weight loss, and smoking cessation. Some providers and patients may feel comfortable with a trial of behavioral modification. Others may recommend medication as the first-line treatment, especially for signs of cardiac hypertrophy, with the possibility of discontinuation if lifestyle modifications are successful.

Baseline laboratory assessment is appropriate. Imaging with chest x-ray and echocardiogram may be considered with smoking history and possible cardiac hypertrophy.

The ability of the patient to take his blood pressure at home should be explored and return visits scheduled for serial assessment.

CASE 5

Clinical Setting: Family Practice Office
Nneka Shore—49-year-old female
CC: Neck pain

Vital Signs

Blood pressure: 148/88

Respirations: 14 per minute

Pulse: 68 bpm

Temperature: 98.4 degrees F

Weight: 142 lbs

Height: 5′3″

CASE 5	
Nneka Shore **49-year-old female** **CC: Neck pain**	
___ Addresses patient by name	
___ Introduces self and explains role	
___ Properly washes hands prior to touching patient	
___ What brings you in today?	My neck hurts.
Chronology/Onset	
___ When did it **start**?	I woke up with it yesterday morning.
___ Any **injury or new activity**?	I probably just slept on it wrong.
___ Have you ever **had this before**?	Yes, it acts up now and then.
___ What have you done for it in the past?	I put a hot pad on it and take some Tylenol.
___ How many milligrams?	325.
___ How many at a time?	Two.
___ How often do you take them?	Twice yesterday and once today.
___ Has it **changed** in any way?	No.
Description/Duration	
___ Can you **describe** the pain?	It's a tight pain.
___ **Where** is the pain?	More on the back, right side of my neck.
___ Does it **radiate** [go] anywhere?	No.
Intensity	
___ How **severe** is it, on a scale from 1 to 10?	Oh, I'd say a 7. (HDO)
Exacerbation	
___ Does anything **make it worse**?	Yes, I can't turn my head the whole way.

Remission	
____ Does anything **make it better**?	The Tylenol helps for a little while and **Jimmy** rubs some ointment into it. (HDO)
____ Who's Jimmy?	My husband. (HDO)
Symptoms Associated	
____ **Fever or chills**?	No.
____ **Swelling**?	No.
____ **Redness or warmth**?	No.
____ **Lights bother the eyes**?	No.
____ **Numbness or tingling**?	No.
____ **Weakness**?	No
____ **Pain in other joints**?	My hands get a little sore now and then.
SMASH FM	
Social History (FED TACOS)	
____ Do you **exercise** routinely?	I chase my three grandkids around. (HDO)
____ Have you ever used **tobacco**?	No.
____ Do you drink **alcohol**?	No.
____ What's your **occupation**?	I do data entry.
___ Does your work bother your neck?	Sometimes.
____ **FDLMP**	When they took out my uterus 3 years ago.
___ What was the reason they took it out?	Fibroids.
____ Do you have any **medical** conditions?	No.
____ History of neck injury?	No.
____ Do you have any **allergies**?	No.
____ Any other **surgeries**?	Just the one.
____ Any prior **hospitalizations**?	Just for that surgery.
____ **Medical conditions** that run in the **family**?	Diabetes.

___ Have you been screened for diabetes?	Everything is fine and I don't eat sweets.
___ Are you on any other **medications**?	No.
Physical Examination	
___ Informs patient that the physical exam is to begin and asks permission	
General	
___ Assess for distress	No apparent distress
___ Position of comfort	Head tilted slightly to the right
Vitals	
___ Repeats blood pressure with correct technique	136/82 right arm
___ Both arms	136/80 left arm
Head	
___ Inspection	NCAT
___ Palpation	Without tenderness
Neck	
___ Inspection	Slight neck rotation and extension, right
___ Range of motion	Active ROM limited in side bending left to 30 degrees and rotation left to 45 degrees
___ Auscultation of carotids	No bruits
___ Assist patient to supine position	
___ Passive range of motion	Side bending L 45 degrees, rotation L 45 degrees
___ Palpation	Increased warmth, bogginess, tender at C5 transverse process. C5 RrSr
Lymphatic	
___ Cervical and axillary	No lymphadenopathy
Cardiac	
___ Auscultation performed on bare skin	Regular rhythm without rub
___ Aortic, pulmonic, tricuspid, and mitral	Without murmur

Respiratory	
____ Auscultation performed on bare skin	Clear to auscultation
____ Complete inspiration and expiration	
____ Symmetrically	
____ Minimally 3 anterior, 2 lateral, and 3 posterior	
____ Assists the patient to seated position for posterior assessment	
Neurologic	
____ Sensory testing upper extremity	Intact to touch, sharp/dull bilaterally
____ Motor strength testing	5/5 throughout
____ Reflexes	2/4 throughout
Assessment	
____ Presents patient with a proposed diagnosis	Cervical somatic dysfunction
	Rule out osteoarthritis
	Elevated blood pressure without diagnosis = of hypertension
Plan/MOTHRR	
____ Medications	Pain management such as NSAID
____ OMM	Myofascial, muscle energy, facilitated positional release, HVLA
____ Testing	Consider imaging
____ Humanistic/Holistic	Patient education for ergonomic workplace
	Offers to provide information for employer
	Avoidance of combination heating pad and topical ointment
____ Return plan	Follow-up visit to reassess and monitor blood pressure
Patient now completes Humanistic Domain Evaluation.	

Case 5 Review

Ms. Shore is 49 years old and presents with neck pain. Review of the patient data sheet reveals elevated blood pressure, which will need to be addressed during the visit. All other vital signs are stable.

As the patient awoke with the pain, trauma is unlikely, but the patient should be questioned about new activities or trauma in the days before onset. She has had similar episodes before and finds some relief with acetaminophen, a hot pad, massage, and ointments. The provider should make a note to discuss avoiding concurrent use of heating pads and ointments, so as to prevent accidental burns.

The pain is located in the posterior, right neck, and does not radiate. In a patient who presents with neck pain it is important to rule out an infectious process such as meningitis. The patient denies fever, chills, and photophobia, which makes an infectious process less likely.

The patient admits limited range of motion of the neck but notes that the limited motion is described as rotation, again turning the provider away from meningitis as a cause, as it more frequently demonstrates limitation in flexion.

No symptoms of radiculopathy are found. Pain in the hands may suggest an arthritic component but may also correlate with the patient's occupation in data entry.

There are multiple areas where the provider needs to follow up with secondary questions to obtain all associated information: medication doses, the mentioning of a name, occupation, and indication for surgery.

There are also several areas that open themselves for expression of humanistic behavior: the level of pain, the involvement of her husband, her grandchildren, and her attentiveness to wellness, to name a few.

On examination, the patient is afebrile and normotensive when the blood pressure is repeated. This finding requires follow-up with sequential readings on separate occasions to rule out hypertension. The patient should be educated that HTN cannot be diagnosed with an isolated reading and that the blood pressure elevation may be a result of her neck pain.

There is increased warmth, bogginess, and tenderness at the C5 transverse process, and C5 is rotated to the right. When active range of motion is limited, passive range of motion should be assessed. These findings help to further rule out an infectious process and point to cervical somatic dysfunction or strain.

The heart, lung, and neurologic examinations lack abnormal findings.

Cervical somatic dysfunction is the most likely diagnosis; however, the provider may consider underlying arthritis, for which an x-ray may be ordered.

Manipulation should be explained to the patient and, after obtaining a verbal consent, performed on the patient. The treatment plan may also include a trial of NSAIDs for pain control, advising the patient of the possible side effects and instructing her to take it with food to protect the stomach.

The patient should be educated about workplace ergonomics and other lifestyle modifications such as stretching exercises to reduce reoccurrences.

Finally, schedule the patient for a return follow-up visit over several weeks to reassess the neck and recheck the blood pressure.

CASE 6

Clinical Setting: Family Practice Office
Fred Train—42-year-old male
CC: Fatigue

Vital Signs

Blood pressure: 165/98

Respirations: 16 per minute

Pulse: 62 bpm

Temperature: 98.4 degrees F

Weight: 315 lbs

Height: 5′11″

CASE 6	
Fred Train **42-year-old male** **CC: Fatigue**	
___ Addresses patient by name	
___ Introduces self and explains role	
___ Properly washes hands prior to touching patient	
___ What brings you in today?	I can't keep my eyes open and if I fall asleep at work one more time, I'm going to lose my job. (HDO)
Chronology/Onset	
___ When did it **start**?	I've been tired for a year, Doc.
___ Have you ever been evaluated for it?	They just say I'm fat and out of shape. (HDO)
___ Has it **changed** in any way?	I seem to fall asleep anytime I sit still for a couple of minutes.
Intensity	
___ Have you ever fallen asleep while driving?	No.
___ Fallen asleep while talking to someone?	Just my wife when we are going to bed. She gets mad. She'll be talking and I'm out in 30 seconds. (HDO)
Exacerbation	
___ Does anything **make it worse**?	I don't see how it can get any worse.
Remission	
___ Does anything **make it better**?	Even if I sleep all night I wake up tired. (HDO)
Symptoms Associated	
___ Do you **snore**?	My wife says I do.
___ Does your wife say you ever **stop breathing**?	I'd bet sometimes she'd like me to. (HDO)
___ Do you ever **wake yourself up**?	I have these dreams I can't breathe and jerk awake.
___ **Problems concentrating**?	Yeah, I'm getting in trouble at work. (HDO)

___ **Depression**?	No. Just frustrated.
___ **Anxiety or panic attacks**?	No.
___ **Mood swings**?	Little things seem to set me off sometimes. Then I feel stupid. (HDO)
___ **Headaches**?	Sometimes in the morning.
___ **Weight gain**?	How much did I weigh today?
___ **315.**	That's about 20 pounds more than I thought.
___ **Shortness of breath**?	No.
___ **Chest pain**?	No.
___ **Changes in bowel movements**?	No.
___ **Changes to your hair or skin**?	No.
___ **Lightheadedness**?	No.
SMASH FM	
Social History (FED TACOS)	
___ Can you describe your **diet**?	I'm a big guy. I eat a lot.
___ What kinds of foods?	Seefood—I see it, I eat it.
___ Do you **exercise** routinely?	I'm too tired to exercise. (HDO)
___ Have you ever used **tobacco**?	No.
___ Do you drink **alcohol**?	I have a couple of beers a night.
___ What's your **occupation**?	Computer repair.
___ Are you **sexually active**?	That's another thing my wife is mad about. It's hard to be interested when you're tired all the time.
___ Do you have any **medical** conditions?	I have low thyroid and high blood pressure.
___ When was the last time your labs were checked?	About six months ago.
___ Do you have any **allergies**?	No.
___ Any other **surgeries**?	No.

___ Any prior **hospitalizations**?	No.
___ **Medical conditions** that run in the **family**?	Weight's a problem for most of us.
___ Are you on any other **medications**?	Atenolol and Synthroid.
___ How many milligrams of atenolol?	I think that's 20.
___ How many times a day?	Once.
___ How many micrograms of Synthroid?	That one, I'm not sure of.
___ How many times a day?	Just once.
Physical Examination	
___ Informs patient that the physical exam is to begin and asks permission	
Vitals	
___ Repeats blood pressure with correct technique	
___ Uses appropriate cuff size	
___ Both arms	166/98 left arm,168/98 right arm
General Appearance	
___ Inspection	Obese, fatigued
Nose	
___ Inspection	Mucosa pink, no septal deviation or masses
___ Palpation	Patent bilaterally
Throat	
___ Inspection	Mucosa pink; no tonsillar or uvula hypertrophy; tongue of normal size
Neck	
___ Inspection	Measures 18 inches in diameter
___ Auscultation of carotids	No bruits
___ Palpation	No palpable thyromegaly

Cardiac	
____ Auscultation performed on bare skin	Distant; regular rhythm without gallop
____ Aortic, pulmonic, tricuspid, and mitral	No murmur
Respiratory	
____ Auscultation performed on bare skin	Distant but clear to auscultation
____ Complete inspiration and expiration	
____ Symmetrically	
____ Minimally 3 anterior, 2 lateral, and 3 posterior	
____ Assists the patient to seated position for posterior assessment	
Abdominal	
____ Helps patient to supine position	
____ Drapes lower extremities with sheet	
____ Inspection: properly exposes the abdomen	Obese, hypoactive bowel sounds
____ Auscultation prior to palpation	NABS × 4, no bruits
____ Palpation watching facial expression	Nontender without pulsatile masses
____ Assists patient to seated position	
Neurologic	
____ Mental status	Alert and oriented × 3
____ Motor strength testing	5/5 throughout
____ Reflexes	1/4 throughout
Extremities	
____ Inspection	No edema
Assessment	
____ Present patient with a proposed diagnosis	Sleep apnea
	Hypothyroidism

	Hypertension
	Elevated BMI
Plan/MOTHRR	
___ Medications	Antihypertensive class change
___ Testing	Sleep study. Laboratory assessment including thyroid function and CBC
___ Humanistic/Holistic	Patient education: symptoms related to sleep apnea, role of thyroid in weight gain
	Offers to provide information to wife
	Diet and exercise
___ Referral	Registered dietician
___ Return plan	Follow-up in next few weeks
Patient now completes Humanistic Domain Evaluation.	

Case 6 Review

Mr. Train is a 42-year-old male presenting to the office complaining of fatigue, which carries a broad differential diagnosis. Hypertension and elevated BMI are noted from the patient data sheet.

At the opening statement we quickly learn that the patient has a lot of anxiety surrounding the issue, with his job being at stake. The provider should recognize this and provide focused empathy and support throughout the visit. Though this has been occurring for some time, it appears to have been attributed only to his obesity and lack of physical fitness.

His falling asleep at work confirms daytime somnolence. Intensity can be assessed through questions regarding falling asleep while driving, watching TV, or participating in conversation with other people. If the patient admits to having a hard time staying awake while driving, the practitioner has an obligation to inform the Department of Motor Vehicles.

Symptoms associated focuses on other symptoms associated with sleep apnea: snoring, apnea, difficulty concentrating, morning headaches, weight gain, and mood swings are all positive. Other symptoms associated are added later after discovering a history of hypothyroidism and hypertension, concentrating on evidence of suboptimal therapy for his hypothyroidism and anemia, frequent causes of fatigue, and consequences of hypertension.

This patient is obese and has poor dietary and exercise habits. These can be addressed as part of the treatment plan, including educating the patient regarding calories from beverages such as beer or pop, which are often disregarded by patients as major sources of calories.

Review of his medications shows the patient is on a beta-blocker, which can also be a causative agent of fatigue. Consideration of antihypertensive class change is appropriate.

After completing the history, sleep apnea appears to be a likely diagnosis.

On physical exam the patient's BP should be

repeated, as the initial screening was high. The patient is not at goal, another reason for consideration of an adjustment in the patient's medication.

The patient is obese and appears fatigued. Inspection of the airways is appropriate. The oral pharynx should be examined for evidence of erythema, large tonsils and uvula, excessive soft tissue, and a prominent tongue, which are associated with sleep apnea. His neck diameter increases his risk for sleep apnea and inhibits adequate palpation of the thyroid.

Otherwise the physical exam is benign, with heart and lung sounds being distant as a result of the patient's obesity.

The patient should be evaluated for sleep apnea but has many possible contributing factors that must also be explored: suboptimal treatment of his hypothyroidism, medications, body mass, and lifestyle behaviors.

Prior to the patient's leaving the office, he should be educated on sleep apnea and the need for lifestyle modifications. Patient education is paramount. Identifying the stress being placed on both his work and his home life, time should be spent with both the patient and his wife to discuss the role sleep apnea is likely playing and the benefits to be expected from appropriate intervention, including weight loss, improvement in blood pressure, increased concentration, mood stabilization, and increase in libido.

The patient should be advised to follow a low-sodium, low-fat diet, with referral to a registered dietician. He should also limit his alcohol intake, avoiding it before bedtime. Exercise should be encouraged.

The patient should be scheduled to return to assess progress and monitor his blood pressure.

CASE 7

Clinical Setting: Family Practice Office
Arthur Falieur—67-year-old male
CC: Cough

Vital Signs

Blood pressure: 110/50

Respirations: 24 per minute

Pulse: 112 bpm

Temperature: 101 degrees F

Weight: 232 lbs

Height: 6′

CASE 7

Arthur Falieur
67-year-old male
CC: Cough

___ Addresses patient by name	
___ Introduces self and explains role	
___ Properly washes hands prior to touching patient	
___ What brings you in today?	I have a cough.
Chronology/Onset	
___ When did it **start**?	It's been building up the last couple of weeks.
___ Have you ever had this **before**?	No.
___ Has it **changed** in any way?	It keeps me up at night now. (HDO)
Description/Duration	
___ Can you **describe** the cough?	It's wet.
___ Are you bringing anything up?	Yes.
___ What color is it?	Whitish yellow.
Intensity	
___ How has it affected your **daily activities**?	I don't get out of the house much.
___ Why's that?	Walking makes me cough and I can't catch my breath. (HDO)
Exacerbation	
___ Does anything **make it worse**?	It's worse at night.
Remission	
___ Does anything **make it better**?	No. Cough medicine didn't help.
___ How often do you take it?	I tried a whole bottle over two days that I picked up at the store and it didn't touch it.

Symptoms Associated	
___ **Runny nose**?	No.
___ **Sore throat**?	Just a little from the coughing.
___ **Fever or chills**?	Haven't taken my temperature but I feel warm.
___ **Chest pain**?	My ribs are a little sore from the cough too. (HDO)
___ **Wheezing**?	No.
___ **Shortness of breath**?	Yes. I get winded just going to the kitchen.
___ **Shortness of breath lying flat**?	That's what I mean by worse at night. I have to sleep in my recliner.
___ **Waking up suddenly short of breath**?	No.
___ **Weight gain**?	I haven't measured myself.
___ **Swelling of your legs**?	Actually, they are swollen.
SMASH FM	
Social History (FED TACOS)	
___ Can you describe your **diet**?	I have high blood pressure so I try to avoid salt.
___ Do you **exercise** routinely?	I used to but now I get too short of breath. (HDO)
___ Have you ever used **tobacco**?	I used to smoke.
___ When did you quit?	Two weeks ago. (HDO)
___ How much did you smoke a day?	One pack.
___ How long have you been smoking?	Since I was about 16.
___ Do you drink **alcohol**?	No. I'm not a drinker.
___ What's your **occupation**?	I retired from sales.
___ Do you have any other **medical** conditions?	Just the high blood pressure.
___ Do you have any **allergies**?	No.
___ Any other **surgeries**?	No.
___ Any prior **hospitalizations**?	Once for pneumonia.

____ When was that?	A couple years ago.
____ **Medical conditions** that run in the **family**?	Some heart problems.
____ Do you know what kind of problems?	Dad had a heart attack at 43.
____ Are you on any other **medications**?	I was started on lisinopril a month ago.
____ How many milligrams?	25.
____ How many times a day?	Twice.
Physical Examination	
____ Informs patient that the physical exam is to begin and asks permission	
Vitals	
____ Repeats blood pressure with correct technique	
____ Uses appropriate cuff size	
____ Both arms	108/50 left arm, 108/52 right arm
____ Repeats pulse	Regular at 112 bpm
General Appearance	
____ Inspection	Mild accessory muscle use
HEENT	
____ Inspection of conjunctiva	Pink
____ Inspection of throat	No erythema or exudate
Neck	
____ Inspection at 45 degrees recumbency	3 cm JVD; no thyromegaly
____ Auscultation	No carotid or thyroid bruits
____ Palpation	No thyromegaly
Cardiac	
____ Inspection: properly exposes the chest	
____ Heave/PMI	No visible heave or PMI

___ Auscultation performed on bare skin	Regular rhythm, S3
___ Aortic, pulmonic, tricuspid, and mitral	No murmur
___ Palpation for PMI	Unable to locate
Respiratory	
___ Inspection	Mild accessory muscle use; no cyanosis; AP:lateral ratio 1:1.5
___ Auscultation performed on bare skin	Diminished basilar breath sounds
___ Complete inspiration and expiration	B/l lower lobe crackles
___ Symmetrically	Mild expiratory wheezes
___ Minimally 3 anterior, 2 lateral, and 3 posterior	
___ Palpation: tactile fremitus	Increased tactile fremitus b/l bases
___ Percussion	Dullness in b/l bases
Extremities	
___ Inspection	2+ peripheral edema
Assessment	
___ Presents patient with a proposed diagnosis	Heart failure
Plan/MOTHRR	
___ Referral	Advises patient of need for hospitalization
___ Humanistic/Holistic	Offers to contact family or support
	Confirms patient has transportation to the hospital.
Patient now completes Humanistic Domain Evaluation.	

Case 7 Review

Mr. Falieur presents with the complaint of cough. Reviewing the patient data sheet shows us that he has an elevated temperature and pulse with a relatively low blood pressure. This patient is ill. With the fever, infectious respiratory processes should be considered.

The cough began slowly over the last several weeks and keeps the patient from sleeping. It is described as being wet; however, "wet" does not mean productive of sputum, and this should be specifically questioned. The patient does have sputum, prompting the provider to ask the patient to describe what the sputum looks like. White, yellow sputum is more often associated with viral respiratory tract infections.

Regarding intensity, cough as a symptom does not scale well, such as, "How bad is your cough on a scale of 1 to 10?" However, intensity can be ascertained by defining how it affects the patient's activities of daily living (ADLs). Here the patient admits to staying at home. The provider should follow this answer with "Why?" By doing so, the provider learns that walking increases the cough, but more importantly causes shortness of breath. At this point, cardiac origins for the cough, such as heart failure, should be considered, as acute precipitations of heart failure may be caused by respiratory infections.

The patient's cough is "worse at night." Initially this may be interpreted as its being worse at the end of the day. We later discover that the patient meant when he lies down his cough and breathing get worse. The finding of orthopnea, along with shortness of breath walking to the kitchen (dyspnea on exertion), suggest heart failure as well. Though he has not weighed himself, he does admit to peripheral edema.

Positives for symptoms associated include mild sore throat and ribs, which the patient attributes to his persistent coughing. The patient should also be questioned about chest pain, as cardiac ischemia is also a common cause of heart failure.

The patient's social history could have misled the provider had the patient's response of "I used to smoke" not been followed up on. When a statement like this is made, the provider must explore it more deeply. Here we learn that the patient quit only two weeks ago after smoking a pack a day for around 50 years. Though the patient should be congratulated, the provider must suspect that once the acute illness has passed, the patient has a high likelihood of returning to smoking, and intervention should be offered.

The patient has a known history of hypertension, which makes his low screening blood pressure of even more concern. We also learn of a prior hospitalization for pneumonia, which should be considered in the differential, along with acute bronchitis associated with his significant smoking history.

Finally, a review of his medications reveals the recent addition of a new antihypertensive medication, an angiotensin-converting enzyme inhibitor, which may cause a persistent dry cough. It does not seem likely to be the primary cause of his cough, and would not account for the fever, but it should be taken under consideration.

On physical examination, the patient's blood pressure and pulse should be rechecked, noting tachycardia and relative hypotension on the patient data sheet. Rechecking the pulse allows the provider to determine if a dysrhythmia is present, such as atrial fibrillation, which is another common cause of heart failure. A regular rhythm is found here.

Moving head to toe, the conjunctiva should be assessed for pallor, as significant anemia may precipitate failure. A mild sore throat prompts examination for signs of upper respiratory tract infection.

The primary area for examination would be the respiratory and cardiac systems. Here we discover 3 cm jugular venous distention (JVD), crackles at the bases of his lungs, an S3, and peripheral edema, all of which point to heart failure. Decreased breath sounds, increased tactile fremitus, and dullness to percussion suggest consolidation associated with pulmonary edema.

Heart failure is a symptom. The etiology is still to be found. As you are in an outpatient setting, you should explain the likely diagnosis of heart failure, possibly related to respiratory tract infection.

The provider should discuss the need for hospitalization, facilitating transport and the involvement of the patient's family or support system.

Other diagnoses to include in the differential during SOAP note documentation may include hypotension (a possible ACEI side effect), cough, elevated BMI, tobacco use disorder, bronchitis, pneumonia, and history of hypertension.

CASE 8

Clinical Setting: Family Practice Office
Alfred Himmer—76-year-old male
CC: Forgetfulness

Vital Signs

Blood pressure: 128/68

Respirations: 12 per minute

Pulse: 72 bpm

Temperature: 98.0 degrees F

Weight: 128 lbs

Height: 5′8″

CASE 8	
Alfred Himmer **76-year-old male** **CC: Forgetfulness**	
____ Addresses patient by name	
____ Introduces self and explains role	
____ Properly washes hands prior to touching patient	
____ How can I help you today?	Well. I'm really getting forgetful and it's concerning me. (HDO)
Chronology/Onset	
____ When did you **first notice** it?	Quite a while ago, probably a year or so.
____ Have you ever had it **before**?	I've always had a tendency to be forgetful, but now it's starting to bother me.
____ Has it **changed** in any way?	I'm noticing it more often now.
Description/Duration	
____ Can you **describe** what you mean by forgetful?	I misplace my glasses all the time and when I'm in a store and run into someone I should know, I can't remember their names. It's embarrassing. (HDO)
____ You recognize them but can't remember their name?	Right.
Intensity	
____ Has it changed your **daily activities**?	Well, no. It just takes me longer to get out of the house when I can't find my keys.
Exacerbation	
____ Does anything **make it worse**?	I seem to make more **mistakes** when I am in a hurry.
____ What kind of mistakes?	Like leaving the lights on or the garage door open.
Remission	
____ Does anything **make it better**?	I'm sharper after a good night's rest.

___ How many hours of sleep do you get?	Usually about six or seven.
___ Any problems sleeping?	I wake up around 4 and sometimes turn on the radio, but then fall back asleep until 6.
Symptoms Associated	
___ **Fever or chills**?	No.
___ **Burning with urination**?	No.
___ **Slurred speech/facial droop**?	No.
___ **Numbness or tingling**?	No.
___ **Weakness** on one side of the body versus the other?	No.
___ **Balance problems or fallen**?	No.
___ **Anxiety or depression**?	No. I'm concerned but not depressed.
SMASH FM	
Social History (FED TACOS)	
___ Could you describe your **diet**?	I've become a pretty light eater.
___ Why is that?	I'm a widower. It's boring to cook for yourself. (HDO)
___ I'm sorry. When did you lose your wife?	Five years ago.
___ How are you coping with it?	I'm OK. I have a lot of friends. (HDO)
___ Do you **exercise** routinely?	Oh yes. I walk 5 miles every day. (HDO)
___ How much **caffeine** is in your diet?	Two cups of coffee in the morning.
___ Have you ever used **tobacco**?	No.
___ Do you drink **alcohol**?	Just a beer on bowling night.
___ What is your **occupation**?	Retired, electrician.
___ Do you have any **medical** conditions?	I used to get the gout now and then but since they told me what to avoid in my diet, I haven't had it since. (HDO)
___ Do you have any **allergies**?	No.

___ Any prior **surgeries**?	Appendix when I was 12.
___ Any prior **hospitalizations**?	Not other than that.
___ **Medical conditions** that run in the **family**?	Alzheimer's. Both my mom and dad.
___ Are they still living?	No. Mom died at 80 and Dad at 79. (HDO)
___ Are you on any **medications**?	No.
___ Herbals or supplements?	I take one multivitamin and one D a day.
Physical Examination	
___ Informs patient that the physical exam is to begin and asks permission	
General Assessment	
___ Inspection	Well developed, thin, in no distress.
Head	
___ Inspection	NCAT
Eyes	
___ Ophthalmoscopic examination	Cup:disc ratio 1:2 with sharp margins
Neck	
___ Inspection	Symmetrical
___ Auscultation of carotids	No bruits
Cardiac	
___ Auscultation performed on bare skin	Regular rhythm without rub or gallop
___ Aortic, pulmonic, tricuspid, and mitral	Without murmur
Respiratory	
___ Auscultation performed on bare skin	Clear to auscultation
___ Complete inspiration and expiration	
___ Symmetrically	
___ Minimally 3 anterior, 2 lateral, and 3 posterior	

Neurologic	
___ Mental status testing	29/30 on Mini Mental Status exam
___ Cranial nerve testing	CNII through XII intact
___ Motor strength testing—bilateral comparison	5/5 throughout
___ Reflexes	2/4 throughout, downgoing Babinski
___ Sensory	Intact to light touch, sharp/dull throughout
___ Cerebellar testing	Intact Romberg, finger/nose, RAM
Assessment	
___ Presents patient with a proposed diagnosis	Healthy male; common forgetfulness, mild anxiety, no signs of dementia
Plan/MOTHRR	
___ Testing	Laboratory analysis: CBC, chemistries, TSH, folic acid, B12, cholesterol
___ Humanistic/Holistic	Patient reassurance and education for monitoring of signs/symptoms
___ Return plan	Follow-up with lab results
Patient now completes Humanistic Domain Evaluation.	

Case 8 Review

Mr. Himmer is a 76-year-old male who brings himself in for forgetfulness, though it is common for family members to bring patients in for memory impairment concerns. The initial differential diagnosis should include Alzheimer's disease, stroke, cancer, infection, depression, and metabolic disturbance. With this introductory statement and throughout the case, empathy should be expressed, as the patient expresses obvious concern and embarrassment over increasing frequency of events.

Description plays a major role in this case. The provider should determine what the patient considers forgetfulness to mean. The patient describes misplacing his glasses and car keys. He also forgets the names of people he meets. This should be pursued more, clarifying that he does recognize their faces but can't place a name.

He admits to increased frequency of what he considers mistakes when he is in a hurry, which is not uncommon. His responding to remitting factors with "a good night's rest" should prompt the provider to inquire about sleeping patterns. Sleep disturbance is common with advancing age and can play a role in forgetfulness.

Intensity should be evaluated based on effect on his ADLs. Very little effect is found, with an apparently active social life with many friends, exercise, and bowling.

Symptoms associated should focus on ruling out common causes of mental status change and dementia. He exhibits no signs of infection (urinary tract infections being the most common cause of confusion in the elderly), cerebral ischemia, cerebellar dysfunction, or depression. There is a possible hint of anxiety.

When exploring the diet in social history, the provider should have noted a relatively low BMI from the patient data sheet. The patient is discovered to be a light eater, preferring not to cook for himself. The provider should express empathy at the loss of his wife and explore how he is coping. We learn he has adjusted well, leading away from depression as the primary diagnosis.

It is only when we get to family history that anxiety may be at the heart of his concern. Both of his parents had Alzheimer's dementia and died near 80 years of age, which he is now approaching.

There is no definite test available to diagnose Alzheimer's disease. The diagnosis is made through historical data, physical and neurologic examinations, and the use of diagnostic criteria.

The patient's vital signs are normal. He regularly exercises and has no significant risk factor for stroke. He should be examined for carotid bruits and papilledema, both of which are negative.

The physical examination should focus on a complete neurologic exam, including a mental status examination. No deficits are discovered.

In this case, reassurance should be offered and the suspicion of association with his parents' diagnosis openly discussed. Laboratory assessment is reasonable to rule out pathology and as health maintenance.

A follow-up appointment should be made to review lab results and reassess his anxiety.

CASE 9

Clinical Setting: Family Practice Office
Paine Shroder—48-year-old male
CC: Shoulder pain

Vital Signs

Blood pressure: 126/70

Respirations: 16 per minute

Pulse: 68 bpm

Temperature: 98.2 degrees F

Weight: 188 lbs

Height: 6′1″

CASE 9	
Paine Shroder **48-year-old male** **CC: Shoulder pain**	
___ Addresses patient by name	
___ Introduces self and explains role	
___ Properly washes hands prior to touching patient	
___ How can I help you today?	My shoulder hurts.
Chronology/Onset	
___ When did it **start**?	A couple weeks ago.
___ Did anything happen at the time?	I was probably just overusing it.
___ In what way?	I'm a roofer.
___ Have you ever had it **before**?	It's gotten sore now and then. Not like this.
___ Has it **changed** in any way?	No. It's just not getting any better.
Description/Duration	
___ Can you **describe** the pain?	It's like a bad toothache. (HDO)
___ **Where** is the pain?	Right here. (Rubs anterior left shoulder.)
___ Does the pain **radiate** [go] anywhere?	A little down into my bicep.
Intensity	
___ How bad is the pain on a scale from 1 to 10?	Like a 5. (HDO)
Exacerbation	
___ Does anything **make it worse**?	It starts to feel better by the end of the weekend, but as soon as I start using it again, it comes right back.
___ Any particular activity?	Lifting buckets of nails.
___ Which arm do you hammer with?	My right.

Remission	
___ Does anything **make it better**?	Icy Hot helps.
___ How often are you using that?	I usually put it on at bedtime.
Symptoms Associated	
___ **Swelling**?	No.
___ **Redness**?	No.
___ **Limited range of motion**?	I did notice it hurts to lift something straight out in front of me.
___ **Numbness or tingling**?	No.
___ **Weakness**?	I don't know if it's weakness or just pain, but I can't lift as much with that arm now.
___ **Neck pain**?	No.
___ **Chest pain**?	No.
___ **Nausea or vomiting**?	No.
___ **Shortness of breath**?	No.
SMASH FM	
Social History (FED TACOS)	
___ Could you describe your **diet**?	I eat pretty healthily.
___ Do you **exercise** routinely?	I play softball.
___ Has this affected your ability to play?	Just batting; I'm right handed.
___ Have you ever used **tobacco**?	No.
___ Do you drink **alcohol**?	A couple beers Thursdays after the game.
___ Do you use any **recreational drugs**?	No.
___ Do you have any **medical** conditions?	No.
___ Do you have any **allergies**?	No.
___ Any prior **surgeries**?	Nothing big. Stitches here and there.

___ Any prior **hospitalizations**?	No.
___ **Medical conditions** that run in the **family**?	Not really.
___ Any heart attacks or strokes?	Not that I know of.
___ Are you on any **medications**?	No.
Physical Examination	
___ Informs patient that the physical exam is to begin and asks permission	
General Assessment	
___ Inspection	Well developed, no apparent distress
Neck	
___ Inspection	Symmetrical
___ Range of motion	Full active range of motion
___ Auscultation of carotids	No bruits
___ Palpation	Nontender
Cardiac	
___ Auscultation performed on bare skin	Regular rhythm without rub or gallop
___ Aortic, pulmonic, tricuspid, and mitral	Without murmur
Respiratory	
___ Auscultation performed on bare skin	Clear to auscultation
___ Complete inspiration and expiration	
___ Symmetrically	
___ Minimally 3 anterior, 2 lateral, and 3 posterior	
Musculoskeletal	
Shoulders	
___ Exposes bilateral shoulders	

___ Inspection	Muscle mass symmetrical without erythema, ecchymosis, edema, or lesions
___ Range of motion—bilateral comparison	Left side hesitant but full AROM
___ Palpation	Point tenderness in left bicipital groove
Special Testing: Speeds and Yergason Tests	Positive
Neurologic	
___ Upper extremity strength testing—b/l	4/5 left elbow flexion with pain otherwise 5/5 throughout
___ Upper extremity reflexes	2/4 throughout
Assessment	
___ Presents patient with a proposed diagnosis	Bicipital tendonitis
Plan/MOTHRR	
___ Medications	NSAIDs
___ OMM	Counterstrain, myofascial release
___ Humanistic/Holistic	Assesses need for work restrictions; offers to involve others in treatment plan, including employer; aggravating factor avoidance; stretching exercises
___ Return plan	Follow-up with lab results
Patient now completes Humanistic Domain Evaluation.	

Case 9 Review

Mr. Shroder is a 48-year-old roofer who presents with left shoulder pain. The patient data sheet shows normal vital signs.

The patient's pain has been occurring for the last several weeks. In cases of possible injury, events occurring at time of onset should be discerned. Though no trauma is noted, he does describe overuse as a possible cause. This prompts the provider to inquire as to what "overuse" is occurring, revealing his occupation as a roofer. He suggests improvement with rest, as the pain is improving by the end of the weekend but returns when he begins working again. Look for specific activities associated with the pain. It may have been assumed that repetitive hammering has caused his injury; however, we find that he actually hammers with his right but lifts pails of nails with his left.

Although the case seems straightforward for musculoskeletal injury, other more serious causes of the shoulder pain must be considered. Your differential diagnosis initially should include musculoskeletal etiology and myocardial infarction. He has had the pain for the past couple weeks and denies chest pain, nausea, and shortness of breath. He does not smoke or have a history of HTN or dyslipidemia, which makes a cardiac cause less likely.

Other symptoms associated point toward musculoskeletal etiology, with limited range of motion and apprehension in lifting.

On physical exam, consider possible etiologies for shoulder pain: The shoulder is primary but also consider cervical radiculopathy. Examination of the neck is benign.

Begin the shoulder examination with proper exposure. There is no asymmetry in muscle mass or evidence of localized inflammation. No bulging mass is seen to suggest bicipital rupture. Though the patient was apprehensive, he was able to move the shoulders through full ranges of motion. If active range of motion is limited, passive range of motion should be assessed.

Palpation reveals tenderness in the bicipital groove. Speeds test, attempted shoulder flexion from 30 degrees with elbow straight and forearm supinated, is positive. Yergason test, attempted pronation of the forearm against resistance with the arm in adduction and elbow bent at 90 degrees, is also positive, suggesting bicipital tendonitis. No other neurologic deficits are found.

The patient should be treated conservatively with therapy localized to the shoulder, such as anti-inflammatory medications. Manipulation may include techniques such as counterstrain, myofascial, and Spencer's.

The effect of the condition on his employability should be discussed. Rest and lifting restrictions should be advised, though it may not be possible for the patient to comply with them if his financial security requires him to work without available sick time or change of duties.

The patient should participate in home range-of-motion exercises. If improvement has not occurred at follow-up, referral to physical therapy should be considered.

CASE 10

Clinical Setting: OB/Gyn Office
Imissa Mimencies—22-year-old female
CC: No period × 3 months

Vital Signs

Blood pressure: 110/60

Respirations: 12 per minute

Pulse: 60 bpm

Temperature: 98.2 degrees F

Weight: 105 lbs

Height: 5′4″

CASE 10	
Imissa Mimencies **22-year-old female** **CC: No period × 3 months**	
___ Addresses patient by name	
___ Introduces self and explains role	
___ Properly washes hands prior to touching patient	
___ How can I help you today?	I haven't had my period.
Chronology/Onset	
___ **First Day Last Menstrual Period** (FDLMP)?	About 4 months ago.
___ Have you ever missed a period **before**?	No.
___ Have your periods **changed** at all before this?	They seemed to be getting lighter, then just stopped.
Gynecologic Hx	
___ Were your periods regular before this?	Yes, until about a year ago, then they started to get a little unpredictable.
___ How many days were they normally?	About 28.
___ How long do they usually last?	About 3 days.
___ Describe the flow as heavy, medium, or light.	Light each day.
___ Age at first period?	11.
Sexual History	
___ Are you sexually active?	Yes.
___ Do you use protection?	Yes.
___ What form of protection do you use?	We use the rhythmic cycle.
___ Have you ever been pregnant?	No.
___ How would you feel about being pregnant?	Do you think I'm pregnant? (HDO)
___ Responds to patient's question.	I'm not sure how I would feel about that.

Symptoms Associated	
___ **Breast tenderness or enlargement**?	They're a little sore after I run.
___ **Discharge from the breasts**?	No.
___ **Nausea or vomiting**?	I'm a little nauseated after I run.
___ **Fatigue, cold intolerance, weight gain**?	No.
___ **Abdominal pain**?	No.
___ **Visual changes**?	No.
SMASH FM	
Social History (FED TACOS)	
___ Could you describe your **diet**?	I'm a vegan.
___ How many calories a day?	About 1500.
___ How much do you run (exercise)?	10 miles a day. (HDO)
___ Have you ever used **tobacco**?	No.
___ Do you drink **alcohol**?	No.
___ Do you use any **recreational drugs**?	No.
___ What is your **occupation**?	I'm a yoga instructor.
___ Do you have any **medical** conditions?	No.
___ Do you have any **allergies**?	No.
___ Any prior **surgeries**?	No.
___ Any prior **hospitalizations**?	No.
___ **Medical conditions** that run in the **family**?	Cancer. My father has prostate cancer and my mother died at 50 from breast cancer. (HDO)
___ Are you on any **medications**?	No.
___ Herbals or supplements?	I take a VegaVit. It's a multivitamin to replace what you would get in meat.

Physical Examination	
____ Informs patient that the physical exam is to begin and asks permission	
General Assessment	
____ Inspection	Alert, thin, appears shy, glancing to the floor often
HEENT	
____ Assess for facial hair	No facial hair
____ Assess peripheral fields	Intact
____ Inspection of teeth for erosions	No erosions
Neck	
____ Inspection	Symmetrical, without masses
____ Palpation	No thyromegaly or masses
Cardiac	
____ Auscultation performed on bare skin	Regular rhythm without rub or gallop
____ Aortic, pulmonic, tricuspid, and mitral	Without murmur
Respiratory	
____ Auscultation performed on bare skin	Clear to auscultation
____ Complete inspiration and expiration	
____ Symmetrically	
____ Minimally 3 anterior, 2 lateral, and 3 posterior	
Abdominal	
____ Helps patient to supine position	
____ Drapes lower extremities with sheet	
____ Inspection: properly exposes the abdomen	Scaphoid
____ Auscultation prior to palpation	NABS × 4
____ Palpation watching facial expression	Nontender without masses

Genitalia	
___ Advises breast exam (not performed)	Nontender without discharge
___ Advises pelvic exam (not performed)	
___ Performed with assistant in the room	
___ Assists patient to seated position	
Assessment	
___ Presents patient with a proposed diagnosis	Secondary amenorrhea
Plan/MOTHRR	
___ Testing	Office pregnancy test; if negative, consider prolactin, FSH
___ Humanistic/Holistic	Educates patient on possible cause of low body mass and exercise; discuss preferences and options for pregnancy prevention; offer to involve others in treatment plan
___ Return plan	Follow-up time based on lab results and need to monitor
Patient now completes Humanistic Domain Evaluation.	

Case 10 Review

Imissa presents with a concern of missing her period for the last three cycles. The differential diagnosis should minimally include pregnancy, thyroid dysfunction, exercise-induced anovulation, and eating disorders.

In this case, the patient presents complaining of no menses for a precise period of time. History of prior menses should be explored, as never having had a menses is considered primary amenorrhea, while having menses that then cease is considered secondary amenorrhea.

Many of the components of CODIERS are not pertinent to the case, such as description, intensity, and exacerbating and remitting factors. Providers should not let this throw them off. Simply consider each component. If it cannot be related to the case, check it off and move on to the next.

Following the standard pattern, the three components of chronology are ascertained: onset, prior history of the same, and changes that have occurred. Here we learn that her menses have been getting lighter. This should prompt the provider to elicit a detailed gynecologic history.

It is important to define menarche (the age at first menstruation), if and when the menstrual cycle became regular, how many days apart the menses occur, and how many days each lasts. In addition, it is also important to quantify the amount of bleeding that occurs, often categorized as light, moderate, or heavy flow. This can be quantified by asking the number of tampons or pads used per day if need be. Often patients will present not with an absent menses but with a change from baseline. Specifically asking how the menses has changed is important.

The most common cause of secondary amenorrhea is pregnancy. Providers are often hesitant to take a sexual history. The topic should be introduced in the same way as inquiring about allergies:

- Do you have any allergies?
- Are you sexually active?

The two questions should sound exactly the same in tone.

In this case, it is likely obvious to the patient why a sexual history should be assessed. If the connection is less obvious, sensitive questions may be introduced through statements such as, "I have to ask you some questions that we ask everyone who comes in with a concern like yours. These questions will help us in making the right diagnosis and treatment plan for you." This tells the patient that you are not judging him/her or implying anything, but simply trying to provide the best possible care. For example, in the male patient who presents with a rectal complaint, the introductory statement may be made, then, at some point, simply asking if anything is ever inserted into the rectum allows the patient to answer as freely as possible.

This patient is sexually active and uses the rhythm method for birth control. In other cases, defining sexual activity may require more explanation. Some people define sexual activity only as having intercourse where penetration occurs. Penetration, however, is not necessary for pregnancy to occur. You may also have to ask if there has been any contact whatsoever to sperm or body fluids. In any case, amenorrhea in females of reproductive age requires evaluation by a pregnancy test.

As the presenting complaint and history do not suggest sexually transmitted infection as a possible diagnosis, the sexual history may be limited in this regard. We are trying to ascertain the likelihood of pregnancy. By asking about the method of birth control, using the "rhythm method" suggests male partners and the possibility of pregnancy. If we had not gleaned this answer, it may have been appropriate to ask whether the patient has sex with men, women, or both, as she may be sexually active but have no chance of pregnancy as her partner is female.

When asking about past pregnancies, the patient asks if she is pregnant. The provider should ascertain how the patient would feel about being pregnant if she were. Would this be a happy occurrence or one of stress? Here the patient should be assured that there are other causes for missed menses that need to be evaluated. The provider must also not allow his/her own prejudices to interfere with patient care. Though you must explore the patient's support system, you should not immediately follow the question of how she would feel about being pregnant with, "Are you married?" implying that she should be.

The symptoms associated focus on symptoms related to pregnancy and the other causes of secondary amenorrhea. Though she has a little breast tenderness and nausea, she relates these to occurring after running. The provider may follow this lead now, obtaining details about her exercise patterns instead of waiting to ask during the inquiry of social history. She runs 10 miles per day.

Symptoms associated with hypothyroidism and pituitary disease, both causes of secondary amenorrhea, are denied. Hypothyroidism should have been considered unlikely with the patient's body habitus and BMI.

The social history reveals a vegan diet with what initially appears to be a good caloric intake; however, we also learn that in addition to running she is a yoga instructor. Her caloric intake may not be supporting her level of activity and may be evident by her BMI. With this caloric intake, anorexia nervosa is not suspected. Suppression of the hypothalamic pituitary access is more likely with her low BMI.

Humanistic domain characteristics should be expressed on learning the patient's family history with the loss of her mother. Is such a loss a driving factor for the patient's level of focus on her own health care, including her level of exercise and diet?

The physical exam focuses on pregnancy and ruling out secondary causes of amenorrhea. Facial hair may have been associated with androgen excess and polycystic ovarian disease, peripheral fields with pituitary adenoma, and tooth erosions with self-induced vomiting and eating disorder.

The patient does not have physical findings suggestive of a thyroid disorder, such as weight gain or thyromegaly. The abdominal exam shows no uterine enlargement. Both a breast exam and pelvic exam would be indicated. There was no galactorrhea or other signs of pituitary disease or pregnancy.

The most likely diagnosis for the patient is secondary amenorrhea due to suppression of the hypothalamic pituitary access from her low BMI. A pregnancy test should be performed, with further testing considered if negative.

Patient education of the cause would reassure her. As she shows astuteness in her own health care, taking a supplement to support her vegan diet, she may be able to increase her caloric intake to meet the demand.

CHAPTER 17

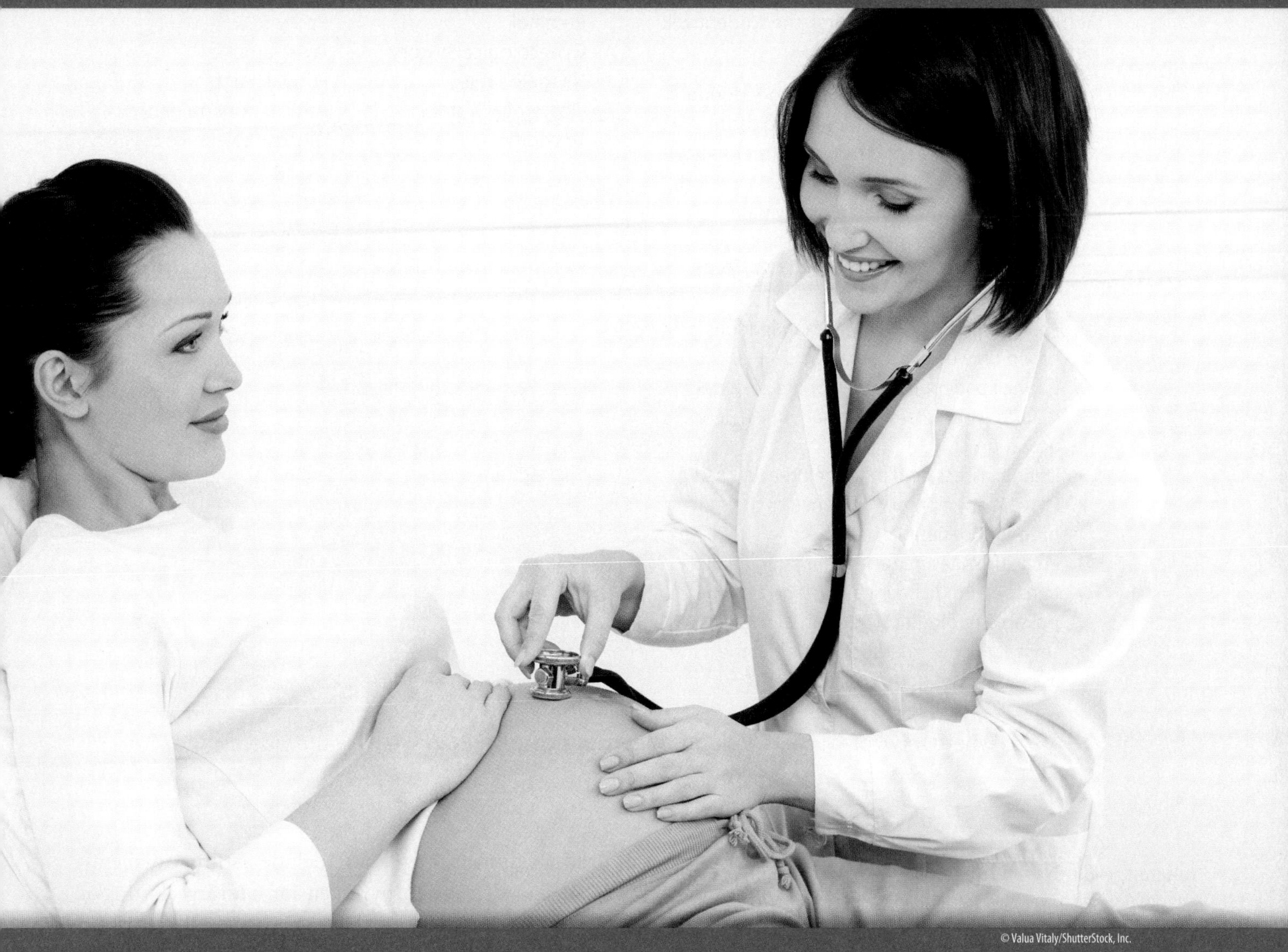

© Valua Vitaly/ShutterStock, Inc.

The Pregnant Patient

Andrea Skomo, DO
Krystle Lappinen, MD

OBJECTIVES

At the conclusion of this chapter, the student will be able to

1. Obtain a complete medical history during the first prenatal visit, identifying those conditions increasing risk to the pregnancy
2. Given the first day of last menstrual period, calculate the estimated delivery date through the use of Naegele's rule
3. Document obstetrical history through the use of TPAL
4. Perform prenatal physical examinations based on weeks of gestation
5. Council patients on appropriate prenatal laboratory assessment based on weeks of gestation
6. Define, assess, and manage preeclampsia
7. Provide anticipatory guidance to the pregnant patient
8. Properly measure fundal height in relation to expected gestational age and provide possible etiologies when variation exists
9. Utilize glucose tolerance testing in the assessment of gestational diabetes

KEY TERMS

Prenatal
Gynecological history
Naegele's rule
Obstetrical history
Gravidity
Parity
Preeclampsia
Fundal height
Anticipatory guidance
Glucose tolerance test

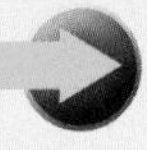

Where this icon appears, visit **go.jblearning.com/HPECWS** to view the video.

Prenatal: period of time from onset of pregnancy to delivery

At the first **prenatal** visit, a thorough history and physical examination should be performed. It is important to gather information about the patient, her family, the father of the baby, and his family. At the subsequent prenatal visits, only a limited physical needs to be performed. This chapter explains the examination of the pregnant patient at each visit.

First Prenatal Visit

HISTORY

Past Medical History

Obtain the history as you would with any patient. Some medical conditions that are important to know about during pregnancy include asthma, diabetes, anemia, depression, hypertension, and any clotting or bleeding disorders. Be sure to ask how well-controlled the condition is, whether the patient has ever been hospitalized for any of her medical conditions, and about any medications she takes for them.

Past Surgical History

Past surgeries that may have relevance during pregnancy include any surgery on the cervix such as a loop electrocautery excision procedure (LEEP), cone biopsy, or cryotherapy, and any abdominal surgery. Also document any problems that the patient may have had with anesthesia during or following prior surgeries.

Past Gynecological History

Begin the **gynecological history** by determining the patient's age of menarche, the number of days between cycles, the number of days her menses typically lasts, when her last menstrual period was, and any irregularities in her cycles. If the patient knows the first day of her last menstrual period and has no history of irregular cycles, her estimated date of delivery can be determined using **Naegele's rule**:

- Take the first day of the patient's LMP — May 25, 2013
- Add one year — May 25, 2014
- Subtract three months — February 25, 2014
- And add one week — March 4, 2014

Ask the patient if she has ever had an abnormal Pap smear. If so, determine what was done in follow-up, documenting procedures such as colposcopy, cervical biopsies, LEEPs, cryotherapy, and cone biopsies. Determine the date and results of the most recent evaluation.

It is also important to know if the patient has any history of any sexually transmitted infections (STIs), as well as their treatments and outcomes. Specifically ask about gonorrhea, chlamydia, herpes, syphilis, and HIV.

Past Obstetrical History

In obtaining the **obstetrical history**, it is important to know the total number of times the patient has been pregnant (**gravidity**) and how many children she has delivered (**parity**). It is also important to know if the patient delivered her previous children at full term or preterm and how many living children she has. Also ask about spontaneous abortions (miscarriages) and elective abortions. This information is recorded in the chart as the patient's gravidity and parity. Gravidity is the total number of times the patient has been pregnant, including the current pregnancy. Parity is separated into term deliveries, preterm deliveries, abortions (spontaneous and elective), and living children (TPAL). Some providers use "F," for full-term delivery, in place of "T" (FPAL).

For example, if a woman who presents for her first prenatal visit has had two full-term deliveries and one miscarriage and has two living children, her gravidity and parity would be written as G3 (three total pregnancies) P2 (two term deliveries) 0 (no preterm deliveries) 1 (one abortion) 2 (two living children): G3P2012.

If the patient has had previous pregnancies and deliveries, ask how many weeks' gestational age she was when she delivered, the route by which she delivered (vaginal or caesarean), and how much the baby weighed. If the patient delivered vaginally, determine whether it was a spontaneous or operative (vacuum or forceps) delivery. Also ask if the patient had any tears and, if she did, what degree of tear she had.

If the previous pregnancies resulted in caesarean section, ask if the patient labored at all and what the reason was for performing the caesarean section. Also ask about plans for delivery of this pregnancy. If the patient would like to try to deliver a baby vaginally after a caesarean section, you must determine the kind of incision that was made on her uterus: classical (vertical) or transverse. If the patient has had two or fewer caesarean sections and had a low transverse uterine incision, she is a candidate for a trial of labor after caesarean (TOLAC). Many patients may not know the direction of incision. Attempt to obtain medical records if this is the case.

If the patient has had a miscarriage, be sure to ask whether she needed to have a dilation and curettage.

Social History

Ask the patient's relationship status—single, married, or divorced—and if the father of the baby is involved. Also ask about support at home. Ask about tobacco, alcohol, and drug use. Patient education will be of utmost importance. Inquire about willingness to quit and how you can assist the patient so that the attempt at cessation is a success.

Medications

List all medications that the patient is currently taking. It is important to know what medications are safe to use during pregnancy. Do not assume that the patient's other providers would have adjusted medications once the patient became pregnant. If you are unsure of the medication's effect on pregnancy, look up each one,

Gynecological history: medical history regarding such information as age at menarche, number of days between cycles, number of days menses lasts, first day of last menstrual period, cycle irregularities, and history of STI

Naegele's rule: estimation of delivery date calculated by taking the first day of last menstrual period, adding one year, subtracting three months, and adding one week

Obstetrical history: medical history regarding such information as attempts at achieving pregnancy, prior pregnancies, and the outcomes

Gravidity: total number of times the patient has been pregnant

Parity: total number of children delivered

Preeclampsia: development of hypertension after 20 weeks of pregnancy in association with protein in the urine

document the effect, and discuss it with the patient. Consultation with her other providers is indicated to coordinate medication changes or cessation.

Advise all women of childbearing age that they should take 0.4 mg of folic acid daily whether planning to conceive or not.

Family History

The family history is very important in the evaluation of a pregnant patient. However, it is also important to learn about the history of the father of the baby and his family as well. Any history of congenital problems is especially important in the evaluation of the pregnant patient.

PHYSICAL EXAM

Height, Weight, and BMI

Measure a baseline height and weight of the patient. Calculate the BMI.

Vital Signs

Assess vital signs including temperature, pulse, respirations, and blood pressure. During pregnancy, a woman's blood pressure is typically lower than her normal blood pressure. Blood pressure reaches its nadir in the second trimester and then begins to return to levels closer to the patient's normal range. It is important to get an accurate blood pressure reading at every visit. Blood pressures greater than 140/90 are concerning for preeclampsia (pregnancy-induced hypertension). However, if a pregnant patient's blood pressure is elevated before 20 weeks, it is likely that she has chronic hypertension. Other causes of elevated blood pressure or **preeclampsia** prior to 20 weeks include multiple gestations and molar pregnancy. After 20 weeks, new onset of elevated blood pressure is more concerning for the development of preeclampsia.

General Appearance

Assess the general appearance of the patient. Look for signs of distress. Emotional distress is common in unplanned pregnancies and may lead to or exacerbate depression and anxiety. As the pregnancy advances, fatigue may become apparent.

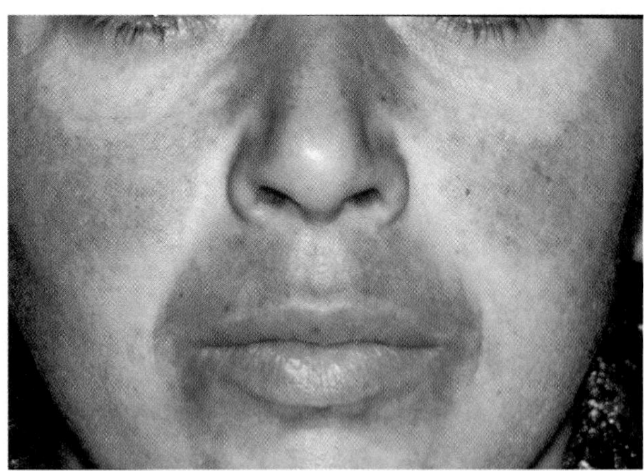

FIGURE 17-1 Melasma.
© BSIP/Photo Researchers, Inc.

Integumentary

A discussion of dermatologic changes at the first prenatal visit will educate the patient on changes that are likely to occur, and will give the provider an opportunity to offer reassurance before the patient has unnecessary concern. Increases in skin pigmentation are very common during pregnancy. Hyperpigmentation of the face is called melasma, or the mask of pregnancy (see **FIGURE 17-1**). The patient should be assured that if it occurs it will typically resolve within one year without treatment.

Stretch marks (striae gravidarum) are also very common, occurring mostly on the abdomen, breasts, and legs (see **FIGURE 17-2**). Patients will often question if there is a way to prevent their occurrence, but no clinical studies have demonstrated effectiveness of preventive treatment. Stretch marks often fade but do not disappear completely.

It is not uncommon for moles to change appearance under the hormonal influence of pregnancy. Advise the patient to be observant for and to alert you to any changes in lesions consistent with melanoma: asymmetry, border irregularity, color variation, or diameter greater than 6 mm. Angiomas are also common.

Scalp hair may become thicker, and facial hair may develop. Patients should be advised that following delivery hair loss is common but not permanent.

HEENT

Sinus and nasal mucosa edema is common during pregnancy. This may lead to sinus pressure, frontal or

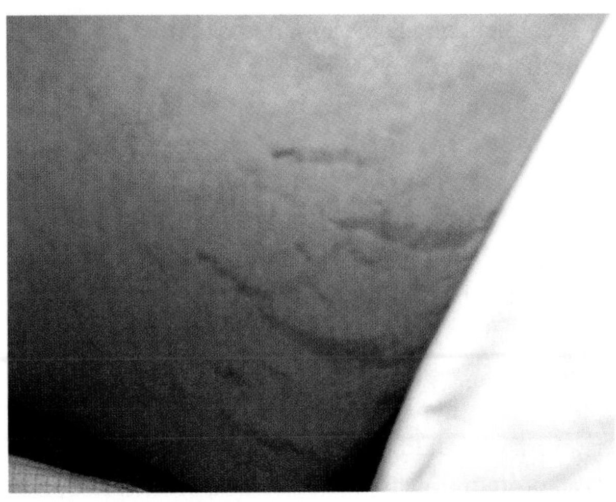

FIGURE 17-2 Striae gravidarum.

facial headaches, and difficulty breathing through the nose. Gingival hypertrophy may also occur.

Cardiovascular

Perform a detailed cardiovascular assessment. The development of systolic ejection murmurs is common in pregnant patients. Document the presence of murmurs at the initial exam and any subsequent development. Varicosities may develop along with palmar erythema and facial flushing.

Respiratory

Note any adventitious sounds. Depth of respirations decreases as uterine height increases late in pregnancy.

Abdominal

Palpate the abdomen for tenderness, masses, and organomegaly. **Fundal height** should be measured if palpable.

Extremities

Inspect for baseline edema, calf tenderness, and erythema.

Genitourinary

Examine external genitalia for lesions that may be transmittable to the fetus at delivery, such as herpes genitalis or condyloma. A speculum exam should be performed and Pap smear obtained if the patient has not had one within the last year. Obtain cultures for gonorrhea and chlamydia, and a wet prep to check for bacterial vaginosis, yeast, and trichomonas.

Fundal height: height of the uterus as measured from the pubic symphysis to the fundus

Perform the bimanual exam, gently palpating the uterus to determine its size and position: midposition, anteverted, or retroverted. Palpate the adnexa for size, shape, masses, and tenderness.

LABORATORY ANALYSIS

Blood work collected at the first prenatal visit includes a CBC with differential, blood type and Rh factor with antibody screen, hepatitis B, HIV, varicella, rubella, TSH, and RPR (syphilis). If the patient is rubella or varicella nonimmune, she should receive the vaccine postpartum.

A clean-catch urine sample should be collected. A point-of-care test, urine dipstick, should be performed to check for glucose, ketones, blood, and protein. A urinalysis should be performed and sent for microscopic analysis and cultures. A pregnant patient with asymptomatic bacteriuria should be treated to prevent the development of pyelonephritis.

If the patient has diabetes or a history of preeclampsia, a 24-hour urine collection for protein should be collected.

GENETIC SCREENING

At the first prenatal visit, discuss the options for genetic testing with your patient. Genetic screening identifies the risk of delivering a child with Down syndrome, trisomy 18, and trisomy 13. The specific tests performed depend on the gestational age of the patient.

First-trimester screening can be performed between weeks 9 and 13. This test includes ultrasound measurement of nuchal translucency, beta hCG, and pregnancy-associated plasma protein (PAPP-A). First-trimester screening does not screen for neural tube defects.

Second-trimester screening can be performed between weeks 15 and 20. This test measures beta hCG, MSAFP, unconjugated estriol, and inhibin A.

Integrated screening is performed in both the first and second trimesters. With this screening test, the patient does not receive any results until all of the

Anticipatory guidance: provision of information surrounding anticipated conditions or findings prior to their occurrence to aid in their identification and preparation of responses

testing is completed. Between 10 and 13 weeks, nuchal translucency and PAPP-A are measured. In the second trimester, between 15 and 18 weeks, unconjugated estriol and inhibin are measured.

Stepwise sequential testing uses the first-trimester portion of the integrated screen (nuchal translucency and PAPP-A). Women whose results show a high risk for having an infant with a chromosomal abnormality are then offered chorionic villus sampling (CVS) for definitive diagnosis. Those who are not high-risk can go on to complete the second-trimester portion of the screening.

PREECLAMPSIA

Preeclampsia is the development of hypertension after 20 weeks of pregnancy in association with protein in the urine, and is one of the most common conditions associated with pregnancy and one of the primary reasons for the recommended frequency of follow-up visits. If blood pressures begin to elevate, a 24-hour urine collection is indicated to assess for protein. A preeclampsia panel should be ordered, which includes CBC with differential, BMP, liver panel, uric acid, and LDH.

The diagnosis of preeclampsia requires two blood pressure readings > 140 systolic and/or > 90 diastolic at least six hours apart and proteinuria of 300 mg in 24 hours. Severe preeclampsia requires blood pressure readings of > 160 systolic and/or > 100 diastolic with two readings six hours apart and proteinuria of 5 grams or more in 24 hours.

Management of mild preeclampsia includes:

- Delivery if full-term
- Non-stress Test (NST) twice weekly
- Biophysical profile every other week

Management of severe preeclampsia includes:

- Delivery
- Considering betamethasone for fetal lung maturity
- Monitoring labs closely (platelets, LFTs)
- Magnesium sulfate

Magnesium sulfate is started for seizure prophylaxis. A 4-gram bolus is followed by infusion at 2 grams per hour and is continued until 24 hours postpartum.

A patient on magnesium needs to be evaluated for signs of toxicity every two hours. Signs of magnesium toxicity include hyporeflexia, respiratory suppression, and cardiovascular collapse. The patient should be advised to report and be frequently assessed for chest pain, shortness of breath, and generalized weakness. Frequent examination of the heart, lungs, and reflexes is required. Hyporeflexia is the first sign of magnesium toxicity. The treatment for magnesium sulfate toxicity is 1 gram of calcium gluconate via IV push.

Chronic hypertension with superimposed preeclampsia should be suspected in women with new-onset proteinuria, hypertension and proteinuria prior to 20 weeks, sudden increase in blood pressure in a normally well-controlled hypertensive patient, platelet count less than 100,000, or elevated liver enzymes.

ANTICIPATORY GUIDANCE

Anticipatory guidance surrounds common concerns at the first prenatal visit, including nausea, exercise, diet, cramping, and sexual intercourse.

Nausea

Advise the patient to eat small, frequent meals and to drink plenty of fluids. Some over-the-counter recommendations include vitamin B6, ginger supplement, and unisom. If none of this is effective, the patient may be prescribed Zofran or Phenergan for unremitting nausea and vomiting.

Exercise

Patients should remain active during pregnancy. Thirty minutes of moderate activity most days of the week is recommended during pregnancy. As the pregnancy progresses, some modifications of the patient's exercise routine may need to be made.

Diet

Advise the patient to eat a well-balanced diet. An additional 300 calories a day is recommended during pregnancy. Expected weight gain is frequently questioned.

Recommended weight gain during pregnancy is based on BMI.

- Low BMI (< 19.8): 28–40 lbs
- Normal BMI (19.8–26): 25–35 lbs

- Overweight BMI (26–29): 15–25 lbs
- Obese BMI (> 29): at least 15 lbs

Cramping

Patients may experience cramping throughout the pregnancy. Typically cramping is not concerning. However, cramping and bleeding together are concerning and patients should be advised to call immediately if they experience either.

Intercourse

Sexual intercourse is safe throughout pregnancy. Advise patients that they may experience light spotting after intercourse because the cervix is more friable during pregnancy, though heavy bleeding is never normal. Patients also may experience cramping after intercourse.

Exam Based on Weeks of Gestation

FIRST PRENATAL TO 28 WEEKS

From the first prenatal visit until 28 weeks, the patient should be seen every 4 weeks. At each visit inquire about vaginal bleeding, discharge, leakage of fluid, cramping, swelling, and fetal movement. Patients typically do not feel fetal movement until about 18 to 20 weeks. Multiparous women may feel movement slightly earlier.

At each visit, it is important to record the patient's height, weight, and blood pressure. Obtain a clean-catch urine sample for protein testing.

At around 10 weeks, fetal heart tones should be obtainable using a Doppler. Normal fetal heart rate is between 110 and 160 beats per minute. If you are unable to find heart tones with a Doppler, the patient should be sent for an ultrasound to assess for fetal well-being.

Between 18 and 20 weeks, the patient should be sent for an anatomy scan to ensure that the fetus is structurally normal. At this time, the sex of the fetus can typically be detected and disclosed if the patient would like to know. Inquire about her perception of fetal movements.

Starting at 20 weeks, the fundal height should be measured and recorded. The measurement is from the top of the pubic bone (see **FIGURE 17-3A**) to the fundus of the uterus (see **FIGURES 17-3B** and **17-3C**). At 20 weeks, the fundus should be at the level of the umbilicus. After 20 weeks, the fundal height should correspond with the gestational age +/– 2 cm. If the difference is greater than 2 cm, the patient should be sent for an ultrasound to assess fetal growth. If the fundal height is greater than the gestational age, there is concern for multiple gestation, macrosomia, and polyhydramnios. If the fundal height is measuring less than the gestational age, there is concern for intrauterine growth restriction and oligohydramnios. Another reason for size greater than or less than dates could be inaccurate dating, and the patient may be further along or not as far along as she thinks she is.

Between 24 and 28 weeks, a one-hour **glucose tolerance test** should be performed. For this test, the patient drinks 50 grams of glucola. One hour after the

Glucose tolerance test: laboratory assessment measuring blood glucose levels following ingestion of oral glucose, which can be used in the diagnosis of gestational diabetes

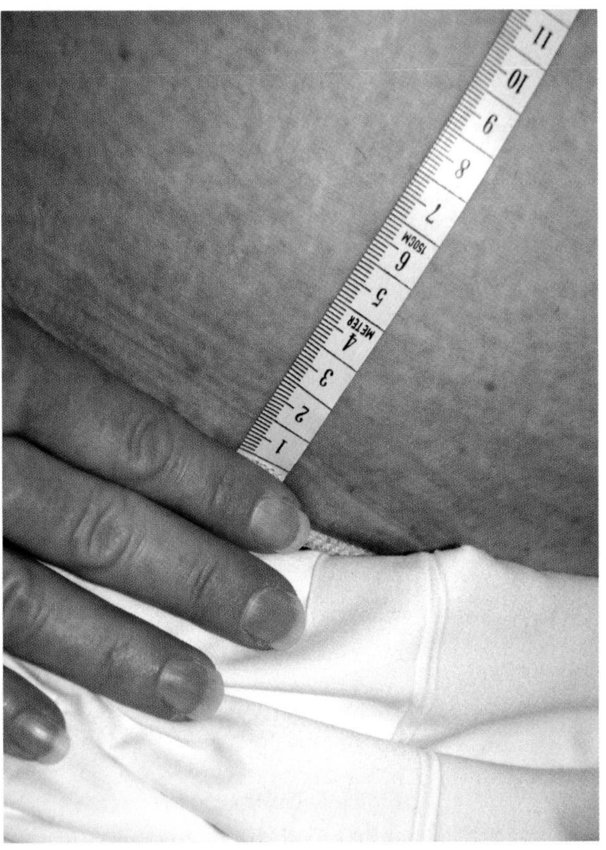

FIGURE 17-3A To measure fundal height, place the zero marker of the tape measure on the pubic symphysis.

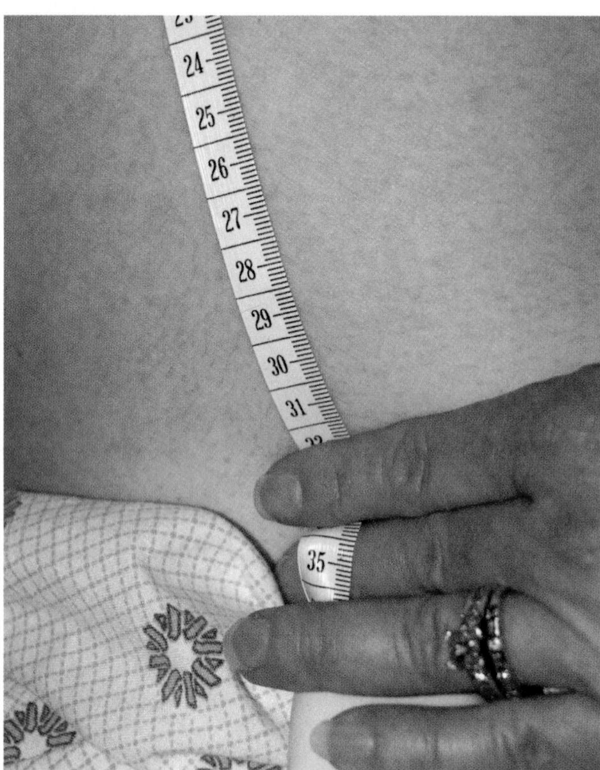

FIGURE 17-3B Stretch the tape measure to the top edge of the uterine fundus.

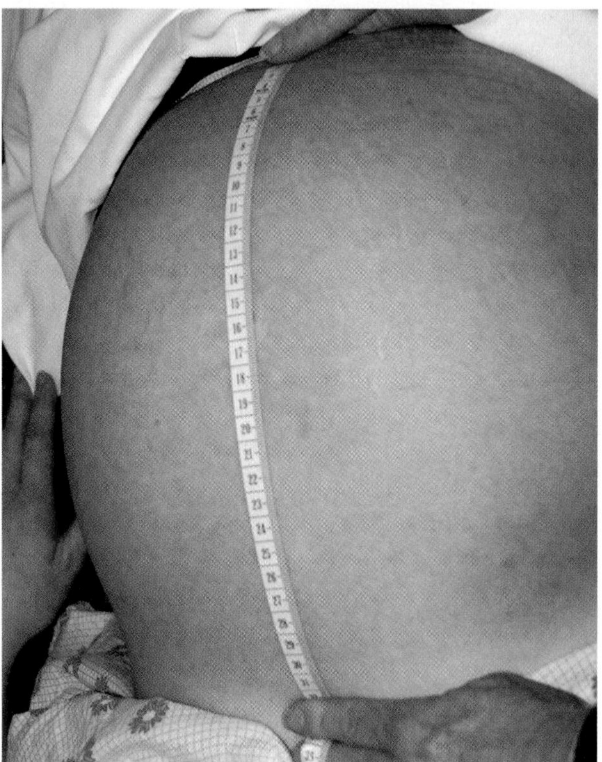
FIGURE 17-3C Measure the total distance to determine fundal height.

drink is finished, the patient has blood drawn. The serum glucose should be < 135–140. If the result of the one-hour glucose tolerance test is > 135–140 (cut-off varies by physician), the patient must then have a three-hour glucose tolerance test. For the three-hour test, the patient's glucose is checked after fasting. The patient then drinks 150 grams of glucola. Her blood glucose level is then checked one, two, and three hours after finishing the glucola.

Normal values for the three-hour glucola are:

- Fasting < 95
- 1 hour < 180
- 2 hours < 155
- 3 hours < 140

If two or more of these values are elevated, the patient is diagnosed with gestational diabetes. The patient should be counseled on diet. She should check her blood sugar four times daily with a goal of fasting blood sugars < 95 and one-hour postprandial levels < 120. If the patient continues to have elevated blood sugars after modifying her diet, then she should be started on insulin treatment. If uncontrolled, gestational diabetes can lead to complications including macrosomia, fetal hypobilirubinemia, operative delivery, shoulder dystocia, and birth trauma. A repeat CBC should also be drawn at the time the one-hour glucose tolerance test is performed.

Common Concerns

Common concerns or complaints at the prenatal visit until 28 weeks include round ligament pain, fetal movement, vaginal discharge and cramping/contractions, swelling, and numbness/tingling in the hands.

Round Ligament Pain.

This is a common complaint around 12–16 weeks as the uterus begins to enlarge and move above the pelvis. It is typically described as an achy pain in the inguinal area and is bilateral. Reassurance is indicated.

Fetal Movement.

If a patient is concerned about fetal movement, advise her to determine kick counts. To do this, the patient should drink juice or eat something sweet. She should then lie down in a quiet room and count the number of times she feels the baby kick in one hour. She should feel at least 10 kicks in an hour. Lesser frequency prompts evaluation.

Vaginal Discharge.

It is normal to have an increase in vaginal discharge during pregnancy due to the increased amount of progesterone. The patient should be concerned only if the discharge is a color other than clear or white, has a foul odor, or causes itching or irritation. If she has any of these complaints, perform a wet mount to look for bacterial vaginosis, yeast, and trichomonas.

Bacterial vaginosis is a common infection during pregnancy. It is not an STI. Treatment of bacterial vaginosis is Flagyl 500 mg BID for 7 days. Yeast infections are also common. Treatment for a yeast infection is Diflucan 150 mg PO × one dose.

Cramping/Contractions.

It is common to have Braxton Hicks contractions near the end of pregnancy. These contractions are painful, but not consistent, and do not cause cervical change. If there is a concern for preterm labor, obtain a fetal fibronectin, monitor contractions, and consider steroids for lung maturity and tocolytics to stop contractions. To obtain the fetal fibronectin (FFN), the gestational age must be between 24 and 33.6 weeks. The patient must not have had intercourse or anything in the vagina in the past 24 hours, as a false positive can result. The FFN has a very strong negative predictive value, and if negative, there is a very small chance of the patient going into labor within the next two weeks.

If the patient is not in preterm labor, consider other causes for the contractions including dehydration, recent intercourse, and infections including urinary tract infections, bacterial vaginosis, yeast infections, trichomonas, gonorrhea, and chlamydia.

Swelling.

As pregnancy progresses, edema becomes more common. Most women complain of swelling at the end of the day after being on their feet. Inquire about swelling in the face and hands and significant rapid weight gain or increase in swelling, which can be signs of preeclampsia.

If the patient has only mild swelling, elevation of the feet whenever possible is indicated. Compression stockings help to decrease the swelling throughout the day.

Numbness/Tingling in the Hand.

Carpal tunnel syndrome is very common in pregnant females due to the increased fluid retention during pregnancy. The excess fluids cause compression of the median nerve, resulting in numbness and tingling in the hand along the median nerve distribution. A wrist splint at night can help improve symptoms. Symptoms typically resolve after delivery as the woman's body returns to its normal state and the fluid volume decreases.

28 TO 36 WEEKS

After the 28-week visit, the patient will return for her prenatal visits every two weeks. During these visits, obtain a clean-catch urine specimen for protein and check blood pressure to monitor for preeclampsia. Fundal height and fetal heart tones are measured at each visit.

Between 34 and 36 weeks, a speculum exam should be performed. During this exam, gonorrhea and chlamydia cultures as well as a group B beta strep culture can be obtained. The gonorrhea and chlamydial cultures are obtained from the endocervix. The patient should be treated appropriately if the gonorrhea or chlamydia cultures are positive. The group B beta strep (GBS) culture is collected from the vagina as well as the anorectal area. If the GBS culture is positive, the patient will need to be treated with penicillin during labor. If the patient has a penicillin allergy, the culture should be sent for sensitivities to determine which antibiotic can be used. The treatment of choice for a penicillin-allergic patient is clindamycin. If the strain is resistant to clindamycin, vancomycin is the treatment of choice.

AFTER 36 WEEKS

At 36 weeks, any patient with a history of genital herpes should be started on suppression therapy with valacyclovir 500 mg daily to prevent an outbreak. On admission to labor and delivery, any patient with a history of herpes simplex virus needs to have a speculum examination to ensure that there are no herpetic lesions. Evidence of any herpetic lesions is an absolute contraindication to vaginal delivery, and the patient must undergo caesarian section.

Between 36 and 40 weeks, the patient should be seen weekly. It is important to ask about contractions, leakage of fluid, and fetal movement at these visits. Also ask about symptoms of preeclampsia including headache that is not relieved with Tylenol, visual changes, epigastric or right upper quadrant pain, and significantly increased edema, especially hand and facial edema. At these visits, Leopold maneuvers can be performed to determine fetal position and estimate fetal weight (see **FIGURE 17-4**). This is also the time period where providers begin examining the patient to check for cervical dilation.

At each visit, review the signs and symptoms of labor with the patient and be sure that she knows when she should call her doctor. Advise the patient to call if she experiences more than five contractions in an hour or one every four to five minutes, leakage of fluid, or vaginal bleeding. Remind the patient that vaginal spotting is normal after a cervical exam, but that she should never experience heavy vaginal bleeding.

Common complaints at the prenatal visits between 36 and 40 weeks include pain, swelling, and contractions. A patient may experience contractions off and on throughout the day for several weeks. She should be advised to call if they become more frequent, regular, or intense.

If the patient has not gone into labor by 40 weeks, discuss the possibility of induction of labor. Pregnancy should not go beyond 42 weeks.

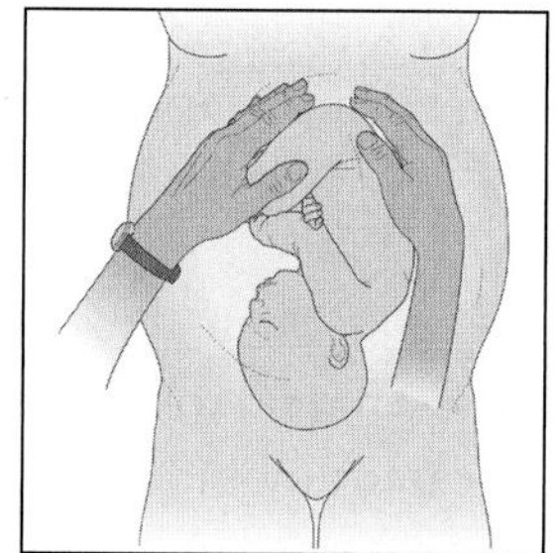

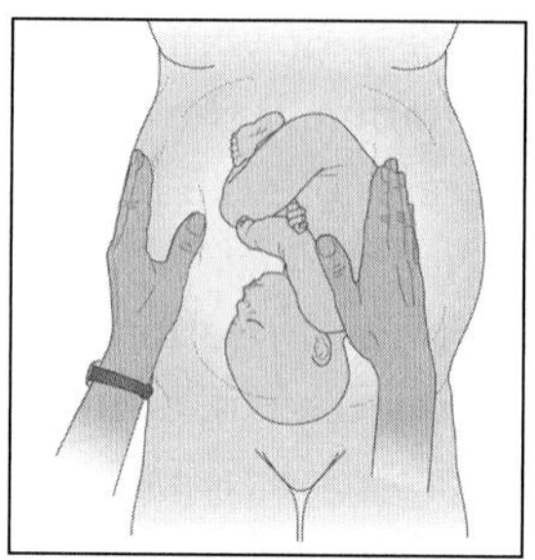

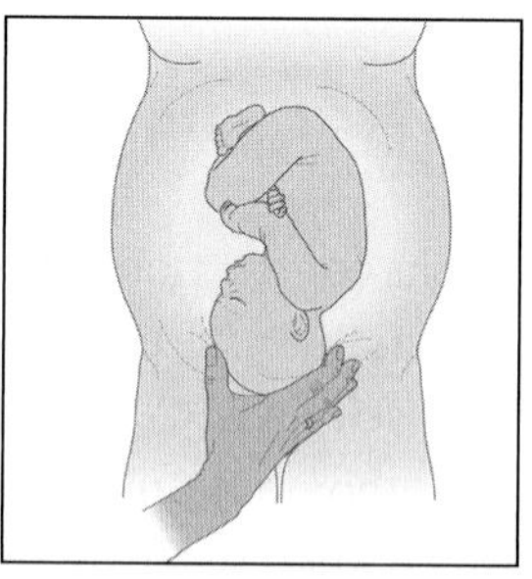

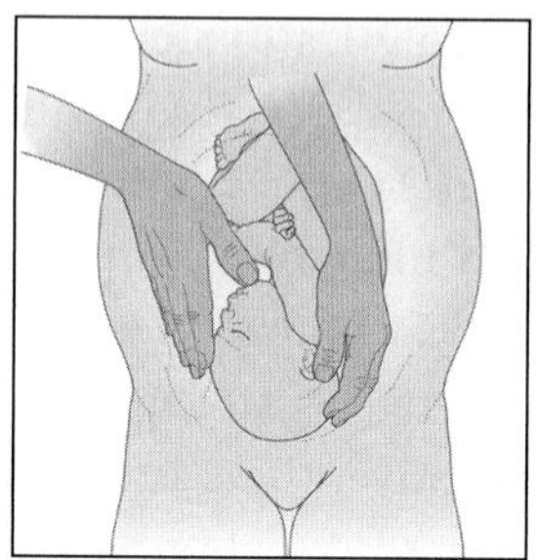

FIGURE 17-4 Leopold maneuvers used to assess intrauterine positioning of the baby.

CHAPTER 18

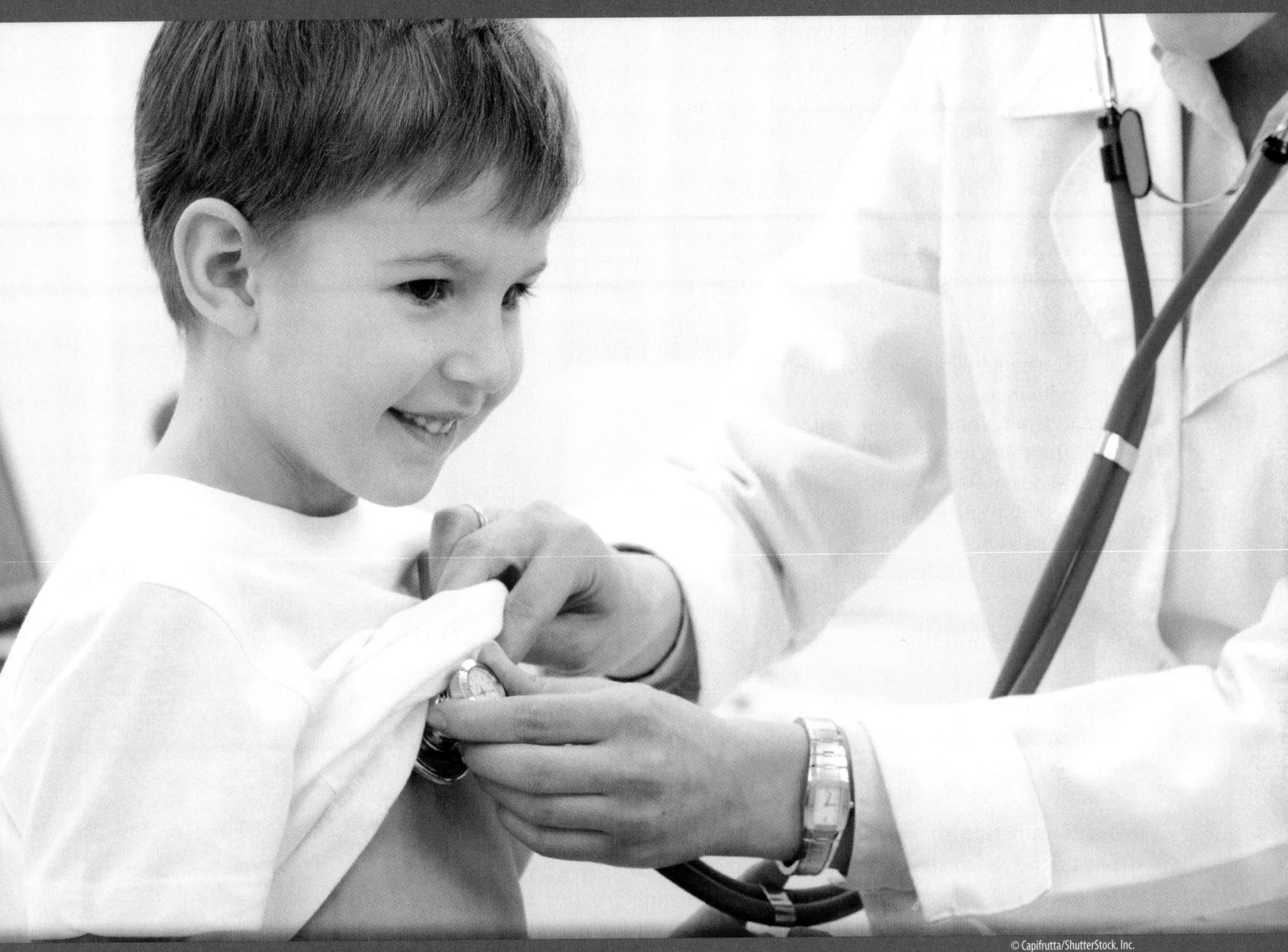

© Capifrutta/ShutterStock, Inc.

Pediatric Patient Examination

OBJECTIVES

At the conclusion of this chapter, the student will be able to

1. Identify key components of the maternal history as related to the newborn assessment
2. Obtain the history of delivery
3. Identify risk factors and perform an evaluation for newborn sepsis
4. Assign APGAR scores to newborns
5. Identify abnormal vital signs
6. Perform pediatric examinations based on patient age
7. Distinguish innocent from pathologic murmurs
8. Identify common pathologic findings on the newborn exam
9. Assess reflexes in the newborn, identifying abnormalities suggestive of pathologic conditions
10. Diagnose hip dysplasia

KEY TERMS

Newborn
Infant
Preschool
School-aged
Adolescence
Newborn sepsis
Vernix caseosa
Lanugo
Fontanelles
Omphalocele
Gastroschisis
Asymmetric tonic neck reflex
Moro reflex
Grasp response
Walking reflex
Hip dysplasia

Where this icon appears, visit **go.jblearning.com/HPECWS** to view the video.

The examination of the pediatric patient ranges from the newborn stage through adolescence, with lessening variation from the adult exam as the child ages. Though various categories exist for physical examinations through the stages of development, these can be generally categorized as:

- **Newborn**—recently born
- **Infant**—from birth to 12 months
- **Preschooler**—from 1 to 5 years
- **School-aged child**—from 6 to 10 years
- **Adolescent**—from 11 to 20 years

Newborn: pertaining to the period of life in close proximity to birth

Infant: pertaining to the period of life from birth to 12 months of age

Preschooler: pertaining to the period of life from 1 to 5 years of age

School-aged child: pertaining to the period of life from 6 to 10 years of age

Adolescent: pertaining to the period of life from 11 to 20 years of age

General Principles of Physical Examination

Assessment of growth and development at each visit should always include height, weight, and BMI. Head circumference should be measured at each visit until the age of 3. Vital signs should include pulse and respiratory rates, with blood pressure starting at the age 2 years. Temperature measurements are generally not indicated during well visit encounters.

In the newborn through preschool ages, history-taking is directed toward the caregivers. As the child becomes cognizant of being examined, the provider should demonstrate techniques of examination on the caregiver first, allowing the child to see that no harm occurred, lessening any hesitancy or fear that they may have. Examination techniques that have the potential to disrupt or cause pain or fear should be performed late in the encounter. Allowing the child to be held by a caregiver during the exam helps the provider perform a detailed physical examination.

As school-aged children progress toward adolescence, the patient should receive the primary focus of the encounter, with the provider attempting to obtain the history directly from the patient, asking for confirmation from the caregiver as needed. The physical exam begins to model that of the adult, working in a head-to-toe pattern and saving sensitive exams, such as assessment of physical maturation that may cause embarrassment, for last.

The Newborn

Screening assessment of the newborn is typically performed immediately after delivery utilizing APGAR scoring and is followed by a comprehensive history—including full maternal, family and prenatal histories—and a detailed physical examination (see **FIGURE 18-1**). Careful analysis of the history, preferably prior to delivery, aids in identifying exposures and risks that could put the normal development of the baby in jeopardy, identifying any abnormality that would alter the normal newborn course, or identifying a medical condition that should be addressed, such as birth anomalies, injuries, hyperbilirubinemia, and cardiopulmonary disorders.

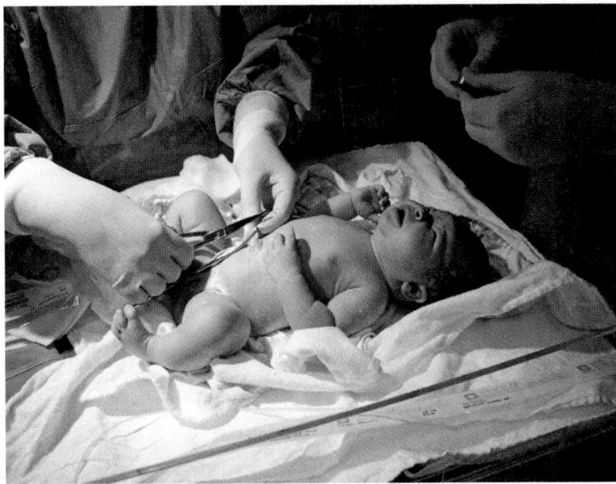

FIGURE 18-1 Newborn.

© Ingvald Kaldhussater/ShutterStock, Inc.

HISTORY

If possible, review of the medical history should occur prior to delivery and begins with maternal progress of the current pregnancy, including screening tests, labor, delivery, and an assessment of the newborn for sepsis. A careful assessment of outcomes from past pregnancies should include history of congenital anomalies, stillbirths, and genetic or syndromic conditions, expanding to include the mother and father, which would guide the provider to search for occurrence in this newborn.

Maternal medical conditions such as diabetes and preeclampsia should be noted. Medications should be reviewed in association with intrauterine effects as well as those that are excreted in breast milk.

The mother's chart usually accompanies her to delivery; if not, she should be asked about results of routinely performed screening tests, which typically include ABO blood type, Rhesus (Rh) type, an antibody screen to detect antibodies potentially causing hemolytic disease of the newborn, rubella status (immune or nonimmune), syphilis screen, hepatitis B surface antigen, hematocrit or hemoglobin to detect anemia, urinalysis and urine culture to detect asymptomatic bacteriuria, group B streptococcal colonization testing, chlamydia, thyroid function, and diabetes.

Screening may have been performed for inherited diseases or birth defects such as Down syndrome or neural tube defects. Results of fetal ultrasounds should also be reviewed. In mothers with substance abuse, maternal toxicology screening should be performed.

Delivery

The history of delivery should include duration of labor, rupture of membranes, mode of delivery, newborn's condition at delivery, and any need for resuscitation.

Risk Factors for Newborn Sepsis

The most common organism causing **newborn sepsis** is group B streptococcus. Between 34 and 36 weeks, a speculum exam should have been performed that included a group B beta strep (GBS) culture to assess for maternal colonization. If the GBS culture was

Newborn sepsis: bacterial infection of the blood in the newborn most commonly caused by group B streptococcus

positive, the mother should have been treated with intrapartum antibiotic prophylaxis (IAP) during labor. This should be noted on the newborn's chart, along with the duration of treatment.

Risk factors for sepsis should be assessed and include:[1,2]

- Evidence of fetal infection such as fever, tachycardia, tachypnea
- Maternal fever
- Maternal group B streptococcus colonization
- Prolonged rupture of membranes of ≥ 18 hours
- Premature delivery at < 37 weeks of gestation
- Chorioamnionitis

Evaluation for Sepsis

Newborns who appear ill require evaluation for sepsis with a complete blood count (CBC) and blood cultures. In addition, asymptomatic infants who have risk factors for sepsis but whose mothers did not receive adequate IAP treatment should also be tested.

If the newborn appears ill or the mother is suspected of or has proven chorioamnionitis, empirical antibiotics should be started. If testing is negative, the antibiotics may be stopped.

PHYSICAL EXAMINATION

APGAR

Immediately at delivery the newborn is assessed utilizing APGAR scoring. This assessment is performed at 1 and 5 minutes.[3] The five categories assessed through the APGAR mnemonic are shown in **TABLE 18-1**.

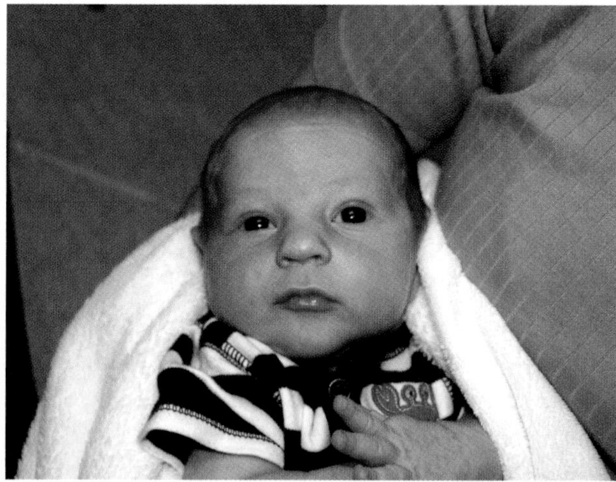

FIGURE 18-2 Exam with child being held.

Each category is given a score of 0, 1, or 2. The scores are then added together for a total score. Infants with APGAR scores of 2 or less are considered to be in poor condition. Those who score between 3 and 7 are considered to be in fair condition and scores 8 or higher in good condition. Neonatal death rates increase dramatically as the APGAR score falls.[4]

The Comprehensive Examination

The newborn examination deviates from the standard head-to-toe approach used in the examination of the adult, though it does begin with general assessment. Before disturbing the baby, observe the newborn in his/her current environment.

If a parent is holding the baby or nursing, ask to be allowed to observe their baby's interactions. Advise the parent that you will perform as much of the examination as possible while the child is being held, and then you will need to move the child to complete any remaining exam (see **FIGURE 18-2**).

TABLE 18-1 APGAR Scoring

Criteria	0	1	2
Appearance (skin color)	Central and peripheral pallor or cyanosis	Peripheral cyanosis	No cyanosis
Pulse rate (heart rate)	No pulse	Less than 100 bpm	Greater than 100 bpm
Grimace (irritability to stimulation)	No response	Weak response	Strong response with cry or withdrawal
Activity (muscle tone)	Absent tone	Some flexion	Flexion against resistance
Respiration (breathing effort)	No respirations	Weak respirations	Strong respirations

Data from: Apgar, V. A proposal for a new method of evaluation of the newborn infant. *International Anesthesia Research Society*. 1953;July–August:260–267. http://apgar.net/virginia/Apgar_Paper.html. Accessed May 25, 2012.

TABLE 18-2 Newborn Vital Signs

Normal Ranges[5]	
Temperature	36.1 to 37 degrees C 97.0 to 98.6 degrees F
Respiratory rate	40 to 60 breaths per minute
Pulse rate	120 to 160 beats per minute

Data from: American Academy of Pediatrics, American College of Obstetricians and Gynecologists. ***Guidelines for Perinatal Care***. 6th ed. Elk Grove Village, IL: American Academy of Pediatrics; 2007.

Keep the baby wrapped and warm, exposing only the area to be examined and then re-covering when completed. Good lighting is essential.

Vital Signs.

Review the infant's documented signs and compare them to your own assessment (see **TABLE 18-2**). Normal temperature measured in the axilla ranges from 36.1 to 37 degrees C (97.0 to 98.6 degrees F).[5]

The normal respiratory rate ranges between 40 and 60 breaths per minute. The normal heart rate ranges from 120 to 160 beats per minute.

Blood pressure is not typically measured in the newborn unless cardiovascular or renal abnormalities are suspected.

Body Measurements.

Review charted body measurements including weight, length, and head circumference. If they have not been performed, consider performing them later in the examination, allowing the baby to remain undisturbed for critical evaluation of the cardiac and respiratory systems.

Body measurements are plotted on standard growth curves to determine the percentile according to gestational age and to assess intrauterine growth. Weight is classified as appropriate, large, or small for gestational age. Length is measured with the infant in the prone position. It may be easier to mark the table paper at the top of the head and bottom of the foot with the leg extended, then move the baby and measure the distance between the marks.

Head circumference is measured at the maximum diameter (see **FIGURE 18-3**). Plotting these measurements may reveal macrocephaly (increased circumference), such as found with hydrocephalus, or microcephaly, such as with neural tube defects or syndromic conditions.

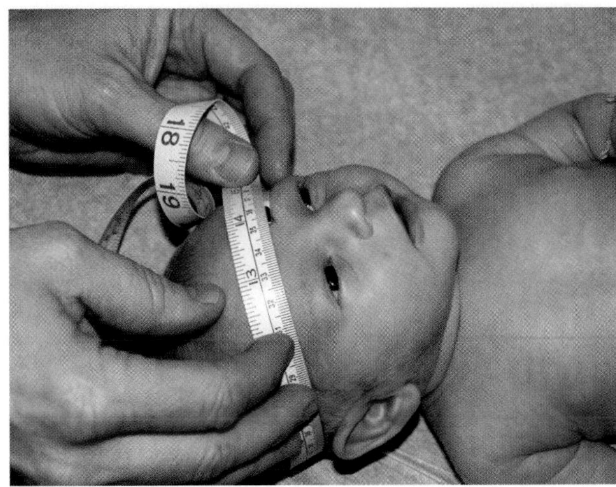

FIGURE 18-3 Head circumference.

General Assessment.

General assessment begins with inspection for obvious developmental deformity, which may indicate the presence of a syndrome.

Nutritional state can be estimated by noting the amount of subcutaneous fat on the anterior thighs and gluteal region and the presence of Wharton's jelly, the mucouslike substance of the umbilical cord surrounding the vessels (see **FIGURE 18-4**).

Assess the respiratory effort. Paradoxical breathing with the abdomen moving outward and the chest inward during inspiration is normal. Inspect for signs of respiratory distress, which include tachypnea, nasal flaring, cyanosis, and use of accessory muscles.

Note body positioning, which reflects how the baby was positioned within the uterus. A position with hips, knees, and ankles flexed suggests intrauterine vertex positioning. Extended legs suggest a breech presentation.

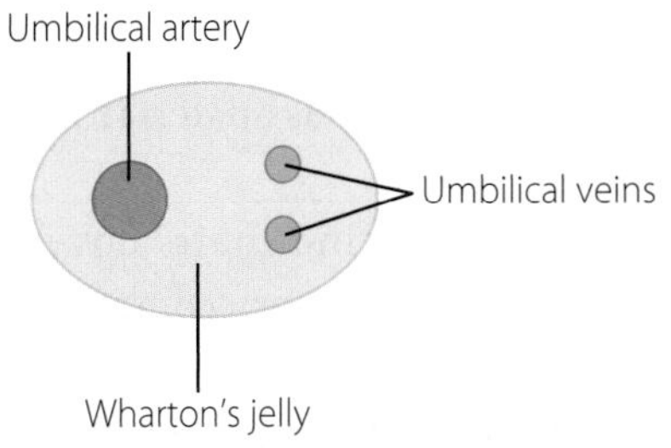

FIGURE 18-4 Umbilical cord with labels.

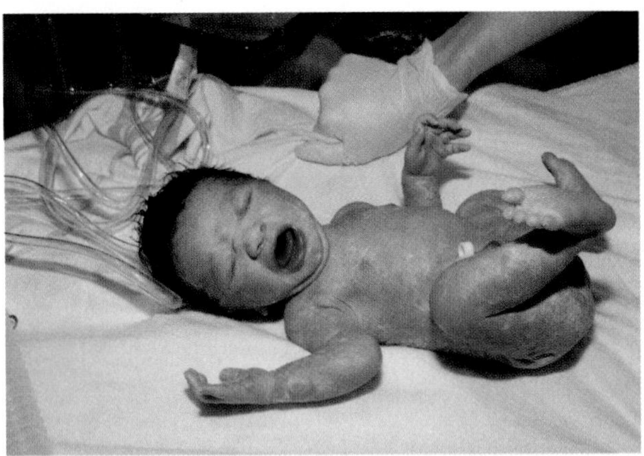

FIGURE 18-5 Cyanosis, and peripheral and vernix caseosa.
© Patricia Marks/ShutterStock, Inc.

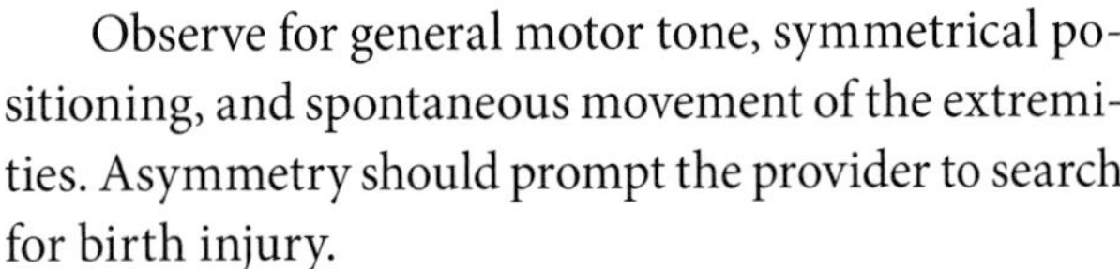

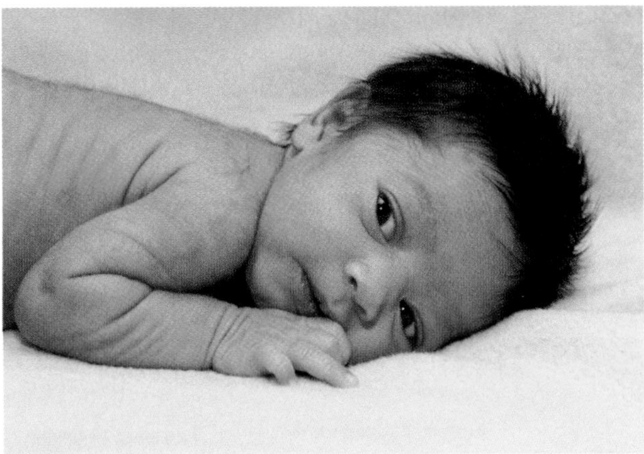

FIGURE 18-6 Lanugo.
© Suzanna Tucker/ShutterStock, Inc.

Observe for general motor tone, symmetrical positioning, and spontaneous movement of the extremities. Asymmetry should prompt the provider to search for birth injury.

Inspect the general color of the newborn. Assess for central cyanosis by looking at the mucosa of the mouth and the tongue, which would indicate the presence of hypoxia. Mild perioral cyanosis and cyanosis of the hands and feet are termed acrocyanosis, a condition common in the first few days of life (see **FIGURE 18-5**).

Examine for ecchymosis, suggestive of trauma. Pallor may indicate the presence of anemia, erythema with polycythemia, and jaundice with hyperbilirubinemia. Meconium staining appears green.

Integumentary.

As with the adult, inspection of the skin is commonly completed concurrently with examination of other body systems.

One of the most common findings in the newborn is **vernix caseosa**, a waxy white coating most commonly in the flexure surfaces and skin creases (see Figure 18-5). This coating is composed of sebaceous material and skin exfoliation.

Vernix caseosa: waxy white coating composed of sebaceous material and skin exfoliation most commonly in the flexure surfaces and skin creases at birth

Lanugo: fine hair covering the body of the newborn more commonly found in prematurity

Lanugo—fine hair covering the body—is more commonly found in premature newborns and will shed in the weeks after delivery (see **FIGURE 18-6**).

Other common integumentary findings of the newborn include milia, which are seen as white papules on the nose and cheeks (see **FIGURE 18-7**). These transient lesions are composed of keratin and sebaceous material in the pilaceous follicles. Parents should be assured that they resolve in the first few weeks of life.

Mongolian spots are macules or patches of dermal melanocytes in blue or brown hues, typically on the back and buttocks (see **FIGURE 18-8**). They are commonly seen in babies of African American and Asian ethnicity. Again the parents should be assured that these lesions resolve spontaneously.

Commonly called "stork bites," nevus simplex are erythematous macules composed of dilated capillaries that may be found on the face and the back of the

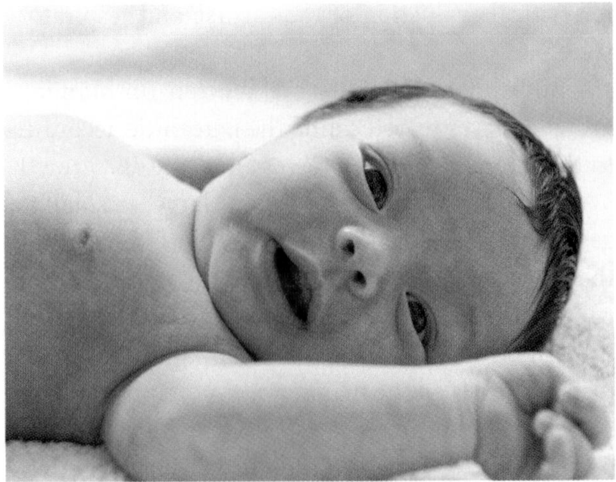

FIGURE 18-7 Milia.
© Michael Pettigrew/ShutterStock, Inc.

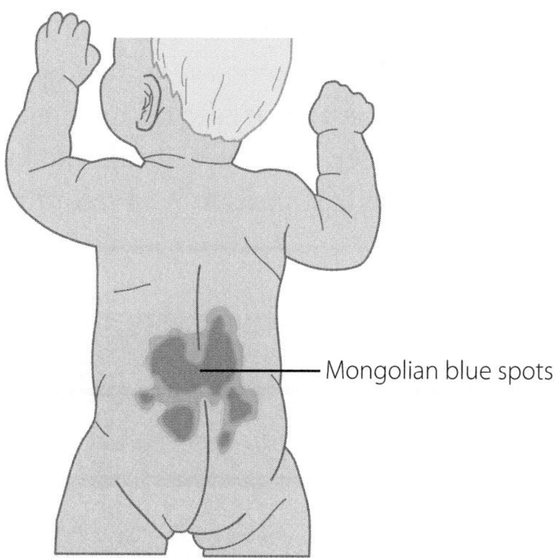

FIGURE 18-8 Mongolian spots.

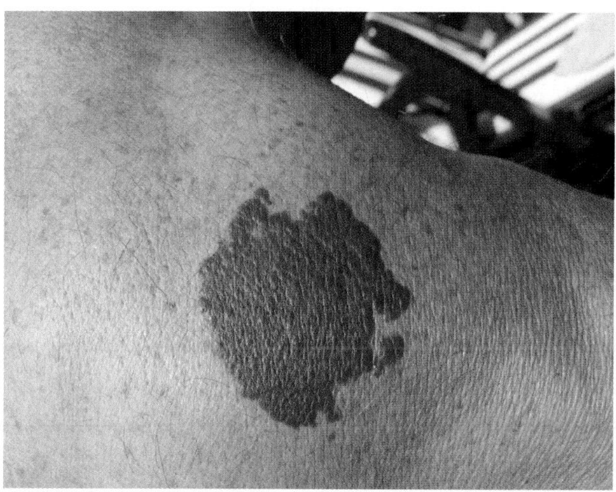

FIGURE 18-10 Port-wine stain.
© guentermanaus/ShutterStock, Inc.

neck (see **FIGURE 18-9**). These commonly resolve by 18 months, though neck lesions may persist.[6]

In contrast, port-wine stains (nevus flammeus), though they are also dilated capillaries, do not resolve spontaneously and may be progressive, resulting in disfigurement or dysfunction if not treated (see **FIGURE 18-10**). In addition, port-wine stains may be evidence of related syndromes such as Sturge-Weber or Klippel-Trenaunay-Weber.

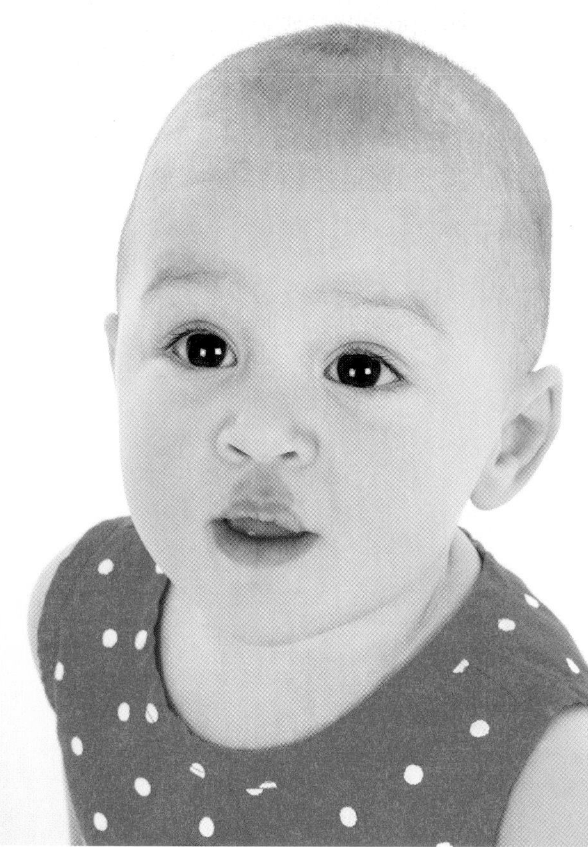

FIGURE 18-9 Nevus simplex (stork bites).
© Jaimie Duplass/ShutterStock, Inc.

Cardiorespiratory Auscultation.

If the baby is quiet, start with auscultation of the heart and lungs using the small-diameter stethoscope head. Warm the stethoscope by rubbing it against your palm and slip it under the clothing to auscultate on bare skin. Later in the examination the thorax will be exposed, but listening first allows for detection of faint abnormalities that might be missed should the baby cry. Assess breath sounds for symmetry, noting any adventitious sounds. Diminished breath sounds of the left lower lobe, often associated with respiratory distress, may indicate diaphragmatic hernia.

Auscultate the heart over each valvular area, axilla, and the back. Identify S1 and S2. Note the presence of any murmurs. Frequently murmurs are present at birth and are most commonly caused by a patent ductus arteriosus (PDA), which closes over time, the murmur resolving. PDA murmurs heard best over the left second intercostal space, with possible radiation down the left sternal border, are continuous and "machinerylike."

Innocent murmurs typically have the following characteristics:

- Intensity less than grade 3
- Heard at left sternal border
- Normal second heart sound

- Crescendo-decrescendo pattern
- Lack of other symptoms

Murmurs outside these parameters suggest pathologic disorders.[7]

Palpate the precordium for the point of maximal impulse (PMI). As opposed to the adult, who has a dominate left ventricle, the right ventricle is dominant in the newborn, meaning the PMI shifts to the left sternal border overlying the right ventricle.

If the baby is crying, attempt calming measures such as rocking and cooing. Continue through other examination techniques, but divert to auscultation of the heart and lungs at any point when calming and crying cessation occurs.

HEAD.

As the baby's face is exposed, examine this next for general color, noting any pallor, cyanosis, or jaundice. Note facial asymmetry, which suggests injury to cranial nerve VII, the facial nerve. This is a peripheral nerve injury often associated with injury from forceps delivery but usually self-resolves. Asymmetry will be most prominent when the infant cries, where the flaccid side of the face reflects injury. As with Bell's palsy, forehead wrinkling will be intact from cross-innervation; however, the lower face may show loss of the nasolabial fold and drooping of the corner of the mouth. CNVII is also responsible for closure of the eye, so that the eye may not be able to close completely with an injury. Complications may include corneal drying and abrasion, prevented by use of eye lubricant and difficulty feeding.

Remove any caps and inspect the head for size, shape, erythema, ecchymosis, and lacerations. Closely examine areas of localized swelling to determine if it crosses suture lines. Swelling that crosses suture lines, termed caput succedaneum, is caused by edema related to the presenting part of the head at delivery and self-resolves. Conversely, a cephalohematoma is an area of subperiosteal bleeding that stops at suture lines. This collection of blood will be reabsorbed but typically takes several weeks or more to do so.

Fontanelles: soft, membrane-covered gaps occurring between the cranial bones of newborns and infants that can be used in assessment of the state of hydration and intracranial pressure

Note retractions of the **fontanelles**, which could reflect dehydration, or bulging, which may suggest increased intracranial pressure as seen with hydrocephalus, subdural hematomas, or meningitis (see **FIGURES 18-11A** and **18-11B**). If head circumference measurement has not been completed, it can be done now, using a disposable tape measure and recording in centimeters.

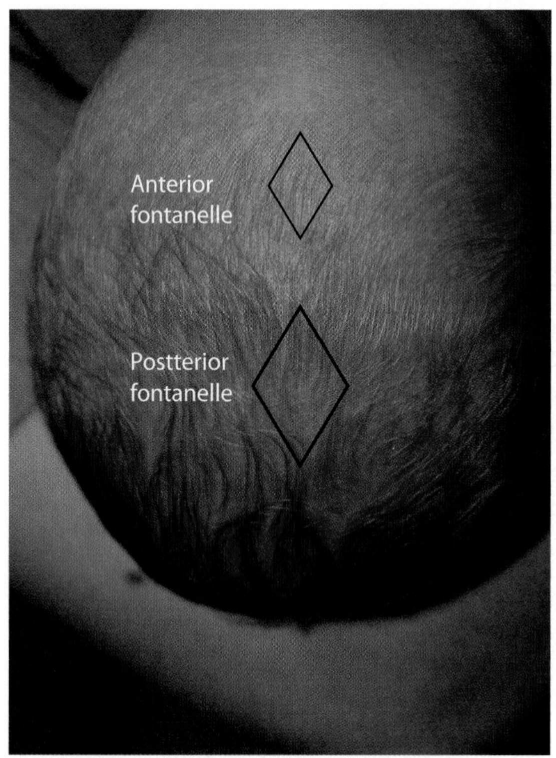

FIGURE 18-11A Fontanelles.

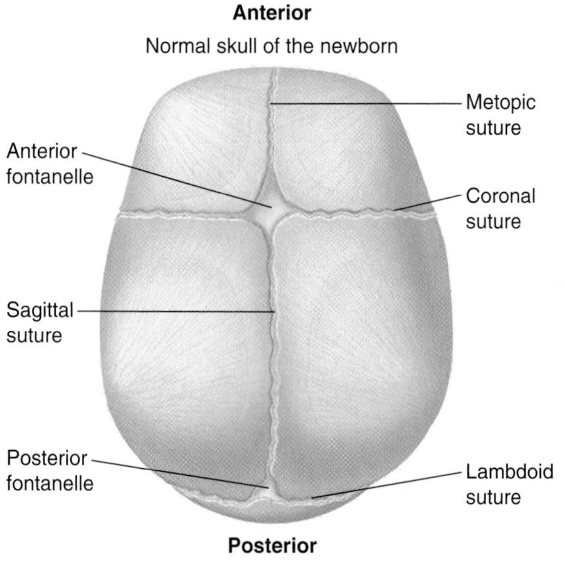

Anterior

Normal skull of the newborn

Metopic suture

Anterior fontanelle

Coronal suture

Sagittal suture

Posterior fontanelle

Lambdoid suture

Posterior

FIGURE 18-11B Fontanelles and sutures.

Reproduced from: AAOS. *Anatomy and Physiology: Paramedic*. 1st ed. Sudbury, MA: Jones & Bartlett Learning; 2004. www.jblearning.com. Reprinted with permission.

Palpate the skull sutures, noting molding and overlapping caused by delivery through the birth canal. Molding typically resolves after several days. Bony deformity may suggest craniosynostosis, premature fusion of a suture line. Increased intracranial pressure may cause widening of the sutures.

Replace the cap to reduce heat loss.

Neck.

Inspect for symmetry, masses, and branchial cleft or thyroglossal duct cysts. A webbed appearance to the neck may be associated with syndromes such as Turner. Contracture of the sternocleidomastoid (SCM) muscle is termed torticollis and may be caused by intrauterine positioning or birth trauma (see **FIGURE 18-12**). Unilateral contracture results in the head being extended and rotated away from the affected side.

Eyes.

Note the positioning of the eyes. Widely spaced eyes should prompt the provider to search for other signs of syndromal conditions.

If the baby's eyes open at any time during the exam, inspect for ptosis. Shine a light at both eyes, noting the light reflection, which should be symmetrical (see **FIGURE 18-13**). Asymmetry is found with eye deviation (strabismus). Large epicanthal folds may give the false appearance of strabismus but should also alert the provider to search for syndromes such as trisomy 21.

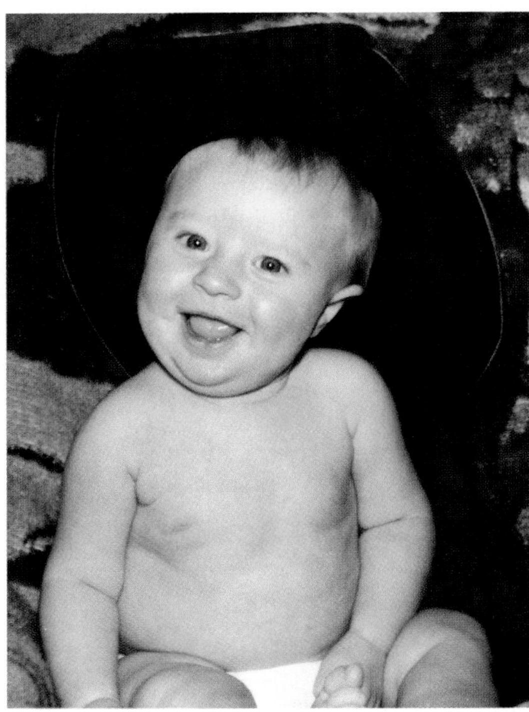

FIGURE 18-12 Torticollis.

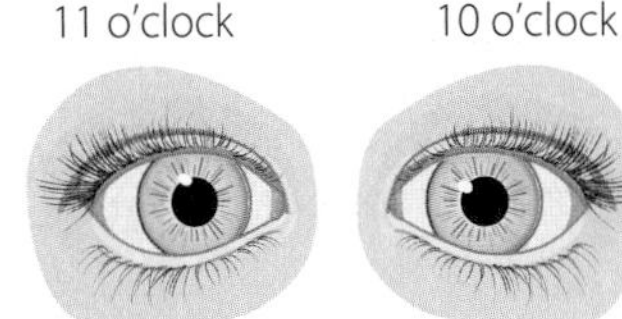

FIGURE 18-13 Light reflex.

Working from the peripheral eye centrally to the pupil, examine the conjunctiva for color, pallor suggesting anemia, erythema, and exudate associated with infection.

Inspect the color of the sclera. Icterus reflects hyperbilirubinemia, the level of which can be estimated as it progresses in a cephalad-to-caudad manner. Icterus reflects an approximate 2 md/dL level of bilirubinemia, jaundice of the face 5 mg/dL, upper thorax 10 mg/dL, and below the umbilicus approaching 20 mg/dL (see **FIGURE 18-14**). If jaundice is suspected, move to an area of natural lighting. Jaundice is unusual in the first 24 hours of life, is almost always pathologic, usually caused by hemolysis, and requires evaluation. Dark blue sclera may be associated with osteogenesis imperfecta.

Moving centrally, work front to back starting with the cornea. Clouding is suggestive of increased intraocular pressure. Observe for obvious lesions. Inspect the iris for defects. Note the shape of the pupil and check for direct and consensual pupillary reaction.

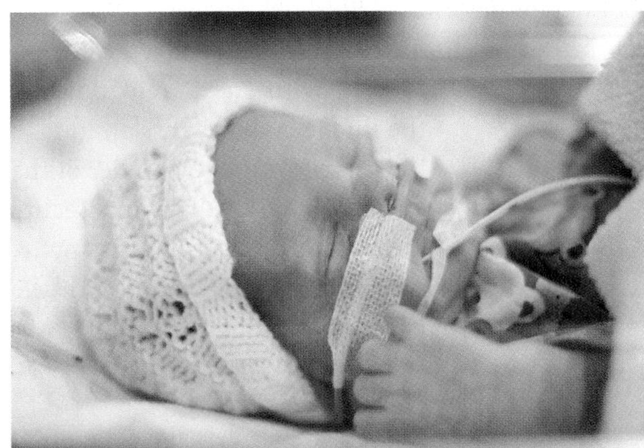

FIGURE 18-14 Jaundice.

© Steve Lovegrove/ShutterStock, Inc.

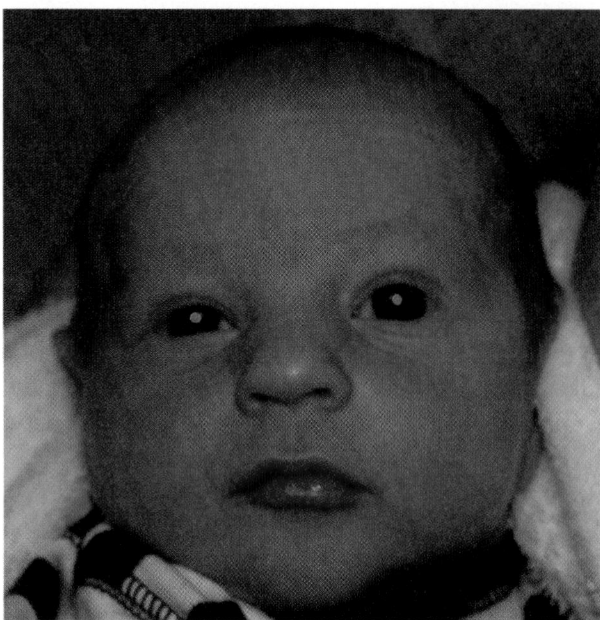

FIGURE 18-15 Red reflex.

Use an ophthalmoscope to detect a red reflex (see FIGURE 18-15). An absence or asymmetrical red reflex may reflect retinoblastoma or congenital disorder such as cataract. Direct observation of the retina through ophthalmoscopy is not typically performed.

At this point the baby will need to be unwrapped but will have on a diaper and typically a onesie, or body garment. Leave these intact and examine the distal extremities for symmetry in development. Note any cyanosis or skin lesions. Assess for symmetry of warmth and palpate the brachial pulses. Asymmetry of brachial pulses may reflect coarctation of the thoracic aorta. Count the number of fingers and toes, looking for deformity.

The exam until this point may have been performed with the parent holding the infant. Ask permission to take the infant for the remainder of the exam, placing the baby in a secure area, often the bedside bassinette, but staying in the room with the parents if possible.

Omphalocele: defect in development of muscles of the abdominal wall allowing viscera to protrude through the umbilicus, being covered with a sac of peritoneum

Gastroschisis: protrusion of abdominal viscera through an abdominal wall defect lacking a peritoneal sac

Thorax.

Remove the undergarment so that the thorax is now exposed. Inspect the chest and abdomen, noting the respiratory pattern with paradoxical breathing—the abdomen moving outward and the chest inward during inspiration. Inspect the chest wall for shape and deformity such as pectus excavatum or carinatum. Inspect the breasts and nipples, looking for supernumerary nipples. Breast enlargement and thin, white discharge is common and secondary to maternal hormones.

Palpation of the thorax should be systematic. Begin by palpating the clavicles for fracture or congenital absence, then work downward over the chest wall.

Abdomen.

Inspect the shape of the abdomen, which is normally rounded. A flat abdomen may indicate a diaphragmatic hernia with abdominal contents shifting into the thoracic space. Distention may reflect intraabdominal ascites, bowel obstruction, or enlargement of the liver, spleen, or kidneys (organomegaly). Protrusion of abdominal contents such as bowel and organs through the abdominal wall is termed an omphalocele or gastroschisis.

An **omphalocele** results from a defect in development of muscles of the abdominal wall, allowing viscera to protrude through the umbilicus, and is covered with a sac of peritoneum (see FIGURE 18-16). In contrast, **gastroschisis** is a protrusion of abdominal viscera through an abdominal wall defect that lacks the peritoneal sac (see FIGURE 18-17). Omphaloceles are more commonly related to other birth defects such as cardiac abnormalities.

Inspect the umbilical cord remnant. Diminished Wharton's jelly suggests poor nutritional state. There should be two umbilical arteries and one umbilical

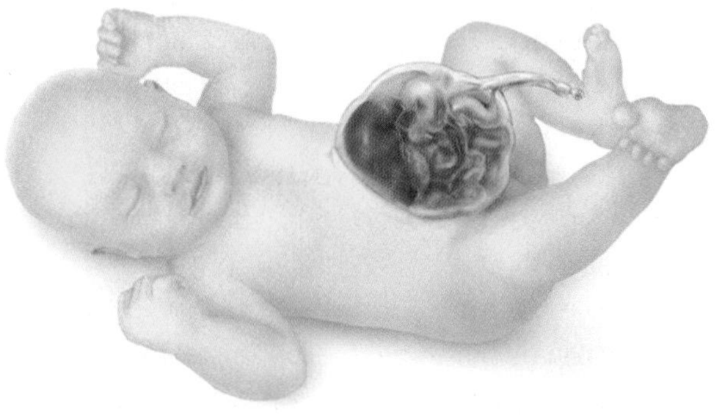

FIGURE 18-16 Omphalocele.
Reproduced from: Centers for Disease Control and Prevention, National Center on Birth Defects and Developmental Disabilities.

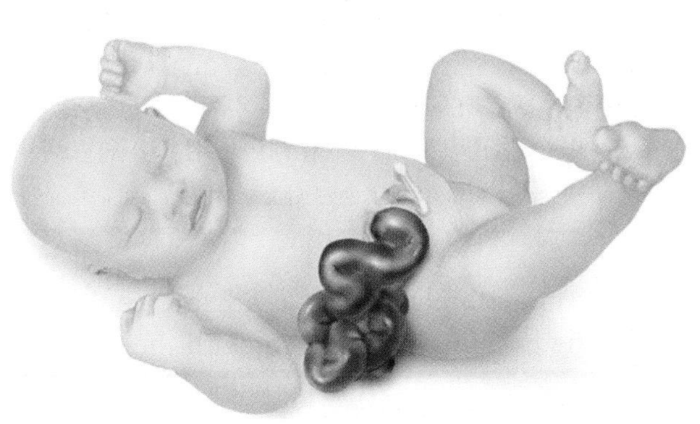

FIGURE 18-17 Gastroschisis.
Reproduced from: Centers for Disease Control and Prevention, National Center on Birth Defects and Developmental Disabilities.

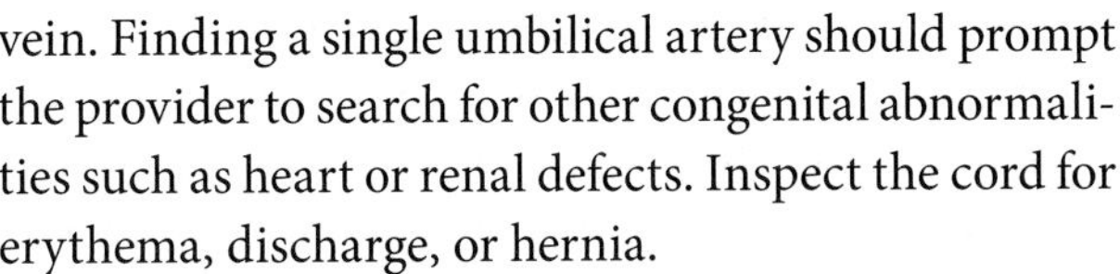

vein. Finding a single umbilical artery should prompt the provider to search for other congenital abnormalities such as heart or renal defects. Inspect the cord for erythema, discharge, or hernia.

Using the small headpiece, auscultate for bowel sounds in each quadrant. Palpate gently for organomegaly or masses. The liver border may be palpable from under the right costal margin. Liver enlargement of greater than a few centimeters should be considered hepatomegaly. Intra-abdominal masses may represent kidney enlargement or tumor, such as teratoma. Percuss the abdomen to assess tympany.

Peripheral Pulses.

Now open the diaper to expose the femoral arteries, palpating for strength of pulse. Diminished femoral pulses may reflect coarctation of the thoracic aorta in the distal arch.

Genitalia.

Male genitalia. Inspect the genitalia. In males, assess for scrotal enlargement, suggestive of a hydrocele or inguinal hernia. If a scrotal mass is present, transillumination should be performed (see **FIGURES 18-18A** and **18B**). Hydroceles will transilluminate whereas hernias will be duller. If encountered, auscultate for bowel sounds.

Palpate each side to identify the testicle. The testicles should be in the scrotal sac or just inside the inguinal canal. Applying slight palpatory pressure above the external ring along the canal may displace the testicle downward, allowing for palpation.

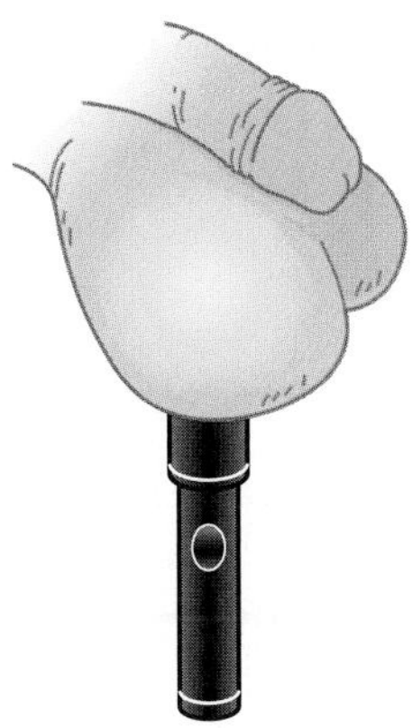

FIGURE 18-18A Hydrocele anatomy.

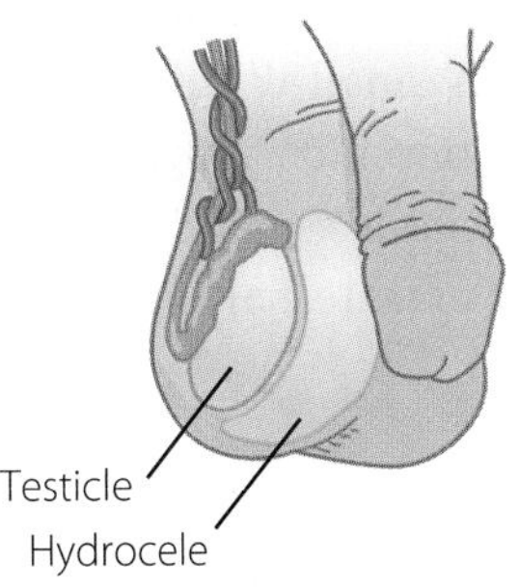

FIGURE 18-18B Hydrocele anatomy.

Inspect the penis. Note the foreskin but do not attempt to retract it, as it is commonly tight. Identify the urethral meatus, which should be located at the tip of the glans. A urethral meatus that opens on the ventral surface is termed hypospadias and is more common (see **FIGURE 18-19**). Dorsal placement is termed

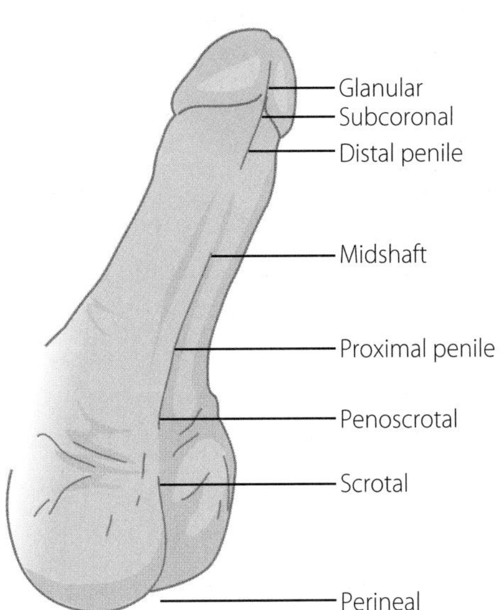

FIGURE 18-19 Hypospadias.

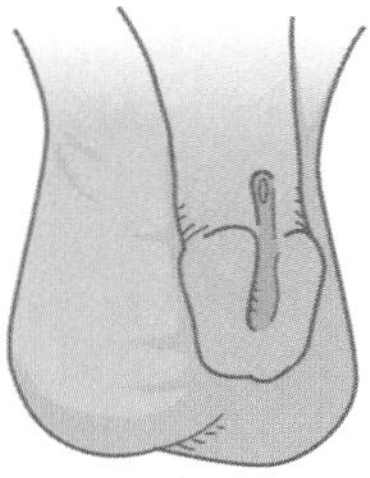

FIGURE 18-20 Epispadias.

epispadias and is frequently associated with bladder exstrophy (see FIGURE 18-20).

Female genitalia. Examine female genitalia, beginning with the labia. Separate the labia to inspect the clitoris and urethral meatus. A small vaginal opening should be present, a lack of which indicates an imperforate hymen. A thin white vaginal discharge may occur under the influence of maternal hormones.

Posterior Thorax.

To examine the back, place a supporting hand under the baby so that both the thorax and the head are supported. Place the other hand over the thorax so that the index and middle finger split, lying on each side of the mandible, then roll the baby onto the hand and distal forearm to expose the back. Inspect from the back of the head down to the anus, noting alignment of the spine, masses, lesions, or dimpling, and paying particular attention to the intergluteal fold, where neural tube defects may be hidden. Masses or lesions overlying the spine may reflect underlying deformities.

Small sacral dimples with intact bases are typically benign (see FIGURE 18-21). Large dimples may reflect neural tube defects especially with associated skin discoloration or hair.

Follow the perineum to the anus, assuring patency. Lack of patency is termed imperforate anus. Secure the diaper.

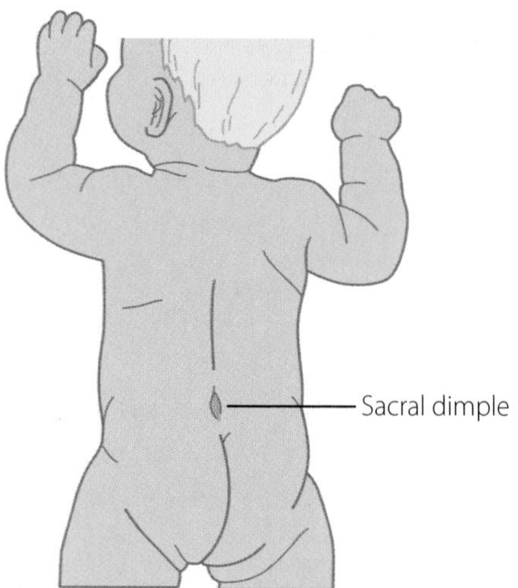

FIGURE 18-21 Sacral dimple.

Ears.

Lay the baby securely on her back. Examine the ears, noting the position in alignment with the eyes. The helix of the ear should line up with the level of the eyes. Ears that are set lower than this may be associated with Down, Turner, or other syndromes. Examine the shape of the external ear, noting any abnormalities such as tags or sinuses. External ear malformations are commonly associated with renal abnormalities. Perform an otoscopic examination by rolling the baby's head to the side and retracting the ear down, back, and out to straighten the canal (see FIGURE 18-22). Visualize the canal to rule out atresia. Do not be overly aggressive in attempting to observe the tympanic membrane, as the narrow canal makes observation difficult.

Nose.

Newborns are obligate nose-breathers. Assess nasal patency by holding a thin wisp of cotton in front of each nares, observing for movement with respiration.

Mouth.

Use a tongue blade to inspect the mouth. Inspect the mobility of the tongue and the palate for clefts. Natal teeth may be present. Glove one hand and stroke the side of the baby's face from the cheek to the corner of

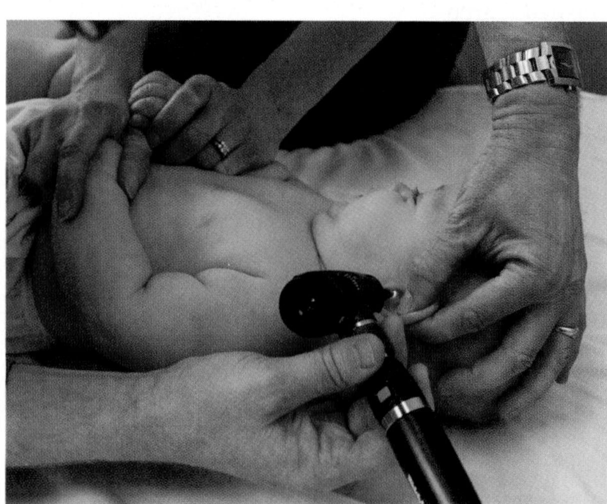

FIGURE 18-22 Otoscopic exam, infant.

the mouth to assess the rooting reflex. With an intact reflex, the lips will move to the side of the finger and the head may turn toward it slightly. Now slip the pinky into the baby's mouth and assess the strength of suckle. Palpate the palate for defects.

MUSCULOSKELETAL/NEUROLOGIC EXAM.

Motor tone. Though you have already noted motor tone during the general assessment, refocus on each extremity, running each through full range of motion. 18-1 As you have already performed the rooting reflex, continue the nervous system examination of newborn primitive reflexes in head-to-toe fashion.

18-2 ***Asymmetric tonic neck reflex.*** To perform the **asymmetric tonic neck reflex**, have the newborn in the supine position and rotate the head to one side. The extremities on the chin side extend while the extremities on the occiput side flex. Persistence of this reflex after 6 months may indicate cerebral palsy.

18-3 ***Moro reflex with palmar grasp response.*** To perform the **Moro reflex**, the provider places his/her thumb pads into each of the newborn's palms. This first step also assesses the palmar grasp response, where lightly touching the palms results in the newborn grasping at the touch area. Placing supporting fingers behind the baby's hand, the provider then lifts the hands upward until the thorax barely lifts and the head begins to flex but does not leave the table. The hands are then suddenly released, imitating a fall. A normal response is seen with extension of the back, extension and abduction of the arms, and fanning of the digits, followed by flexion and adduction of the arms, and closing of the fingers as in a motion of trying to cling. The infant may cry as part of the reflex as well. The reaction should be symmetrical. If not, consider peripheral nerve injury or cerebral palsy. If present after 6 months of age, cerebral palsy should be considered.

18-4 ***Plantar grasp reflex.*** Complete the **grasp response** by tapping the plantar surfaces of the feet. Again the feet should grasp. Persistence of grasp reflexes after 1 year may be seen with birth injury and developmental delay.

18-5 ***Babinski reflex.*** Now stroke the bottom of each foot from the heel, laterally along the side and across the ball of the foot. A positive Babinski reflex should be seen, with extension and fanning of the toes.

Walking reflex. To assess the **walking reflex**, lift the baby with the thumbs over the anterior chest, hands under each axilla, and fingers wrapped around the back. Hold the baby over the table and lower until the feet are just above it. Touch the feet lightly to the table. A normal walking reflex results when the baby attempts to walk across the surface.

Placing reaction. Similarly, holding the infant upright and touching the anterior distal tibia against the edge of the table should cause the infant to lift the foot, flexing the hip and knee as if attempting to step up onto the table surface. Absence at birth may indicate brain damage.

HIP DYSPLASIA.

Finally, examine for **hip dysplasia** by performing the Ortolani and Barlow maneuvers with the newborn in the supine position.

18-6 The Ortolani maneuver assesses for posterior dislocation of the hip. To perform the test, the provider flexes the infant's hips and knees to 90 degrees bilaterally with the pads of the index and middle fingers on the greater trochanters and the thumbs medially on the distal femurs (see **FIGURE 18-23**). With anterior pressure on the fingertips against the trochanters, the legs are slowly abducted using the thumbs (see **FIGURE 18-24**). Audible or palpable clicking indicates that the femoral head had been in a position of posterior dislocation and has now been replaced into the acetabulum.

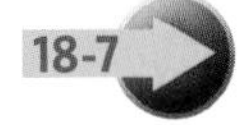

The Barlow maneuver results in posterior displacement of an unstable hip. This test

Asymmetric tonic neck reflex: reflex where rotation of the head is accompanied by extension of the extremities on the side of the chin with flexion of the extremities on the occiput side

Moro reflex: extension and abduction of the arms with fanning of the digits, followed by flexion and adduction of the arms with closing of the fingers when the hands of an infant under slight traction are suddenly released, imitating a fall

Grasp response: grasping of the hands or feet in the newborn when the palmar or plantar surfaces are tapped

Walking reflex: appearance of a baby attempting to walk when held over a flat surface allowing the feet to lightly touch

Hip dysplasia: anatomic abnormality in the development of the hip joint

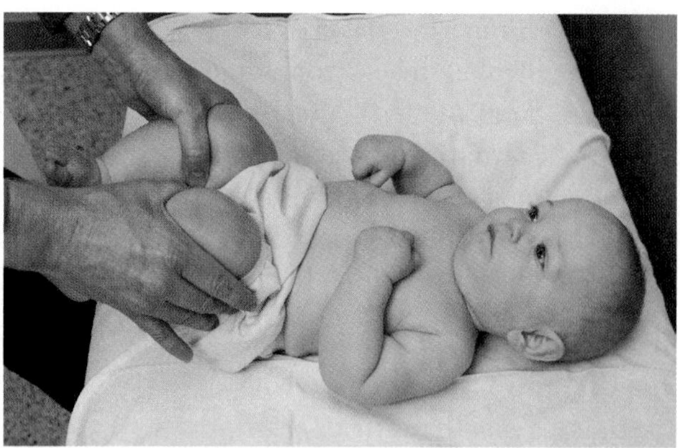

FIGURE 18-23 Ortolani hand placement.

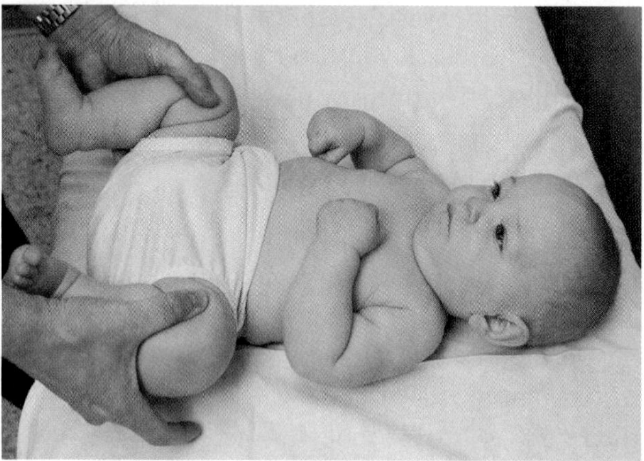

FIGURE 18-24 Ortolani abduction.

is performed with the same hand positioning and the infant's hips and knees bent at 90 degrees; however, the exam begins with the hips in abduction (see **FIGURE 18-25**). Keeping the hips and knees flexed, the legs are then adducted, bringing them together at midline while applying light pressure through the leg toward

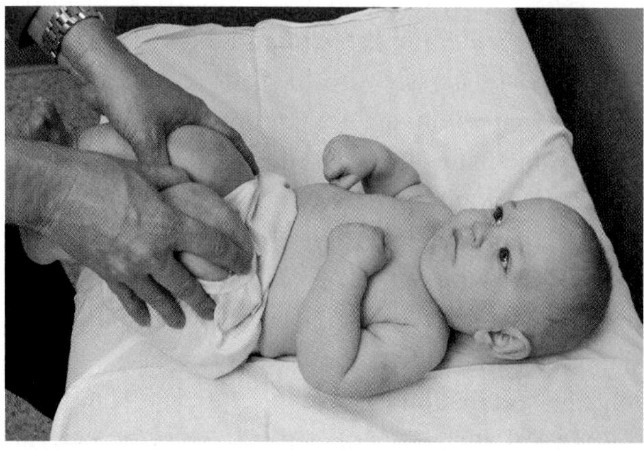

FIGURE 18-25 Barlow abduction.

the back. An audible or palpable click indicates posterior dislocation has occurred, with the femoral head slipping posteriorly out of the acetabulum.

As you have completed the examination, assure a clean diaper, re-dress the baby, and wrap securely. If taken from the parents to perform the exam, return her and reassure the parents that the exam will be discussed with the attending, or take the time to discuss your findings as appropriate to your level of training.

A second full physical examination should be performed prior to discharge of the newborn.

Infant Well Visit

As with any patient visit, the provider should review the chart prior to entering the room. This allows for name recognition, identification of the purpose for the visit, the demographics of the patient, and review of the screening vital signs. When the chart review has been completed, knock and enter when invited. When opening the door, do so slowly, as little fingers may be on the floor right inside it.

HISTORY TAKING

Historical assessment during the infant well visit is provided by the caregiver and focuses on his/her concerns and exploration of the development and attainment of milestones. Many caregiver report screens are available. With this type of screen, the caregiver answers questions relating to observed actions of the child. Developmental milestone screening should occur at approximately the 9, 18, and 24, or 30-month visits, as well as every well visit after 30 months of age.[8]

At well visits, CODIERS will not be employed; however, SMASH FM should be reviewed and should include components of the social history:

- Food/Diet—what the diet consists of, amounts eaten, frequency of feeding, and any concerns
- Exercise—functional ability of the child
- Tobacco—exposure to environment with smokers, including home and vehicles

Historical data concerning the diet should be compared with plotted growth charts from the physical examination. Inconsistencies between reported feeding habits and body size should draw the provider's attention.

Sleeping patterns should also be documented, showing number of hours typically slept during the night and the number and length of naps taken.

PHYSICAL EXAMINATION

As with any examination, the provider should wash his/her hands before touching the infant. The infant exam, from birth to 12 months, is performed in a similar sequence to the newborn exam, performing critical auscultatory techniques such as auscultation of the heart and lungs early on while saving the most distressing exams, such as the otoscopic, mouth, abdominal, and hip exams, for last.

Body measurements of height, weight, and head circumference should be plotted on growth charts (see **FIGURES 18-26** and **18-27**).[9]

Infants should be put into examination gowns or undressed with only the diaper remaining as long as the room is warm. The child can sit on the caregiver's lap for as much of the examination as possible.

General Assessment

Inspect for the general level of nutrition and development. Note the infant's level of alertness, attentiveness to surroundings, and activity. Observe social interactions between the infant and caregiver.

Cardiorespiratory

Auscultation of the heart and lungs should occur early in the sequence of examination while the infant is calm, using the pediatric or small-diameter head of the stethoscope.

Auscultate the four valvular areas of the heart. Identify the S1 and S2. S2 is often split. Though it is difficult to get an infant to take a deep breath, a normal S2 split would disappear with deep inspiration. An S3 may also be encountered and, lacking others signs of heart failure, is a normal finding. Identify any murmurs, noting anatomic location, radiation, timing during the cardiac cycle, shape, and quality. Grade the murmur for intensity, palpating for a thrill if a murmur is identified.

Palpate the PMI, which should have transitioned from the dominant right ventricle of the newborn to the left ventricle.

Inspect the breathing pattern, noting the respiratory rate and effort. In acute illness observe for signs of respiratory distress including cyanosis, nasal flaring, and use of accessory muscles.

Auscultate as you would in an adult, symmetrically side to side, to allow comparison of comparable lobes. Minimally, auscultate at three levels anteriorly and posteriorly, two levels laterally. Note the presence of adventitious breath sounds.

While examining the thorax, complete the examinations of the breasts and back. If breast enlargement from maternal estrogen was present at birth, follow for spontaneous resolution. Note the alignment of the spine.

Abdomen

Inspect the shape of the abdomen, noting any distension. In the postnatal period, observe the umbilicus for signs of infection or hernia. The umbilical cord remnant is typically gone within the first two weeks of birth.

Auscultate bowel sounds. Palpate for organomegaly or masses. Percuss to assess pattern of tympany.

Genitalia

In the male infant, inspect the penis, noting location of the meatus. If circumcision was performed, inspect for appropriate healing and signs of infection. Inspect the scrotum for signs of enlargement. If enlargement is found, transilluminate the scrotal sac to distinguish between hydrocele and hernia. Palpate the testes on each side.

In the female infant, inspect the anatomic structures, noting any discharge.

Head

The HEENT exam has been delayed until now as it can upset the infant. Inspect the head for symmetry. For those infants not yet sitting, an area of mechanical alopecia will be noted on the back of the head from the pressure exerted while lying on the back. This should be in midline. Areas that are not midline may suggest asymmetry or rotation of the head, as in torticollis.

Palpate the fontanelles. The posterior fontanelle closes first, by approximately 2 months of age. The anterior fontanelle closes over a range of between approximately 4 months and 2 years.

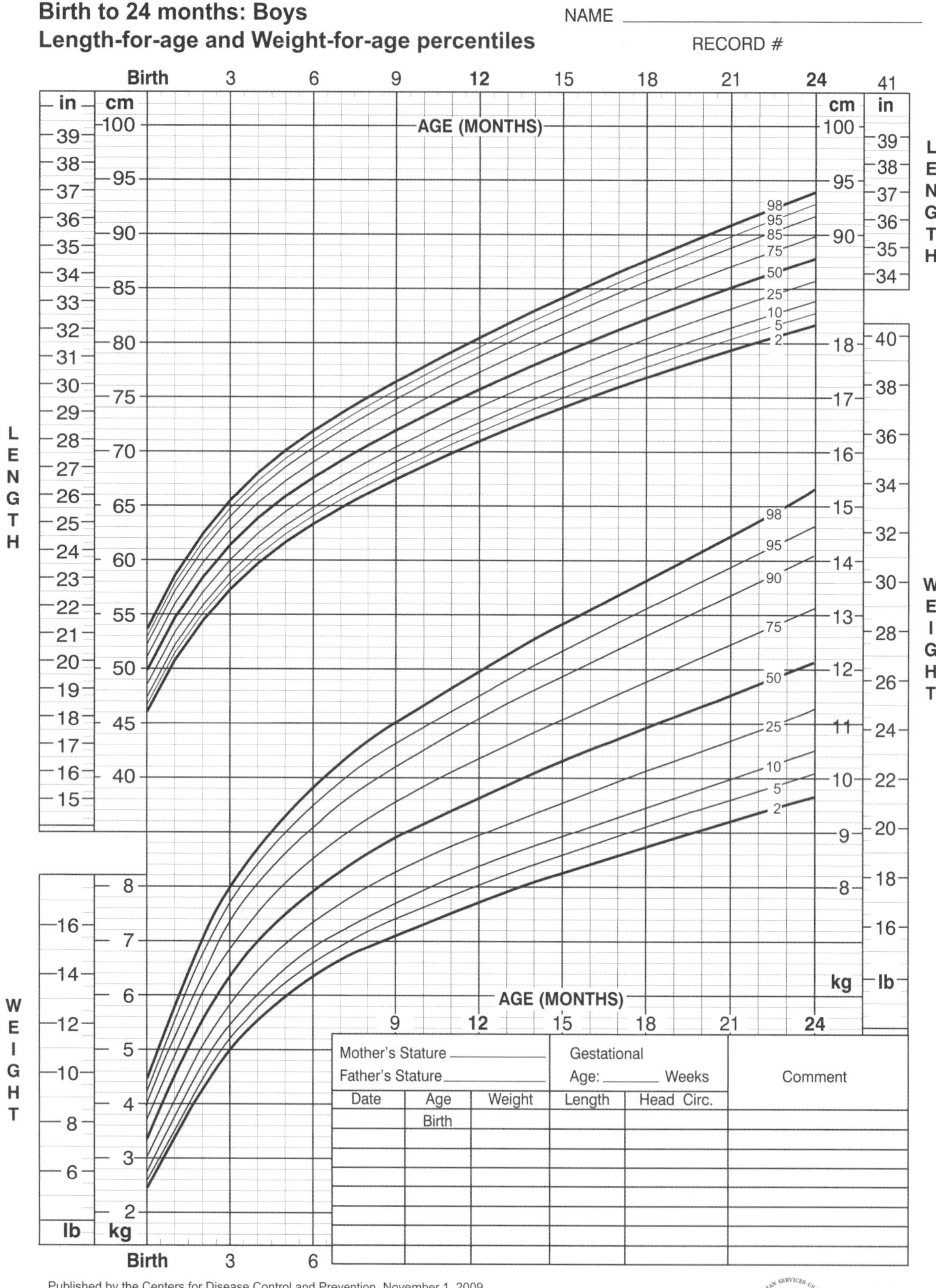

FIGURE 18-26 Birth to 24 months: boys.

Reproduced from: WHO. *Child Growth Standards*. Centers for Disease Control and Prevention; 2009. http://www.who.int/childgrowth/en. Accessed December 13, 2012.

Birth to 24 months: Girls
Head circumference-for-age and
Weight-for-length percentiles

NAME ______________________

RECORD # ____________

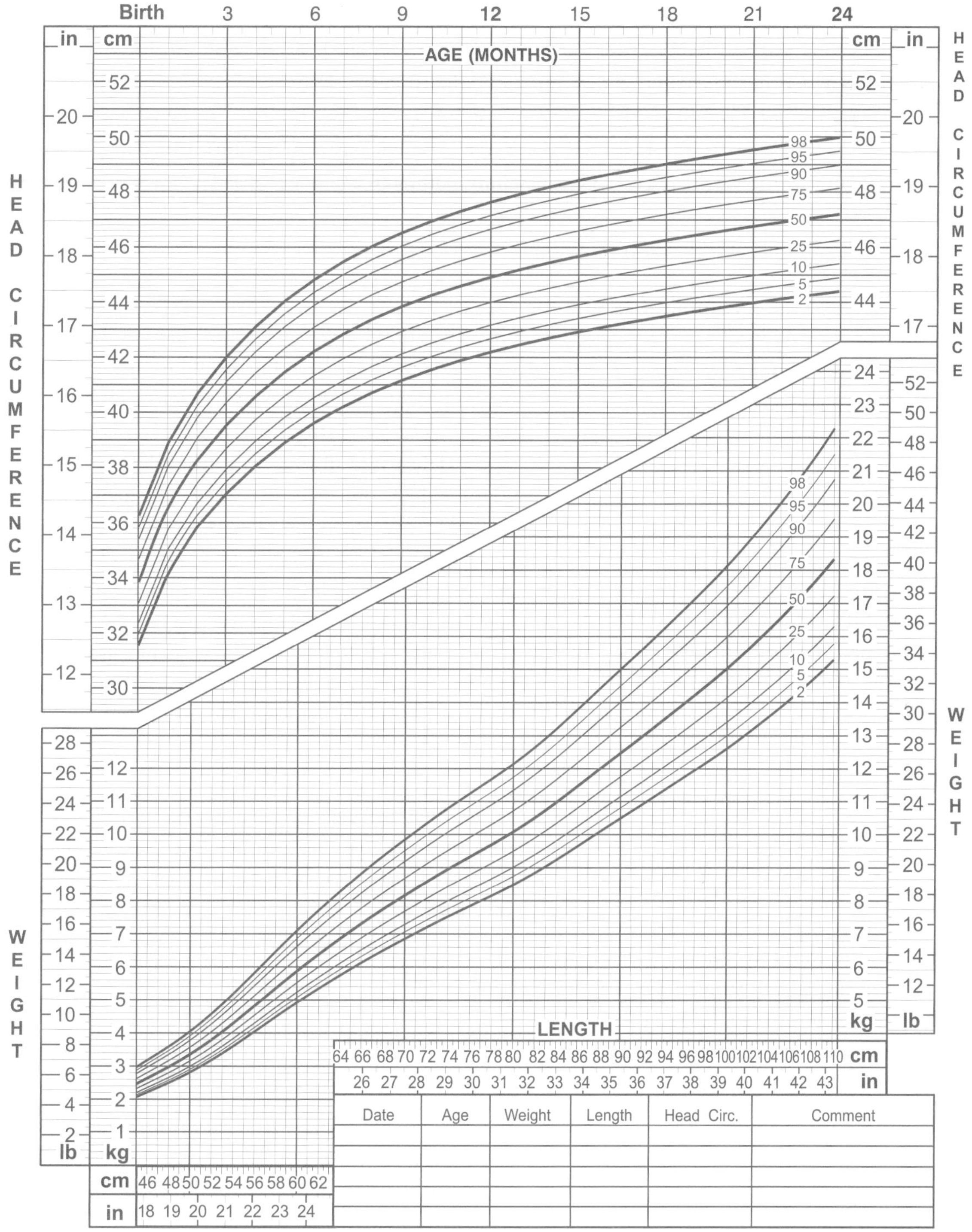

Birth 3 6 9 12 15 18 21 24

AGE (MONTHS)

HEAD CIRCUMFERENCE

in: 12 13 14 15 16 17 18 19 20

cm: 30 32 34 36 38 40 42 44 46 48 50 52

Percentiles: 98 95 90 75 50 25 10 5 2

WEIGHT

kg: 1 2 3 4 5 6 7 8 9 10 11 12 13 14 15 16 17 18 19 20 21 22 23 24

lb: 2 4 6 8 10 12 14 16 18 20 22 24 26 28 30 32 34 36 38 40 42 44 46 48 50 52

LENGTH

cm: 46 48 50 52 54 56 58 60 62 64 66 68 70 72 74 76 78 80 82 84 86 88 90 92 94 96 98 100 102 104 106 108 110

in: 18 19 20 21 22 23 24 26 27 28 29 30 31 32 33 34 35 36 37 38 39 40 41 42 43

Date	Age	Weight	Length	Head Circ.	Comment

Published by the Centers for Disease Control and Prevention, November 1, 2009
SOURCE: WHO Child Growth Standards (http://www.who.int/childgrowth/en)

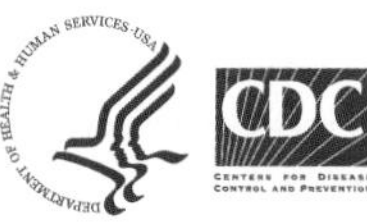

FIGURE 18-27 Birth to 24 months: girls.

Reproduced from: WHO. *Child Growth Standards*. Centers for Disease Control and Prevention; 2009. http://www.who.int/childgrowth/en. Accessed December 13, 2012.

Eyes

From several feet in front of the infant, inspect for ptosis. Shine a light into the eyes, noting the position of the light reflex to identify strabismus. Assess for asymmetry of the red reflex using the ophthalmoscope. A squeaky toy is helpful to assess both hearing and extraocular movements. Ask the caregiver to gently hold the chin in midline. Hold the toy directly in front of the infant at eye level. Squeak the toy to draw attention to it if needed. Once it has been identified, move the toy to each of the six cardial positions of gaze to assess the EOM.

Moving closer, inspect the anatomic structure of the eye to include the conjunctiva, sclerae, cornea, irides, and pupils. Excessive tearing may indicate obstruction of the nasolacrimal duct and can be unilateral or bilateral. This typically self-resolves by the age of 1 as the infant grows.

Ears

Inspect the position and shape of the ear. Perform an otoscopic exam by pulling the ear down, back, and out to straighten the canal. The caregiver can be asked to hold the infant, chest to chest, turning and stabilizing the head to one side then the other. The provider's extended digit should anchor the ophthalmoscope to prevent injury to the tympanic membrane with sudden movement of the head. Identify the TM which may be flushed if the infant is crying.

Nose

The ethmoid sinuses are the only sinuses present at birth, with frontal and maxillary sinuses developing later. Inspect the nose for position. Observe the nasal mucosa and position of the septum. Assess patency by pressing the nares closed, one at a time.

Throat

A tongue blade and light source are required for adequate examination of the mouth and throat. Inspect the structures of the mouth and throat. Teeth typically begin to develop at 6 months of age. The central and incisors erupt first, followed by other teeth in a lateral and back order.

Musculoskeletal/Nervous System

Inspect the neck for symmetry, and position and palpate for masses. Perform passive range-of-motion testing on the neck and then the extremities, working distally through each major joint, noting motor tone and palpating each joint.

Primitive reflexes typically resolve by six months of age as bicep, brachioradialis, and tricep reflexes begin to appear.

Early Childhood (1 to 4 Years)

Early childhood presents a time when children may become fearful of the tall, funny-looking person in the white coat. Providers whose practice involves frequent encounters with pediatric patients should dress appropriately and utilize child-friendly examination equipment. White coats may be left outside the room. Animated characters on clothing such as men's ties draw the child's attention away from the exam. Penlights housed in rubber fish encourage children to open their mouths to let the fish see in.

Special care should be taken to avoid causing pain during the examination, as children quickly learn when something is painful. Successfully looking in an ear with an otoscope without causing pain desensitizes the child for the next exam.

As the child ages, the examinations should move from the caregiver's lap to the exam table with the caregiver sitting close by. Again, have the child in a gown with only a diaper or underwear on. Review the vital signs. Blood pressure assessment should begin at the age of 2.

PHYSICAL EXAMINATION

General Assessment

As with the adult, begin the exam in the seated position, performing a general assessment for distress, color, and development. Assess nutritional state and hygiene for evidence of neglect.

Cardiorespiratory

Auscultation of the heart and lungs should continue to be performed early in the sequence of the exam in younger children, moving more toward the sequential head-to-toe examination, as in the adult exam, as they age.

One technique to aid in auscultation of the heart is for the provider to ask, "Do you know what your heart says?" When the patient answers, say, "I can hear what your heart says with my stethoscope. Do you want me to tell you what it says?"

Ask the child to be very quiet because the heart talks very quietly, then place the stethoscope on the first valvular area. Here the provider must have a little knowledge of classic children's favorites or current fads. While listening to a little girl's heart, slowly say something like, "Your heart says you . . . like . . . Dora. Who's Dora?" You've likely gained a smile if not a trusted friend.

If the child seems apprehensive of an exam technique, perform the exam on the caregiver first.

Abdominal

Advise the child that you next need to examine her belly and need her to lie down. Using child-appropriate language is important. Then assist the child to the supine position. Perform the abdominal exam with gentle palpatory techniques. The liver edge may be palpated just below the right costal margin but no more than 1 to 2 cm.

Musculoskeletal/Neurologic

Complete the musculoskeletal and neurologic exams, including the neck and all extremities, while the patient is still in the supine position. As the child ages, these exams will move to the seated and standing positions. Assess range of motion, strength testing, and reflexes of the extremities.

When the child is able to stand, a screen for scoliosis should be performed. Standing behind the patient, ask the child to "stand as tall as you can" keeping the arms loosely at the sides (see **FIGURE 18-28A**). Observe the distance between each elbow and the side of the thorax. Asymmetry may aid in detecting slight curvature. Inspect and palpate the spine for curvature. Ask the child to "touch your toes" (see **FIGURE 18-28B**) followed by "bend back toward me" to complete examination in three positions: erect, flexion, and extension. Scoliosis may present with either "s" or "c" shaped curvatures (see **FIGURE 18-28C**).

While the child is in the standing position, observe for angulation of the knees. Some valgus deviation is a normal finding in this age group. Inspect the feet for pes planus.

Genitalia

Advise the caregiver of the need to examine the genitalia. Open the diaper to perform the exam. If the child has underwear on, ask the caregiver to remove it. The caregiver should also sit beside and touch the child if reassurance is needed.

The testicles should be fully descended into the scrotum by the age of 1 year. Undescended testicles increase the risk of developing testicular cancer, and referral to a specialist should be made.

HEENT

For younger children finish the exam by looking in the ears and mouth while the child is still in the supine position. If the child is able, he/she should return to the seated position for these last exams.

Inspect the eyes for alignment using the light reflex and the cover-and-uncover test. To perform this test, draw the attention of the child to an object, such as a squeaky toy, while placing one hand in front of one of the child's eyes. As the object is held in the gaze, uncover the eye, watching intently for the eyes to shift to refocus on the object. Repeat in the other eye. If a shift occurs, the child should be assessed for strabismus.

In this age group, the otoscopic exam may be the most difficult exam to perform. Several techniques can be used to gain cooperation of the child. In addition to performing the exam on the caregiver first, you can also touch the tip of the light otoscope to the finger of the child. The finger will glow red but not cause pain. Another technique is for you to hold the otoscope with the tip into your own ear, cupping the head of the otoscope so that it cannot be pushed into the ear, and then ask the child to look in your ear: "I think there's a bird in my ear—can you check?" followed by, "Is there a bird in your ear? Can I look?"

Maxillary sinuses form by the age of 4 years. Transillumination can be performed if indicated.

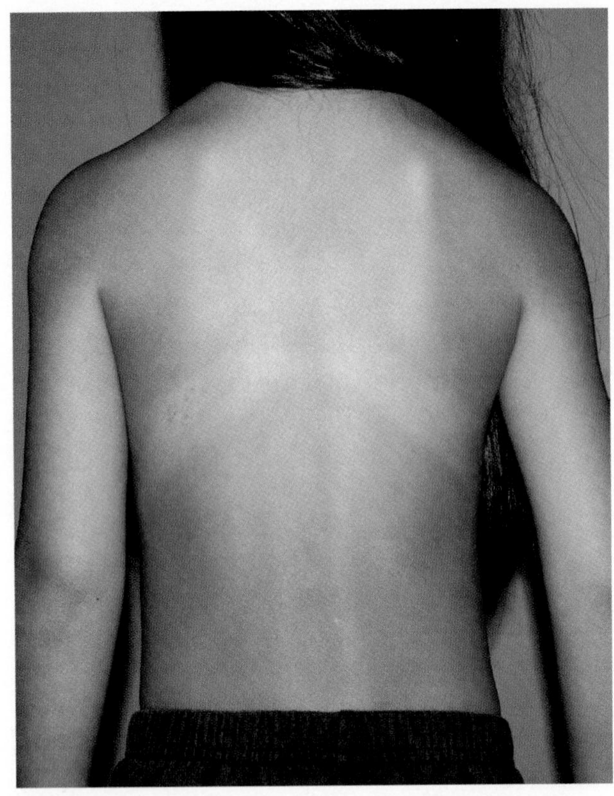
A

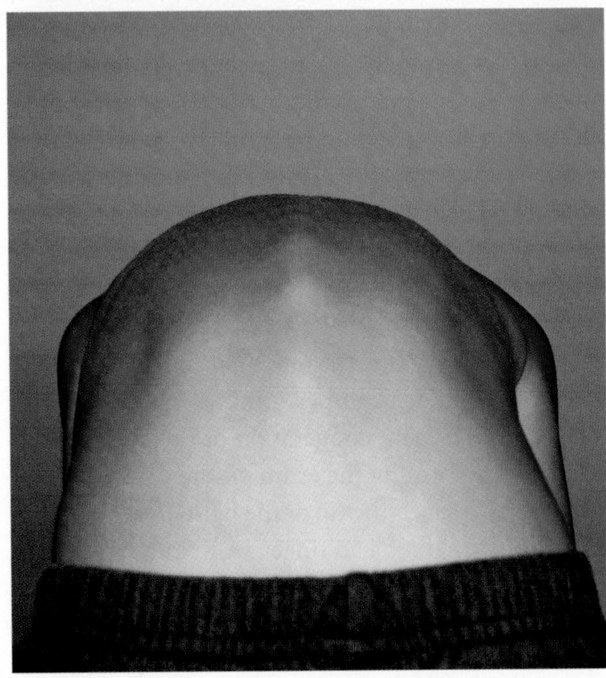
B

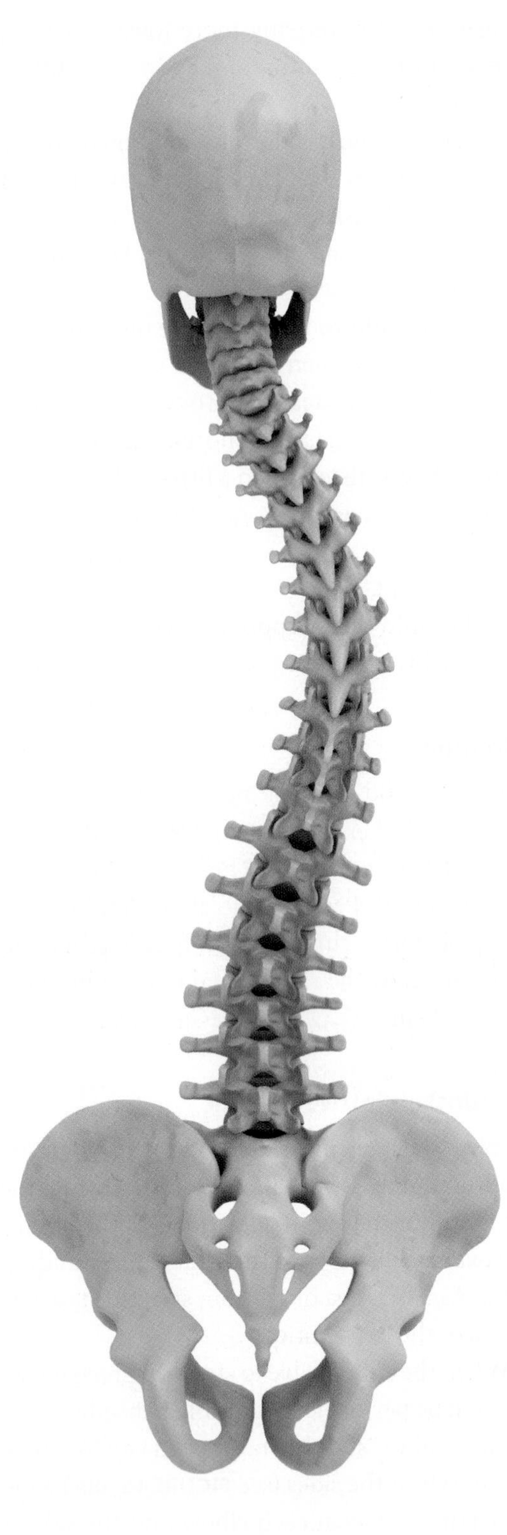
C

FIGURE 18-28 Scoliosis exam.

© Sebastian Kaulitzki/ShutterStock, Inc.

Middle Childhood Through Adolescence

Once the child reaches the age of 5 years, the exam follows the sequence of adult examination. Children over 5 typically cooperate well with the examination. If a child seems fearful or reluctant, even with the caregiver in the room, the provider should consider prior bad experiences during examinations as well as abuse as possible causes.

As the child moves toward adolescence, the visit should be directed more and more toward the patient as the primary provider of historical data.

Caregivers should be asked about their preference regarding the provider's sharing information about sensitive topics such as tobacco, alcohol, and drug use, sexual behavior, and bullying. It is preferable to reserve a few minutes during the visit to interview the patient alone to assess these areas, as few adolescents, with the caregiver present, would volunteer that they are experimenting with drugs.

The conversation with the caregiver can be shared with the patient in the room and should identify that as adolescence is nearing, the development of a trusting patient/provider relationship is optimal. Attaining this relationship allows the provider to offer education and anticipatory guidance. Caregivers should be assured that no physical examination will be completed without their permission and an assistant will be in the room. Ascertain if any topics should or should not be discussed. For example, as part of anticipatory guidance, you would typically include expected changes that accompany sexual development and educate the patient about sexual activity, the avoidance of pregnancy, and sexually transmitted infections. These topics are typically part of school curricula and you would expect the patient to have some knowledge of the topic. In determining caregiver preference, however, you find that the patient is home-schooled and that the caregiver does not want any discussion of sexual issues until the age of 18.

The discussion may run something like this:

- Mrs. Beasley, your daughter is coming to the age where it is important for her to start developing a solid patient/provider relationship. It's an opportunity to ask her questions related to things like tobacco, alcohol, drugs, and sexual issues. Sometimes talking about these things is hard to do in front of parents. I like to take a few minutes out of each visit to talk with patients your daughter's age without the parent in the room. I don't do any examination, and if you prefer, I can have an assistant in the room. Would that be all right with you?

Then add,

- Are there any topics you want me to discuss? Are there any topics you don't want me to discuss?

When you begin the interview, be sure to stress to the patient that your visit is confidential and that unless required by law, you will not be sharing information he/she gives you with anyone else. The provider will need to have knowledge of local and state ordinances.

- Sarah, I know it's hard to talk about some things in front of your parents. For me to take care of you the best I can, I need to ask you some questions. Whatever you tell me will be kept between us unless I am required to report it, such as if you would have any plans to hurt yourself or others, or if you are being abused. Otherwise, our conversation will be between us. If I think we should get your parents involved, I will tell you so and ask your permission before I do so. How does that sound?

You may then begin your questions, asking the least sensitive first—i.e., dietary habits that may suggest eating disorders; reflection of self-image; social interactions including bullying; exposure to and experimentation with tobacco, alcohol, and drugs; anticipated changes in the body with sexual maturity; and sexual behavior.

The physical examination is then conducted in the same manner as the adult exam.

References

1. Rudolph AM, Rudolph CD, eds. *Rudolph's Pediatrics.* 21st ed. New York, NY: McGraw-Hill Medical Publishing Division; 2003. STAT!Ref Online Electronic Medical Library. http://online.statref.com/document.aspx?fxid=13&docid=57. Accessed July 9, 2012.

2. DeCherney AH, Nathan L, Laufer N, Goodwin TM, eds. *Current Diagnosis & Treatment Obstetrics & Gynecology.* 10th ed. New York, NY: Lange Medical Books/McGraw-Hill Medical Publishing Division; 2007. STAT!Ref Online Electronic Medical Library. http://online.statref.com/document.aspx?fxid=30&docid=323. Accessed July 9, 2012.
3. American Academy of Pediatrics, American College of Obstetricians and Gynecologists. *Guidelines for Perinatal Care.* 6th ed. Elk Grove Village, IL: American Academy of Pediatrics; 2007.
4. Finster M, Wood M. The Apgar score has survived the test of time. *Anesthesiology.* 2005 Apr;102(4):855–857.
5. American Academy of Pediatrics, American College of Obstetricians and Gynecologists. *Guidelines for Perinatal Care.* 6th ed. Elk Grove Village, IL: American Academy of Pediatrics; 2007.
6. PubMed Health. A.D.A.M Medical Encyclopedia. *Stork Bite.* http://www.ncbi.nlm.nih.gov/pubmedhealth/PMH0002364. Accessed November 2, 2012.
7. Sondheimer JM, Levin MJ, Deterding RR, Hay Jr. WW, eds. *Current Diagnosis & Treatment in Pediatrics.* 19th ed. New York, NY: Lange Medical Books/McGraw-Hill Medical Publishing Division; 2009. STAT!Ref Online Electronic Medical Library. http://online.statref.com/document.aspx?fxid=33&docid=303. Accessed July 9, 2012.
8. Council on Children With Disabilities, Section on Developmental Behavioral Pediatrics, Bright Futures Steering Committee, Medical Home Initiatives for Children With Special Needs Project Advisory Committee. Identifying infants and young children with developmental disorders in the medical home: an algorithm for developmental surveillance and screening. *Pediatrics.* 2006;118(1):405. http://pediatrics.aappublications.org/content/118/1/405.full. Accessed July 10, 2012.
9. Kuczmarski RJ, Ogden CL, Guo SS, et al. 2000 CDC growth charts for the United States: methods and development. *Vital Health Stat 11.* 2002 May;(246):1–190.

CHAPTER 19

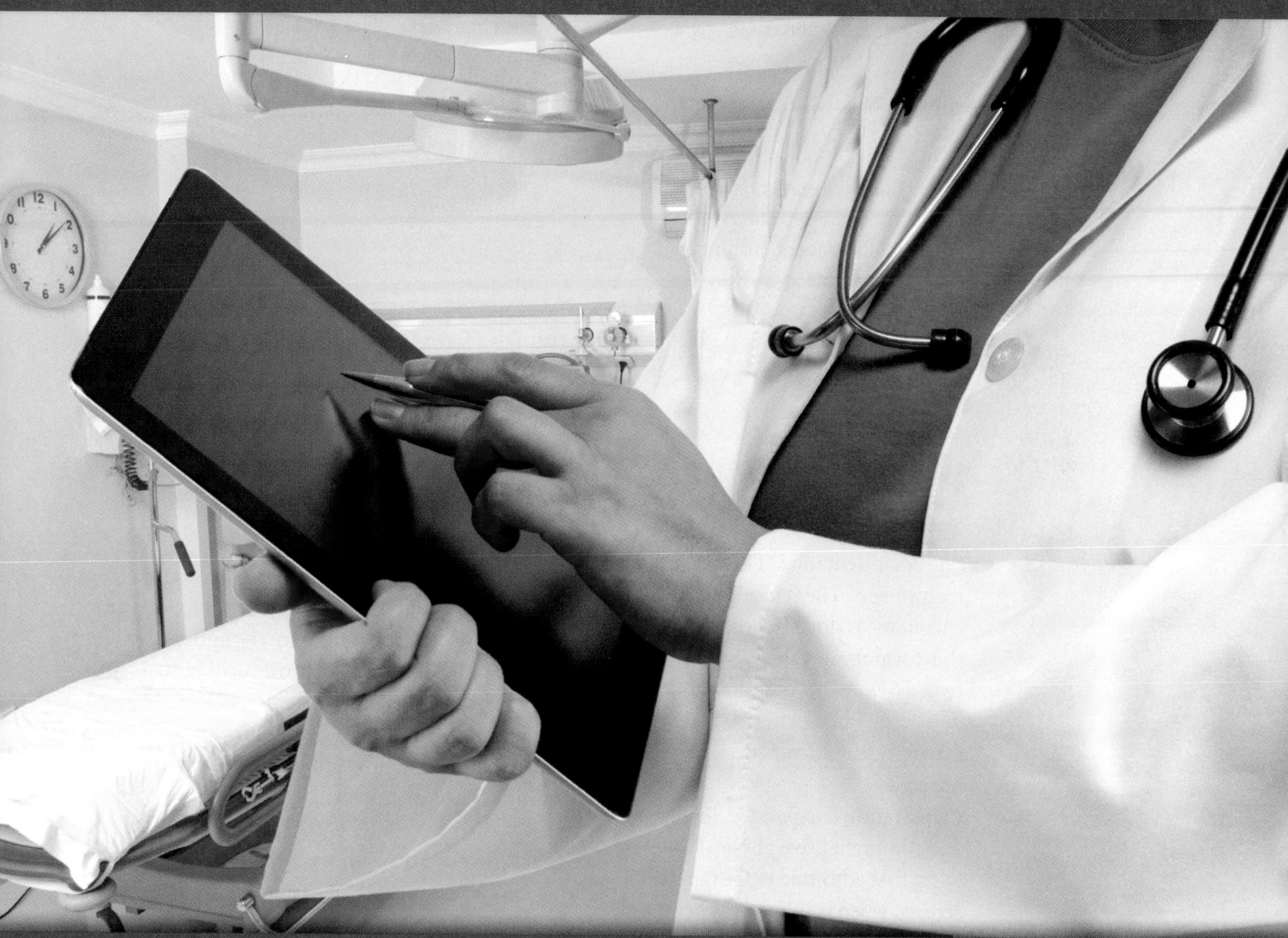

© Levent Konuk/ShutterStock, Inc.

Patient Encounter Documentation

OBJECTIVES

At the conclusion of this chapter, the student will be able to

1. Understand the components of each section of the SOAP note
2. Organize the subjective section of the SOAP note to provide a concise, chronological account of the history of present illness
3. Accurately document the patient encounter utilizing the SOAP note format

KEY TERMS

History and physical examinations (H&Ps)
SOAP note
Subjective
Objective
Assessment
Plan

Where this icon appears, visit **go.jblearning.com/HPECWS** to view the video.

History and physical examinations: evaluation of the patient through attainment of a complete medical history and the performance of a comprehensive physical examination

SOAP note: standardized documentation format for patient encounters consisting of four sections: subjective, objective, assessment, and plan

All patient encounters require accurate documentation. This comes in many forms. The typical outpatient encounter is documented utilizing the format of subjective, objective, assessment, and plan (SOAP note). The same pattern when used for daily inpatient encounters is referred to as a progress note. Patients require expanded histories and comprehensive physical exams when first admitted to the inpatient setting, when being seen as new patients at outpatient clinics, or routinely at age-appropriate intervals. These comprehensive evaluations are called **history and physical examinations** (H&Ps).

SOAP Note Documentation

Every patient encounter requires documentation not only to preserve the event as related to the care and future reference for the patient, but also for billing and legal purposes. The **SOAP note**, most frequently used in outpatient documentations, records the history obtained, the physical examination performed, the assessment in the form of a differential diagnosis, and the plan for investigation and treatment.

WRITING THE SOAP NOTE

Legibility in documentation is very important and is made easier through the advancement of electronic medical records (EMRs). Even though providers may follow the standard of care in diagnosis and treatment of the patient, when charts are reviewed where bad outcomes have been encountered, illegible notes appear sloppy and allow for misinterpretation to occur: Sloppy writing translates to sloppy patient care.

Each note must begin with the date and time of the encounter—a medical, legal, and coding necessity. A well-written note becomes an accurate account of the patient's current illness followed by his/her general medical history. This is followed by your findings from the physical examination. Your assessment is a list of possible diagnoses that demonstrate your thought processes and interpretation of the history and exam. You finish the document with what you plan to do for the patient, not only immediately but in the long term as well.

The note should be complete and concise, providing a reader unfamiliar with the case with a detailed, easily understood picture of the patient encounter. Only appropriate abbreviations should be used within the SOAP note. Avoid nonstandard abbreviations.

Subjective (S):

Date:
Time:
Chief complaint:
HPI (CODIERS): Demographics followed by CODIERS in paragraph form
SMASH FM (bulleted format)

- Social Hx (FED TACOS)
  - Food (diet)
  - Exercise
  - Drugs
  - Tobacco
  - Alcohol
  - Caffeine
  - Occupation
  - Sexual history
- Medical Hx
- Allergies
- Surgical Hx
- Hospitalizations
- Family Hx
- Medications

Objective (O): Head-to-toe system exam (bulleted format)

- Vitals
- General Assessment
- HEENT–follow with other systems examined

Assessment (A): Differential diagnosis in order of likelihood

1) Primary diagnoses
2) Rule out (r/o) diagnoses
3) Doubtful diagnoses

Plan (P): (MOTHRR)

1) Medications
2) OMM
3) Testing
4) Holistic/Humanistic
5) Referral
6) Return plan

Legible signature

FIGURE 19-1 The standard SOAP note format contains four sections: subjective, objective, assessment, and plan.

SOAP NOTE FORMAT

The standard SOAP note format with components is shown in **FIGURE 19-1**.

Subjective

The **subjective** section of the SOAP note contains only the history that was obtained from the patient encounter. This is the patient's story, collected through the CODIERS SMASH FM mnemonic tool. By carefully interviewing the patient, you will try to obtain the most thorough and accurate information possible. You may quote the patient directly. Phrases such as "fluid on the lungs" or "a cancer in the belly" are acceptable once you have done your best to obtain more precise information: heart failure and gastric carcinoma. By the same token, the patient's ability to recall dates may not be precise. Patients may only remember that they had a tonsillectomy "as a child" or that they had asthma that "went away in

Subjective: section of the SOAP note containing the chief complaint, patient demographics, and history obtained from the patient encounter

high school," and you may record the information as it is presented to you.

The subjective section always begins with the chief complaint and should be concise, describing the symptoms, diagnosis, or other reasons for the encounter, and in the patient's own words as often as is practical. The following is an example of how chief complaints should be documented:

Subjective 7/21/09 1310

CC: Nasal congestion and frontal HA × 5 days

After the chief complaint the CODIERS portion of the history is recorded in paragraph form. Start with the patient demographics, giving the patient's age, race, and gender: "19 y/o CF complaining of . . . " The rest of the history of the present illness should complete a paragraph giving all of the pertinent information from CODIERS.

Subjective 7/21/09 1310

CC: Nasal congestion and frontal HA × 5 days

S: 19 y/o CF (demographics) presents c/o nasal congestion with thick green rhinorrhea × 5 days. Also c/o b/l frontal HA × 3 days, increased with bending over, postnasal drainage, and cough with green sputum production, especially in the am. Rates HA with a 5/10 intensity. No prior history of the same. Denies sore throat, fever, chills, sob, ear or neck pain.

When you first start writing SOAP notes, it may be difficult to decide exactly which information to include. You may start by following the CODIERS questions very closely, converting the answers to declarative sentences. As you gain skill in creating the narrative of SOAP notes, you should find that you are thinking ahead to the assessment and plan while writing down the subjective material. With practice, the SOAP will become a cohesive story from start to finish.

Once you are able to decide in advance what you want to express in the assessment and plan, you will have a better idea of what will be needed in your subjective to support it. For example, if you believe that a patient with coughing, sneezing, and a runny nose has a cold, you should carefully describe the symptoms that convinced you of the diagnosis (pertinent positives) and then include all of the factors that helped you decide that the patient did not have other conditions associated with each of those symptoms, such as allergies or sinusitis (pertinent negatives).

The SMASH FM information should consist of short lists of information in outline format. The individual initials do not have any specific meaning in the world of medical documentation so you need to write out the words they stand for or use an accepted abbreviation. Documenting "M: Diabetes" will not be intelligible to anyone, so you should write out "Medical History: Diabetes."

Once again it is important to include the negative information. You may know that the patient has never been hospitalized, but no one else will until you write it out. It is also important to remember to be very specific in asking patients their history to be sure to get the exact information you are seeking. A perfectly compliant patient might tell you that he/she has no medical conditions, no medications, and no surgeries and then tell you that he/she has been hospitalized for pneumonia twice in the last year, but only if you ask.

Subjective 7/21/09 1310

CC: Nasal congestion and frontal HA × 5 days

S: 19 y/o CF presents c/o nasal congestion with thick green rhinorrhea × 5 days. Also c/o b/l frontal HA × 3 days, increased with bending over, postnasal drainage, and cough with green sputum production, especially in the am. Rates HA with a 5/10 intensity. No prior history of the same. Denies sore throat, fever, chills, sob, ear or neck pain.

Social Hx:	**Tobacco: ½ ppd × 4 years**	**(SMASH FM bulleted)**
	Alcohol: None	
	Occupation: College freshman	
	FLDNMP: 1 week ago	

Medical Hx: Otitis media—childhood

Allergies: None

Surg Hx: B/L ear tubes at 4 y/o

Family Hx: No contacts with similar symptoms

Medications: Birth control pill

A frequently seen error is putting CODIERS under Subjective and SMASH FM under Objective, where the physical examination belongs, and then completely omitting the physical exam from documentation. Avoid this mistake.

Objective

Under **objective**, begin with documenting the vital signs provided to you from the patient data sheet. If you repeat any vitals, mark them as such: "Repeated vitals: BP 132/76 Right arm."

The next lines should contain the problem-specific physical examination in outline format with headings for each part of the system exam. Unless the chief complaint is very minor and the patient extremely healthy (a splinter in the finger of a 12-year-old child), assessment of the heart and lungs is almost always included.

Your examination should be written up in the following format:

Objective

WDWN CF in no apparent distress

T-99.0F, P-88, R-16, BP-160/94, Repeated BP-136/82 R arm

Skin—warm and dry w/o rash

Head—NC, frontal sinus tenderness to palp and percussion b/l

Ears—TMs gray b/l with good light reflex

Nose—mucosa edema and erythema with green exudate

Pharynx—minimal erythema, green PND. No tonsillar hypertrophy.

Neck—w/o lymphadenopathy

Lungs—CTA w/o wheezes, crackles

Heart—RRR w/o murmur, rub, or gallop

An ideal physical examination would include every positive finding that helps confirm the most likely diagnosis and any negative findings that help to exclude other items in the differential. Be very careful not to write anything in the physical exam that you did not actually do. It is preferable to write "not assessed" rather than "deferred," which has some ambiguity. If a patient refuses part of the examination, it should be noted as "refused" or "declined by patient."

Assessment

The **assessment** is the differential diagnosis and should be numbered in order of likelihood. For our patient with coughing, sneezing, and runny nose, you could write simply:

Assessment

1. **URI**
2. **Rule out rhinosinusitis**
3. **Doubt seasonal allergies**

The first item in the differential should be the most likely and should never be preceded by "rule out." If the diagnosis is not known, the presenting symptoms can be documented. For example, if a patient presents with a cough of unknown etiology, the first diagnosis would be "cough," not "rule out pneumonia." If, however, through your physical findings you identify pneumonia as the cause of the cough, your first entry would be "Pneumonia."

Additional suspected diagnoses that require further investigation can be entered with "rule out" or "R/O."

If there is no actual complaint in the reason for the patient's visit, you should list preexisting medical problems, health maintenance issues, or risk factors appropriate to the patient's age and reason for the visit. For example, a 50-year-old diabetic male presents for a yearly physical examination that is required for him to drive a school bus. He smokes, has an allergy to bee stings, and is noted to have a mild elevation of his blood pressure with no history of prior elevation. Your assessment might include items such as:

Assessment

1) **Diabetes mellitus** (preexisting medical condition)
2) **Tobacco use disorder** (risk factor)
3) **Elevated BP without diagnosis of hypertension** (risk factor)
4) **Bee sting allergy** (preexisting condition)
5) **Colorectal cancer screening** (health maintenance issue)

Objective: section of the SOAP note documenting the finding of the physical examination performed on the patient

Assessment: section of the SOAP note documenting the differential diagnosis derived from the patient encounter in order of likelihood

Plan: section of the SOAP note documenting the proposed treatment plan for the patient

Plan

The first priority in the **plan** section should be to give a well-thought-out course of treatment for the diagnosis you believe is most likely and to include as many elements of proper medical care as possible. You may also rule out secondary diagnoses as appropriate. For example, in a patient with a likely URI, strep pharyngitis could be addressed and ruled out effectively with a simple notation of "throat culture" in the plan.

MOTHRR.

Using the mnemonic "MOTHRR" covers all of the elements needed to construct a complete plan for the patient. MOTHRR stands for:

- Medicines
- Osteopathic treatment
- Testing
- Holistic/Humanistic items
- Referrals
- Return plan

Not every aspect of this mnemonic is required for every case, but you should at least think of each category as you decide on the appropriate treatment for your patients. Remember also that the letters used in the mnemonic are not standard medical abbreviations, requiring you to either write out the individual headings or simply number the items that address each of the categories. Do not write out the initials M-O-T-H-R-R as headings.

Medications. Document the drug name, dose, frequency, amount dispensed, number of refills, and specific instructions that were shared with the patient.

- Ibuprofen 600 mg PO three times a day with food, Disp #30, 1 refill.

Osteopathic treatment. For each diagnosis consider if osteopathic manipulation is appropriate. If so, be certain you have documented the dysfunction necessitating manipulation within the physical examination and the differential. Document the intervention, noting areas of treatment, techniques, and outcome on reassessment.

Testing. Testing includes all of the tests you want to order to confirm the diagnosis, rule out less likely diagnoses, and guide your treatment plan. This includes such things as blood work, radiological studies, and specialized tests performed by other providers.

Holistic/Humanistic. Holistic/Humanistic items show your concern for the patient as a whole and demonstrate that you are thinking of the patient as a person rather than as a simple diagnosis. Classic examples include asking if the patient would like to include a relative, friend, or other support person in the discussion of diagnosis and building of a treatment plan, or asking questions that indicate that you are thinking about how the current illness is affecting the patient's life by interfering with work or the activities of daily living. These questions should be asked of every patient. Writing in your plan that you are going to take steps to overcome these problems allows you to give concrete evidence that you have considered these matters carefully.

Referral. Referral is another area where you will not always have anything to add. If you are convinced that you need the help of a specialist to take care of the patient, then by all means ask for one, but do not order excessive consultations simply to have something to put in this category.

Return Plan. The return plan is the last thing to address. If the patient is to be admitted to the hospital, a return plan may not be appropriate until the outcome of the admission is known. In all other instances, you should indicate the follow-up plan to see the patient. Whether a day or a year later, as a dedicated provider who is committed to making certain the patient has received optimal care, you will need to follow up with the patient.

Plan

Medications: Amoxicillin 500 mg tid × 14 days

OMM: Frontal sinus drainage techniques applied b/l

Holistic: Increase fluids, return to work in 2 days

Return Plan: Nursing to call in 3 days to reassess. Patient to call earlier with increase in headache, fever, change in vision, no improvement.

The complete SOAP note may be similar to this example.

Subjective 7/21/09 1310

CC: Nasal congestion and frontal HA × 5 days

S: 19 y/o CF presents c/o nasal congestion with thick green rhinorrhea × 5 days. Also c/o b/l frontal HA × 3 days, increased with bending over, postnasal drainage, and cough with green sputum production, especially in the am. Rates HA with a 5/10 intensity. No prior history of the same. Denies sore throat, fever, chills, sob, ear or neck pain.

Social Hx: **Tobacco: ½ ppd × 4 years**

Alcohol: None

Occupation: College freshman

FLDNMP: 1 week ago

Medical Hx: Otitis media—childhood

Allergies: None

Surg Hx: B/L ear tubes at 4 y/o

Family Hx: No contacts with similar symptoms

Medications: Birth control pill

Objective

WDWN CF in no apparent distress

T-99.0F, P-88, R-16, BP-160/94, Repeated BP-136/82 R arm

Skin—warm and dry w/o rash

Head—NC, frontal sinus tenderness to palp and percussion b/l

Ears—TMs gray b/l with good light reflex

Nose—mucosa edema and erythema with green exudate

Pharynx—minimal erythema, green PND. No tonsillar hypertrophy.

Neck—w/o lymphadenopathy

Lungs—CTA w/o wheezes, crackles

Heart—RRR w/o murmur, rub or gallop

Assessment

1. **Sinusitis**
2. **URI**
3. **Doubt seasonal allergies**
4. **Tobacco use disorder**

Plan

Medications: Amoxicillin 500 mg tid × 14 days

OMM: Frontal sinus drainage techniques applied b/l

Holistic: Increase fluids, return to work in 2 days

Return Plan: Nursing to call in 3 days to reassess. Patient to call earlier with increase in headache, fever, change in vision, no improvement.

Complete History and Physical Examination

The full history and physical examination follow essentially the same format as the SOAP note, with expansion of details (see **FIGURE 19-2**). The subjective section is replaced by the terminology "History of Present Illness" but contains the exact same components of CODIERS. Though symptoms associated with the CC are still present in the HPI, an additional screening called the review of symptoms (ROS) is a general survey of all body systems and is not based on the presenting complaint. SMASH FM is expanded to include more details in the social history, medical history with immunizations, and surgical, hospitalization, and family history. Assessment and plan remain the same.

Patient Name:
Date: 01/12/2013
Time: 0234

CC: "In the patient's own words" × duration

HPI: Demographics—Age, race, sex, presents (CODIERS)

- **Social History (FED TACOS):**

Food (diet)	Alcohol
Exercise	Caffeine
Drugs	Occupation
Tobacco	Sexual history

- **OB/GYN History:**

Gravida Para	Menstruation: Frequency, duration, flow, FDLMP
Menarche	Menopause

- **Medical History:**
- **Immunizations:**
- **Allergies:**

Food with reaction
Drug with reaction
Environmental with reaction

- **Surgical History:**

Procedure Date

- **Hospitalizations**

Cause Date

- **Family History:** Living/deceased Medical conditions Cause of death

Mother
Father
Siblings
Children
General

- **Medications:** Name Dose Frequency

- **Review of Systems:**

Constitutional	Genitourinary
Integumentary/breast	Musculoskeletal
Eyes	Neurologic
Ears, nose, mouth, and throat	Psychiatric
Cardiovascular	Endocrine
Respiratory	Hematologic/lymphatic
Gastrointestinal	Allergic/immunologic

FIGURE 19-2 History and physical examination format.

Physical Exam:

• **General:**

Nutrition
Development
Alertness
Hygiene
Appearance to the stated age
Distress
Position of comfort

• **Vitals:**

BP / L arm position
/ R arm position
Respirations Rhythm and rate/minute
Pulse Rhythm and rate/minute
Temperature Degrees

• **Integumentary:**

Skin:
- Inspection:
  - Color:
    - Diffuse
    - Localized
  - Lesions:
    - Primary
    - Secondary
- Palpation:
  - Temperature
  - Texture
  - Moisture
- Turgor

Hair:
- Inspection:
  - Distribution
  - Infestations
- Palpation:
  - Texture

Nails:
- Inspection:
  - Color
  - Condition
  - Lesions
  - Clubbing
- Palpation:
  - Capillary refill

FIGURE 19-2 History and physical examination format. *(Continued)*

- **HEENT:**

Head:
- Inspection:
  - Shape
  - Trauma
  - Lesions
- Palpation:
  - Tenderness
- Percussion:
  - Tenderness

Eyes:
- Visual acuity
- Inspection:
  - Periorbital areas
  - Extraocular movements
  - Eyelids
  - Alignment—light reflex
  - Sclera
  - Conjunctiva
  - Cornea
  - Iris
  - Anterior chamber
  - Pupil
  - Pupillary reaction
  - Ophthalmoscopic exam
    - Retina
    - Vessels
    - Optic nerve
    - Cup/disc ratio

Ears:
- Auditory acuity
- Inspection:
  - External ear
  - External canal
  - Canal
  - Tympanic membrane

Nose:
- Inspection:
  - External
  - Internal
- Palpation:
  - Nasal patency

Throat:
- Inspection:
  - Teeth
  - Gingiva
  - Tongue
    - Lesions
    - Protrusions
  - Floor of the mouth
    - Salivary ducts
  - Buccal mucosa
    - Parotid ducts
  - Hard palate
  - Soft palate
  - Uvula with phonation for deviation
  - Posterior pharynx

FIGURE 19-2 History and physical examination format. *(Continued)*

Neck:

Inspection:

Symmetry

Range of motion

Jugular veins

Auscultation

Carotid

Thyroid

Palpation:

Muscoloskeletal

Trachea

Thyroid

Carotid

Lymphatics:

Palpation:

Cervical

Axillary

Inguinal

Respiratory:

Inspection:

Accessory muscle use

Chest wall

AP:lat ratio

Auscultation

Palpation:

Symmetry in rise and fall

Tenderness

Percussion:

Lung fields

Diaphragmatic excursion

Cardiovascular:

Heart:

Inspection:

Precordium

Point of maximal impulse (PMI)

Heaves

Auscultation:

Rhythm

Valve closure—S1, S2

Extra heart sounds

S3, S4, opening snap, ejection click, murmur

Palpation

PMI

Thrills

Extremeties:

Inspection:

Lesions

Edema

Varicosities

Hair loss

Clubbing

Palpation:

Peripheral pulses scaled 0 to 4

Capillary refill

FIGURE 19-2 History and physical examination format. *(Continued)*

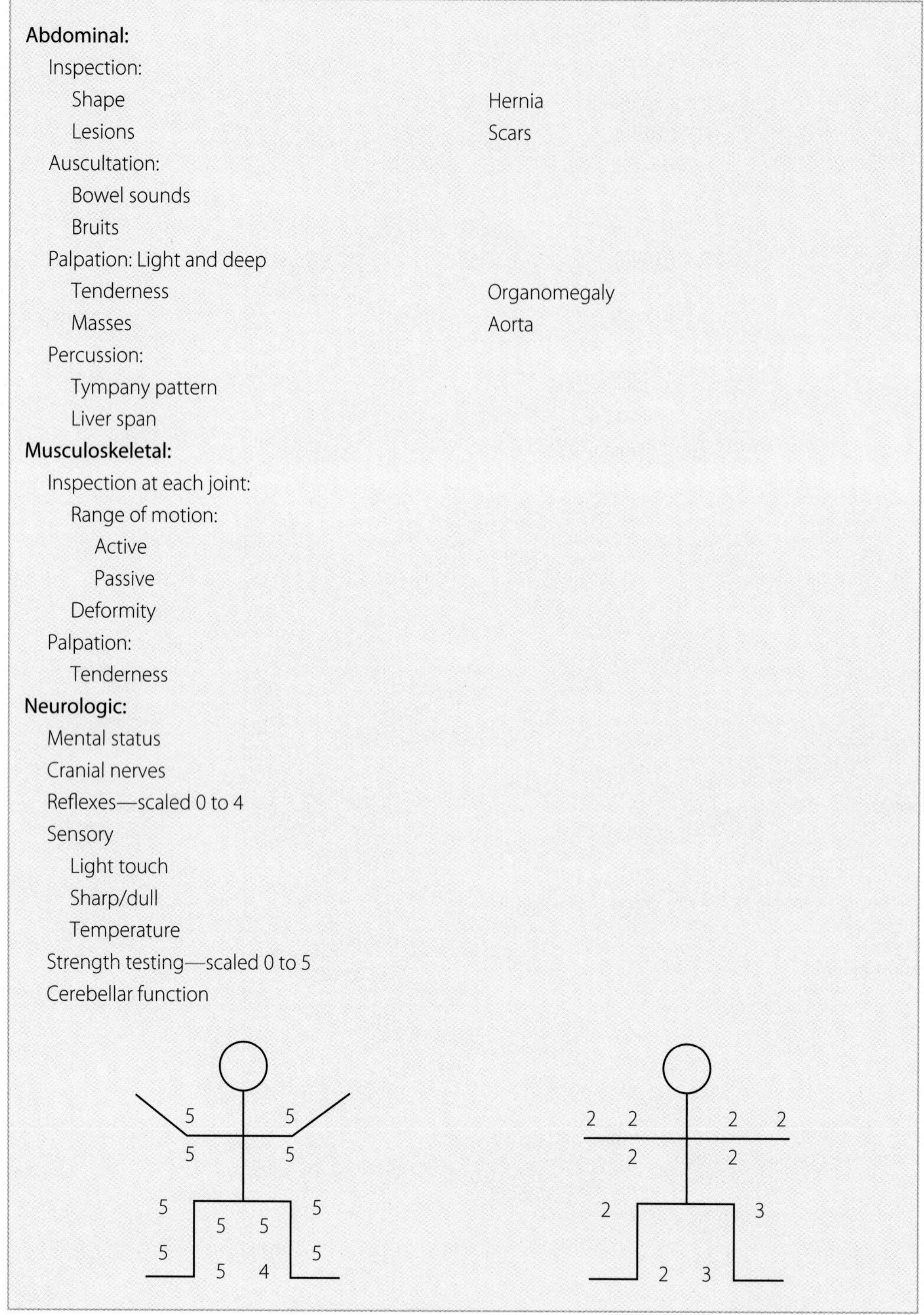

Abdominal:

- Inspection:
  - Shape — Hernia
  - Lesions — Scars
- Auscultation:
  - Bowel sounds
  - Bruits
- Palpation: Light and deep
  - Tenderness — Organomegaly
  - Masses — Aorta
- Percussion:
  - Tympany pattern
  - Liver span

Musculoskeletal:

- Inspection at each joint:
  - Range of motion:
    - Active
    - Passive
  - Deformity
- Palpation:
  - Tenderness

Neurologic:

- Mental status
- Cranial nerves
- Reflexes—scaled 0 to 4
- Sensory
  - Light touch
  - Sharp/dull
  - Temperature
- Strength testing—scaled 0 to 5
- Cerebellar function

FIGURE 19-2 History and physical examination format. *(Continued)*

Breast:

Inspection:

- Symmetry
- Tanner stage
- Skin changes
- Nipple direction
- Discharge

Palpation:

- Masses
- Discharge
- Tail

Female genitalia:

Inspection:

- Mons pubis
- Labia majora
- Labia minora
- Perineum
- Clitoris
- Urethral orifice
- Vaginal opening:
  - Discharge
  - Skene's glands
  - Bartholin's glands
- Vaginal outlet
- Speculum:
  - Vaginal walls
  - Cervix
  - Os

Bimanual palpation:

- Vaginal wall
- Cervix and fornices
- Uterus
- Adnexa

Rectovaginal palpation:

- Rectal walls
- Posterior vaginal wall

Male genitalia:

Penis:

- Inspection:
  - Prepuce
  - Glans
  - Urethral meatus
  - Shaft
- Palpation:
  - Glans
  - Shaft

Scrotum:

- Inspection:
  - Skin
  - Contour
  - Testes
  - Masses
- Transillumination with masses
- Palpation:
  - Testes
  - Epididymis
  - Spermatic cord with vas deferens
  - External ring

FIGURE 19-2 History and physical examination format. *(Continued)*

Rectum:
- Inspection:
  - Sacrococcygeal
  - Perianal
- Palpation:
  - Perianal
  - Sphincter tone
  - Rectal wall
  - Masses
  - Tenderness
  - Prostate:
    - Lobes
    - Median sulcus

Assessment/Plan:

Signature:

FIGURE 19-2 History and physical examination format. *(Continued)*

Patient Name: Gail Stoner
Date: 01/12/2013
Time: 0236
Historian: Patient–reliable

CC: "My stomach hurts" × 2 days
HPI: 46 y/o female presents to the ER with abdominal pain. Pain started approximately 2 days ago with gradual onset. Pain is described as an "ache" that is constantly present. Intensity started at 2/10 and built to current level of at 8/10 with wax and wane from 6 to 10. Pain is localized in the RUQ with radiation to the back during exacerbations. Took 4 chewable antacids at midnight without relief. Nothing makes the pain worse. Denies association with particular foods. Admits two prior occasions of similar pain, six months and one month ago, which remitted without treatment or seeking intervention. Admits nausea, fever (no actual temperature taken), and chills. Vomited × 2 at approximately 10 PM and 1 AM consisting of about a cup each of food-like emesis without blood or bile. States husband told her that her eyes looked a little yellow. Denies jaundice, cough, dyspepsia, diarrhea, change in color of stools, tea-colored urine, hematuria, or flank pain.

- **Social Hx:**

Diet: Avoids milk (lactose intolerance)

Exercise: Walks 2 to 3 days a week × 30 minutes

Drugs: Denies

Tobacco: Denies

Alcohol: Occasional beer (1–2 per week)

Caffeine: Denies

Sexual Hx: Monogamous with husband × 20 years. No hx of STD.

Occupation: Actor

Travel: Traveled to Mexico 2 weeks prior. Diarrhea during trip resolved.

- **OB/GYN Hx:** G3P3003, menarche 12, FDLMP 1 week ago.
- **Medical Hx:** High cholesterol
- **Allergies:** Denies food, drug, and environmental allergies
- **Surg Hx:** Appendectomy—12 y/o. Left ankle fracture—24 y/o
- **Hospitalizations:** Only for appendectomy
- **Family Hx:** Mother living at 66—HTN, colonic polyps
  Father—deceased at 68—MI, hyperlipidemia, smoker
  Brother—deceased at 23, MVA
  Brother—living at 43, hyperlipidemia
  Daughter—14—good health
  Daugther—11—Asthma
- **Medications:** Statin (name unknown), 1 daily, started within last month, dosage unknown
  Fish oil OTC, bid
  ASA 81 mg daily

FIGURE 19-3 Sample of a complete history and physical examination. *(continues)*

- **Review of Systems:**

Constitutional: (+) Fever, chills
(–) Weight loss or gain, night sweats, fatigue
Eyes: (–) Blurred or loss of vision, double vision, eye pain, injection, discharge, deviation
Ears, nose, mouth, and throat: (–) Ear pain, discharge, hearing loss, epistaxis, nasal congestion, lesions, tooth pain, dysphagia, tinnitus, sore throat
Cardiovascular: (–) Palpitations, chest pain, peripheral edema, claudication, irregular heartbeats, murmur, orthopnea
Respiratory: (–) Shortness of breath, dyspnea on exertion, coughing, wheezing, chest pain, paroxysmal nocturnal dyspnea, hemoptysis
Gastrointestinal: (+) Nausea, vomiting, abdominal pain, eructation, lactose intolerance
(–) dyspepsia, diarrhea, constipation, bloating, hematemesis, hematochezia, change in caliber of stools, bright red blood per rectum, melena
Genitourinary: (–) Hesitancy, flank pain, dysuria, hematuria, urgency, frequency, decrease in force of stream, vaginal discharge or bleeding, dyspareunia
Muscoloskeletal: (–) Arthralgia, myalgia, bony deformity, weakness, range of motion limitation
Integumentary/breast: (–) Changes in pigmentation or texture, rashes, lesions, pruritus, hair loss or change in hair texture, nail changes, dimpling of the breast, change in direction of the nipples, discharge
Neurologic: (–) Facial asymmetry, memory loss, paresthesias, weakness, slurred speech, imbalance, changes in gait, dysphagia
Psychiatric: (–) Depression, anxiety, suicidal or homicidal ideation, hallucinations, phobias,
Endocrine: (–) Polyuria, polyphagia, polydipsia, heat or cold intolerances
Hematologic/lymphatic: (–) Easy bruising or bleeding, anemia, transfusion history, syncope, lymphadenopathy
Allergic/immunologic: (–) Allergies, recurrent infections, eczema, nasal polyps

Physical Exam:

- **General:** WNWD, alert, well kept, CF who appears the stated age, in moderate distress, seated on stretcher flexed toward R abd
- **Vitals:** BP–110/64 L arm seated, Resp–32/min, Pulse–reg at 62 bpm, Temp 101.4 F, Wt 138 lb, Ht 5'6"
- **Integumentary:**
  - Skin: Tan w/o jaundice, cyanosis, pallor, or erythema. Warm, smooth, & slightly diaphoretic. Well-healed 10-cm vertical surgical scar of the RUQ. Turgor intact. No edema.
  - Hair: No alopecia or hirsutism. Smooth to palp. No suspicious lesions.
  - Nails: Pink, cuticles, nail folds intact. No lesions or clubbing. Capillary refill <2 seconds throughout.
- **HEENT:**
  - Head: Normocephalic, atraumatic, w/o infestation, lesions, or rashes. Sinuses nontender to palp and percussion.
  - Eyes: Left–20/20, Right–20/40 by handheld chart. PERRLA, EOMI. Possible mild icterus. No nystagmus, ptosis, strabismus, injection, lesions, hemorrhage, pallor, exudates, or shallow anterior chamber. Cornea w/o clouding. Retina without A/V nicking, copper or silver wiring, exudates, or hemorrage.
  - Ears: Hearing intact to whispered word at 24 inches b/l. External ear w/o lesions, canal w/o exudate.
  - Nose: Without deformity, lesions, or exudates. Nasal patency intact b/l.
  - Throat: Teeth in good repair. Gingiva without bleeding, retractions, hypertrophy, or lesions. Mucosa moist without lesions, Erythema, or exudates. Tongue distends midline, pink, moist w/o lesion. Uvula raises midline. Pharynx without lesions, exudates, or postnasal drainage.

FIGURE 19-3 Sample of a complete history and physical examination. *(Continued)*

- **Neck:** Symmetrical, trachea midline. Full ROM. No bruits, masses, thyromegaly, or JVD.
- **Lymphatics:** No cervical, axillary, or inguinal lymphadenopathy.
- **Respiratory:** Symmetric rise and fall. No bony abnormalities or accessory muscle use. AP:lat ratio 1:2. Ausc: clear to auscultation without wheezes, rubs, rhonchi, or crackles. Palpation without tenderness. Percussions symmetrical and resonant throughout. Diaphragmatic excursion 6 cm R, 5 cm L.
- **Cardiovascular:**
  Heart: Inspection w/o visible PMI or heaves. Regular rhythm w/o murmur, rub, or gallop. Palpation w/o thrills. PMI 5th ICS MCL.
  Extremities: w/o lesions, edema, varicosities, hair loss, clubbing, or cyanosis. Capillary refill < 2 seconds throughout.

	Br	Rad	Fem	Pop	DP	DT
R	2	2	2	2	1	1
L	2	2	2	2	1	1

- **Breast:** Patient declined exam
- **Abdominal:** Rounded, symmetrical w/o distention, lesions, hernia, or scars. Normoactive BS, no bruits.
  Nontender to palp w/o masses or organomegaly. Abd aorta 2 cm. No bruits. Percussion tympanic at gastric bubble. Liver span 6 cm R MCL.
- **Musculoskeletal:** TMJ w/o click. Full AROM throughout upper & lower ext b/l. Nontender. Fingers w/o nodes.

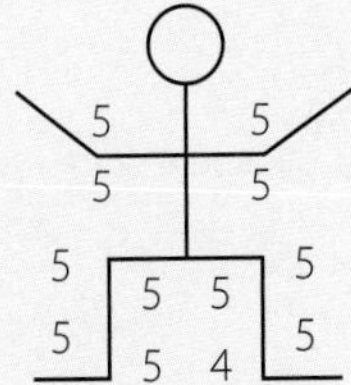

- **Neurologic:** Oriented × 3. CN II–XII intact. Reflexes 2/4 throughout. Light touch & sharp/dull intact throughout. No cerebellar function deficits. Babinski downgoing b/l. Romberg test neg.

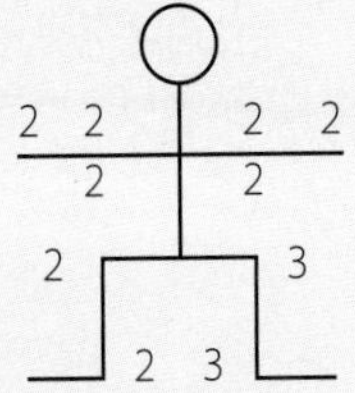

- **Genitalia:** Patient declined exam.
- **Rectal:** Sphincter tone intact. Heme negative.
- **Osteopathic:** Chapman's points with tissue texture change T6 transverse process R

Assessment:
1) Cholelithiasis r/o common duct obstruction
2) R/O hepatotoxicity secondary to statin
3) R/O hepatitis A infection

Plan:
1) US of gallbladder and bile ducts
2) CBC w/diff, CMP, hepatitis panel, pregnancy test, coags
3) Consult surgery
4) NPO
5) IV hydration
6) Pain management
7) Possible admission based on evaluation

Steward Dent, OMSI

FIGURE 19-3 Sample of a complete history and physical examination. *(Continued)*